WATERLOGGED

THE SERIOUS PROBLEM OF OVERHYDRATION IN ENDURANCE SPORTS

Tim Noakes, MD, DSc

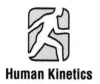

Human Kinetics

Library of Congress Cataloging-in-Publication Data

Noakes, Timothy, 1949-
  Waterlogged : the serious problem of overhydration in endurance sports / Tim Noakes, MD, DSc.
    p. cm.
  Includes bibliographical references and index.
  ISBN 978-1-4504-2497-4 (soft cover) -- ISBN 1-4504-2497-X (soft cover)
  1. Endurance sports--Physiological aspects. 2. Water intoxication. I. Title.
  RC1220.E53N63 2012
  613.7'1--dc23
                                2011052800

ISBN: 978-1-4504-2497-4 (print)

Content Developer: Christine M. Drews; **Developmental Editor:** Laura E. Podeschi; **Assistant Editor:** Claire Marty; **Copyeditor:** Jan Feeney; **Indexer:** Alisha Jeddeloh; **Permissions Manager:** Martha Gullo; **Graphic Designer and Graphic Artist:** Bob Reuther; **Cover Designer:** Keith Blomberg; **Photographer (cover):** Enrico Calderon/Aflo/Getty Images; **Photo Asset Manager:** Laura Fitch; **Photo Production Manager:** Jason Allen; **Art Manager:** Kelly Hendren; **Associate Art Manager:** Alan L. Wilborn; **Illustrations:** © Human Kinetics, unless otherwise noted; **Printer:** Total Printing Systems

Human Kinetics books are available at special discounts for bulk purchase. Special editions or book excerpts can also be created to specification. For details, contact the Special Sales Manager at Human Kinetics.

Printed in the United States of America   10 9 8 7 6 5

The paper in this book is certified under a sustainable forestry program.

Human Kinetics
P.O. Box 5076
Champaign, IL 61825-5076

Website: www.HumanKinetics.com

In the United States, email info@hkusa.com or call 800-747-4457.
In Canada, email info@hkcanada.com.
In the United Kingdom/Europe, email hk@hkeurope.com.

For information about Human Kinetics' coverage in other areas of the world,
please visit our website: **www.HumanKinetics.com**

E5689

This book is dedicated to the memory of Cynthia Lucero, PhD,
and all those who have died from the encephalopathy
caused by exercise-associated hyponatremia.

I wrote it also for those who yet grieve,
that others may be spared your unimaginable sorrow.

This book is the culmination of an investigation that took 30 years,
each moment of which was shared with my most special friend
and inspiration, Marilyn Anne, to whom it is also dedicated.

Cynthia Lucero
August 28, 1973 to April 17, 2002
2002 Boston Marathon bib number 15611

The Spirited Runner

While the world mourns for your departure
Your spirit lives on
You showed us how to live
And how to give
Four miles more you were only a Boston finisher
Four miles short you became a heroine
A legend
May you guide us
Through the clouds to heaven

Alan Lam
Reprinted courtesy of Alan Lam.

All royalties from the sale of this book will be donated to the
Tim and Marilyn Noakes Trust for Sports Science Research
and the Dr. Cynthia Lucero Center for Health Psychology.

CONTENTS

FOREWORD

Tim Noakes doesn't do anything halfheartedly. In his youth, he ran marathons and ultramarathons and had many finishes in South Africa's two most famous races: the 36-mile Two Oceans and the 54-mile Comrades ultramarathons. Years later, when he turned to book writing, Noakes, a physician thoroughly versed in all aspects of running and exercise physiology, produced the astonishing *Lore of Running*, which is certain to remain the definitive evidence-based running book for decades to come. Running—it's a simple subject, but one worthy of deep exploration in the hands of a curious and inexhaustible mind.

Now Tim has turned his attention to water, another simple subject. And once again he has dug deep to produce a remarkable account. In *Waterlogged*, he explains how the commercial world came to exaggerate our need for daily fluid consumption.

I found myself immersed in this world nearly 15 years before I first met Tim. In 1968 I was invited to be a subject in an experiment comparing the effects of no fluids, water, and Gatorade on endurance performance. This study was designed by exercise physiologist David Costill, PhD, one of the first serious investigators in the physiology of endurance athletes. Gatorade was a new product then, concocted by Dr. Robert Cade to help the massive, out-of-shape, University of Florida Gators football team at their steamy first practices in August.

Costill, from Ball State University in Muncie, Indiana, had received a grant from the then-corporate owner of Gatorade, Stokely Van Camp. He wanted to see if the beverage would benefit highly fit, heavy-sweating, marathon runners. I readily accepted his invitation to participate in the study. Like most distance runners, I was eager to learn more about the physiology behind my performance.

Costill picked me up in Detroit at the NCAA Indoor Meet, where I had just been nearly lapped by Jim Ryun and Gerry Lindgren. I fell asleep in his car as he drove the 240 miles to Muncie through the middle of the night. On three of the following four days (I got one rest day), Costill asked me to run 20 miles on his laboratory treadmill at a pace of 6 minutes per mile. One day he gave me water to drink, one day Gatorade, and one day nothing.

After I finished the two runs with fluids, he snaked a long plastic tube through a nostril all the way down to my stomach. This enabled him to siphon off any unabsorbed fluids. I gagged on the tubing. "It's simple," he insisted. "Just pretend you're swallowing a strand of spaghetti." That helped a little, but not much.

I distinctly remember that I felt best the day I drank nothing. I had grown up in distance running without ever drinking water or anything else. I had run dozens of midsummer New England road races that began at high noon in July and August, and at none of those races had the runners been offered water. What's more, the old veterans of New England racing warned that cold drinks would cause stomach cramps. "Don't drink while you're running," they counseled. I did as I was told, and everything worked out fine.

When I tell this story to today's runners, they look at me as if I'm a visitor from a distant, unenlightened land. They can't imagine a time when races started at noon (in summer!) or how anyone could finish a 5K, 10K, or longer race without drinking copiously at almost every opportunity.

Back to the Costill experiment. On the two days when I received fluids (according to scheduled protocol), my stomach sloshed like the Pacific Ocean in a tsunami, and I felt nauseated. When I drank nothing, I felt fine. Two months later, Costill showed up at the 1968 Boston Marathon to weigh us before and after the 26 miles. At the start of the race I weighed 138 pounds. There were no water stops on the course then, just young children handing out orange slices. After a warm, sunny race to downtown Boston, I weighed 129 pounds.

According to physiology textbooks, I should have been near death after a weight loss that dramatic. I wasn't. Quite the opposite: I was celebrating my victory in the race.

That day marked the beginning of my interest in—and skepticism about—fluid consumption, health, and endurance performance. Two decades later, I was stunned to see how many of my co-workers clutched at their 2-liter water bottles from dawn to dusk as if they were oxygen tanks on the moon. In 5K road races, some runners spent as much time at the water stops as they did moving forward. Marathoners dragged canteen belts to the start line, looking like Lawrence of Arabia on a desert campaign.

The magazine I edited, *Runner's World*, carried advertisements warning that an athlete could lose up to 6 pounds of water per hour of exercise. That was technically true. I had actually attended a scientific presentation about a tennis player who sweated this prodigiously. But the researchers admitted the poor fellow was a genetic freak, like the 8-foot tallest man on Earth. The rest of us had nothing to learn from the "6 pounds of water" story. But of course it frightened many into thinking they'd better have another big gulp of fluid.

Fascinated by the hoopla, but also confused by it, I spent several months in 2003 looking into the research on water consumption. I found no support for exaggerated claims about human needs. As far as anyone could tell, the human body had evolved an exquisite system to regulate water consumption. It's called thirst. When you're thirsty, you need to drink. When you're not thirsty, you don't.

Now I'd be the first to admit that we don't always pay a lot of attention to our thirst. Not when we're dashing through our busy lives, shuttling from work to family life to daily chores. Sometimes we get distracted, and sometimes we don't find ourselves near a water faucet. No problem. As it turns out, the body is wonderfully equipped to deal with transient dehydration, which lasts from 4 to 8 hours. It's only chronic dehydration, lasting for days on end, that leads to health problems. (The classic example of this is an elderly person trapped in an overheated apartment during a summer heat wave.)

Similarly, when we run marathons, we might not pay as much attention to our thirst as we should. But that's okay, because a marathon is transient. It's normal to get dehydrated during a marathon. When you reach the point of 2% dehydration, you probably will get thirsty and start looking for water. If you don't find any water, you might slow down a little. That's not the end of the world. You'll have plenty of time to rehydrate after you finish.

In the past decade, I'm happy to note, many runners, physiologists, and fitness experts have started to come to their senses. In early 2012, I interviewed a top American female runner, Mary Coordt, who has qualified for four U.S. Olympic Marathon Trials and also holds a master's degree in nutrition. I asked her about nutrition secrets of the top marathoners. She said, essentially, that there are none. A serious commitment to training is what makes Olympians, not quick diet fixes.

Naturally, I asked Mary about fluid replacement during a marathon. "That's one of the few areas where we have advanced beyond the old routines," she replied. "We used to be so afraid of dehydration that we told runners to drink before they got thirsty. Now we understand that when you run long distances, a certain amount of dehydration is part of the process. And you don't need to start sipping fluids until you feel thirsty. The days of chugging water are over."

This is what Tim Noakes has been telling us for decades. Without his persistent voice, we might never have changed course.

I doubt that Tim is fully satisfied yet. After all, old habits and unproven truisms often last far longer than they should. But Tim has almost single-handedly turned the tide, a Herculean task for which he deserves our credit and our acclaim.

Amby Burfoot

ACKNOWLEDGMENTS

Eleanor Sadler's letter describing her experiences in the 1981 Comrades Marathon projected me into an exciting academic odyssey that would not otherwise have happened. Atlanta physician Bob Lathan, who correctly concluded that he had developed exercise-associated hyponatremic encephalopathy (EAHE) because he drank too much (24 liters in just over 10 hours) during the 1983 Chicago 100-kilometer Ultramarathon, was the first to support our heretical opinions. Drs. Doug Hiller and Bob Laird, who both believed otherwise, were never other than respectful and gentlemanly in their opposition—the proper behavior in scientific discourse.

Dr. Tony Irving entrusted his academic future to my tutelage and applied his gentle mind and diligent manner to performing the first study proving that athletes with EAHE are indeed "waterlogged" because they consume fluids in excess during prolonged exercise. Tony showed that athletes with EAHE are not suffering from a sodium deficiency. By simple logic, his 1988 study also proved that the ingestion of extra sodium either before or during exercise cannot prevent EAHE in those who overdrink.

Dr. Dale Speedy performed a series of definitive studies in New Zealand triathletes, including the first intervention trial in the 1998 New Zealand Ironman Triathlon, thereby proving that the incidence of EAHE and exercise-associated hyponatremia (EAH) can be reduced simply by ensuring that athletes drink moderately and not to excess during prolonged exercise. Dale taught me that it is possible to study 700 athletes in a single endurance event.

This knowledge inspired our own studies expertly managed by Dr. Karen Heath (Sharwood), which challenged the industry-inspired dogma that any weight loss during exercise can have catastrophic consequences. Rather, those studies confirmed a historical observation: The best athletes in any endurance event finish the race with the highest levels of dehydration because they sweat the most and drink only sparingly when running the fastest. They also complete those races with the highest body temperatures.

Dr. Tamara Hew-Butler witnessed the inappropriate management of patients with EAHE and decided to study why the condition was so prevalent in the Houston Marathon. Her unwelcome discoveries forced her to seek solace in Cape Town, where I was privileged to add focus to her boundless energy, unbridled enthusiasm, and dogged determination to make a difference. She organized the First International Consensus Conference on EAH in Cape Town in March 2005. And there I met Drs. Arthur Siegel, Carlos Ayus, and Joe Verbalis, legendary North American colleagues, from whom I learned of the role that the inappropriate secretion of the hormone arginine vasopressin must play in the development of EAHE and the importance of using hypertonic sodium chloride infusions in the treatment of EAHE.

Another conference attendee, Dr. Lulu Weschler, offered expert understanding of the mathematics of sodium balance in the body. This taught us why only a minority of those who overdrink during exercise develop either EAH or EAHE.

Few but the most fortunate scientists in developed countries can fulfill their creative urges and so maximize their productivity exclusively by undertaking publicly funded research that improves the human condition. Thus, virtually all creative scientists in the 21st century are faced with a classic conflict of interest. To fulfill their inventive drives, they must undertake commercially driven research, whether or not it also advances truth. As a scientist working in developing countries, I am especially vulnerable because the level of government funding of research is even more limited than in Europe or North America. Unless one researches the scourges of developing nations—HIV/AIDS, malaria, and tuberculosis—it is extremely difficult to build a world-standard research program without industry support. Our group has undertaken research sponsored by a number of commercial companies, including those that produce sports drinks and nutritional supplements.

My involvement began with the Leppin company, then a wholly owned South African business, who developed the Leppin FRN sports drink and sports supplement line. The acronym FRN refers to the surnames of Bruce Fordyce, Bernard Rose, and me, the three South Africans who helped in the initial development of these products. At the time of my initial involvement, the company was not publicly listed. I am indebted to Nils and Til Hanneman, who provided the initial funding (10 R100 notes in a brown envelope) to reimburse research subjects in one of our very first studies. Their financial support when we had little else helped Drs. Vicki Lambert, Andrew Bosch, John Hawley, Holden MacRae, and Sandy Weltan develop expertise in the study of carbohydrate metabolism during exercise. This research became the basis of all our subsequent research.

It was a special privilege to work with Bernard Rose and Bruce Fordyce during that period. We shared a great friendship and some wonderful memories, especially during Bruce's nine victories in the 90-kilometer Comrades Marathon as well as the 1984 and 1985 London-to-Paris Triathlons. Neither Nils nor Til ever asked me or any of my staff to say or write anything about their products that was scientifically indefensible. This attitude continues as a requirement in all our dealings with the commercial funders of our research.

When the Hannemans sold their company, we began to work with the Bromor Foods company. I thank that company for honoring our scientific independence and for using their marketing prowess to ensure that their sports drink, Energade, became the official drink of the 90-kilometer Comrades Marathon, South Africa's unique foot race. They also supported our campaign to ensure that South African athletes drink according to thirst (ad libitum) during exercise and not as much as tolerable. The incidence of EAH and EAHE has been negligible in the Comrades Marathon since 1990, which is a direct result of our ability to establish a credible contrary message, first in South Africa and New Zealand and then in the rest of the world.

More recently, another South African company has acquired Bromor Foods, and our collaboration with Bromor has ended. Collaborating with DSM (manufacturers of nutritional products), Drs. Andrew Bosch and Vicki Lambert have continued our research into athletes' use of supplements.

The major sponsor of my work and that of the Sports Science Institute of South Africa (SSISA) is the health insurance company Discovery Health, which has supported our primary function to undertake studies that improve the health and physical fitness of all South Africans.

Through their contributions, the Medical Research Council of South Africa, the University of Cape Town, and the National Research Foundation, especially through the THRIP program, have made it possible for me to undertake research of an international standard in a developing nation.

It is a pleasure to acknowledge the independent thinking of Professors Frank Marino and Paul Laursen from Australia, Sandra Fowkes-Godek and Jonathan Dugas from the United States, Drs. Chris Byrne and Yannis Pitsiladis from England, Dr. Jason Lee and Professor Fabian Lim from Singapore, and Andrew Edwards (together with Dale Speedy) from New Zealand, all of whom were unwavering in their support of our once heretical ideas.

Equally important was the support of two scientific journals, *Clinical Journal of Medicine* and *British Journal of Sports Medicine,* whose respective editors, Winne Meeuwisse and Karim Khan, were fiercely independent and never hesitant to take on these controversial issues. Without their principles of integrity and honesty, this story could not have been told. Professor Khan's friendship for the past two decades has been one of the joys of my scientific career.

I am especially indebted to my colleagues and students at the UCT/MRC Research Unit for Exercise Science and Sports Medicine and the Sports Science Institute of South Africa, who contributed the bulk of the work described in chapter 3, which forms the scientific basis for this book. All showed personal courage in undertaking work that would bring them into conflict with a majority of their international peers.

My personal assistant, Megan Lofthouse, manages my daily work plan, ensuring that at least most of the time I know where I am meant to be and what I should be doing. To the book she contributed thousands of hours typing, managing the reference material on which the book is based, inserting the references into the text, and tracking down crucial but elusive material. Her calm demeanor never faltered; she is another of the group of women who have made my life journey a pleasure and whose contribution made the production of this book a continual source of joy. I thank Amanda Sables for contributing hours of typing my handwritten corrections to many of the 26 drafts from which the final manuscript eventually materialized for submission to the publisher, Human Kinetics.

I was privileged to discover the artistic ability of Sigal Chives more than a decade ago. Since then she has produced every academic slide or figure that I have ever used. Her special ability is to precisely visualize my always cryptic and inadequate explanations. Sigal produced all the original figures, which were then skillfully finalized for inclusion in this book.

This book would not have happened without the support of an extraordinarily committed group of people working for Human Kinetics (HK). When I completed what I considered to be the final (27th) draft of this book, I was still without a publisher but was hopeful that Human Kinetics, the publisher of my book *Lore of Running*, might be interested. With some apprehension, I e-mailed a 1,300-page manuscript that contained everything I know about fluids and exercise.

A few weeks later Ted Miller, vice president of acquisitions for Human Kinetics, phoned to confirm that, yes, his company was interested but the information could not be published as I had presented it. It would require a major overhaul for HK to produce a book that would do proper justice to the topic. Were I willing, he would be happy to appoint Chris Drews as editor to bring focus to my wordy and sometimes derisive detail.

For the next 7 months Chris worked tirelessly to turn my manuscript into a work of focused beauty. The scale of her contribution cannot be overstated. Without Chris' involvement, there would have been no final book; the product of 30 years of work would have languished as a brooding academic tome, unknown to the wider public. Although the words in this book remain mine, they have been carefully selected and reorganized in a way that I, because of my subjective involvement with the material, could not ever have achieved.

Thanks, Chris. It was a great privilege and joy to have worked with you on this book. Your extraordinary commitment to producing the best possible work based on your mystical ability to choose only what is necessary was at all times humbling. I know that the magnitude of your effort went way beyond considerations of financial reward. I trust that presenting the truth will always be the more satisfying reward.

Laura Podeschi was responsible for putting the final product together by selecting and sourcing the photographs, finalizing the permissions, and ensuring that the painstaking job of copyediting was skillfully done within the required time frame by Jan Feeney. To her and all at Human Kinetics who worked so diligently to produce this book, a huge thank-you. Your contributions have all been flawless. Could an author ever wish for more?

Ultimately it is one's family who provides the time and the support required to produce a work of importance. Marilyn has been my sole and constant companion since we first met on 9 December, 1966. Now in our 41st year of marriage, she has provided the foundation for all that I have achieved during that time. She remains as fresh, as beautiful, as vibrant, and as unique as she was when, at 15 years old, she first captivated me. Our children, Travis Miles and Candice Amelia, now our friends, are a constant source of pride, joy, knowledge, and fascination.

To all of these people I am sincerely indebted. My hope is that this book honors all of you, your contributions, and your sacrifices.

INTRODUCTION

When I began running in 1969, completing my first 42 km (26 mile) marathon in September 1972, we were advised to drink sparingly, if at all, during exercise. As I recall, that race provided only one "refreshment" station at 32 km (20 miles); there, our running times were also recorded, perhaps as proof that we had indeed been present at least at one point on the race course.

This approach had been followed ever since marathon running became an official event in the first modern Olympic Games in Athens in 1896. Until the 1970s, marathon runners were discouraged from drinking fluids during exercise for fear that it would cause them to slow down. For some, drinking during marathon running was considered a mark of weakness. My childhood running hero and subsequent friend, Jackie Mekler, five-time winner of the 90 km (56 mile) South African Comrades Marathon, described the drinking philosophy of runners with whom he had competed before his retirement in 1969: "To run a complete marathon without any fluid replacement was regarded as the ultimate aim of most runners, and a test of their fitness" (Noakes, 2003, p. 252).

Marathon runners were not alone in this belief. Cyclists in the race that was considered the ultimate physical challenge—the Tour de France—were advised similarly: "Avoid drinking when racing, especially in hot weather. Drink as little as possible, and with the liquid not too cold. It is only a question of will power. When you drink too much you will perspire, and you will lose your strength." As a result only "four small bottles for a long stage (of the Tour), it was frowned upon to drink more" (Fotheringham, 2002, p. 180).

There is no evidence that this advice was especially dangerous, produced ill health or death, or seriously impaired athletic performance. Indeed, the most rapid improvements in marathon running performances occurred from 1920 to 1970 (figure 1, page xiv) in the period when athletes were not drinking much during races and were generally ignorant of the science of distance running, including the value of specific diets (Noakes, 2003).

A plateau in running times occurred after 1970. This effect is most apparent in the 42 km marathon, suggesting that all human runners, marathoners especially, are rapidly approaching the physical limits of human running ability. Note that in the period of 1900 to 1970, marathon runners were actively discouraged from drinking during exercise. The introduction and encouragement of frequent drinking after 1976 were not associated with any sudden increase in world-record performances in the marathon. Rather, an opposite trend is apparent (figure 1). The same trend exists also at the shorter–distance races, during which athletes do not usually drink.

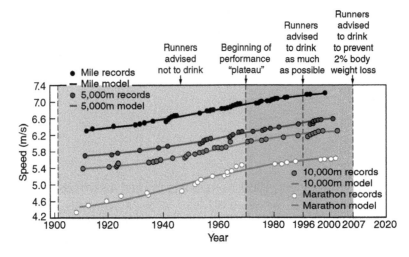

FIGURE 1 The progression of world running records at the mile (1.61 km), 5,000 m, 10,000 m, and 42 km marathon distances from 1900 to 2000 shows an acceleration in record-breaking performances at all distances from 1900 to 1970 and a definite slowing (plateau) thereafter.

Adapted, by permission, from A.M. Nevill and G. Whyte, 2005, "Are there limits to running world records?" *Medicine & Science in Sports & Exercise* 37(10): 1785-1788.

The notion that athletes should drink during exercise took hold rather slowly. In November 1976 the prestigious New York Academy of Sciences (NYAS) held a conference titled "The Marathon: Physiological, Medical, Epidemiological and Psychological Studies" (Milvy P., 1977). The conference coincided with the first running of the New York City Marathon through the five boroughs of the Big Apple.

The race was a major success, launching the concept of the big-city marathons and stimulating an unprecedented growth in marathon running in particular and endurance sport in general. Thus, entrants in the New York City Marathon climbed from fewer than 2,000 in 1976 to more than 10,000 in 1980, reaching 30,000 by the late 1990s. Similar rates of growth were seen in the Boston and London Marathons, among many others (figure 2a).

No speaker at the NYAS conference on the marathon spoke exclusively on the role of fluid ingestion during exercise. Fluid balance during exercise was discussed only fleetingly because it was considered to be of little scientific relevance.

James F. Fixx, a writer from Riverside, Connecticut, who had begun running in the late 1960s—in the process losing 27 kg (60 lb) and completing six Boston Marathons—was an especially attentive attendee at the 1976 NYAS marathon conference. He came to acquire the medical and scientific information necessary for completing a book titled *The Complete Book of Running* (Fixx, 1977) that he had begun writing in April 1976. When published a year later, the book became an instant phenomenon, topping the *New York Times* best-seller list for 11 weeks and selling over a million copies. It was subsequently translated into all the major languages.

In *The Complete Book of Running*, Fixx wrote the following: "Drink lots of water while you're exercising. It used to be considered unwise to drink while working out.

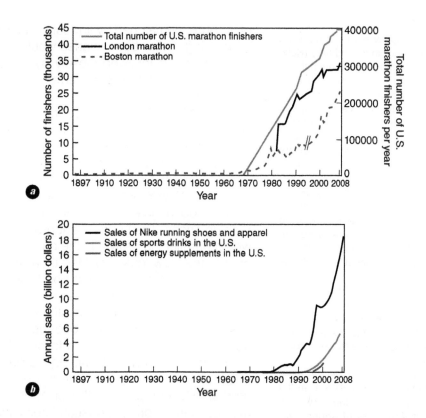

FIGURE 2 *(a)* Participation in individual marathons increased from only a few hundred entrants each year to over 30,000 in big-city marathons, with a total of 400,000 runners competing in marathons in the United States in 2008. *(b)* Three industries that benefited from the growth in interest in physical activity after 1976 were Nike and the sports drink and sports supplement industries, especially in the United States. All showed impressive growth at the same time that marathon running was becoming a global phenomenon.

Recent studies have shown, however, that athletes, including runners, function best when allowed to drink *whenever they want to* [my emphasis]. A 5 percent drop in body weight can reduce efficiency by 15 percent, and 6 percent is about the maximum you can comfortably tolerate" (p. 146).

Perhaps Fixx's summary of the "state-of-the-art" guidelines gleaned from the 1976 NYAS marathon conference was that runners should drink according to the dictates of their thirst ("drink whenever you want to") and should not lose too much weight during exercise since this causes an impaired "efficiency." Interestingly, he made no reference to any dangers caused by dehydration in those who drank little and lost substantial amounts of weight during exercise. Rather, he reported that a loss of up to 6% of body weight could be "comfortably tolerated." This confirms that Fixx did not hear anything at the NYAS conference or elsewhere proposing that runners should drink as much as tolerable in order to prevent any weight loss during exercise.

The sudden global growth in the number of marathon runners in Europe and North America soon generated a potential market for those selling products used by runners. James Fixx was himself perhaps the first to benefit through the sales

1 The Nike company born in 1972 soon became the maverick in the industry (Katz, 1994), selling not simply equipment but also an emotion. In 1978 the company published an ad claiming that excessive pronation (inward rotation) of the subtalar (ankle) joint was the cause of most running injuries to the lower limb. Naturally, Nike alone produced the solution to the problem—specially designed antipronation shoes. Sports doctors, including me, became disciples of this received wisdom (Noakes, 2003). In our naïvety we failed to question whether the advice was designed to sell more running shoes. Perhaps the fact that I received free running shoes from Nike South Africa for many years blunted my appetite for serious interrogation of their claims.

Only later (when my supply of free Nike running shoes ran out) would I begin to question whether excessive pronation is the cause of most running injuries. Indeed, it may play little role at all (see Noakes, 2003, pp. 767-770).

Writing this book has made me more aware of the effects of accepting even the most innocuous gifts from industry. How could a few dozen pairs of shoes over decades possibly influence my thinking? But it did. Because I was (and still am) a Nike guy. And Nike guys don't question the hand that is feeding them the myth.

of his book, unmatched by any subsequent book on running. Other beneficiaries would be Nike running shoes[1] followed closely by the sports drink and nutritional supplement industries (figure 2b).

I visited New York in 1976 to attend the NYAS marathon conference and to run the marathon. I wished also to take home some Nike running shoes, then unavailable in South Africa. To do this, I was forced to travel the length and breadth of New York City. Eventually I found the single shop in the entire city that specialized in running shoes. The subsequent growth of Nike would parallel the growth in the number of runners in the New York City Marathon (figure 2). It predated the growth in the sports drink and nutritional supplement industries by some years.

Until then, there had been little incentive to study endurance exercise because the only sports with money were the professional sports such as American football, basketball, and baseball and, to a lesser extent, golf. Sports medicine encompassed the orthopedic and medical care of professional athletes injured in those sports. The physiological needs of endurance athletes were not considered particularly important. Frank Shorter, the American winner of the 1972 Munich Olympic Marathon and the person held accountable for the subsequent growth of marathon running especially in the United States, wrote at the time that people expressed their disbelief whenever he referred to himself as a "professional marathon runner." What sort of profession was that? they wondered.

But the tipping point occurred after 1976 with the sudden explosion in the number of marathon runners entering races, especially in the United States. This would provide a massive new market not just for running shoes but for a novel product, a sports drink for use during exercise, which had been developed in the late 1960s by a renal physician, Dr. Robert Cade, working at the University of Florida.

Already by 1976 his product had become a runaway commercial sensation in the United States, soon establishing itself as an essential ingredient for success in American football. The product also claimed medicinal properties. While it could enhance athletic performance, it could also prevent and cure dehydration, heatstroke,[2] and muscle cramps. Before long, its manufacturers would begin to eye the much greater numbers of the physically active, including this new population of joggers aspiring to become marathon runners.

But Dr. Cade's product faced some significant challenges. First, if drinking during exercise was so important, then why should a product that contains no unique molecules (i.e., a product that was *not* discovered in an ultrasophisticated laboratory after decades of intensive research including thousands of heart-wrenching failures) ever be taken seriously, especially if its core ingredients are chemicals present in even the most rudimentary kitchen—glucose, salt, water, and a dash of lemon? Second, how does one advance substantive medical claims in the absence of proof of efficacy?

Thus, the challenge faced from the outset by those manufacturing Dr. Cade's product was to sell a drink consisting of common kitchen chemicals on the basis of scientific evidence that did not exist in the 1960s and that some would argue still does not exist even today. The commercial success of Gatorade confirms the effectiveness of modern marketing tactics and the strength of a unique, positive product image.

2 If heatstroke is caused by not drinking, then many runners must have developed this condition in that period before 1976 when they were discouraged from drinking during exercise. In addition, those cases should have disappeared after marathon runners began to drink more copiously after the introduction of new drinking guidelines beginning in the late 1970s. As you will learn in chapters 3 and 5, heatstroke historically has been rare in endurance sport. Of nearly 2,000 cases of heatstroke reported in the medical literature, only 6 have occurred in marathon or longer running races, including 3 since 1976, whereas many occur each year in short-distance running races (5 to 15 km, or 3 to 9 miles), which are over well before the athletes can become dehydrated. Thus, something other than dehydration causes heat stroke.

"Advertisers have dispensed with the idea of promoting a product's attributes in favour of marketing the product's image. This image is conceived by marketing psychologists quite independently of the product itself, and usually has more to do with a target market than the item being sold" (Rushkoff, 2000, p. 19).

Indeed, the marketing of drinks claiming medicinal properties, of which Coca-Cola was the first global success, led to the following conclusion: "Patent medicine makers were the first American businessmen to recognise the power of the catchphrase, the identifiable logo and trademark, the celebrity endorsement, the appeal to social status, the need to keep 'everlastingly at it.' Out of necessity, they were the first to sell image rather than product" (Pendergrast, 2000, p. 11). Thus, "Like all great love affairs ours depends to a large extent on creating a set of illusions, feelings that we are special. We are who we are because we are all things to all people all the time everywhere" because "we're selling smoke. They're drinking the image, not the product" (p. 443). So it was that a drink, with ingredients that are freely available and cheap, became iconic.

One might argue that this is simply the reality of the modern world and that we are naïve to expect otherwise. But it is disturbing that incorrect advice to the public and the public's own susceptibility to effective promotional efforts resulted in a novel medical condition that affected thousands of soldiers, hikers, runners, cyclists, and triathletes, causing some to die (appendix A). Sadly, this phenomenon and the deaths that apparently resulted from it were preventable.

This story also is a cautionary tale about how a movement can take hold and manifest itself into something unhealthy and potentially very harmful. As bad as water restrictions and required ingestion of salt tablets were during the 1960s, so too is the current nearly universal notion of drinking despite a lack of thirst. Today, athletes, parents, coaches, and even many professionals in medicine, fitness, and sport science push the intake of fluid far beyond the bounds of what solid research suggests. Indeed, tens of millions of athletes and fitness enthusiasts are waterlogged in that the hydration practices to which they religiously adhere adversely affect their health and performance.

The driving force in writing this book is a desire to reposition the commonly held belief of proper hydration so that it is consistent with the research and more effective for today's and future athletes and fitness enthusiasts. I do so by presenting the facts. And I do, based on that evidence, present guidelines for intake of water and sports drinks that should replace the general "drink until you can't take another sip" hydration practices that prevail today.

My days as a marathoner might have ended years ago, but I continue to enjoy running, in part because I train and race smarter today than I did even a decade ago. *Waterlogged* affords you the same opportunity to make intelligent, informed decisions regarding hydration. Drink it up.

CHAPTER 1

Perspectives on Human Physiology and Hydration

Distance running was revered because it was indispensable; it was the way we thrived and spread across the planet. You ran to eat and to avoid being eaten; you ran to find a mate and impress her, and with her you ran off to start a new life together. You had to love running, or you wouldn't live to love anything else. And like everything else we love—everything we sentimentally call our "passions" and "desires"—it's really an encoded ancestral necessity. We were born to run; we were born because we run. We're all Running People, as the Tarahumara have always known.

Christopher McDougall (2009, pp. 92-93)

April 15, 2002, dawned as a very special day for 28-year-old New York-born Cynthia Lucero, who grew up in Guayaquil, Ecuador, before returning to the United States to pursue her graduate studies.

Cynthia was to run her second 42 km (26 mile) marathon at the 106th Annual Boston Marathon over the most famous running path in the world—from the town of Hopkinton, Massachusetts, to the finish line outside the Boston Public Library.

Three days earlier, Lucero, a clinical psychologist working as an intern at the Center for Multicultural Training in Psychology at the Boston Medical Center, had submitted her PhD thesis to the Massachusetts School of Professional Psychology (MSPP) for examination. Its title reflected her recent interest in the effects of marathon running on the psyche: "Effects of a Marathon Training Program on Family Members and Friends of Cancer Patients."

Her thesis included the personal stories of some of the runners with whom she had trained for the 2002 Boston Marathon. Her Spanish surname, meaning beam of light, foretold her effervescent personality and her friendly and cheerful attitude about life. As she wrote in the introduction to her 100-page dissertation, she chose the marathon because "At first, running a marathon sounds too demanding, if not absolutely impossible to accomplish. But I believe this is not only a realistic goal to accomplish but also an excellent coping mechanism that helps runners and many cancer patients and their families" (Arnold, 2002).

Lucero survived a near-fatal car accident in 1998, which instilled a new appreciation of the transience of life. So she dedicated herself to the service of others. She chose to spend more time working for charities; she would build her life on service—on giving and caring. For her volunteer work she counseled psychologically damaged women at the Shelter for Battered Women, the Cambridge Health Alliance, the South End Community Health Alliance, and the Big Sister program. She worked with families who lost loved ones at Logan International Airport after the September 11 terrorist attacks the previous year. A friend, Rick Wasserboehr, who trained with her for the Boston Marathon, recalled that when asked how people can best contribute to society, Cynthia replied, "That's simple . . . just be nice to people" ("From Rick Wasserboehr," n.d., paragraph 2). Lucero believed that by giving more and expecting less, she could make a difference in the world. She was guided by five tenets: "Remove all worry from your mind; remove all hatred from your heart; live simply; give more; expect less" (Massachusetts School of Professional Psychology, 2004, p. 9). Unknown to her family, in 1999 she signed a card authorizing the donation of her organs in the event of her death (Hohler, 2005).

So as she lined up with race number 15611 on Main Street in Hopkinton, Massachusetts, at noon on April 16, 2002, she had every reason to believe that her life was blessed. It was, she said to a friend, "an extraordinary time," her "week of triumph," one of the few moments in her life when "everything comes together" (Arnold, 2002, p. A1). Her run would raise money for the Massachusetts chapter of the Leukemia and Lymphoma Society. The weather, too, was especially kind. The air temperature at the start was 51 °F (11 °C), the relative humidity (RH) was 96%, a fresh side wind was blowing from the northwest at a speed of 7 mph (11 km/hr), and there was 100% cloud cover.

But her immediate challenge was to complete the 26 miles from Hopkinton through Ashland, Framingham, Natick, Wellesley, and over the Newton Hills to the finish in Copley Square where her parents, who recently traveled from Ecuador to attend her PhD thesis colloquium at MSPP, would witness her triumph. There they would share her extraordinary dual joy of completing her doctoral thesis and the Boston Marathon in the same week. They had little reason for apprehension; their daughter had conquered this challenge before, completing the 2000 San Diego Rock 'n' Roll marathon in 5 hours 19 minutes.

Her parents' certainty was strengthened by the knowledge that for 5 months before the Boston Marathon, Cynthia had trained with an experienced coach and 150 other aspiring marathon runners. She might have been told that it is essential, even life-saving, to drink continuously during the race in order to prevent dehydration, fatigue, and heat illness. Perhaps she had even seen the advertisement placed by the Gatorade Sports Science Institute (GSSI) in the January 2002 issue of *New York Runner* magazine. On the race number of a lean, bare-bellied, athletic female runner was the warning "Research shows that your body needs at least 40 oz of fluid every hour, or your performance could suffer."[1]

The advertisement claimed that this advice was based on the results of "thousands of tests" that "have been run on thousands of athletes to gain a solid understanding of your needs. To help meet those needs, Gatorade offers specifically formulated products." Since her training was in psychology, not exercise physiology, Dr. Lucero could not know whether those claims were true. But why would they not be?

Or perhaps she, her coach, and her fellow trainees had absorbed the message of the advertisement that the GSSI had placed in the January 2002 issue of *Runner's World*, North America's leading running publication. The advertisement, titled "Drinking 101," had presented the following information under the heading "Important Fluid Guidelines From the Gatorade Sports Science Institute":

> **1** The 40 was printed five times larger than the surrounding text. Forty oz/hr equals 1,200 ml/hr, the same rate of fluid ingestion first tested by Costill, Kammer, and colleagues in the first Gatorade-funded study in 1970 and later by Montain and Coyle in their Gatorade-funded study published in 1992. These studies did not evaluate whether such high rates of fluid ingestion either improved or impaired exercise performance. But the 1970 study of Costill and colleagues did show that runners attempting to drink fluid at such high rates developed a feeling of intestinal fullness and refused to ingest any more fluid after about 75 minutes of exercise. A subsequent Gatorade-funded study (Below, Mora-Rodriguez, et al., 1995) of even higher rates of fluid intake makes no reference to any intestinal discomfort experienced by the athletes. Our study using similarly high rates of fluid ingestion (Robinson, Hawley, et al., 1995) found a high prevalence of intestinal symptoms sufficiently severe to affect the cycling performance of a significant number of the subjects we tested.

1. Drink early and often. Two hours before a run, drink 16 to 20 ounces [i.e., 480-600 ml] of water or sports drink. Take in between 7 and 10 ounces every 10-20 minutes during the run [i.e., 600-1680 ml/hr].
2. Always drink sports drinks on long runs. Performance is significantly improved when sports drinks are consumed during hour or longer workouts. . . . electrolytes [in sports drinks] help reduce the risk of muscle cramps, fatigue, and hyponatremia.
3. Don't wait until you feel thirsty. You don't often feel thirsty early in a run, but that's exactly when you need to start drinking.
4. Rehydrate after the run. Drink between 20 and 24 ounces [i.e., 560-800 ml] of sports drink for every pound of body weight lost during exercise.
5. Beware of hyponatremia. Hyponatremia, or "water intoxication," could happen during long, hot runs, when a runner loses a lot of sodium through sweat and consumes a great deal of water. This can dilute sodium levels in the blood, causing an electrolyte imbalance.

   Warning signs mimic those of dehydration,[2] including confusion, disorientation, muscle weakness, and vomiting. To help maintain blood sodium levels, consume sports drinks, rather than plain water, on runs over an hour.

> **2** The symptoms of exercise-associated hyponatremia are not the same as those of dehydration. In fact, they are distinctly different (see chapter 11, table 11.1, page 348). For a start, the dehydration that develops during exercise has only one symptom: thirst. Confusion arising from this distortion has resulted in the inappropriate treatment of athletes suffering from hyponatremia.

So Cynthia would have been taught that she should not wait to become thirsty before she began to drink. Instead, she must drink to stay ahead of her thirst at each of the fluid replacement stations placed every mile (1.6 km) along the marathon course. And because she did not wish to develop "water intoxication" during or after the race, she consumed large quantities of the race sponsor's official sports drink, Gatorade. This drink, she had been assured, would "maintain [her] blood sodium levels" regardless of how much she drank during the 26 miles (42 km) of the 2002 Boston Marathon.

From the start, Cynthia ran with unfettered abandon. Her name written in bold letters on her leg evoked the support of the crowds lining the course. Running through Wellesley after 14 miles, she high-fived all the Wellesley College women at the road side.

At mile 19 (31 km), where the Newton Hills begin, she was running fast enough to pass a friend. He called her Dr. Lucero, congratulating her on her recent academic achievement. When asked in what discipline her doctoral thesis was granted, Cynthia replied, "Psychology . . . and I need all of it today! ("Carole," n.d., paragraph 6). Then she ran ahead.

Shortly before 5:00 p.m., Cynthia entered the Cleveland Circle—still 4 miles (7 km) from the finish. She complained that she felt "dehydrated and rubber-legged." Soon she became unsteady, wobbled briefly, and fell to the ground. By the time the paramedics reached her, Lucero was already unconscious although her pulse and blood pressure were in the expected range. The paramedics drove her to Brigham and Women's Hospital, where she was admitted to the emergency room within the hour.

A blood sample drawn at 6:07 p.m. established that she was suffering from a markedly reduced blood sodium concentration (113 mmol/L) compared to the normal value of 135 to 145 mmol/L that would have been present when she began the race. As the advertisement had warned, she had indeed "diluted" her blood sodium levels, even though she had drunk large quantities of Gatorade, which the sponsor's advertisement had stated would help prevent the development of hyponatremia (fluid intoxication).

Other results showed that her serum arginine vasopressin (AVP) concentration was inappropriately elevated at 6.2 pg/ml (normal 1.0-13.3 pg/ml); her urine osmolality was 329 mOsm/kg (normal 390-1093 mOsm/kg), and her urine sodium concentration was 81 mmol/L (data courtesy of Dr. Arthur Siegel, Harvard Medical School), all indicating the presence of syndrome of inappropriate ADH secretion (SIADH). A chest x-ray showed that her lungs were filled with fluid (pulmonary edema).

3 AVP/ADH is one of the most powerful hormones in the body. It is measured in picograms (pg) per milliliter; one picogram is one trillionth of a gram. At a concentration of 4 pg per milliliter (4 pg/ml) of blood—equivalent to 4 trillionths (10^{-12}) of a gram of the hormone in each ml of blood—the hormone will restrict the rate of urine production to about 50 ml/hr; at a concentration of 1 pg/ml, urine production will be about 200 ml/hr. To allow an adequate urine production in an athlete who overdrinks by 500 to 1,000 ml/hr, the blood ADH/AVP concentrations must be suppressed to less than 0.25 of a trillionth of a gram of hormone per ml of blood and so is essentially undetectable.

The clinicians entrusted with her care likely would have diagnosed exercise-associated hyponatremic encephalopathy (EAHE) causing noncardiogenic (not heart caused) pulmonary edema. (The EAHE was likely due to SIADH.) The immediate cause of her condition was an abnormal increase in the amount of water in her body caused in part by an abnormally elevated concentration of the hormone arginine vasopressin (AVP) in her blood. This hormone, secreted when the body's water store (the total body water, or TBW) is reduced, causes the kidneys to retain water and to excrete sodium into the urine; hence, it is also known as antidiuretic hormone (ADH).[3] The concentration of this hormone (AVP/ADH) increases normally in the blood of runners who run fast and sweat profusely, causing them to lose body water if they drink less than they sweat, as is the more usual practice (Hew-Butler, Noakes, et al., 2008).

But in a person moving quite slowly in moderate environmental conditions—Cynthia had jogged and walked at about 7 km per hour in an air temperature that peaked at 52°F (11°F) at 3:00 p.m. with air humidity that ranged from 89% to 96% with wind speeds that varied from 6.9 to 9.2 mph (11-15 km/hr)—and who is drinking excessively, the production of AVP/ADH by the brain must cease in order to allow the excretion by the kidneys of the excess fluid that is being ingested, a process known as (kidney or renal) diuresis. But the presence of inappropriate blood concentrations of AVP/ADH causes fluid retention, leading to water intoxication if the rate of fluid intake is excessive in those who, like Cynthia Lucero, have been advised to drink as much as tolerable in order to stay ahead of thirst (ACSM, 2004; Armstrong, Epstein, et al., 1996; Convertino, Armstrong, et al., 1996).

Dr. Lucero was suffering from abnormal fluid retention causing an increase in the TBW with a dilution of her blood sodium concentration. The presence of sodium in her urine ("sodium wasting") when her blood sodium concentration was so low (in which case sodium retention should occur) confirmed that her TBW was increased as a result of inappropriate secretion of the water conserving-hormone AVP/ADH. This condition is known as the syndrome of inappropriate ADH secretion (SIADH).

Whether an athlete critically ill with EAHE lives or dies hinges not on a single correct or wrong decision but on a sequence of choices that together become either life saving or life ending. Through no personal fault, Dr. Lucero had already made a series of potentially fatal, incorrect choices; her error was to believe that the conventional wisdom about hydration during exercise had to be correct. But once she fell unconscious in the Cleveland Circle, the probability that she would survive depended on the knowledge of those into whose care fate had delivered her.

The first critical decision was taken by the paramedics who transported Cynthia to the hospital, the next was by the emergency room physician under whose care she was admitted to the hospital. Critical would be their understanding of fluid balance and kidney function during marathon running. Dr. Lucero still had one chance at life as she was wheeled into the emergency room at Brigham and Women's Hospital (box 1.1, page 6).

Some hours after Cynthia's hospital admission, a brain scan showed evidence of swelling due to EAHE. While she was unconscious, the attending physicians used an electrocardiogram (EEG) to determine whether there was evidence for electrical activity in Cynthia's brain. When the EEG showed no such activity, Dr. Lucero was declared brain dead. Her documented wish that her organs—her kidneys, heart, liver, pancreas, lungs, and corneas— be used to sustain life in five other critically ill women (Hohler, 2005) was respected.

* * *

The hunt is easier in the winter months after the rains have turned the Kalahari Desert of Southern Africa into a temporary paradise, because the tracks are easier to follow. And the African antelopes—the duiker, the steenbok, and the gemsbok—find it more difficult to run on a giving surface. Their split hooves sink into the soft soil, splaying with each step. In a few hours they become too sore to continue. And so finally they can be approached and killed with spears thrown from close range by their chasers, the !Xo San hunters, the ancestral South Africans.

BOX 1.1   Predicted Physiological Cascade in Cynthia Lucero

I do not know what decision the attending emergency room physician made. Cynthia's chance at life depended on the doctor's knowledge of the correct treatment for EAHE, already published in 2000 in the *Annals of Internal Medicine* by Dr. Ayus and colleagues (2000), who had proven that infusion of a 3% saline solution could safely return most patients suffering from EAHE from the brink of death. Perhaps the attending physician made the wrong choice. Or perhaps Cynthia's fate had already been determined by the volume of fluid she had ingested during the race and perhaps compounded by the treatment she might have received in the hour after her collapse and before her admission to the hospital.

When Cynthia Lucero began the 2002 Boston Marathon, her blood sodium concentration would have been ~140 mmol/L. This is because the blood sodium concentration is rigorously controlled, in physiological terms "defended," within a narrow range. If the value is too high because the TBW is too low, the cells become parched; if the value is too low, the cells take up water and increase their volume, becoming waterlogged. The cells of the brain that regulate all human functions are more resistant to shrinkage than to swelling. As the blood sodium concentration falls, the brain cells swell and their function becomes progressively impaired. Ultimately the soggy brain cannot be constrained within the confines of the rigid skull. A small part herniates through the opening at the base of the skull—the foramen magnum—making death inevitable.

Since we can guess Cynthia's approximate weight and we know her blood sodium concentration when she was admitted to the hospital, it is possible to determine exactly what actions caused her to collapse and why she died on 15 April, 2002. The only factor we need to guess is her blood sodium concentration at 5:05 p.m. when she collapsed in the Cleveland Circle. Since most athletes with EAHE become unconscious at a blood sodium concentration below ~125 mmol/L, I have used that value in these calculations (table 1.1). An hour later at 6:05, we know that her measured blood sodium concentration was 113 mmol/L. Table 1.2 on page 8 shows the environmental conditions during the 2002 Boston Marathon.

To make these calculations, we need only to estimate her likely sweat rate and her sweat sodium concentration. The average sweat rate of athletes finishing a 42 km marathon between 4:30 and 6:00 p.m. in the cool conditions in which the 2002 Boston Marathon took place is typically a maximum of 500 ml/hr (Twerenbold, Knechtle, et al., 2003); the sweat sodium concentration is typically ~32 mmol/L (Weschler L, unpublished data), and the sweat potassium concentration is typically ~4 mmol/L (Weschler, unpublished data). Even if these estimates are incorrect by a reasonable amount, they will not greatly affect the conclusions.

Thus, when Cynthia Lucero collapsed at the Cleveland Circle at 5:05 p.m. with an estimated blood sodium concentration of 125 mmol/L, she would have lost about 2.5 kg of sweat containing ~90 mmol of osmotically active electrolytes, sodium, and potassium. Had she drunk nothing at all during the race, these changes would have caused her blood sodium concentration to increase to 150 mmol/L since she had lost more water than electrolytes from her body, causing her body fluids to become more concentrated and so to have a higher osmolality.

The effect of this increased tissue osmolality would have caused Cynthia to become thirsty; the loss of 2.5 kg of body water carries no health risks (chapter 3) and is routinely measured in marathon winners (figure 3.7a, page 71) who run much faster (19-20 km/hr) than Cynthia Lucero did (~7 km/hr). The loss of 90 mmol of electrolytes in sweat does not cause exercise-associated hyponatremia (EAH) as has been claimed; rather, in those who do not drink during exercise, it causes the opposite response—a rise in the blood sodium concentration (chapter 4, table 4.2, page 129). Thus, the absence of drinking and a failure to replace electrolytes lost in sweat could not have caused fatal EAHE to develop in Cynthia Lucero.

Instead, we know that she drank large quantities of Gatorade during the race; the medical report of her autopsy concluded that she died because she drank "too much fluid," including "large amounts of Gatorade" (Smith, 2002).

TABLE 1.1 **Predicted Fluid and Sodium Balance in Cynthia Lucero**

Time	Weight (kg)	TBW (L)	Blood [Na+] (mmol/L)	Water lost as sweat (kg)(L)	Electrolyte (Na+ plus K+) deficit or surplus (mmol)	Fluid excess to explain measured blood [Na+] (L)	Additional electrolyte deficit to explain measured blood [Na+] (mmoles)	Rate of fluid intake (L/hr)
12:00 noon	57	34.2	140	0	0	0	0	0
5:05 p.m.								
Drinking Gatorade	60.5*	37.7*	125	2.5	+52	3.5	0	1.20*
Drinking water	59.8*	37.0*	125	2.5	−90	2.8	0	1.06*
Drinking nothing	54.5	31.7	150	2.5	−90	0	0	0
6:05 p.m.								
Drinking Gatorade	61.5†	40.2†	112	2.5	+206††	6.0 L	−280†††	2.5 ††††

Assumptions: Body weight 57 kg. Total body water (60% of body weight) 34 L (34 kg). Sweat rate 500 ml/hr. Sweat sodium concentration 32 mmol/L. Sweat potassium concentration 4 mmol/L. Sodium concentration in Gatorade 18 mmol/L.

* At this time there could have been an additional 1.5 L of unabsorbed fluid in the intestine. If correct, this would increase the TBW and weight by 1.5 kg and the rate of fluid intake by 0.30 L/hr.

† Assuming the intravenous infusion of 1 L of 0.9% sodium chloride (NaCl) and the absorption of 1.5 L of unabsorbed fluid present in the intestine.

†† Due to the infusion of 1 L of 0.9% sodium chloride (NaCl), which contains 150 mmol of Na+.

††† Due to osmotic inactivation on circulating sodium (Na+) and subsequent storage in an intracellular site (chapter 4).

†††† Due to the addition of 1 L of fluid infused intravenously and 1.5 L of intestinal fluid reabsorbed in the first hour after collapse.

For a complete explanation, check the text. Data based on calculations provided by Dr. Lulu Weschler.

(continued)

BOX 1.1 Predicted Physiological Cascade in Cynthia Lucero *(continued)*

TABLE 1.2 Environmental Conditions During the 2002 Boston Marathon, 15 April, 2002

Time	Air temperature (°C)	(°F)	Humidity (%)	Cloud cover (%)	Wind speed (mph)	(kph)	Wind direction (°)
11:00 a.m.	51.1	10.6	96	100	8.1	13.0	310
12:00 noon	51.1	10.6	96	100	6.9	11.1	330
1:00 p.m.	51.1	10.6	92	100	5.8	9.4	360
2:00 p.m.	52.0	11.1	80	100	3.5	5.6	20
3:00 p.m.	52.0	11.1	89	100	8.1	13.0	90
4:00 p.m.	50.0	10.0	93	88	9.2	14.8	130
5:00 p.m.	48.2	9.0	93	25	9.2	14.8	120
6:00 p.m.	48.2	9.0	93	88	11.5	18.5	110
7:00 p.m.	48.0	8.9	93	50	8.1	13.0	100

Although there was no rain, fog was present for most of the day, reducing visibility to less than 2 miles for most of the race. Data are for the Boston Logan International Airport, which is 6 km from the race finish.

Information purchased from www.findlocalweather.com on 20 March, 2009.

Table 1.1 shows that to lower her blood sodium concentration to 125 mmol/L while drinking Gatorade, Cynthia would have had to increase her TBW by 3.5 L. Since our calculations show that she would have lost 2.5 L as sweat, to increase her TBW by that amount, she would have needed to drink 6.0 L (202.9 fl oz) of Gatorade during 5 hours of exercise. Her rate of intake (1.2 L/hr, or 40.6 fl oz/hr) was precisely the rate recommended by the advertisements published in *New York Runner and Runner's World* three months earlier (January 2002). Interestingly, the sodium she had ingested in Gatorade would have placed her in a positive electrolyte balance at the end of the race. These calculations show that Cynthia Lucero did not need a sodium deficit to explain why she collapsed at 5:05 p.m. with EAHE. Thus, her condition would not have been prevented by ingesting even more sodium during the race.

Had Cynthia drunk only water during the race, at the moment she collapsed her sodium deficit would have been 90 mmol (since she had not replaced that deficit by drinking an electrolyte-containing sports drink). It would have required a slightly lesser whole-body fluid excess (+2.8 L) to lower her blood sodium concentration to 125 mmol/L. She would have achieved this by drinking 5.3 L of water (1.06 L/hr) during the race. This drinking rate falls well within the GSSI guidelines. It also shows that to develop EAHE, an at-risk athlete would need to drink at a rate of about 140 ml/hr more (1.2 vs. 1.06 L/hr) if she chose to drink Gatorade rather than water during the race. But the much easier way to prevent the condition would be simply to drink less.

Three mechanisms could explain why Cynthia's blood sodium concentration could drop a further 12 mmol/L to 113 mmol/L in the 60 minutes between her collapse and her admission to the hospital:

1. *Absorption of unabsorbed fluid present in the gut.* Using data from Armstrong, Curtis, and colleagues (1993), Dr. Lulu Weschler was able to calculate that there could be

as much as 1.5 L of unabsorbed water in the intestine of athletes who overdrink for a prolonged period during exercise. Adding this volume of fluid to the TBW would drop the blood sodium concentration to 119 mmol/L. To have accumulated this additional volume of fluid during the race, Dr. Lucero would have had to ingest fluid at a rate of 1.5 L/hr for 5 hours during the race.

2. *Infusion of normal (0.9%) saline intravenously.* Almost certainly, Cynthia would have received some fluids intravenously after she collapsed. However, the infusion of even 3 L of fluid in this way would not have lowered her blood sodium concentration further since the infused fluid had a higher sodium concentration than her blood sodium concentration at that time. However, the added fluid would have increased her TBW and therefore the extent to which her brain was "waterlogged."

3. *Osmotic inactivation of blood sodium.* Even if Cynthia's TBW had increased by 5.5 L by 6:05 p.m., it would have reduced her blood sodium concentration to "only" 119 mmol/L. To lower her blood sodium concentration further to 113 mmol/L, she would have had to lose a substantial additional amount of sodium. The only possible avenues are in urine or in a complex and poorly understood phenomenon known as osmotic inactivation of circulating (extracellular) sodium. This possibility is discussed more fully in chapter 4.

Dr. Lucero's urine contained substantial amounts of sodium (81 mmol/L) when she was in the hospital, but we do not know the volume of urine that she passed in the 6 hours before her hospital admission. Thus, we cannot calculate how much sodium she lost in her urine. However, it must have been very little because the calculations in table 1.1 presume that she did not pass any urine during the race. If she had indeed passed urine, her fluid intake would have had to be even higher during the race. This seems highly improbable. Also, her blood AVP/ADH concentrations were substantially elevated, reducing urine production to a minimum.

In summary, these data show that the only way Cynthia Lucero could have reduced her blood sodium concentration from 140 mmol/L at the start of the race to 113 mmol/L 6 hours later was by increasing her TBW by at least 3.5 L. This required that she drink Gatorade at a rate of at least 1.2 L/hr for 5 hours. Then she required two additional biological predispositions (SIADH) and osmotic inactivation of circulating sodium to cause such severe EAHE.

Her case shows that the ingestion of a sports drink in excess of thirst cannot prevent the condition of EAHE.

But when the summer comes and the semi-desert has returned, it is more difficult for the hunters. Then it is the time to hunt the larger antelope—the eland, the kudu, the hartebeest, the zebra, and the wildebeest—who can run all day without tiring. Except when it is hot, very hot, more than 40 °C (104 °F), at the end of the dry season, when the sun shines from a clear sky and the animals, less nourished, have been weakened by the biting of the !oam insect.

Like the Tarahumara in Mexico (McDougall, 2009), the Paiutes and the Navajo in the southwestern United States, and the Australian Aborigines (Watanabe H., 1971), the !Xo San of the Kalahari have been chasing large mammals, especially antelope like the kudu and the eland, to the animals' exhaustion for thousands of years. This ability as a distance runner is highly regarded in certain cultures. The !Xo San culture requires that to become a man, each adult male must first kill a large male and female antelope. Scars on both forearms, left for a male and right for a female, indicate that a young man has achieved the transition to adulthood—that he is able to capture antelope either by running the animal to its exhaustion or by stalking it with a bow and arrow and therefore provide meat for his community.

There are now only a few remaining !Xo San hunters. Their remarkable abilities have been captured in an award-winning documentary, *The Great Dance*,[4] filmed by the Foster brothers from Cape Town, South Africa, and in the scientific (2006) and popular (1990) writings of Dr. Louis Liebenberg.

4 *The Great Dance* can be viewed at www.senseafrica.com.

Louis Liebenberg, PhD, began his study of the !Xo San hunting phenomenon in July 1985 and has followed nine "persistence" hunts in which the antelope are run to their exhaustion without the use of poisoned arrows or spears. He discovered that the most important factor determining the successful outcome of a hunt is the midday temperature. So the !Xo San hunters must wait until the midmorning temperature exceeds 40° C (104 °F).

At lower temperatures, the antelope can run without tiring for 6 or more hours; the evening brings cooler temperatures, allowing the chased antelope to escape. But at higher temperatures, the superior human physiology acts in the hunter's favor. Then the antelope's advantage in all other conditions—a superior sprinting speed—cannot match the human's superior ability to maintain a safe body temperature when jogging persistently for 4 or more hours in air temperatures in excess of 40 °C. Of all creatures, *Homo sapiens* is the best adapted for prolonged running in extreme dry heat. No other mammal comes close.

So when the weather promises to be sufficiently hot, the hunters begin by drinking as much water as they can tolerate. Then as a group they run toward their chosen antelope. As they approach too closely, the antelope sprint away before stopping out of sight to rest in the shade. The hunters must now follow their tracks and travel sufficiently fast so that they reach the chased antelope before its body temperature has cooled as it pants while standing still in the shade. This process is continued until one of the chased antelope becomes too hot to continue. In this state, the animal becomes paralyzed and can be killed by spears thrown to pierce its heart at close range. Although many chasers may begin the hunt, usually only one is able to outlast the antelope.

Fewer than a dozen hunts have ever been followed. The recorded hunts lasted from 2 to more than 6 hours in air temperatures ranging from 32 to 42 °C (89.6-107.6 °F), covering distances from 17 to 35 km (10.6-21.7 miles) at running speeds ranging from 4 to 10 km/hr (2.5-6.2 mph) (Liebenberg, 2006). The chasing speed is influenced by the heat of the day, the condition of the surface (slower in soft sand), and the difficulty of tracking an individual animal that may use different methods to mislead the tracker. A hunted animal may circle back onto its own tracks, forcing the tracker to decide which tracks to follow. Unsuccessful hunts usually occur when the tracks are lost, not because the hunter becomes exhausted.

The basis for successful hunting is the ability to track while running at speed. Hence, tracking skills are at least as important as running ability; but without either it is not possible to hunt effectively. The expert hunter must identify the weakest antelope and track it from among many others; he must anticipate the actions of antelope that he cannot see, and he must keep running without drinking or eating regardless of how thirsty he may become. Then when the antelope has been killed, the hunter must return home with the dried and partially cooked meat.

This requires that a reserve of energy be retained so that the hunters are able to navigate back to their home base, often at night and before they have quenched the thirst generated by the hunt.

When the !Xo San hunter Karoha Langwane was filmed while he ran in the Kalahari Desert for 6 hours in 40 to 46 °C (104-114.8 °F) with no cloud cover but low humidity, covering approximately the same distance as had Cynthia Lucero in the 2002 Boston Marathon but over a more demanding surface, he drank a total of about 1 L of fluid. Yet he did not die from either dehydration or heatstroke. Nor did he describe any significant symptoms, other than thirst.

* * *

In this book, I attempt to explain why one human running in cool conditions with free access to all the fluid she could probably wish tragically died, whereas another could run without incident even when he drank perhaps one-sixth of the volume of fluid he lost during 6 hours of exercise in much hotter conditions.

The Catastrophe Theory of Human Physiology

To some scientists, Cynthia Lucero's story might seem to prove the tragic failure of the human body to survive activity that pushed it beyond its capabilities. But how, then, do we explain the !Xo San hunter's ability to outlast an antelope in a 6-hour hunt in extreme environmental conditions and the completion of marathons, ultramarathons, and Ironman triathlons by hundreds of thousands of participants who have not died of heatstroke while training for or participating in such events?

According to the catastrophe model of human physiology, normal physiological processes occur without control until a catastrophic physiological failure occurs, ultimately leading to death. In this view, a person might continue exercising without anticipating the future danger of the failure of heat loss and without controlling homeostasis until the body suddenly collapses from heatstroke due to thermoregulatory failure. According to this catastrophe model, the body cannot accommodate even small increases in body temperature during exercise, nor can it adjust to the fluid and sodium deficits that develop as it loses both in sweat during exercise. Instead, when exposed to exercise under demanding conditions, the body will simply continue without control until eventually a catastrophic physiological failure must inevitably develop.

Some physicians and exercise scientists have been taught to view every exercising human as a catastrophe about to happen—they have presumed that all are equally at risk of developing heat illness, heatstroke, muscle cramping, EAH, and EAHE during exercise. As it relates to the topic of this book, this has led to recommendations that all exercisers must avoid dehydration at all costs and that the only way to do so is to ignore built-in control mechanisms, most especially thirst, because all these controls are hopelessly inadequate. Only by overriding these natural controls will it ever be possible for us to avoid catastrophic collapse, especially during more prolonged exercise.

As you will see in the chapters to come, there is an overwhelming body of evidence showing that humans alter their behaviors to ensure that body temperature is homeostatically regulated regardless of the stresses, either internal (e.g., the level of dehydration) or external (e.g., the environmental temperature) experienced. Humans do this by lowering their metabolic rates (slowing down) well before heatstroke occurs. Thus, the brain acts in anticipation to ensure that its temperature remains within an acceptable range regardless of the environmental conditions.

In addition, the body has strong biological controls to maintain sodium and fluid balance even in the face of sodium deficits or states of fluid loss or even when fluid overload threatens in those who overdrink during exercise. The body is designed to regulate the blood sodium concentration always within a narrow range. It does this by regulating the amounts of sodium and water stored in the body. When sodium or water is lost from the body, for example, the brain can direct the kidneys to retain either more or less sodium or water from the urine, or it can cause the mobilization of sodium from internal body stores so that the blood sodium concentration remains within its normal range. When the fluid intake exceeds the requirement, urine production should also increase as it normally does, provided the subject does not have SIADH, as Cynthia Lucero did in the 2002 Boston Marathon. Of course, all these controls are directed by the subconscious parts of the brain; they do not need any additional override from conscious actions.

It is when we do not listen to our bodies and override our biological instincts with advice from external sources that we run into problems that can, in fact, lead to catastrophe.

The classic story of Pablo Valencia (box 1.2) illustrates the ability of a human to survive under extreme conditions.

BOX 1.2   Pablo Valencia in the Yuma Desert

One of the most remarkable examples of prolonged survival in the desert without water was reported by McGee in 1906 (McGee, 1988). The story centers on Pablo Valencia, a 40-year-old Mexican man weighing 70 kg (154.3 lb) and standing 170 cm (67 inches). On the early morning of Tuesday, 15 August, 1905, Pablo and his friend Jesus set out on horseback to prospect in the desert. By midnight, Jesus returned to camp, having left Pablo 56 km (34.8 miles) away with a single 2-gallon (7.6 L) canteen of water and the reassurance that Jesus would return the following day.

After resting for a few hours, Jesus set out at 3:30 a.m. on Wednesday, 16 August, returning the following morning at 7:00 with the news that he was unable to find Pablo. A second rider was then dispatched 3 hours later with extra water and the instructions "to go to the limit of the horse's endurance and then to his own limit beyond" (McGee, 1988, p. 231) in order to find Pablo. The rider reached the point where Pablo had last been seen and then followed Pablo's tracks for 7 more miles without success, returning to camp at midday on Friday, 18 August, in a state of "speechless exhaustion" (p. 232). Convinced that Pablo must be dead by this time since "Pablo had already been out over three days with only one day's water—and most of those who die from desert thirst expire in less time" (p. 232), no one made any further rescue attempts.*

Five days later on the dawn of 23 August, the impossible happened—a roar like that of a wild animal was heard and an unidentifiable human crawled into the camp. It was Pablo back where he had left 8 days earlier:

Pablo was stark naked; his formerly full-muscled legs and arms were shrunken and scrawny; his ribs ridged out like those of a starveling horse; his habitually plethoric abdomen was drawn in almost against his vertebral column; his lips had disappeared as if amputated, leaving low edges of blackened tissue; his teeth and gums projected like those of a skinned animal, but the flesh was black and dry as a hank of jerky; his nose was withered and shrunken to half its length; the nostril-lining showing black; his eyes were set in a winkless stare, with surrounding skin so contracted as to expose the conjunctiva, itself black as the gums; his face was dark as a negro, and his skin generally turned a ghastly purplish yet ashen gray, with great livid blotches and streaks; his lower legs and feet, with forearms and hands, were torn and scratched by contact with thorns and sharp rocks, yet even the freshest cuts were as so many scratches in dry leather, without trace of blood or serum; his joints and bones stood out like those of a wasted sickling, though the skin clung to them in a way suggesting shrunken rawhide used in repairing a broken wheel. From inspection and handling, I estimated his weight at 115 to 120 lbs [52-54 kg]. We soon found him deaf to all but loud sounds, and so blind as to distinguish nothing save light and dark. The mucus membranes lining mouth and throat were shrivelled, cracked, and blackened, and his tongue shrunken to a mere bunch of black integument. His respiration was slow, spasmodic, and accompanied by a deep guttural moaning or roaring—the sound that had awaken us a quarter of a mile away. His extremities were cold as the surrounding air; no pulsation could be detected at wrists, and there was apparently little if any circulation beyond the knees and elbows; the heartbeat was slow, irregular, fluttering, and almost ceasing in the longer intervals between the stertorous breathings" (McGee, 1988, p. 233). With careful feeding he recovered fully within a week.*

McGee concludes that Pablo was in the desert for 8 days and nights with one day's water, during which he walked and crawled perhaps 160 km (99.4 miles). Half of those who die in the desert do so within the first 36 hours; another quarter die within 48 to 50 hours and nearly all within 70 to 80 hours. Yet Pablo survived without water for 160 hours. He survived by eating insects and drinking his own urine until the final two days when his kidneys were no longer producing urine. His bowels stopped working on the third day. His total weight loss was about 18 kg (39.7 lb), or about 25% of his body weight. He survived because "he was obsessed with the desire for revenge against Jesus, the dream of casting himself in the Tule Well, and the delusion of death—yet he never lost his trail-sense, and apparently squandered little vitality in those aimless movements that commonly hasten and harden the end of the thirst-victim" (McGee, 1988, p. 242).

A more recent survival story suggests that the reports on Pablo were not exaggerated. In 1994, Mauro Prosperi went missing in a sandstorm during the 160-mile (256 km) Marathon des Sables in the Sahara Desert. During an 80 km stage on the fourth day of the event in an ambient temperature of 46 °C (114.8 °F), Prosperi lost his way but found shelter in a Muslim shrine where he survived for 9 days by moving only when it was cool, eating bats, and drinking his own urine. The doctors at the Algerian hospital where he was brought "reported that the desert wanderer had lost about 33 pounds (15 kg) and that 16 liters of intravenous fluids were needed to replace his water loss. His kidneys were barely functioning, his liver was damaged, and he was unable to digest food. His eyes had sunk back inside his sockets, and his skin was dry and wrinkled. He looked like a tortoise. But he would survive" (Kenney, DeGroot, et al., 2004, p. 481).

*Reprinted from W.J. McGee, 1906, "Desert thirst as disease," *Interstate Medical Journal* 1-23.

The Survival Theory of Human Physiology

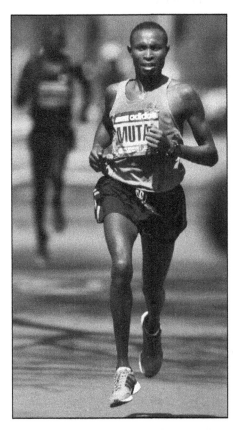

Bipedalism, little body hair, unequaled sweating capacity, and the ability to resist the effects of thirst and water loss make humans the premier hot weather runners.

AP Photo/Steven Senne

The catastrophe theory of human physiology cannot explain why people survive and even thrive in extreme circumstances. It does not explain how the !Xo San hunter and modern marathoner can survive endurance exercise in the heat with little fluid intake. But the fact is that we do survive these activities. Our biological controls are so robust that humans can scale the heights of Mt. Everest; swim at the North Pole; bike the Tour de France, the Race Across America, or even the more grueling Tour d'Afrique (12,000 km, or 7,500 miles) from Cairo to Cape Town; and complete 100 km (60 mile) ultradistance running events.

Nothing in nature is wasted; everything has a purpose. So it is that every human characteristic makes us more competitive as individuals and as a species, better able to cope with the unsafe and hostile environment of the African savannah on which we developed. Humans differ from other mammals and especially the chimpanzees in a number of important ways. The common feature of many of these physiological differences is that each provides for our species' ability to run long distances at a moderate pace and to maintain a safe body temperature when exercising in extreme dry heat. So just as the entire biology of the lion is designed for stalking, sprinting, and dispatching large prey, it seems that humans are the best hot-weather distance runners.

This unexpected conclusion invites this intriguing question: What competitive survival advantage do humans have? To answer this question, we need to study those specific anatomical and biological features that differentiate humans from the great apes.

■ Humans stand erect and walk on two legs (bipedalism).

A period of marked climate change caused the replacement of tropical rain forests with open grasslands in east and southern Africa to the east of the Great Rift Valley. One explanation is that the uplifting of the Rift Valley highlands produced a rain shadow to its east with preservation of heavily wooded areas to the west and the progressive development of grasslands mixed with shrubs and some trees to the east (Hanna and Brown, 1983).

Our human ancestors found themselves on the edge of "the widest possible expanse of open plain devoid of forests, fruits and nuts but abounding in a greater degree with dangerous beasts than any other country in the world" (Dart, 1953). Bipedalism allowed us to explore and even thrive in these conditions.

The savannah is much hotter than the tropical rain forests, especially at midday when the sun shines directly overhead and bakes everything it touches. Without the shady protection of the forest trees, the most effective way to reduce the radiant heat load carried in the sun's rays is to stand and walk upright. Bipedalism reduces the surface area exposed to direct solar radiation.[5] In addition, it raises the body into a cooler microclimate where there is increased air flow. Here it is possible to lose more heat by convection, the process by which the cooler air coursing over the skin is heated up, thereby removing heat from the body.

5 The rays of the sun transfer heat to all bodies that are at a lower temperature. This process is known as (solar) radiation. This solar heat load experienced by any body is determined by the area of that body exposed to the sun's rays. As the sun rises more than 40° above the horizontal, a biped exposes less surface area to the sun than a quadruped does. As a result, at midday when the sun is directly overhead, a biped has 60% less surface area exposed to the sun than does a quadruped of the same mass (Wheeler, 1993).

At typical savannah air temperatures of 35 to 40 °C (95-104 °F), early humans could forage for food at all times of the day without needing to cool down by resting in the shade (Wheeler, 1988). Were we quadrupedal (walking on four legs), we would be forced to seek shade in the midday heat in order to cool down. Bipedalism allowed humans to collect food at midday. In contrast, because they are quadrupedal and also have an inferior capacity to regulate their body temperatures (thermoregulation) since they do no sweat, large, nonsweating predators, such as leopards and lions, must seek shade and avoid exercising (hunting) in the midday heat.

Bipedalism also allows us to walk up to 15 km a day while losing only about 1.5 L of fluid as sweat, whereas a quadrupedal human of the same mass (were such an animal to exist) would lose about 2.5 L of sweat to cover the same distance (Wheeler, 1991a; Wheeler, 1993). So bipedalism provided a significant thermoregulatory advantage, first for exploring and scavenging and later for running on the African savannah in scorching midday heat. Bipedalism alleviates "the most stressing problem of open equatorial environments: heat gain from direct solar radiation" (Wheeler, 1984, p. 97).

■ Humans sweat more profusely than any other living creature.

Relatively few mammals sweat. Those that do include the horse, the donkey, the camel, the baboon, and certain large African antelope such as the eland and the oryx (gemsbok). Sweat removes body heat and therefore acts in maintaining a safe body temperature in these larger mammals either when they are resting in a hot or humid environment or when they exercise, especially in dry heat.

But no mammal sweats as much as humans do (box 1.3, page 16). Comparative studies show that horses can sweat at a rate of 100 gm/m²/hr,[6] camels at 250 gm/m²/hr, but humans at rates in excess of 500 gm/m²/hr (Folk, 1966). This requires that the concentration of sweat glands in human skin be substantially greater than in any other sweating mammal.

So sweating allows humans to survive without distress in conditions that are fatal for apes. For example, chimpanzees cannot survive in air temperatures greater than 38 °C (100.4 °F) (Hanna and Brown, 1983), whereas humans are able to exercise moderately vigorously for many hours under these conditions provided the air humidity is low.

6 The measurement g/m²/hr means the number of grams (ml) of sweat excreted per hour relative to the total body surface area measured in square meters (m²).

BOX 1.3 Relative Advantages of Sweating and Panting

When mammals exercise, they generate heat in proportion to their body masses and the speeds at which they travel. One advantage of being small is that at any running speed, smaller mammals generate less heat and so need to lose less water by either panting or sweating to maintain a safe body temperature. This helps to explain why elite distance runners are inevitably small—about 50 kg (110 lb) for both men and women—and how being lighter by even a few kilograms can produce a large competitive advantage when running in the heat (Dennis and Noakes, 1999; Marino, Mbambo, et al., 2000).[7]

There are four ways by which mammals transfer heat from the site at which the heat is produced in their exercising muscles to where it is absorbed by the environment at the skin surface (figure 1.1): convection, radiation, conduction, and sweating or panting (i.e., humans do pant but do not transfer a significant amount of heat via rapid breathing).

Humans involved in persistence hunting, or marathon running for that matter, lose heat by evaporation from the skin surface (sweating) or the respiratory tract (equivalent to panting), by convection, by radiation, and to a lesser extent by conduction. As exercise begins, the blood flow to the muscles increases. As it passes through the muscles, the blood is heated. The heat is then distributed throughout the body but

[7] Smallness provides a decisive advantage in distance running in the heat. At any running speed, the rate of heat production is greatest in the heaviest runners since it is a function of body mass. Thus, when both run at the same speed, smaller runners produce less heat than larger runners. To maintain a safe body temperature, a smaller runner would need to sweat less than a heavier runner. Larger mammals have a larger TBW and can lose more water before becoming substantially dehydrated. But the challenge is not so much the extent of the water loss but rather the rate at which the heat produced by exercising humans can be soaked up by a hot, humid environment.

The key determinants of the safety of sustained exercise in any environment are the rate at which the athlete will be generating heat (Dennis and Noakes, 1999) and whether that environment can absorb that heat sufficiently rapidly. As the temperature and humidity increase, less heat can be absorbed by that environment. Instead, the athlete will naturally slow down, as dictated by the control centers in the brain, which, detecting this imbalance between heat production and heat loss, will ensure that dangerous hyperthermia is avoided.

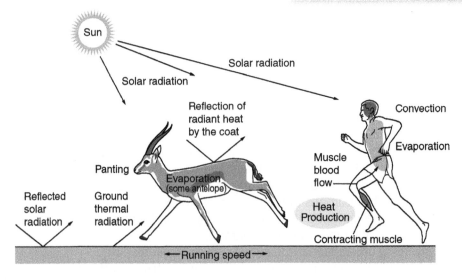

FIGURE 1.1 Factors involved in heat loss and heat gain by a persistence hunter and antelope. In this race, the human hunter holds the thermoregulatory advantage.

especially to the skin as blood flow to the skin is increased in exercising mammals. The increased blood flow to the skin raises the skin temperature. Circulating air currents waft air over the skin; this air is usually cooler than the skin temperature of 33 to 35 °C. The (hotter) skin then offloads its heat by warming the cooler air in contact with the skin. This form of heat transfer is known as convection. The more quickly the unwarmed air traverses the skin, the greater the convective heat losses from the skin.

Any nearby body whose surface temperature is lower than that of the skin—for example, trees or the road surface—will attract this heat, which travels by electromagnetic waves in a form of heat transfer known as radiation. In contrast, the large radiant heat load from the sun especially at midday heats the body, again emphasizing the advantage of bipedalism. The development of a prodigious sweating response not only offsets the disadvantage posed by an increased radiant heat load on the shadeless African savannah but it provides us with a thermoregulatory system more advanced than any present in any other large African mammal. This provided early humans with a competitive advantage, potentially exploitable during prolonged exercise in the midday heat.

A lack of fur increases heat gain from radiation but improves the efficiency of heat loss by sweating, which also lowers the skin temperature. (The coat of the hunted antelope reduces its heat gain from radiation.) The main source of heat gain during exercise is the (inefficient) energy production by human muscle, in which 75% of the energy released is wasted as heat, not as athletic endeavor.

Conduction is the transfer of heat between two bodies that are in direct contact. This occurs within the human body during exercise as the hotter exercising skeletal muscles conduct heat directly to the overlying skin.

The skin is also cooled and heat is lost from the body when the thin film of sweat secreted by the sweat glands onto the skin surface evaporates in the process known as evaporation of sweating. The production of sweat by the sweat glands does not cause heat loss from the body; vaporization of that water film into steam causes the heat loss.

The majority of nonhuman mammals do not sweat. Instead, they regulate their body temperatures by panting, in which they accelerate their breathing rates, vaporizing water from the respiratory tract. Panting is the main source of heat loss in antelope, although some large antelope like the desert-dwelling oryx (gemsbok) and eland can also sweat. Panting also lowers the brain temperature. But panting is a less effective method of cooling the brain than sweating is from most of the skin surface. As a result, humans are better able than most antelope to maintain safe brain temperatures during prolonged exercise in extreme dry heat.

Following are the advantages of panting (Richards, 1970; Taylor, 1977):

1. Panting does not lower the skin temperature as sweating does. The disadvantage of a lower skin temperature is that heat is more easily absorbed from the surrounding environment (by radiation) if the environmental temperature is higher than the skin temperature. Thus, at an environmental temperature of 47 °C (116.6 °F), twice as much heat flows by radiation and convection into a sweating human than into a panting animal (Taylor and Rowntree, 1973) because of the lower skin temperature of the sweating mammal. Conversely, because the skin temperature of panting animals is higher, their capacity to lose heat by the reverse movement of convection from the (hotter) skin to the (cooler) surrounding air is also increased.

One of the key adaptations shown by African hunting dogs and other desert dwellers like the oryx and the camel (Schmidt-Nielsen, 1964) is that all maintain higher-than-expected body and skin temperatures when exposed to heat. This aids heat loss from the skin by

(continued)

BOX 1.3 **Relative Advantages of Sweating and Panting** *(continued)*

8 !Xo San hunters use this biological peculiarity to their benefit even though they may not fully understand the physiological principles. Hunters will camp at a water hole and repeatedly prevent those antelope that they wish to hunt from drinking. They will keep this up for 24 to 48 hours or until they expect that the antelope is about to leave the area and move to another watering hole. The dehydrated antelope will respond by raising its body temperature in order to conserve water during the day. As a result, when the hunt begins, the antelope's body temperature is already elevated so that less exercise is required to raise the body temperature to that at which paralysis occurs. Thus, the hunt will be shorter.

convection and radiation while lowering the need for heat loss by panting—that is, the capacity to maintain a higher body temperature is a water-conserving mechanism.[8]

2. Panting animals lose little salt in their expired air. In contrast, because human sweat contains sodium chloride (salt) in varying amounts depending on the habitual diet and the level of heat acclimatization, sweating removes sodium chloride from the body. Theoretically at least, sweating could cause substantial salt losses from humans. Chapter 4 contains the scientific evidence that disproves this popular myth.

3. Panting generates its own wind speed across the evaporative surfaces, thereby aiding heat loss. In contrast, mammals who sweat must generate a wind speed across the evaporative surface (the skin) by either standing in the wind or by walking or running.

In contrast, sweating from the skin surface produces the following advantages:

1. Sweating occurs from a much larger surface area (most of the body surface) than panting does (the upper respiratory tract). In addition, sweating animals lose heat both from their respiratory surfaces (as do panters) and from their skin surfaces. Thus, their potential for heat loss is much increased.

2. Sweating occurs independently of the respiratory cycle and can be modulated to increase to very high levels when required. In contrast, the amount of heat lost from panting can increase only to the extent to which the animal is prepared to pant.

3. Sweating animals can eat and cool at the same time, whereas panting animals like the cheetah and lion cannot. Rather, they must pant first to lower their body temperatures before they can eat.

4. Efficiency of heat loss by sweating is increased by the lack of fur or hair. Wind traveling over a coat of fur >2 cm thick at the speeds at which humans run (10-20 km per hr, or 6.2-12.4 mph) does not disturb the layer of air caught in the hair or fur and thus does not lower the skin temperature.

An absence of hair and the ability to sweat make humans particularly adept at regulating their body temperatures when running in hot, dry conditions that favor heat loss by sweating. The effectiveness of heat loss falls as the air humidity rises because it impairs the capacity to lose heat by sweating.

Thus, humans are not as well adapted for exercising in the type of heat present in forests or jungles, in which the humidity is high (~100%). But bipedalism and our unmatched sweating capacity allow for exceptional performance in hot, arid conditions.

The cost of sweating is that it removes water from the body, promoting fluid loss and causing what has been termed *voluntary dehydration.* For each individual there is a level of dehydration that causes physical incapacitation and ultimately death.[9] In a very hot, sunny environment typical of the desert in which there is also little shade, humans can usually survive usefully for 24 hours, becoming increasingly disabled thereafter; death usually occurs on the third day. There have been some notable exceptions, including Pablo Valencia, whose story appears in box 1.2 (page 12).

Our capacity to sweat profusely when exposed to desert heat prevents us from being true desert-dwelling mammals like the oryx or the kangaroo rat, both of which can survive in the desert without access to free-standing water (Schmidt-Nielsen, 1964). On exposure to heat, humans sweat in order to maintain a whole-body but specifically a brain temperature below ~40 °C; sweating progressively reduces body water stores, reducing the duration of survival without water.

9 The level of dehydration at which humans become physically disabled and at risk of dying is central to the debate of how much athletes should drink during exercise. Before the development of the world's first sports drink, this topic drew little discussion. Rather, it was assumed that humans could safely exercise for perhaps 8 to 10 hours in the heat while requiring little fluid replacement.

But with the development of the world's first sports drink, the concept arose that athletes should drink as much as tolerable to ensure that they do not lose any weight during exercise. I have termed this the zero % dehydration rule. More recently it has been suggested that a weight loss of less than 2% of body weight during exercise is safe and will not impair exercise performance (Sawka, Burke, et al., 2007). The arguments for and against these ideas are presented more fully in later chapters.

Our species' great capacity to sweat profusely severely limits our ability to survive without water in hot conditions. This means that sweating must provide some decisive survival advantage.

The ability of humans to stand upright aided by an effective sweating mechanism allowed humans to survive exposure to the large radiant heat load on the hot, shadeless African savannah (Newman, 1970). The loss of hair is a disadvantage that is offset by sweating as an additional and more effective method of heat loss. But our sweating capacity far exceeds that required just to offset the thermoregulatory disadvantage of the lack of hair.

■ Humans have very little body hair.

Like clothing, hair traps a thin layer of air next to the skin. The body soon heats that trapped layer of air to the temperature of the skin. This insulating air layer prevents a continual heat loss from the body when the skin temperature is higher than the surrounding air temperature. The optimal skin temperature that allows humans to maintain thermal balance at rest is about 33 °C (91.4 °F) compared to the usual core body temperature at rest of 37 °C (98.6 °F). Like sweating, the main function of body hair is thermoregulatory, so this reduction in body hair has produced a decisive thermoregulatory advantage.

When the Earth cooled, woodlands and savannah replaced the equatorial rain forests east of the Great Rift Valley (the continuous geographic trench, approximately 6,000 km, or 3,700 miles, in length, that runs from northern Syria in Southwest Asia to central Mozambique in Southeast Africa). The tropical rain forest that the savannah replaced has the following characteristics: a daily maximum temperature of about 28 to 32 °C (82.4-89.6 °F), very little air movement, and a very high humidity (up to 100%) caused by the water expired by plants as they convert sunlight and carbon dioxide into oxygen and the chemicals necessary for their growth. But in the tropical forest, there is little exposure to radiant heat from the sun since the leaves of the jungle canopy absorb that energy.

Provided they do not exercise too vigorously, the large primates—the gorillas and chimpanzees—can comfortably exist in the tropical rain forest under these conditions since their skin temperatures (~34 °C) are always higher than the air temperature in the forest. As a result their bodies are able to transfer heat by convection from the skin surface to the cooler surrounding air, thereby cooling the primates.

However, the open savannah poses a different thermal challenge because solar radiation is much more intense on the savannah than in the tropical forest. The sun's direct rays add a substantial amount of radiant heat to creatures that venture beyond the shade provided by the forest canopy. This added heat load is the equivalent of an effective 7 °C (12.6 °F) increase in air temperature.

But air moves more freely on the savannah across open spaces, unimpeded by forest vegetation. This increases the rate at which heat can be convected away from the (hotter) skin by the (cooler) air passing over it. This effect increases as an exponential function of the wind speed (Adams, Mack, et al., 1992; Saunders, Dugas, et al., 2005). Convection cools the body very effectively, even during vigorous exercise.[10]

In addition, the air on the savannah has a much lower water content (humidity) because there is limited vegetation to add water to the air. The efficiency of heat loss by sweating is greatly increased at low humidity but falls steeply as the humidity rises. Thus, sweating is a more effective method for heat loss on the savannah than in the more humid jungle environment.

A coat of hair that reflects most of this radiant heat is the best protection against solar radiation, better even than an upright body posture. Thus, the coats of the African antelopes, the eland, and the hartebeest reflect 70% of the radiant heat carried in the sun's rays (Finch, 1972). The light-colored coat of the oryx, the only true desert-dwelling antelope, is so reflective that the oryx does not need to seek shade at midday but can continue grazing. Those oryx with the lightest-colored coats have penetrated the farthest into the desert (Taylor, 1969). Camels with full coats sweat less in desert heat than when they are shorn (Schmidt-Nielsen, 1959), proving the efficacy of the camel's coat in reflecting radiant heat.

Humans' thermoregulatory disadvantage of a reduced capacity to reflect radiant heat from the sun caused by the lack of hair must be offset by some other more valuable thermoregulatory advantage. The key advantage is probably the ability to lose heat more effectively by sweating since profuse sweating provides humans with the greatest heat-losing capacity of any mammal. And this advantage becomes greatest

10   This effect is well known to professional cyclists who feel very hot as they climb steep mountain passes at slow speeds (but at high rates of heat production) and then become icy cold when they speed down the other side of the mountain at very high speeds (but low rates of heat production). The high wind speeds they generate as they descend increase their rates of convective heat loss as an exponential function of how fast they travel, thus producing a large cooling effect. Convective heat losses must be taken into account when conducting laboratory studies to determine optimal rates of fluid ingestion during exercise.

in hot, dry conditions—the exact conditions present on the African savannah east of the Rift Valley.

While hair is an effective reflector of radiant heat, it traps a layer of (warm) air within the fur, a few millimeters from the skin surface. This reduces the efficiency of sweating since sweat is evaporated from the surface of the fur, not from the skin itself. Sweating from a hairy surface fails to cool the skin directly while drawing some of the heat needed to evaporate the sweat from the air itself, not from the skin surface. Loss of hair increases the efficiency of heat loss by sweating, reducing the magnitude of the sweat loss required to cool the body (Wheeler, 1992). Provided humans can sweat profusely from the entire skin surface area, the amount of heat they can lose by sweating far exceeds that needed to offset the extra radiant heat gain resulting from the lack of a reflective fur coat (Wheeler, 1985).

Because they have a sweating capacity much inferior to humans', primates are unable to regulate their body temperatures when exercising in a savannah-type environment and cannot survive in air temperatures greater than 38 °C (100.4 °F). In addition, their coat of hair provides a significantly greater barrier to heat loss by convection than the hairless skin of humans (Johnson and Elizondo, 1979).

The result is that the lack of hair and a much superior capacity to lose heat by sweating allows exercising humans to maintain body (and brain) temperatures safely below ~40 °C even while they perform vigorous physical activity in air temperatures of 29 to 35 °C—precisely the conditions faced on the African savannah.

■ Humans do not selectively cool their brains to the same extent as some mammals do.

Some mammals (but not primates or humans) have developed methods of maintaining their brains at cooler temperatures than the rest of their bodies (Wheeler, 1988; Wheeler, 1984; Wheeler, 1993). They achieve this by panting, which cools the nasal passages and the blood present in an extensive network of veins in the muzzle (figure 1.2, page 22). This acts as a radiator, cooling the venous blood draining from the face as its returns to the heart. The arterial blood vessels taking blood to the brain form a plexus (or network), the carotid rete, which intertwines with these veins near the base of the brain. In this way, the hotter (arterial) blood traveling to the brain from the center of the body is cooled by a transfer of heat to the (cooler) venous blood draining from the face.

Primates and humans do not contain either a radiator or a carotid rete, nor are they designed to lose substantial amounts of heat by panting. Instead, humans have the most advanced cooling mechanism of any living creature—profuse sweating from the surface of the whole body. In this way, humans are able to maintain whole-body temperatures cooler than the "critical" temperature at which brain function is impaired and the brain is at risk of being "cooked." In addition, humans exhibit behavior modifications to ensure that they never exercise at intensities that will produce an excessive rise in body temperature when exercising in the heat. Finally, if this behavior change fails for any reason and the brain temperature reaches a dangerously high level, humans become temporarily paralyzed—unable to move in any coordinated fashion—and therefore unable to continue exercising.

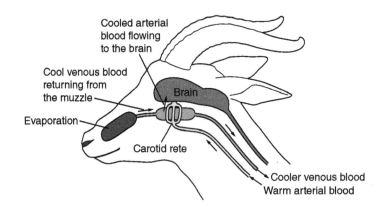

FIGURE 1.2 The "radiator" in the nasal passages of some mammals, such as African antelopes, allows venous blood to be cooled and thereby cool the hotter arterial blood traveling to the brain. This allows them to maintain their brains at temperatures cooler than the rest of their bodies.

Wheeler (1988) concludes, "It is probably no coincidence that today the mammal with the most developed brain is also the species that possesses the most powerful and effective cooling system [sweating from the whole body] to protect it" (p. 65). For example, the temperature of the blood perfusing the brain of an antelope running to escape a chasing cheetah may be only 41 °C when its body temperature, increased by the heat produced by the vigorous muscular activity of an all-out sprint, may be 45 to 46 °C[11] (Taylor and Lyman, 1972).

Human biology uses a different solution, a larger radiator in the form of an overwhelming sweating response able to maintain a safe brain temperature by keeping the body temperature below that at which brain damage occurs. The advantage is that this allows humans to maintain body (and brain) temperatures within a safe range even when exercising vigorously in midday heat.

Further, to prevent exercising too vigorously in the heat, humans also have a subconscious controller that ensures a reduced pace (Tucker, Marle, et al., 2006; Tucker, Rauch, et al., 2004) when the environmental conditions are excessively hot and in which uncontrolled exercise might overwhelm even humans' superior cooling ability, causing dangerously high brain temperatures.

11 The evolutionary explanation for the development of different methods of cooling the brains of antelope and humans would seem to be the different physical stresses experienced by antelope and early humans as they carved out their specific ecological niches on the hot African savannah. The key difference is the modern antelope's need to keep its brain cool while it sprints all out for about 40 seconds to escape the pursuing cheetah or lion. In contrast, our human ancestors needed to maintain a low brain temperature while they chased antelope for hours in midday heat. Sweating was the only solution for the thermoregulatory challenges faced by early humans. The point is that the speed that animals, including humans, can sustain during prolonged exercise is ultimately determined by the size of the "radiator" that they possess. Sweating provides humans with the largest radiator of any mammal. Panting does not produce anything like the same cooling capacity. As a result, humans have the greatest capacity of any mammal to run in dry heat (Dill, 1938; Schmidt-Nielsen, 1964).

■ Humans have an insulating layer of fat immediately below the skin—the subcutaneous layer of fat.

The loss of body hair in humans increases both radiant heat gain during the day but also heat loss from the body when the environment cools at night. However, a thin layer of fat below the skin increases insulation, reducing heat loss. Clothing, the use of fire, and behavioral changes like huddling together further improve cold tolerance at night.

During exercise, the insulating effect of the subcutaneous layer of fat can be bypassed by sweating and by increased blood flow to the skin. The increased blood flow raises the skin temperature, increasing heat loss by convection. The presence of an insulating subcutaneous layer of fat does not alter the efficiency of either of these mechanisms.

■ Humans have a linear design and are taller than 1 meter.

Whereas bipedalism minimizes the surface area of the body that is exposed to radiant heat from the sun, a greater vertical height (linearity) increases the total surface area of the skin, enhancing the capacity to lose heat by convection and reducing the need to lose heat by sweating. Thus, bipedalism and increased vertical height maximize the total surface area of the skin for evaporation and convection but minimize the area exposed to direct solar radiation. Increased linearity, like bipedalism, is a water-conserving adaptation for humans living in hot, arid environments. But in extreme heat (>35 °C, or 95 °F), when the environmental temperature exceeds that at the skin surface (~33 °C), this benefit is lost as heat is transferred to the body from the surrounding air.

A tall, linear *Homo sapiens* has a greater capacity than smaller species to lose heat by convection while still exposing less of his total skin surface to the sun's rays. The same absolute area of skin might be exposed to the sun's rays, but *Homo sapiens* would have two distinct advantages: First, a greater body mass associated with this increased height increases the total body water (TBW) content. Second, a greater total skin surface area increases the capacity for convective and evaporative heat losses (Wheeler, 1993), resulting in a savings of water.

Finally, the vegetation on the African savannah is 25 to 150 cm tall (Wheeler, 1991a; 1991b). Thus, an important benefit of being tall is that air movement is greater and the air temperatures lower ~150 cm above the ground.

■ Humans are heavier than the nearest primate relatives.

The weights of female and male chimpanzees and bonobos are 30 and 40 kg (66.1 and 88.2 lb), respectively, somewhat smaller than modern sub-Saharan Africans. A greater body mass increases total surface area of the skin, increasing capacity to lose heat by convection and sweating, which allows for further travel away from home base before becoming debilitated by a dehydration of more than 5%.

■ Humans have shorter arms than apes and arms that are shorter than their legs. The reverse applies for the great apes.

Longer arms and fingers are used for climbing but shorter arms and fingers, longer legs, and a foot with an arch and five forward-pointing toes clearly allow for running.

■ Humans have long legs with built-in springs that increase efficiency while running.

Relative to body weight, humans have the longest legs of any species. We also have springs in the lower limbs that conserve energy while running. In addition, we have a subconsciously controlled brain mechanism that activates leg muscles immediately before the feet touch the ground (Nummela, Heath, et al., 2008; Nummela, Paavolainen, et al., 2006). This further increases and regulates the springiness of the legs. Humans also have thinner legs than other hominins, and the most successful distance runners in the world usually have extremely thin legs. Thin, light legs reduce the energy cost of moving the lower limb back and forward when running.

The increased springiness of our lower limbs allows energy to be stored when our feet land on the ground as we run. As the foot leaves the ground, the spring stretches, releasing this temporarily stored energy. This adaptation is of no value in walking because little energy can be stored and returned during the walking stride. Rather, this adaptation specifically improves efficiency as long-distance runners (Bramble and Lieberman, 2004; Carrier, 1984; Lieberman and Bramble, 2007). This is the first piece of compelling evidence suggesting that long-distance running ability was critically important in the development of *Homo sapiens*. Similarly, shorter toes reduce the forces required to sustain running and further reduce mechanical cost of running (Rolian, Lieberman, et al., 2009).

■ Humans have large buttock muscles (gluteus maximus).

Compared to all the primates, "being endowed with prominent rounded buttocks is the unique privilege of humans" (Jouffroy and Médina, 2007, p. 135). Interestingly, the gluteus maximus muscle is essentially inactive when standing or when walking on a level surface. As a result, humans in whom the gluteus maximus is paralyzed are able to walk on a flat surface without any obvious difficulty.

Activities that require the action of the gluteus maximus muscle include jogging, running, sprint starting, leaping, climbing stairs, and walking up a slope. In these activities, the muscle acts to extend the hip and to control the side-to-side balance of the trunk (Lieberman, Raichlen et al., 2006). The muscle also acts to slow the rotation of the trunk in the throwing motion. By slowing the trunk rotation, the angular momentum is transferred to the arm, increasing the speed at which an object can be thrown. Thus, this muscle is highly active in baseball pitching (Watkins, Dennis, et al., 1989). In addition, the muscle is active when straightening up from a stooping, squatting, or crouching position. The gluteus maximus muscle is integral to the biomechanical demands of jogging and running, including the stabilization of the side-to-side movements during faster running, the capacity to throw objects with force, and the ability to straighten up from the crouching position when living at ground level.

■ Humans are able to counterrotate the upper body on the pelvis while keeping the head still.

This adaptation is essential for maintaining balance when running and is perhaps the second piece of compelling evidence suggesting that *Homo sapiens* was on the road to becoming a superior long-distance runner. When running, but not when walking, the center of gravity transfers from one side of the body to the other as we land on alternate feet with each stride. It is not possible to balance when only one foot is on the ground (as occurs in running but not in walking) other than by rotating the upper body and arm in the opposite direction while keeping the head still. Chimpanzees and other great apes are unable to run because they lack this ability to rotate their upper bodies while keeping their heads still.

This ability to rotate the upper body while keeping the head still also provides humans with an ability to throw an object and to strike with an implement; these skills are the basis for human sporting ability in all hitting sports (including golf, tennis, and hockey) and in combined throwing and hitting sports (like cricket and baseball).[12]

■ Humans have larger brains and smaller intestines than primates.

Modern humans have an average cranial capacity of about 1,300 cubic cm (cc), whereas fossils of hominids show much smaller brain sizes: 200 to 250 cc for *Ardipithecus ramidus,* 450 to 500 cc *Australopithecus africanus,* and 1,000 cc for *Homo erectus.* Increased brain size may have allowed *Homo erectus* to hunt effectively by keeping "the task constantly in mind for several days and to anticipate the results well into the future" (Krantz, 1968, p. 450).

In addition, the skull surrounding the human brain is thicker and the general robustness of the skeleton is increased. Both adaptations favor successful hunting—skeletal robustness to increase the power of the muscles used in throwing and to absorb any blows received from the horns and bodies of large animals injured in the hunt (Brace and Montagu, 1977).

12 By rotating the pelvis, a torsional force is generated in the upper body and arms, allowing a weapon held in the hand to be accelerated and to become potentially lethal. This ability to rotate the upper body and to either throw or strike may have provided the method of dispatching animals before cutting weapons became available (Dart, 1953). Charles Darwin (1877) recognized the importance to human evolution of this "capacity to stand still and to transform the immobilised feet into a rock-like base from which the whirling body can operate as a whole" (p. 53).

Primates need very long intestines to digest food, the predominant constituents of which are plants with low energy content. But a high-energy diet containing mainly protein and fat (and also perhaps more salt to sustain a larger body water content) could be accommodated by a smaller intestine. And the smaller intestine allows for a metabolically expensive larger brain, since, relative to its weight, the brain is the most metabolically active organ in the human body (Aiello and Wheeler, 1995).

With a smaller intestine comes a smaller abdomen. So while apes show a barrel-shaped chest and protruding belly to accommodate the intestines, modern humans have a smaller, rounder chest and pelvis and a smaller abdominal cavity, allowing the appearance of a waist.

An interesting consequence of a high-energy diet is that it reduces the frequency of defecation, different from the "typical primate eating pattern which is that of the more-or-less uninterrupted snack, followed by a similar output of the day-long defecation" (Brace and Montagu, 1977, p. 314).

13 The human kidneys have a limited capacity to excrete a fluid load. The human intestine can absorb fluid faster than the kidneys can excrete the absorbed fluid. We have shown that the maximum rate at which the kidneys can excrete a fluid load is less than 1,000 ml/hr (Noakes, Wilson, et al., 2001), even in 70 to 80 kg males, and probably is closer to 800 ml/hr. In smaller (50-60 kg) females, it is likely to be even less, perhaps as low as 600 ml/hr.

This has important implications for the amount of fluid that humans can safely ingest or receive via intravenous injection. If fluid is ingested or infused at rates faster than the kidneys can excrete that fluid, it must be retained, causing an expansion of the TBW and a progressive fall in the blood osmolality and sodium concentration, leading ultimately to hyponatremic encephalopathy and death from respiratory arrest.

A reduced intestine makes better physiological sense than reduced muscle mass or kidneys. Adequate muscle mass provides the strength and endurance for hunting and scavenging for the high-energy diet, and large, metabolically expensive kidneys allow humans to survive in a dry environment in which water is not always freely available.

Human kidneys can excrete a moderately salt-concentrated urine but not as concentrated as the urine of desert-dwelling animals like the kangaroo rat, camel, and oryx, all of which can survive for either prolonged periods (camel) or indeed indefinitely (oryx) without the need to ingest free-standing water. All these mammals excrete a urine that is 2 to 3 times more concentrated than the maximally concentrated human urine[13] and is also 1.5 to 2 times more concentrated than seawater (Schmidt-Nielsen, 1964).

As a result, all these mammals can survive by drinking seawater (whereas humans cannot), although the magnesium sulphate in seawater is a laxative and will produce diarrhea if large volumes are ingested. In contrast, the maximum concentrating capacity of the human kidney is only about two-thirds the salt concentration of seawater. As a result, if humans ingest seawater, they must excrete additional water to lose the extra salt ingested in the seawater (Schmidt-Nielsen, 1964).

The functional capacity of the human intestine and kidney has been described as "enough, but not too much" (Diamond, 1991). Within the constraints imposed by a dietary energy supply that was also enough but not too much, humans developed the most efficient physiology that would perform those functions that provided the biological advantage to ensure survival as a species (box 1.4).

Several other characteristics ensure that a reduced capacity for intestinal absorption would not interfere with the ability to exercise in dry heat during profuse sweating:

- Humans have large posterior semicircular canals in the middle ear and well-developed posterior neck muscles that stabilize the head when running.
- Humans can adapt (acclimatize) so that they are better able to exercise in the heat. The key adaptations are the ability to increase already generous sweat rates and to maintain lower body temperatures while placing less demand on the heart and circulation.
- Humans actively regulate the amount of sodium chloride (salt) lost in sweat and urine to equal the amount ingested in the diet.
- Humans drink frequently in small amounts and delay the full correction of any fluid deficits generated by exercise.

BOX 1.4 Maximum Absorptive Capacity of the Human Intestine

Many of those advising athletes about how much they should drink during exercise have assumed that there is no limit to the rate at which the human intestine can absorb fluid. Thus, they have presumed that any rate of fluid ingestion that they prescribe, however great, will always be less than the maximum rate at which the human intestine can absorb that fluid. As a result, the fluid will be rapidly absorbed; it will not accumulate in the intestine and cause the symptoms of nausea and intestinal fullness, leading ultimately to diarrhea and the vomiting of clear fluid. Given the high frequency of the symptoms of nausea and intestinal fullness and the number of athletes who vomit clear fluid during or after exercise, it seems that this assumption is probably not correct—especially when athletes are encouraged to sustain drinking rates of up to 1.2 L/hr or even 1.8 L/hr for many hours of exercise.

One study that directly measured the maximum rate of intestinal fluid absorption reported a maximum value of 600 ml/hr, or 20.3 fl oz/hr (Palma, Vidon, et al., 1981). When fluid was infused at rates in excess of this maximum value, most tested subjects began to develop diarrhea (figure 1.3). The authors also calculated that the intestine can store perhaps as much as 1.2 L of fluid before diarrhea develops.

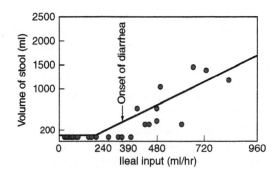

FIGURE 1.3   In a study by Palma and colleagues (1981), diarrhea occurred when the ileal input exceeded 6.3 ml/min (arrowed). This occurred when the rate of fluid infusion was about 10 ml/min (600 ml/hr).

With kind permission from Springer Science+Business Media: *Digestive Diseases and Sciences*, "Maximal capacity for fluid absorption in human bowel," 26(10), 1981, 929-934, R. Palma, N. Vidon, and J.J. Bernier, figure 1. © 1981 Digestive Disease Systems, Inc.

Interestingly, those humans who have not been told to drink as much as tolerable during exercise generally drink fluid at rates of about 400 to 800 ml/hr during exercise (Noakes, Adams, et al., 1988), suggesting that this freely chosen rate of fluid ingestion might indeed be influenced also by their maximum rates of intestinal fluid ingestion since drinking at higher rates would be increasingly likely to produce the symptoms caused by the accumulation of unabsorbed fluid in their intestines. These authors suggest that the maximum amount of fluid that humans can ingest each day is about 8 L (270.5 fl oz). In contrast, other studies suggest that intestinal fluid absorption rates may be as high as 1.3 L/hr (Duchman, Ryan, et al., 1997) to 1.6 L/hr (Shi, Summers, et al., 1994).

A larger intestine would allow humans to drink larger volumes of fluid before satiation. As a result, we would be able to drink more during exercise and therefore minimize the extent to which any water deficit (caused by sweating) would develop during exercise. Instead, our smaller intestine allows for the ability to secure food by hunting in dry environmental conditions where water is not abundant and where small amounts of water would satisfy.

The reduced size of the human gut, including the small size of the stomach leading into the intestine, means that humans are unable to ingest very large volumes of fluid quickly. Rather, we tend to drink enough to fill our stomachs (~500 ml, or 16.9 fl oz); we then wait until the stomach has emptied that volume (requiring 15-20 minutes) before we are again able to drink another large volume. Alternatively, we can ingest small volumes more frequently (sipping). The result, however, is the same: Humans are less able than most other mammals of equivalent size to drink large volumes of fluid quickly.

This uncoupling of thirst from fluid loss would have delayed the desire and indeed the need to drink until evening when our ancestors returned to their home base where stored fluid would have been more freely available. Some believe that this development of the "home base with daily foraging" was a major factor influencing subsequent human social evolution (Hanna and Brown, 1983, p. 263). Had this not occurred, they would have spent their days searching for water, not for edible foods.

Our species' inability to drink large volumes rapidly, due to our large brains and small intestines, has promoted the pejorative concept that humans are poorly adapted for exercise in the heat because we are reluctant drinkers (Szlyk, Hubbard, et al., 1987) who develop an undesirable condition of voluntary dehydration in which there is a "delay in complete rehydration following water loss" (Greenleaf and Sargent, 1965, p. 719).

Thus, it is argued that human physiology is inferior, indeed fatally flawed, since we are unable to completely replace a fluid deficit as it develops; whereas camels, donkeys, and dogs can. In the words of Adolph and Dill (1938), "No other animal than man has been studied in which the amount of water taken at one time is insufficient to restore permanently the water balance. It is not known what factors of alimentary capacity or of rapidity of passage of water through the alimentary tract may be concerned with this difference" (p. 377). These authors noted that they had observed this phenomena in a previous study (Dill, 1938) and that the explorer J. Smeaton Chase had also described how he drank most of his fluids at night as he rode through the Mojave Desert in the early 1900s (Smeaton Chase, 2004).

Since voluntary dehydration develops only in humans, this proves to scientists who hold to the catastrophe theory that humans are incapable of safely managing their fluid balances during prolonged exercise in the heat. As a result, humans can exercise safely only if they are told exactly when and how much to drink during exercise, especially if it is in the heat. When left to their own devices, humans will not drink enough during exercise, becoming dehydrated with potentially fatal consequences. This conclusion ignores the fact that dogs especially and, to a somewhat lesser extent, donkeys and camels (since both sweat) are quite unable to match humans' exceptional capacity for exercising in the heat.

So the truth is that even though we are less able to replace our (larger because we sweat) water deficits as they develop during exercise, we are better adapted for prolonged exercise in the heat than those mammals who do not develop voluntary dehydration. That this conclusion seems improbable is a measure of the extent to which the doctrine has been promoted that fluid balance is *the* critical factor determining human exercise performance in the heat. But if voluntary dehydration has little effect on human exercise performance, then the paradox disappears.

In addition, salt loss in sweat could occur as a mechanism for delaying drinking and so it acutely dissociates the extent of the water loss from the thirst that it produces. This could then be corrected as soon as food is available and the appropriate thirst response is reactivated.

For all the reasons subsequently described, the commercial success of the world's first sports drink in the 1990s was driven at least in part by the development of the zero % dehydration rule, which holds that any level of voluntary dehydration that develops during exercise is profoundly undesirable, indeed dangerous, and could be fatal. Instead, to prevent this potentially catastrophic "disease," exercising humans are taught to replace their sweat losses as they develop. But this advice ignores all the evidence that humans have an unmatched capacity to sweat profusely specifically so that they can better regulate their body temperatures during exercise. Of course, this produces the potential that high levels of fluid loss (dehydration) could also develop. Hence, the need to develop a physiology that favored delayed drinking.

Another feature of humans not frequently remembered is the ability to adapt to a low fluid intake by reducing water losses in both sweat and from the respiratory tract at rest and during exercise (Grande, Taylor, et al., 1958). Thus, "water restricted groups showed marked decreases of sweating during work and of insensible losses during sleep. When water was given ad libitum sweat and insensible loss rose and when the normal diet was reinstituted they rose still further" (p. 202). Humans exhibit the same responses as the oryx and camel and are able to regulate the amount of water they lose in sweat in relation to their ease of access to fluid. This also means that sweat rates during exercise in humans who drink liberally are in excess of the requirement.

Why We Run

The evidence presented here clearly establishes that *Homo sapiens* developed as long-distance runners with a superior capacity to regulate body temperature when exercising in hot conditions. The capacity to sweat profusely, the reduction of body hair, and a greater body size were the three most important adaptations that produced a species better able to exercise more vigorously and for longer in dry heat than any other species, even when access to water and perhaps salt was limited.

It is my hypothesis that the key selective factor driving the subsequent evolution of humans was the need to run long distances in the heat to hunt and capture energy-dense mammals including fleet-footed antelope. Although I view these as adaptations from an evolutionary perspective, one does not need to embrace evolutionary theory to appreciate our ability and history as a species to run long distances in hot environmental conditions and the biological controls that allow us to do so.

Once the process toward ground-based bipedalism had begun, it was irreversible. The thermoregulatory advantages of standing upright and walking on two legs followed naturally.

In his book first published in 1900, Charles Morris noted, "Change of diet or of the mode of obtaining food is the most potent influencing cause of change of habit in animals" (p. 60). The change in diet from vegetable to animal food "would certainly demand a more active employment of the arms as agents in capture" (p. 61).

While advancing his similar hypothesis 24 years later that "Man was differentiated from the anthropods by becoming a hunter" Professor Carveth Read (1925, p. 1), paid appropriate tribute to the ideas of Charles Morris. He concluded that the adoption of a flesh diet was an important development and proposed that the ultimate goal of the erect gait was for "running down our prey" (p. 19).

Like Morris, Read was so certain that early hominids used weapons to kill prey that he, too, overlooked the possible implications of the other defining characteristics of humans—our ability to thermoregulate more effectively than any other mammal of similar size. Instead, he considered that the sole advantage of a reduction in hairiness was purely hygienic. Although hair does provide a favorable home for ticks and lice so that its loss would be hygienic, his conclusion was not the most correct.

An Australian-born professor at a South African university, Raymond Dart, would be the next to advance the theory that humans evolved as "barbaric" hunters. Dart (1953) proposed the ultimately incorrect idea that the southern apes that he discovered, *Australopithecus africanus,* were not only meat eaters but also armed hunters. It now appears that the fossils discovered in those caves were mostly the remains of hominids that had been predated by leopards and the other large cats that then dominated the African savannah (Brain, 1981; Hart and Sussman, 2005). Their bones were found among those of other animals also predated by these large cats (Brain, 1981).

But Louis Leakey, Kenneth P. Oakley, and Bernard Campbell had collectively decided that humans needed first to develop the intelligence to fashion weapons before they could kill large prey. Thus, they proposed that early hominids, including the southern ape, existed solely by scavenging.

Slowly scientists began to ponder the other physiological adaptations that distinguish humans from the great apes and what these might tell of the behaviors that influenced human evolution.

Brace and Montagu (1977) were among the first to propose that humans have a thermoregulatory advantage when running in the midday heat: "More importantly, however, is the fact that large furry quadrupeds are less well provided with heat-dissipating mechanisms than are humans with their hairless skin richly endowed with sweat glands. . . . Of all the major predators in the world, humans alone function exclusively in broad daylight" (p. 312).

In 1968, Grover Krantz suggested that the increase in brain size in *Homo erectus* came about because hominin was "a successful big game hunter as well as a gatherer" (p. 450). He proposed that *Homo* evolved as a successful persistence hunter and that this method of capturing animals was later replaced by the use of projectile weapons, including arrows and spears. He noted that the Tarahumara of Mexico were known to chase deer for up to 2 days and never less than a day: "The Indian chases the deer until the creature falls from exhaustion, often with its hooves completely worn away" (p. 450). He noted that the Bushmen use the same tactic in part because the absence of vegetation in the semi-desert makes stealth and concealment difficult. But he argued that hunting required a large brain since hunting requires "the ability to keep the task constantly in mind for several days and to anticipate the results well into the future" (p. 450).

Krantz conceived that human hunting produced the high-energy diet that allowed the size of the brain to increase. This, in turn, produced the intellectual capacity to become increasingly more adept at hunting, acquiring more food and thus allowing the clever brain to become even bigger and cleverer.

In 1972, Stern proposed that the development of the upper part of the human gluteus maximus muscle, which functions principally to control the side-to-side balance of the trunk during fast locomotion, including jogging and running, might have developed as the result of persistence hunting similar to that undertaken by the !Xo San Bushmen. The resulting changes in the site of the insertion of that muscle into the pelvic bone, the ilium, shown in the fossil hominin record "may be important osteological evidence of well established hunting behavior" (p. 329).

While a doctoral student at the University of Michigan, David R. Carrier (1984) began where Darwin, Morris, and Read had left off. He reaffirmed that the feature differentiating early hominins from the primates from which we evolved is not a large brain size but "the set of characteristics associated with erect bipedal posture and a striding gait" (p. 483). He again proposed that the ability to walk and run, not brain size, is the defining difference between humans and primates. But Carrier's innovative idea was his realization that the energy cost of human walking and running is about twice as high as that of other running mammals and birds.

Carrier also noted the energy cost of traveling a certain distance is independent of the speed of travel in humans but not in other mammals that have been studied, including horses. Thus, it matters not how fast a human finishes a foot race of any distance. Since the distance run by all finishers is the same, the total energy cost is the same whether the athlete finishes first or last.

In contrast, horses (Hoyt and Taylor, 1981) have a specific speed at each locomotor pattern (walking, trotting, cantering, and galloping) at which their energy cost is least and about 50% lower than that of humans (100 ml vs. 200 ml O_2/kg/min/km) (figure 1.4). Thus, Carrier wondered, "What is it about humans that detaches the cost of running from speed?" and "What advantages or disadvantages does this unusual situation create for running humans?" (p. 486). His key conclusion was that humans are not constrained to run at only one or two optimal speeds; rather, they can run at many different speeds depending on requirement.

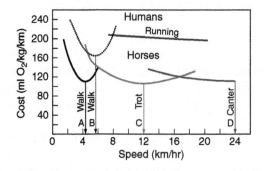

FIGURE 1.4 When expressed relative to body weight and distance traveled, the energy cost of walking (top curve, left) or running (top line, right) in humans is substantially higher than in horses (bottom three curves).

From D.R. Carrier, 1984, "The energetic paradox of human running and hominid evolution," *Current Anthropology* 25(4), 483-495. © 1984 by The Wenner-Gren Foundation for Anthropological Research. Adapted by permission of University of Chicago Press.

The conclusion is that while bipedal humans have a higher cost of transport, they have the ability to run at a much greater range of speeds. Carrier proposes that this would be particularly advantageous for humans hunting animals constrained to run at only certain specific speeds within each gait pattern. By forcing the chased animal to move at a speed that it does not naturally choose, the human would likely force the hunted animal to tire prematurely.

Carrier argues that quadrupedal mammals are constrained to breathe only once with every stride, because they must alternately inhale when the body is in flight and exhale when landing. In contrast, smaller bipedal humans can breathe once, twice, or even three times with each stride, depending on how fast they run. Since the demand to breathe is set by the muscles' metabolic activity, by breathing either more or less frequently per stride, humans can run with a much wider range of metabolic rates (i.e., running speeds) without changing their basic locomotor pattern of walking or running. In contrast, quadrupedal mammals can run only as fast as their one-breath-per-stride breathing will allow within each locomotor pattern.

The result is that while quadrupedal animals must run at a restricted range of speeds for each locomotor pattern, bipedal humans can run at a wide range of speeds without changing to a different form of locomotion other than from walking to running when their speed rises above ~6 km per hour.

Furthermore, nonsweating running mammals, like most medium-sized antelopes that modern humans still hunt, lose heat through their respiratory tracts because the air they expire has a higher temperature than the inspired (ambient) air. This is analogous to panting. Their capacity to lose heat in this way is also constrained by the same factors that limit their breathing rate to one breath per stride.

In contrast, running humans can increase their capacity to lose heat from the respiratory tract by running faster and breathing more frequently. In addition, humans are better equipped to lose heat by sweating and to match rates of heat loss and heat production across a much wider range of running speeds in more severe environmental conditions.

In short, humans can choose a running speed that their prey finds the most inefficient.

Carrier (1984) also describes other biological advantages enjoyed by sweating humans. First, the human sweat glands are under nervous control. This allows a very wide range of sweating rates to be achieved by humans during exercise—from as little as 200 ml/hr in marathon runners competing in arctic conditions (Stuempfle, Lehmann, et al., 2003) to about 3000 ml/hr in large (~160 kg, ~353 lb) American football players (Fowkes Godek, Bartolozzi, et al., 2005). This represents a 15-fold range in the capacity of humans to lose heat by controlled sweating. This exceeds by a wide margin the sweat rates required to maintain a safe body temperature during hunting in the dry heat conditions on the African savannah.

In addition, humans have the capacity to store carbohydrate in the form of glycogen in their muscles. Glycogen is the optimal fuel for endurance exercise but requires a carbohydrate-rich diet to maximize storage. In addition, when glycogen is stored in liver and muscle, it attracts water molecules, which are released as the glycogen is used during exercise. In this way, additional water is released as that fuel is used during exercise. This water can offset some of the sweat losses.

Thus, by 1984, Carrier had proposed that humans evolved as diurnal predators who "depended upon an exceptional endurance in hot (midday) temperatures to disable swifter prey animals" (p. 489).[14]

Paralysis of Profound Hyperthermia

Even if *Homo sapiens* had a superior ability to thermoregulate when hunting in extreme dry heat, the intellectual challenge that remains is to explain how early hominid hunters killed their prey given their small size, relatively weak arms, and likely absence of offensive weapons other than perhaps a crude hand tool that assisted in opening the skin and dissecting the carcass. Exercise physiologists happened upon the solution relatively recently.

In 1993, a group of Danish scientists (Nielsen, Hales, et al., 1993) showed that when humans exercise at a work rate fixed by the experimenter, they choose to terminate the exercise when their bodies reach a temperature predictable for each individual. This research has concluded that an elevated body temperature acts on those brain centers (the motor region of the cerebral cortex) that normally activate the limb muscles during exercise. Inhibition of those centers causes a motor paralysis, terminating exercise when the body temperature reaches the critical temperature.

Of course, this explanation is simplistic because mammals suffering from the paralysis of hyperthermia are not actually paralyzed; they can still walk and do other usual activities. They simply cannot continue to exercise at high rates until their body temperature has cooled. It is difficult to understand how such a partial paralysis can be so easily explained. This phenomenon was well described in other mammals long before it was first appreciated in humans.

It has been suggested that at some time in the past, hominids learned that certain mammals chased for a short distance would soon overheat and could be caught relatively easily. With experience, hominids would soon begin to chase even larger mammals. Improved thermoregulation and endurance running ability would assist in catching larger prey.

Further Development of the Hunting Hypothesis

Comparative thermal physiologist Bernd Heinrich, formerly of the University of Vermont, was perhaps the next to extend this line of argument. Heinrich spent his life studying heat balance in insects, producing some of the finest science writings in the modern literature (Heinrich, 1993; Heinrich, 1996; Heinrich, 2001). But it was only when he wished to become a world-class runner that he became interested in thermal balance in humans.

14 Less well known is how David Carrier came upon his unusual theory in 1984. He recalled to me that when he ran in his home town of Salt Lake City, Utah, in the winter, he could not keep pace with this dog. But in the summer heat, his dog became a listless, ineffective runner. In a moment of inspiration, he wondered, *why?* Why are humans so much better able to run in the heat than are dogs? Could it be possible that a superior capacity to run in the heat gave humans an evolutionary advantage over other mammals?

This moment of inspiration led to Carrier's paper proposing this hypothesis. Yet the response to his article was largely one of ridicule—similar to the response to Raymond Dart's proposal that *Australopithecus africanus* was a prehuman. As a result, Carrier lost interest in his theory (his next paper on the subject would be published only 20 years later). In 2004, a major new work by Dennis Bramble and Daniel Lieberman published in *Nature* rediscovered Carrier's original theory.

15 My ego is not sufficiently secure that I was able to resist including exactly what Professor Heinrich wrote: "I also believe in antelopes. They would not have missed a trick when it comes to running speed and endurance. . . . I had never heard of one doing much more than eating and running. However, if I had read modern exercise literature, such as the excellent book by McArdle, Katch and Katch, or the *Lore of Running* by Tim Noakes, I might have done not only stretching, speed training, and weight lifting, but also warmups and cooldowns" (Heinrich, 2001, p. 235). I have been Professor Heinrich's most ardent supporter ever since!

16 In fact, humans accumulate a heat load very reluctantly. Rather, according to the central governor model, all mammals anticipate the thermoregulatory strain associated with any environment. As a result, they modify their behavior, either slowing down or speeding up, specifically to ensure that they do not accumulate an excessive heat load before they complete the exercise bout. Paula Radcliffe's collapse during the 2004 Athens Olympic Marathon can be explained because her competitive drive was such that she willfully overrode these controls, so strong was her desire to win the Olympic Marathon. Yet she did not die. Thus, her central governor did not fail her.

In 1980, at age 40, Heinrich decided to attempt the world age-group record for the 100 km (62 mile) foot race. To do so, he could find no training guides.[15] Instead, he decided that a study of the physiology of the great athletes in the animal kingdom would direct his training.

At the end of his odyssey, which saw him set a new age-group world record of 6:38:21 for 100 km, Heinrich (2001) concluded the following: "The fact that we, as savannah-adapted animals, have such a hypertrophied [overdeveloped] sweating response implies that if we are naturally so profligate with water, it can only be because of some very big advantage. The most likely advantage was that it permitted us to perform prolonged exercise in the heat. We don't need a sweating response to outrun predators, because that requires relatively short, fast sprinting, where accumulating a heat load is, like a lactic acid load, acceptable.[16] What we do need sweating for is to sustain running in the heat of the day—the time when most predators retire into the shade" (p. 174).

"By about two to three million years ago, they had a leg and foot structure almost identical to our own, and it's reasonable to assume that they walked and ran like we do. While other predators rested, I was able to continue, albeit slowly, because we humans have one major physical advantage: We can sweat, copiously, which allows us to manage our internal temperature and extend our endurance. Most animals have no such mechanism. Through the ages and across the continents there are examples of men actually chasing down beasts that are much faster. In fact, there are modern reports of the Paiutes and Navajos of North America hunting pronghorn antelope on foot, patiently running down a stray until it drops in its tracks from exhaustion and there reverently suffocating the animal by hand. . . . Now we chase each other rather than woolly mammoths" (Heinrich 2010, pp. 96-97).

Bramble and Lieberman (2004) have extended the argument, first proposed by Carrier, that humans evolved for endurance running. They propose that endurance running may have played a role in helping early humans obtain "protein-rich resources such as meat, marrow and brain" (p. 351). Their conclusion was that humans evolved to run, not to walk, since humans show a multitude of traits in the human body, many described earlier in this chapter, that are essential for running but not for walking.

Summary

The biological record appears to give a consistent answer: Humans developed as long-distance runners especially well adapted to run in extreme dry heat in the middle of the day while drinking infrequently and conserving body sodium stores.

Humans are bipedal, reducing the radiant heat gain from the midday sun. Through evolution, we have developed adaptations that allow both superior thermoregulation and the ability to run economically for prolonged periods. The key adaptation that allows superior thermoregulatory capacity is the massive increase in the number of sweat glands in human skin. As a result of this superior sweating capacity, humans enjoy a critical thermoregulatory advantage when hunting nonsweating mammals in the heat.

A potential disadvantage of sweating is that it reduces body water content, causing dehydration. But by delinking thirst from the actual water requirement during exercise, humans were able to exercise in the heat while delaying the need to drink until after exercise when, in the safety of their home base and with access to a more abundant water source, they could leisurely replace the fluid deficit generated by their daily activities in the heat. This adaptation also allowed the development of a smaller stomach and intestine, leading to a more linear design, further reducing heat gain in the midday heat and allowing more efficient running.

Humans must also have a capacity to resist any detrimental effects of such fluid loss (Nolte et al., 2011) if, like the !Xo San hunter Karoha Langwane, they are able to run for 6 hours in 45 °C while requiring minimal fluid replacement. If humans truly are made to run for prolonged periods in extreme dry heat while drinking little or nothing, we must question the advice to drink at high rates and to ingest sodium during exercise regardless of the duration of the exercise or the environmental conditions in which it is performed.

CHAPTER 2

Thirst as a Signal for Fluid Intake

> Discovery consists in seeing what everyone else has seen and thinking what no one else has thought.
>
> **Albert Szent-Gyorgyi, winner of the 1937 Nobel Prize for Medicine for his discovery of the mechanism of action of vitamin C**

Heinrich Harrer, who in 1937 was a member of the first team to summit the vertical north face of the Eiger mountain in the Bernese Oberland, Switzerland, later ascribed their success to an inevitable fate: "A man's nature and way of life are his fate, and that which he calls his fate is but his disposition" (Harrer, 1959, p. 23). To explain his team's pioneering success that came after the first two attempts caused six climbers to lose their lives, Harrer concluded, "Perhaps all four of us were the fortunate owners of a disposition which was the basic factor in our successful climb; training, scientific preparation and equipment being only necessary adjuncts."

My interests lie in medicine, science, and sports, not necessarily in that order, for which there is no apparent ancestral precedent. Both my maternal and paternal grandfathers as well as my father were involved in commerce in the northwest English seaport of Liverpool. My father's commercial interests[1] brought him to Zimbabwe in 1946, immediately after the end of World War II, three years before I was born. In 1954 we relocated to Cape Town, South Africa, where I began my schooling. I have lived in Cape Town ever since.

1 My grandfather owned a company in Liverpool, England, called R.W. Noakes Pty Ltd. As far as I can gather, the company imported tobacco into England, probably originating from the southern tobacco-growing states of the United States as well as Rhodesia (Zimbabwe) and Malawi. At the end of World War II my father and mother, together with my one-year-old sister, emigrated to Zimbabwe, where I was born. There my father established the Rhodesian (Zimbabwe) Leaf Tobacco Company, originally named R.W. Noakes Pty Ltd after my grandfather, which my father later sold to the Universal Leaf Tobacco Company (Richmond, Virginia, USA) in about 1954.

The evidence that tobacco causes lung cancer was first established by Nazi scientists already in the 1930s but achieved a more global acceptance only after 1954 with the publication of a landmark study by a team of epidemiologists at Oxford University headed by Professor Richard Doll. Thus sometime after the mid-1960s my father, an intelligent and well-read man, would have been faced with the truth that tobacco smoking causes lung cancer (among many other negative health consequences). While I was being trained as a doctor in the 1970s (at my father's expense), we tended to avoid debating the issue. Once, he said to me, "I did not do much good, so you must." Perhaps that is the real reason I wrote this book.

My fate was to begin my medical training and a postadolescent interest in endurance sports in 1969, when the prevailing belief was that humans should not drink during exercise. Drinking during exercise, we were taught, was a sign of weakness. And should we succumb to our weakness, we would immediately feel discomfort and our pace would slacken. Our knowledge came from those whose wisdom, forged in the heat of athletic competition, had yet to be tested in the laboratory.

At the time, I was learning to row, not yet to run long distances. In training for rowing, we seldom ran farther than 3 km and then always at maximum pace. But one day when the wind was so strong that we could not venture onto the water, I opted to run around the lake on which we trained. That run was decisive: After 40 minutes I experienced the runner's high, seemingly touching heaven. I knew then that one day I would run a long-distance race, most especially the uniquely South African ultradistance running event, the 90 km (56 mile) Comrades Marathon. But that would happen only 4 years later.

In between these bouts of running, I rowed without ever considering whether or not drinking before, during, or after exercise was of any importance. We drank only after each workout, guided by our thirst. Our coach did not restrict our daily fluid intake to 1 L as happened to the Oxford rowing crew of 1860 whose "outraged human nature rebelled against it; and although they did not admit it in public, there were very few men who did not rush to their water bottles for relief, more or less often, according to the development of their conscientiousness and their obstinacy" (Hughes, 1861/2008, p. 108). Perhaps the author of those English classics *Tom Brown's Schooldays* and *Tom Brown at Oxford* understood that thirst is an extremely powerful sensation not easily overridden or ignored, for the body knows what it needs better than the coach.

Later I discovered that a century ago marathon runners received essentially the same advice: "Don't take any nourishment before going seventeen or eighteen miles. If you do, you will never go the distance. Don't get into the habit of drinking or eating in a marathon race: Some prominent runners do, but it is not beneficial" (Sullivan, 1909, p. 39).

The advice of American Joseph Forshaw, who finished third in the 1908 London Olympic Marathon in 2:57:10, was the same: "As to the taking of stimulants during the race, I will say that I know from actual experience that the full [marathon] race can be covered in creditable time without so much as a single drop of water being taken or even sponging of the head—I have done it myself. This of course is when in perfect trim" (Martin and Gynn, 1979, p. 45; Sullivan, 1909, p. 73). He continued, "I do not believe in eating during the race, as it can scarcely benefit one, as no nourishment can come from the food till digested, and the race will be finished before the food would be digested" (p. 73). We now know that this part of his advice is wrong: Eating does aid performance during prolonged exercise, at least in part because the digestion of food is not impaired during prolonged exercise.

Forshaw also wrote, "To cool the head and the blood in general on a hot day, sponge the head with bay rum, as its rapid evaporation produces a cool sensation, but be careful not to get it in the eyes" (p. 73).

Another U.S. runner, Matthew Maloney, who established a world record of 2:36:26 in the 1908 *New York Evening Journal* Christmas Marathon, wrote, "As to what I use when in a Marathon race: I only chew gum. I take no drink at all, but it is well to have a little stimulant on hand, such as beef tea, should it be needed and when I am running I try to get some competent men as handlers on the track, as good ones are needed there" (Martin and Gynn, 1979, p. 45; Sullivan, 1909, p. 57).

The man who reinvigorated interest in ultramarathon running in the 1920s, South African resident Arthur Newton, who won the Comrades Marathon five times and set world records at distances from 48 to 160 km (30 to 100 miles) as well as the world 24-hour running record, had a similar opinion: "You can't lay down a hard and fast rule (about fluid ingestion during exercise, my addition). Even in the warmest English weather, a 26-mile run ought to be manageable with no more than a single drink or, at most, two" (Newton, 1948, p. 15).

From his experiences in the 1928 and 1929 5,510 km (3,422 mile) American Transcontinental races between New York and Los Angeles (Berry, 1990), Newton noticed that the runners focused more on eating than on drinking during the race: "as big a breakfast as they could tuck away immediately before the start" (Newton, 1947). Only after 24 km (15 miles) would they begin to drink "highly sweetened drinks . . . every 4 or 5 miles to keep them going" (pp. 2 and 19).

This advice had not changed by 1957 when Jim Peters, former world-record holder in the 42 km (26 mile) marathon and arguably the greatest marathoner of all time, wrote, "[in the marathon race] there is no need to take any solid food at all and every effort should also be made to do without liquid, as the moment food or drink is taken, the body has to start dealing with its digestion and in so doing some discomfort will invariably be felt" (Peters et al., 1957, p. 114). Indeed a special conference on nutrition and sport held in London before the 1948 London Olympics included no reference to any need to drink during exercise (Abrahams, 1948; Leyton, 1948).

South African Jackie Mekler, who won the 90 km (56 mile) Comrades Marathon on five occasions and set world records at 48 km (30 mile), 64 km (40 mile), and 80 km (50 miles) in 1954, confirmed that Peters spoke for all runners: "In those days it was quite fashionable not to drink, until one absolutely had to. After a race, runners would recount with pride, 'I only had a drink after 30 or 40 km'" (Noakes, 2003, p. 252) (box 2.1, page 40).

In the 60 years between 1921 and 1981 that Comrades Marathon runners adopted this approach and before drinking stations were provided at increasingly frequent intervals after the mid-1970s, there were no cases of exercise-associated

BOX 2.1   Drinking Advice of Ultramarathon Champion Jackie Mekler

Jackie Mekler won the Comrades Marathon on five occasions and set world records at distances from 48 to 80 km in 1954. In response to my question of what and how much he drank during those races, he provided the following comments:

> To begin with my main drink was lemon squash [Oros or similar] diluted with water with added glucose powder and salt—a pleasing taste the only test. No scientific evaluation of the merits and demerits of this was available to me then.
>
> The other drinks were Coke and salt, or water or hot sugar-sweetened black tea. I recall that when Wally [Hayward] did his 24 hour record in London [256.4 km in 24 hours at Motspur Park, England, on 20th November 1953], he drank a lot of hot sweet black tea. He kept telling [Arthur] Newton [who, like both Hayward and Mekler, also won the Comrades Marathon five times and set numerous world ultradistance running records] the tea was not hot enough. He had lost his ability to differentiate the temperature.
>
> In addition I would take about 8 salt tablets during Comrades or a long run. The quantum was a guesstimate. It was a common belief amongst runners then that because sweat tastes salty, one needed salt. I always believed that it was necessary to take salt to prevent cramps.
>
> Drinks were taken *as and when one felt thirsty* [my emphasis]. In the Comrades up run for instance I would never have a drink before Pinetown [~20 km]. I always drank three-quarters up a hill, this helped me to look forward to this respite. In my "time" each runner had his own second [a second was a support person]—there were no feeding tables nor water points. Each runner had to organize his own drinks. Initially cars were allowed to follow the race but this became more difficult in the '60s as the number of entries increased. In my latter Comrades races [late 1960s] it was essential for the leaders to have a motor cycle attendant as well as a car. None of us worked out that a thermos flask would be a great source of cold water! All the water we drank was tepid, accessed at various garages en route. Ditto other drinks.
>
> My general philosophy always was to train in all temperatures, hot, cold and rain, only to try and become so much more able to withstand the negatives which might apply during the race. This applied to drinking too. I drank when I could, usually half a cup [~125 ml] and obviously the longer the race or the hotter the more frequently the drinks. It was common amongst runners that drinking was seen as a "sign of tiredness"—thus if any other was seen to be drinking frequently or excessively his opponents would interpret it as a sign of weakness. Thus many would boast about how long in a race they went without drinking!

J. Mekler, e-mail correspondence, July 11, 2008. Used with permission.

hyponatremia (EAH) or exercise-associated hyponatremia encephalopathy (EAHE) in Comrades runners. Nor is there any recorded evidence that a large number of runners had to be treated for dehydration or heat illness after the Comrades Marathon in those years. Only *after* the introduction of frequent (every 1.6 km) drinking stations in 1981 did it become increasingly necessary to provide medical care at the finish of that and other marathon and ultramarathon races to treat the growing proportion of collapsed runners seeking medical care for "dehydration" and "heat illness."

The most likely reason that treatment was necessary was the changing nature of the runners entering marathon and ultramarathon races. Before the running boom that began after 1976, only those who were reasonably trained would ever consider entering those races. But the culture became very different thereafter. The new generation of runners was not told to train more to ensure that they did not suffer harm during those races.

Instead they were advised to *drink* more.

Soon drinking, especially a sports drink, would be marketed as the universal panacea. A failure to drink properly during competition became the runner's convenient explanation for why he ran less well than expected; certainly in this new era of entitlement it could never be because of something that was under the runner's personal control, specifically that he had simply not trained enough. Doctors, too, would use this reason to rationalize the dramatic increase in the number of athletes seeking medical care at the end of marathon and ultramarathon races and Ironman triathlons. Surely these ill runners had simply drunk too little during these races. If only they could be encouraged to drink more, the problem would surely disappear.

To fully understand what happened to Cynthia Lucero and the hundreds of others who have suffered from EAH and EAHE (appendix B), we must first understand how the body processes fluid during physical activity.

Fluid Processing During Physical Activity

Water is the major constituent of the human body, accounting for about 60% of body mass. Dependence on water is such that most humans will die within 3 to 6 days if denied water. For this reason, humans have evolved complex behavioral responses to ensure that water is always easily accessible and that we drink just the correct amounts when needed—not too much, not too little. These controls are for the most part not under our direct conscious control. They are the result of the long evolutionary road that humans have walked since the first appearance of life on earth between 2.7 and 3.5 billion years ago. In contrast, the growth of the large human brain, in particular the parts associated with our advanced intellectual capacity, is an extremely modern event, about 0.5 to 1 million years old. As far as we know, the majority of the creatures on this planet are able to regulate their fluid intakes without the need for conscious brain controls. Nor do they need to be told exactly how much they should drink.

The origin of our need to drink begins in a subconscious part of the brain, the hypothalamus, which informs the conscious brain with the development of the sensation of thirst. In response, we begin to seek out and to ingest fluid. The ingested fluid passes down the esophagus, where its volume is likely monitored by processes yet to be fully understood. The fluid then enters the stomach, where its passage to the small intestine is briefly interrupted as it is stored for a time in the stomach. Here its volume may again be measured. In the stomach the ingested fluid is mixed with stomach secretions before being released into the upper reaches of the small bowel, the duodenum (figure 2.1, page 42). The rate at which the ingested fluid is released from the stomach is determined principally by the volume of fluid in the stomach—the more fluid ingested, the more quickly the fluid is released—and its composition. Large volumes of pure water are more rapidly emptied than are energy-rich carbohydrate-, fat-, and protein-containing solutions, for example.

Generally, about two-thirds of any volume of water ingested is emptied within the first 10 minutes; two-thirds of what remains is then emptied within the next 10 minutes. In contrast, as little as about 25% of an energy-rich solution would be emptied in the same time. This process continues—for each specific solution, the same percentage of the fluid present at the start of the measurement period

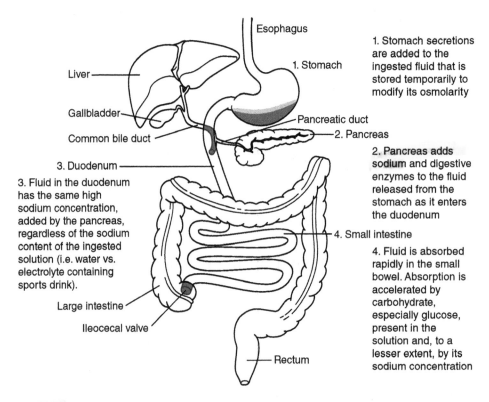

1. Stomach secretions are added to the ingested fluid that is stored temporarily to modify its osmolarity

2. Pancreas adds sodium and digestive enzymes to the fluid released from the stomach as it enters the duodenum

4. Fluid is absorbed rapidly in the small bowel. Absorption is accelerated by carbohydrate, especially glucose, present in the solution and, to a lesser extent, by its sodium concentration

3. Fluid in the duodenum has the same high sodium concentration, added by the pancreas, regardless of the sodium content of the ingested solution (i.e. water vs. electrolyte containing sports drink).

FIGURE 2.1 The sequence of ingested fluid as it passes through the stomach into the duodenum where its sodium concentration is altered by the addition of pancreatic secretions before absorption occurs.

empties in the next 10-minute period (~67% for pure water and ~25% for an energy-rich solution)—until all the fluid has passed into the intestine.

As the fluid passes through the upper reaches of the upper bowel, it receives the secretions of the liver and pancreas, which enter the bowel through the bile duct. This adds electrolytes, especially sodium, increasing the osmolality of the solution; the added electrolytes increase the rate at which the fluid can be absorbed across the intestinal wall. The amount of sodium that is added is clearly regulated to optimize the sodium concentration of the ingested fluid, but the nature of that control is not yet fully understood.

The result is that it matters not whether the ingested solution contains a great deal of sodium or none at all; by the time the solution passes the site of the small intestine where the bile duct enters, all ingested solutions, whether pure water or an electrolyte-containing sports drink, will have identical sodium concentrations. This was first shown by studies funded by the sports drink industry in the United States (Gisolfi, Summers, et al., 1998). Since the rate at which solutions are absorbed by the bowel is in part a function of their sodium concentrations, this finding suggests that adding sodium to an ingested fluid will not increase the rate at which it is subsequently absorbed by the intestine. This has since been confirmed also in studies funded by the U.S. sports drink industry (Gisolfi, Summers, et al., 1995). The authors concluded that "this study suggests that adding sodium to fluid replacement beverages may not be a factor in fluid absorption"

(p. 1414). However, carbohydrate increases the rates of both sodium and water absorption in the bowel, explaining why fluids designed to maximize fluid absorption must contain carbohydrate; the pancreas will add the necessary sodium.

Once the ingested fluid has been conditioned by this addition of sodium, it is ready to be absorbed in the small intestine. Water absorption occurs as a passive process in response to the active, energy-requiring absorption of the glucose and sodium. Thus water absorption from a sports drink does not occur without the absorption of either glucose or sodium, or both.

Once absorbed, the fluid enters the veins, draining the intestine, and becomes part of the fluid compartment lying outside the cells, the extracellular fluid (ECF). The volume of the ECF is usually about 14 L in a 70 kg (154 lb) human, whereas the volume inside the cells, the intracellular fluid (ICF), is about 28 L. The cells that separate the ECF from the ICF allow the free passage of water, which moves in response to any differences in the concentration of solutes, the osmolality, in either compartment. The predominant solute of the ECF is sodium, the content of which is the key determinant of its volume, whereas potassium is the dominant solute in the ICF and the content of which therefore sets the ICF volume.

The volume of fluid in the body is not measured directly; rather, the brain infers the correct volume by comparing the solute concentration or osmolality of the ECF with a known ideal value. If the osmolality is different from this ideal, a series of corrective mechanisms is activated to return the value to its ideal set point. This process is known as homeostasis. Included in these mechanisms are thirst and sodium and water conservation by the kidneys, all activated by a rise in the solute concentration of the ECF. In contrast, excessive fluid consumption will cause an expansion of the ECF (and ICF) with a reduction in the osmolality of the ECF. This will cause an inhibition of thirst and increased water excretion, as urine, by the kidneys (that is, if all the controls act appropriately). Unfortunately, this control does not work perfectly in everyone who overdrinks; EAH and EAHE occur when these controls are faulty.

Dehydration and the Protection Offered by the Thirst Mechanism

Dehydration is a physiological term indicating a reduction in the total-body water content. Once the reduction in body water causes the solute concentration, especially the sodium concentration (actually the osmolality), of the blood to rise, the brain detects the change and develops the symptom of thirst (figure 2.2, page 44). This is a normal biological response that has evolved in all creatures to ensure that they maintain a constant body water content at least once each day, usually after the evening meal (see figure 2.5, page 56).

When fluid is lost from the body, either in sweat as a result of exercise or from the gastrointestinal tract in diseases like cholera or typhoid, the concentration of solutes, especially sodium in the blood, rises, causing the blood osmolality to increase. This rise stimulates receptors in a special part of the brain, the hypothalamus (nuclei 1 to 3 in figure 2.2), which in turn interact with three other nuclei (4 to 6), which increase secretion of the hormone AVP/ADH (arginine vasopressin, also known as antidiuretic hormone), whose function is to increase water reabsorption

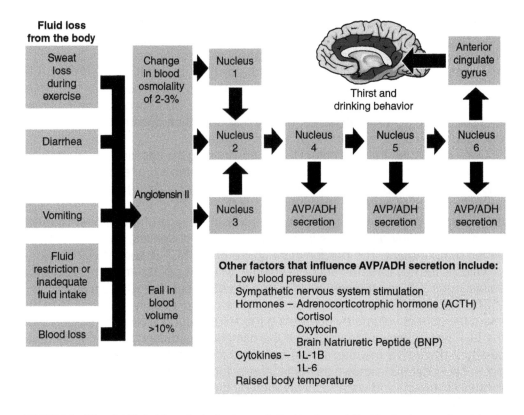

FIGURE 2.2 When fluid is lost from the body, changes in the blood osmolality, blood volume, and angiotensin II concentrations stimulate a sequence of nuclei in the hypothalamus in the brain, and with the release of AVP/ADH and stimulation of the anterior cingulate gyrus, thirst is produced and increases drinking behavior. *Key:* Nucleii 1 to 6 are named respectively: (1) subfornical organ; (2) medial preoptic; (3) vascular organ of the lamina terminalis; (4) lateral preoptic area/lateral hypothalamus; (5) supraoptic; (6) paraventricular.

by the kidney. In response to the action of AVP/ADH, the kidney reduces the amount of fluid secreted. As a result, urine flow into the bladder is reduced. Nucleus 5 also stimulates the cells in another part of the brain, the cingulate gyrus, which increases thirst. As a result, the desire to drink is increased and water (and sodium through the action of aldosterone) is reabsorbed by the kidneys. The result is that the blood osmolality returns to its homeostatically regulated value, switching off the desire to drink (Hew-Butler, Collins, et al., 2007; Hew-Butler, Verbalis, et al., 2006). Osmolality is explained more fully in chapter 4.

Thus the only symptom of dehydration is thirst. If, however, the thirst cannot be quenched because fluid is unavailable, as occurs in those stranded in the desert, then the body activates a series of emergency adaptations that prolong life for a period but ultimately cause death when all the major bodily organs fail, leading probably to cardiovascular collapse.

The remarkable achievement of the sports drink industry was that it convinced recent generations that these control mechanisms do not exist. Instead all athletes must drink to insure that they do not lose *any* body weight during exercise. But there are no known receptors that regulate thirst by monitoring the extent of the body weight lost or gained. In addition, this myth also convinced exercisers that they could become dangerously dehydrated not just when lost in the desert for more than 48 hours but when running for a few minutes in, for example, a big-city marathon, during which they have unrestricted access to as much fluid as they might wish. I am unaware of any other human activity in which so much fluid is freely available as in a modern big-city marathon. How is it possible under these circumstances to become dehydrated except according to a definition that has no proper biological basis?

In response to the body's pure fluid loss, the usual human living in a Western society with easy access to fluid will develop the sensation of thirst and will usually drink fluid as a result. Receptors in the back of the mouth and the esophagus, but particularly in the stomach, then detect how much fluid has been ingested. Once the stomach is filled, the desire to drink is temporarily curtailed but resumes as the stomach empties, especially if food is eaten at the same time. Eventually enough fluid (and sodium) has been ingested to return the solute concentration of the ECF back to the normal range. Since the ECF (and hence whole body) osmolality is then within the homeostatically regulated range, the symptom of thirst is switched off; as a result, most people will stop drinking.

The biological mechanisms controlling thirst have been properly understood only quite recently. It was originally thought that the sensation of thirst arose simply from a dry mouth. But in a study published in 1976, David Dill and colleagues noted that blood osmolality increased in those who did not drink during exercise but stayed within the normal range in those who drank ad libitum, or at one's own discretion (Dill, Soholt, et al., 1976). As a result, they were amongst the first to conclude that "the stimulus to drink is increased osmotic pressure" (p. 241) so that "one drinks enough water to maintain the sodium chloride concentration near the normal value" (Bock and Dill, 1933, p. 443) or "for maintaining a constant osmotic pressure" (Dill, Soholt, et al., 1976, p. 292). Since ECF osmolality, not body weight, is the regulated variable, and since the total-body water content cannot be regained until all the solutes lost from the ECF (sodium) and the ICF (potassium) are also replaced, Bock and Dill (1933) also wrote the following in 1933: "The body weight is not regained until the salt debt is (re)paid" (p. 443). Indeed, the best predictor of the body's state of hydration is the blood (ECF) osmolality (Cheuvront, Ely, et al., 2010), which is understandable since the ECF osmolality is the regulated variable. Since the ECF osmolality is the regulated variable, it is reasonable to conclude that it will be the single best measure of the level of water loss from the body, that is, the level of bodily dehydration.

The result is that as shown in figure 2.2 the only symptom of dehydration is thirst, which is simply a self-correcting biological signal that ensures that healthy humans do not develop a fluid deficit sufficient to cause illness. This thirst mechanism will ensure that all modern athletes competing in long-distance running, cycling, and triathlon events in which they have free access to all the fluid they could possibly desire cannot develop life-threatening dehydration unless they so choose.[2]

2 One athlete who so chose was the female winner of the 1984 Comrades Marathon. She was participating in one of our studies of renal function during exercise (Irving, Noakes, et al., 1990). She chose to drink very little during the race in which she lost 5 kg, or 11%, of her starting body weight (45 kg). She did not pass any urine for some hours after the race and showed evidence of transient acute renal failure that recovered partially after she had received 2 L of fluid intravenously. Evidence for continuous mild renal dysfunction was present for the 14 days after the race at which she was studied.

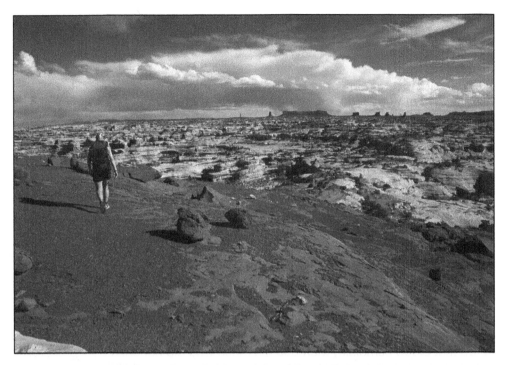

Sweating during exercise causes water loss, which stimulates thirst. When fluid is available humans can drink enough to satisfy their thirst. Only when little or no fluid is available, for example when lost in the desert, is there the risk that humans may drink too little and compromise their health.
Brand X Pictures

Symptoms of Inadequate Fluid Ingestion

When athletes sweat during exercise, they lose both water and electrolytes, especially sodium, in varying amounts. Because sodium is the dominant solute lost in sweat, and since the sweat sodium concentration is always less than its concentration in the ECF, sweating will always cause a greater loss of water than solute from the ECF. As a result, in the absence of any fluid ingestion, sweating must cause the ECF solute concentration to rise. Ultimately this will change enough to stimulate thirst in everyone. However, this response is highly individualized—some athletes will become thirsty at quite low levels of weight loss, whereas the thirst of others allows them to lose up to 12% of body weight during ultraendurance exercise as in the Ironman Triathlon without developing any more severe symptoms of homeostatic failure. To understand the real symptoms that develop when people drink less than their thirst dictates, we need to look at those studies in which participants are forced to exercise for prolonged periods while they have access to less fluid than their thirst dictates. These people develop both an unquenched thirst and additional symptoms caused by a progressive biological failure due to a falling total-body water content. One of the original studies to define these symptoms was performed in the Nevada Desert during the early years of World War II.

The Nevada Desert study[3] reported the sequence in which symptoms of unreplaced water losses, since conveniently termed "dehydration," developed. Of course, one can equally argue that some of these symptoms are due to an absence of drinking and the knowledge that drinking will be allowed only when the activity is completed. We now appreciate that the brain responds not just to biological stimuli but also to what it anticipates will happen in the future. Knowing that a demanding activity must be performed without fluid replacement will cause all symptoms to be experienced more intensively.

Adolph (1947b) wrote, "The order of appearance of the signs and symptoms is particularly characteristic. Thirst is noticeable very early, but does not increase much in intensity as the water deficit continues to increase. Vague discomfort, not experienced by controls who drank water, gradually becomes defined in the flushing of the skin, heat oppression, weariness, sleepiness, impatience, anorexia and dizziness. At about the time that the walking pace can no longer be maintained, dyspnea, tingling, and cyanosis, as well as a suggestion of tetany, appear. Still later, a man cannot stand alone, either because of impaired coordination or fainting" (pp. 228-229). Adolph also recognized that the inability to stand was due to the development of a low blood pressure, postural hypotension: "The inability to continue muscular work (exhaustion) seems to be a consequence of circulatory inadequacy. Temporarily, the movements themselves help in some degree to improve the return of blood to the heart. When the movements stop, failure is suddenly imminent; some persons faint at this point. Lying down promptly relieves the circulation and the symptoms" (pp. 235-236).

[3] Scientists working with the American military produced the classic studies of exercise in the heat that came out of World War II. In particular, they wished to answer this question: How far and for how long can military personnel walk in desert heat before they become incapacitated when they either did or did not ingest fluids? Working in the Nevada Desert between 1942 and 1945, these scientists showed that the distance soldiers could walk in the desert was quite short: ~30 km during the cooler night hours before they became incapacitated by the severe thirst associated with more marked levels of dehydration (>8%). Once that level of dehydration (and associated thirst) was achieved, soldiers became dispirited and disinterested even though their physiology was not too greatly disturbed.

There appeared to be no long-term sequelae: "We do know that a man can suffer a water deficit so incapacitating that he can neither walk nor stand; yet he recovers his walking ability within a few minutes of water ingestion and his feelings of well-being within half an hour or less after he begins drinking. Within a meal or two intervening, his recovery is practically complete in 6 to 12 hours" (Brown, 1947a, p. 225).

Subjects reached exhaustion at very high heart rates and rates of ventilation but at quite low rectal temperatures (below 40 °C). At the extremes of water deficit that two soldiers were able to sustain (9-10%), their rectal temperatures reached only 39.5 °C (figure 11.13 in Adolph, 1947a). The conclusion must be that exhaustion occurred before the rectal temperature reaches dangerous levels, the concept of "anticipatory regulation" to protect body temperature homeostasis that is discussed further in chapter 6.

Similarly, Brown (1947b) described his experiences: "Aside from thirst, the symptoms of dehydration were in large part indications of impending collapse. A vague, generalized discomfort and a feeling of restlessness followed closely the stage of 'mouth thirst.' There was a great desire to sit or lie down. Drowsiness was often noted. A feeling of heat oppression was a frequent complaint; it was often more serious than thirst. Muscular tiredness grew more acute progressively, although manual coordination was not measurably altered. Among the signs of approaching collapse, the most reliable were a rising pulse rate and a rising rectal temperature. Sometimes there was a noticeable dyspnea. Frequently, the subject was cyanotic and his face became flushed. In the exhausted state, tingling in hands, arms, and feet occurred in some cases" (p. 216).

So described are the real symptoms that develop when people exercise in extremely hot conditions without any chance to replace their fluid losses appropriately. Of course this is not what happens in modern marathon races in which athletes exercise usually for relatively short periods of a few hours in much cooler conditions while they have access to unlimited amounts of fluid. This is the precise opposite of what happened in the Nevada Desert experiments, or what happened to 40 troopers of Company A of the 10th Cavalry of the United States Army in 1877 (box 2.2).

The extensive research of the Nevada Desert research group established a range of findings that subsequent research has not contradicted. Not all these findings have received equal exposure over the years. Those findings that dehydration may not be quite as dangerous as the dehydration myth proposes (chapter 3) have not been as widely propagated as those supporting the value of fluid ingestion during exercise. The principal findings were as follows:

- Even when given free access to adequate fluids, people drank less than they lost in sweat or urine. Hence they developed "voluntary dehydration," which was corrected only after exercise and when food was eaten, especially at the evening meal.
- In the experiments in which groups of soldiers either drank freely or not at all during day-long marches in desert heat, a much greater percentage of those who did not drink during exercise were likely to terminate the exercise bout prematurely.
- Subjects in the groups who did not drink during these marches usually stopped when they had lost 7% to 10% of their starting body weights. In this state they experienced postural hypotension (EAPH), but after they experienced the symptoms of fainting caused by EAHP, they recovered rapidly within minutes of lying down and ingesting fluid.
- Dehydration did not reduce either the sweat rate or the rate of urine production during exercise. However, the rectal temperature and heart rate rose as linear functions of the level of dehydration. The body temperature rose about 0.2 to 0.3 °C for each 1% level of dehydration.
- There were no immediate health risks associated with the level of dehydration of 7% to 10% present at the termination of exercise in those who did not ingest any fluids during exercise. The authors considered that only at very high levels of dehydration (15-20%) was there a serious risk of organ failure.

These studies, which clearly established the value of fluid ingestion during exercise, had little impact on the athletic community. Instead, for at least the first two decades after the publication in 1947 of the book describing these studies (Adolph, 1947b), athletes continued to be advised not to drink at all during exercise. Only after the development of Gatorade and the publication of the studies of Pugh and colleagues (1967) and Wyndham and Strydom (1969) was proper attention finally paid to the use of fluid ingestion during exercise.

BOX 2.2 The Nature of Desert Thirst

A report from 1878 describes how powerful the symptom of thirst is and the signs of near-fatal dehydration.

At 1300 hr on 26 July, 1877, 40 troopers of Company A of the 10th Cavalry of the United States Army broke camp at Fort Concho, Texas, in pursuit of a "band of hostile Indians" (King, 1878). The troopers followed the Indian tracks across the "Staked Plains" of Texas until evening, when they camped without finding water. The following day they persisted but were again without water. The heat was "excessive"; two troopers developed "coup de soleil" (sunstroke) and all were severely affected by thirst: "Many were faint and exhausted; some fell from their saddles" (p. 406). That evening a guide was dispatched to find water. He was not seen alive again. The decision was taken to return to base in urgent search for water.

The following day, the third without water, the troopers were in dire condition: "The desire for water now became uncontrollable. The salivary and mucous secretions had long been absent; their mouths and throats were so parched that they could not swallow the government hard-bread; after being masticated it accumulated between the teeth and in the palate from where it had to be extracted with the fingers. . . . The sensibility of the lingual and buccal mucous membranes was so much impaired that they could not perceive that anything was in their mouths. . . . Vertigo and dimness of vision affected all; they had difficulty in speaking, voices weak and strange-sounding; and they were troubled with deafness, appearing stupid to each other, questions having to be repeated several times before they could be understood; they were also very feeble and had a tottering gait. Many were delirious (p. 406).

"At this stage they would in all likelihood have perished had they not resorted to the use of horse-blood. As the horses gave out they cut them open and drank their blood. The horses had been so long deprived of every kind of fluid that their blood was thick, and coagulated instantly on exposure; nevertheless, at the time it appeared more delicious than anything they had ever tasted. . . . Their own urine, which was very scanty and deep coloured, they drank thankfully, first sweetening it with sugar. . . . A few drank the horses' urine. . . . Their fingers and the palms of their hands looked shrivelled and pale" (p. 406).

On the morning of the fifth day after three and a half days without any fluid other than blood and urine, they finally reached water. But ingesting water was of little help initially since, "As they kept filling themselves with water, it was vomited up; the same thing occurred when they endeavoured to eat dry food. Warm coffee was the only thing they had that revived them at all (p. 406).

"Although water was imbibed again and again, even to repletion of their stomach, it did not assuage their insatiable thirst, thus demonstrating that the sense of thirst is, like the sense of hunger, located in the general system, and that it could not be relieved until the remote tissues were supplied" (p. 406).

In the end all but four of the troopers survived, confirming the ability of humans to survive profound levels of dehydration. Other classic reports of desert thirst are contained in a chapter (Brown, 1947a) in Adolph's classic book.

But the real relevance of these stories is that when severe body water loss is present, it is not difficult to recognize it. Perhaps in the future the diagnosis of severe loss of body water, known as dehydration, in marathon runners should include the following symptoms:

- An uncontrollable desire for water
- Inability to detect the presence of fluid or food in the mouth
- Inability to masticate food
- Uncontrollable desire to ingest any fluid, even blood or urine

Then at least we would know that we were dealing with a real, not a fictitious, condition.

Another set of U.S. Army studies occurred soon after American troops began to fight in jungle heat in Burma during World War II. It soon became apparent that on first exposure to conditions of high temperatures and suffocating humidity (caused by the transpiration of water from the leaves of the jungle vegetation), soldiers were essentially incapacitated but began to adapt within a few days (Eichna, Bean, et al., 1945). To study the special physiological challenges posed by jungle heat, a special research group was established at Fort Knox, Kentucky, where a "hot room" was built in which the environmental conditions present in either the desert or the jungle could be reproduced. These studies showed that the major cause for incapacitation on first exposure to both desert and jungle heat was the develop- ment of exercise-related postural hypotension (EAPH), beginning the moment the exercise bout terminated (Eichna and Horvath, 1947). This disappeared within a few days of repeated heat exposures. An important contribution of these studies was to establish the condition of EAPH as a cause of postexercise collapse and to show that this condition was not simply due to dehydration as would become the industry-driven mantra after the 1980s.

Dr. Eichna's group was also interested in the psychological effects of exer- cising in the heat without fluid replacement. Thus they wrote the following: "An important change which the chart does not show was the actual condition of the men, their low morale and lack of vigor, their glassy eyes, their apathetic, torpid appearance, their 'don't-give-a-damn-for-anything' attitude, their uncoordinated stumbling, shuffling gait. Some were incapable of sustained purposeful action and were not fit for work. All they wanted to do was rest and drink" (Bean and Eichna, 1943 p. 155). This shows that the symptoms of dehydration are largely of a psychological nature, the goal of which is to stop the athletes from continuing to exercise. It is a built-in mechanism to prevent bodily damage.

Scientists at the United States Army Research Institute of Environmental Medi- cine (USARIEM) have conducted a study to evaluate the influence of unreplaced fluid losses on the development of various symptoms (Engell, Maller, et al., 1987). The study used fluid restriction and exercise to produce four levels of loss of body weight (0%, 3%, 5%, and 7%) and showed that the intensity of sensations of thirst, tiredness, weakness, lightheadedness, weariness, and dizziness increased lin- early with increasing levels of weight loss (figure 2.3). But thirst was the symptom that was felt with the greatest intensity.

The study is important for two reasons. First, it shows that thirst is the symptom that best indicates the presence of a fluid deficit caused by exercise and fluid restriction. This conflicts with the myth developed in the 1990s that thirst is an inadequate guide to the fluid needs of the body. Rather in this study, a weight loss of 7% produced near-maximal thirst sensations. Second, during competition, some athletes develop levels of weight loss in excess of 7% without developing the same intensity of symptoms experienced by the participants in this study. This shows the individuality of the thirst response. Athletes who lose substantial amounts of weight during exercise without becoming as thirsty either prevent a large increase in the solute content of their ECF (as a result of internal relocation of body sodium stores) or because their brains are less sensitive to any large changes in ECF solute concentrations. These individuals are, in fact, dehydrated because they have lost total-body water; however, this water loss is easily replaced by drinking normally, often with a meal, after the race. It does not lead to myriad

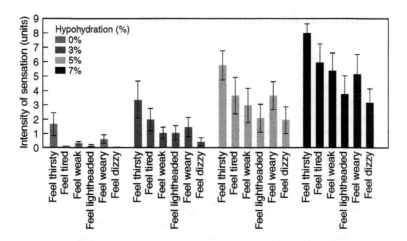

FIGURE 2.3 The extent to which six symptoms develop in response to increasing levels of weight loss produced by fluid restriction and exercise. Note that thirst is the symptom that is felt with the greatest intensity at all levels of weight loss. A score of 9 on this scale indicates the maximum intensity.

Adapted from *Physiology & Behavior*, 49(2), D.B. Engell, O. Maller, M.N. Sawka, et al., "Thirst and fluid intake following graded hypohydration levels in humans," 229-236, copyright 1987, with permission from Elsevier.

ill effects, as the sports drink industry would like us to believe (box 2.3, page 52). In fact, the best endurance athletes in the world are typically those who lose the most weight during exercise, who have the least thirst, and who run the fastest when they are quite markedly dehydrated, perhaps because the weight loss is beneficial to performance, just as the avoidance of thirst must have been an advantage to early hominid persistence hunters.

More recently, the studies of Armstrong and colleagues (Armstrong, Maresh, et al., 1997; Maresh, Gabaree-Boulant, et al., 2004), also affiliated with the USARIEM, further confirm that the sensations of thirst are always sufficient to ensure proper hydration both before and during exercise. Participants who began exercise in a dehydrated state (−3.4% BW) drank 5.3 times as much fluid (1.65 L; 1.1 L/hr) during 90 minutes of exercise than when they started exercise normally hydrated such that, provided they were able to drink during exercise, it made no difference whether subjects began exercise dehydrated or normally hydrated; by the end of exercise their core body temperatures, heart rates, blood osmolalities, and thirst ratings were the same.

Why Runners Collapse

Why would anyone expect the symptom of thirst to be present in collapsed runners? Thirst is such a powerful urge that any thirsty marathon runner suffering from dehydration during a race will simply stop at the next refreshment station and drink until her thirst is slaked. Simple.

The basis for the belief that collapsed runners were suffering from dehydration began with the explosive growth in the number of marathon runners after 1976 (figure 2a, page xv). This produced a massive increase in the number of runners requiring medical care at the finish of those races. Logically, the

BOX 2.3 Fabricating Dehydration as a Disease

This book provides many reasons that explain why an epidemic of EAH and EAHE struck global endurance sports beginning in 1981 before reaching a plateau in about 2002 (see figure 10.1a on p., page 295). One highly influential dogma actively promoted by Gatorade and the GSSI scientists is that dehydration and overhydration cause the same symptoms. As a result, the symptoms of EAH and EAHE mirror those of dehydration. If true, these would explain why doctors often treat patients incorrectly, thinking they are dehydrated when they are really overhydrated.

This misconception helped to sustain the dogma that dehydration is a disease that has a specific set of symptoms, which can be diagnosed and so prevented (by ingesting more sports drink during exercise) or treated by infusing copious volumes of fluid intravenously until the symptoms of dehydration disappear. Of course, if a patient's symptoms are not due to a reduction in the total-body water, then those symptoms caused by some other condition will not disappear when the patient is either told to drink more or is treated with intravenous fluids after exercise. Rather, these treatments are more likely to cause or exacerbate the underlying condition. Thus, a ream of articles have repeatedly described the following overlapping symptoms of EAH, EAHE, and dehydration: confusion, dizziness, headache, lack of coordination, nausea, severe fatigue, swollen hands and feet, vomiting, wheezy breath, bloating, cramping, and fainting. But what are the facts?

As shown in figure 2.2 (page 44), the only symptom of dehydration is thirst. As seen in later chapters (see especially table 11.1, page 348), other conditions cause the myriad symptoms often attributed to dehydration. The essential point is that dehydration is not a medical condition; that is, it is not a disease that produces a complex of unique and iden-tifying symptoms. Rather, dehydration is an associated feature of some diseases such as infantile diarrhea, cholera, or typhoid, all of which cause an accelerated rate of fluid loss from the gastrointestinal tract.

In contrast, the symptoms of disease are caused by pathological changes within the body. They are not self-correcting but require some intervention by the body's own defenses often aided by an external agent such as the use of prescription drugs or a surgical intervention, among many other possibilities. Thus, if an otherwise healthy athlete who seeks medical care is not thirsty, it is unlikely that a reduction in the total-body water content (dehydration) is the cause of any illness or symptoms that may be present at the same time. Not surpris-ingly, thirst is an uncommon complaint in athletes treated during and after endurance events in which fluid is freely available. Indeed, the symptom of thirst is so uncommon in athletes running in marathon races that it is not even listed as a symptom of dehydration by those who have promoted it as a disease.

Certainly unreplaced fluid losses, for example, in those lost in the desert for more than three days will cause death as the result of failure of multiple organs, most especially the kidneys. But the unfortunate travelers so lost have one characteristic symptom that I have never encountered in collapsed athletes treated at the end of endurance events. It is an overpowering, all-consuming thirst that dominates their every conscious thought.

collapse of an athlete *after* rather than *during* a sporting event cannot be due to dehydration, since dehydration, which allegedly impairs circulation, must cause the athlete to collapse *during* the race when the strain on the heart and circulation is the greatest. This cannot happen immediately after the exercise terminates when any stress on the heart and circulation is falling. But this simple logic was ignored. Instead, it was concluded that all these collapsed athletes were suffering from dehydration, and their symptoms were caused by that dreaded disease.

But the truth is that athletes who collapsed *after* endurance events develop very low blood pressure only when standing (exercise-associated postural hypertension, or EAPH). This is caused by physiological changes that begin the moment the athlete stops running or walking after exercise and to which dehydration does not contribute. We know this because the moment these collapsed athletes lie flat, or better, with their legs and pelvis elevated above the level of the heart ("head down"), their symptoms instantly disappear.[4] Thus, if the symptoms occur in athletes who are not thirsty and can be reversed instantly without fluid ingestion, the condition cannot be due to dehydration. Rather, EAPH must be due to the relocation of a large volume of blood from the veins in the chest and neck (which fill the heart and ensure its proper functioning) to the veins of the lower legs (which lie below the level of the heart) and therefore fill whenever an athlete stands.

One of the physiological costs of bipedalism is that it made it more difficult for exercising humans to regulate blood pressure when standing, because more than 60% of the blood in circulation is contained in large veins that are situated below the level of the heart. If this volume increases abruptly at any time, especially on cessation of exercise, it will cause EAPH to develop. Two factors cause this translocation

4   While serving as medical consultant at the 1998 Ironman Hawaii Triathlon, I attempted to introduce the concept of elevating the base of the bed to treat the low blood pressure (postural hypotension) that, in my opinion, is by far the most common cause of postrace collapse in athletes. Lifting the base of the bed cures the symptoms of postural hypotension and reduces the need to give intravenous fluids (inappropriately) for this condition.

This I showed at least to my own satisfaction in one elderly (>70-year-old) finisher whom I was called to see because he was deathly pale. The attending doctor could not detect a measurable pulse or blood pressure. I immediately lifted the base of the bed. Within seconds the patient's pulse became palpable, color returned to his face, and he was miraculously "cured."

Years later, scientific papers written by some of the doctors I had interacted with showed that some lessons had been learned. Dr. Robert Sallis, who had been my close companion in the medical tent in 1998, wrote an article on the GSSI website acknowledging the value of this simple intervention. In that article he wrote, "The most common benign cause of collapse is low blood pressure due to blood pooling in the legs after cessation of exercise (as in postural hypotension, heat exhaustion, or syncope). This condition is treated by elevating the feet and pelvis until symptoms improve" (Sallis, 2004, p. 1). In the article, Dr. Sallis lists dehydration as a "non-serious" cause of collapse in athletes, which seems to conflict with the message of both the ACSM and the GSSI.

immediately after the exercise terminates. First, the muscles in the calf, the contraction of which empties blood from the leg veins pumping it toward the heart, stop working. As a result, the action of this "second heart" is lost, causing blood to pool in the legs. Second, exercise impairs the bodily responses to any sudden reduction in blood pressure. This response requires the rapid activation of the sympathetic nervous system, which raises the blood pressure by increasing the resistance to blood flow in many organs, including the muscles of the legs. But endurance training reduces the sensitivity of the sympathetic nervous system to respond to such sudden stresses.

Those athletes who do not develop EAPH are able to prevent this relocation of blood volume from the center of the body to the legs, which begins the moment exercise terminates, in part because they activate an appropriate response of their sympathetic nervous system the moment they stop exercising.

The symptoms of EAPH are caused by this sudden onset of a falling blood pressure, which results in an inadequate blood supply to the brain (cerebral

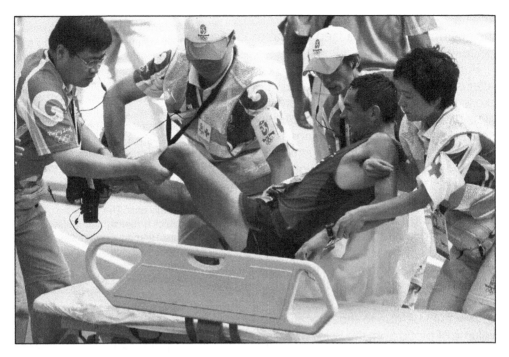

Athletes who collapse immediately after exercising almost always have exercise associated postural hypertension (EAPH). Dehydration does not cause EAPH.

AP Photo/Kevin Frayer

ischemia). The symptoms of cerebral ischemia are dizziness, nausea leading perhaps to vomiting, and a transient loss of consciousness (fainting). These symptoms persist until the blood flow to the brain is restored by an increase in blood pressure. Usually this occurs when the athlete falls to the ground and lies flat, thereby relocating a large volume of blood from the legs (and intestine) back to the center of the body. This sudden return of blood to the heart rapidly improves heart function and restores blood pressure to the appropriate postexercise value ($^{100 \text{ to } 120}/_{60 \text{ to } 80}$ mmHg), which is usually slightly lower than the accepted normal ($^{110 \text{ to } 140}/_{60 \text{ to } 90}$ mmHg) for resting humans who have not recently exercised.

The point is that dizziness, fainting, and nausea are the symptoms not of dehydration but of an inadequate blood supply to the brain. People who die from profound fluid loss when they are lost in the desert for three or more days without water also become confused. But this is not because of an inadequate blood supply to the brain—one of the body's most protected physiological functions—but because they develop multiple organ failure, including heart, kidney, and liver failure. The heart failure reduces blood flow to the brain, while kidney failure and liver failure cause the accumulation of certain toxic chemicals in the body that interfere with brain functioning, causing confusion and ultimately coma and death.

Experienced sport physicians are unable to determine the extent of dehydration (or volume of depletion) on the basis of the methods taught in medical school, that is, by examining the turgor of the skin, the state of hydration of the mucous membranes in the mouth, the presence of "sunken eyes," the ability to spit, and the sensations of thirst (McGarvey, Thompson, et al., 2010). The only way accurately to determine the level of an athlete's state of hydration after prolonged exercise is to measure the body weight before and after exercise and, better, to measure the change in body water. The use of urine color, much promoted by some scientists, is of no value (Cheuvront, Ely, et al., 2010), because it is a measure of the brain and kidneys' response to changes in blood osmolality. It does not tell us exactly what the blood osmolality is and whether it is raised, lowered, or normal. As we will show, athletes with EAH typically excrete a dark urine even though they are severely overhydrated with blood osmolalities that are greatly reduced.

Fluid Loss and Performance

If fluid loss leads to thirst, why do some of the best competitors finish endurance races in quite advanced states of fluid loss? Time and again, studies, even those by researchers expecting different outcomes, have shown that the runners who are the most dehydrated, as measured by percentage of body weight loss, run the fastest. As two examples, notice the results in figure 2.4, from the 2000 and 2001 South African Ironman Triathlons and the 2004 New Zealand Ironman Triathlon.

The largest body weight loss in these studies was 12% in an athlete who finished the race in ~720 minutes (arrowed in figure 2.4a). The five fastest finishers in the South African Ironman all finished in less than 9 hours and all lost 6% to 8% of their body weights during the race (arrowed in figure 2.4a). Three years

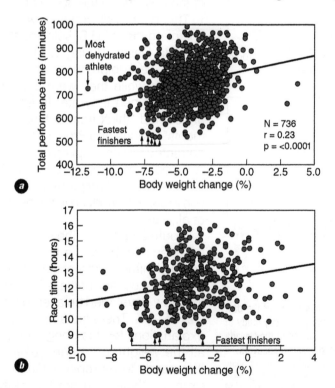

FIGURE 2.4 Results from two studies using data from *(a)* the 2000 and 2001 South African Ironman Triathlon and *(b)* the 2004 New Zealand Ironman Triathlon show a linear relationship with a positive slope between percentage of body weight loss and total performance time.

(a) Reproduced from *British Journal of Sports Medicine*, K.A. Sharwood, M. Collins, J.H. Goedecke, G. Wilson, and T. Noakes, 38(6), 718-724, 2004, with permission from BMJ Publishing Group Ltd. *(b)* Reprinted, by permission, from P.C. Wharam, D.B Speedy, T.D. Noakes, et al., 2006, "NSAID use increases the risk of developing hyponatremia during an Ironman triathlon," *Medicine & Science in Sports & Exercise* 38(4): 618-622.

later, this relationship was confirmed in finishers in the 2004 New Zealand Ironman Triathlon (figure 2.4b).

Why would the fastest endurance performers exhibit the highest percentages of body weight loss during their winning performances? Perhaps clues exist in the phenomenon that has been termed voluntary dehydration. Exercising humans do not drink to maintain a constant body weight every moment of the day. Rather, we develop a water deficit termed **voluntary dehydration** by drinking less than the amount of weight (assumed to be due entirely to water loss) that we lose as sweat during exercise. Only at mealtimes do humans increase water intakes and so correct exactly the fluid loss developed in the hours between meals.

Dill and Adolph (1938) described this phenomenon during a 30-day study of one subject, probably Edward F. Adolph himself (figure 2.5a). The data presented are the average values measured at different hours of the day during the 30-day trial.

This pattern of behavior was also apparent in a group of U.S. soldiers studied in the Nevada Desert during World War II (figure 2.5b). Like Adolph, these soldiers drank the most not while they were exercising in the heat but when they ate. In effect, they had uncoupled "thirst from actual water requirements" (Hanna and Brown, 1983, p. 262) and corrected this uncoupling only when they ate. A modern study from USARIEM scientists confirms that eating promotes fluid consumption in soldiers working in the heat (Szlyk, Sils, et al., 1990).

Figure 2.5c shows the same phenomenon in seven members of a tank crew during 48 hours of maneuvers that included a few hours of a simulated tank battle. After the tank battle, the crew developed an average body weight loss of ~3%. There are a number of probable explanations for this phenomenon. First, not all the weight lost during exercise is fluid that needs to be replaced immediately. For example, there is an inevitable loss of weight caused by the fuel, either fat or carbohydrate, that must be burned in order to provide the energy needed for the exercise. The analogy

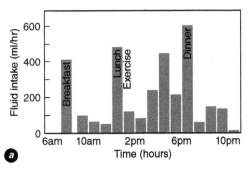

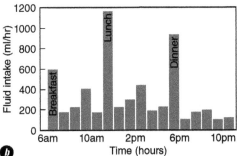

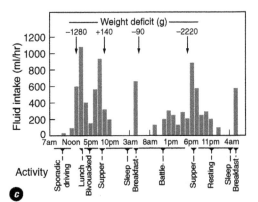

FIGURE 2.5 Fluid intake at various hours of the day, showing a correction at mealtimes: (a) 30-day study of one subject, (b) one U.S. soldier studied in the Nevada desert, (c) and a tank crew during desert maneuvers.

(a) Adapted, by permission, from E.F. Adolph and D.B. Dill, 1938, "Observations on water metabolism in the desert, *American Journal of Physiology* 123(2): 369-378. (b) Adapted from A.H. Brown, 1947, Fluid intakes in the desert. In *Physiology of man in the desert*, edited by E.F. Adolph (New York: Interscience Publishers), 111. (c) From A. Rothstein, E.F. Adolph, and J.H. Wills, 1947, Voluntary dehydration. In *Physiology of man in the desert*, edited by E.F. Adolph (New York: Interscience Publishers), 255. Reprinted by permission of the author.

would be the fuel in a motor car that is burned as the car travels—the result is that, until it is again filled with fuel, the car loses weight in direct proportion to how far it travels.

An additional factor is not covered by this car analogy. It is that the carbohydrate that is burned during exercise may be stored in the muscle and liver in a complex that includes a substantial mass of bound water. It has been argued for some years that each gram of carbohydrate used during exercise releases up to 3 grams of water. This water acts as a fluid reserve that is restored only when the body's carbohydrate stores are again filled 12 to 36 hours after exercise. Because the body can store 500 grams of carbohydrate (Noakes, 2003) (with an associated 1,500 grams of water), this would explain why humans might lose at least 2000 grams of weight during exercise without any real water loss. Indeed, in our studies of this problem (Nolte, Noakes, et al., 2010; Nolte, Noakes, et al., 2011a; Nolte, Noakes, et al., 2011b), we have shown that exercising humans can lose at least 1,000 grams without a measureable change in their total-body water content.

Thus the term *voluntary dehydration* may not accurately describe what happens in athletes who lose less than 1 kg during exercise because they may not have lost any body water and hence are not dehydrated. But athletes who lose more than 3 kg during prolonged exercise probably do show a reduction in total-body water content and hence are likely to be voluntarily dehydrated to varying degrees. The explanation for this phenomenon is that already given—either they prevent a large change in ECF solute concentration in response to quite large changes

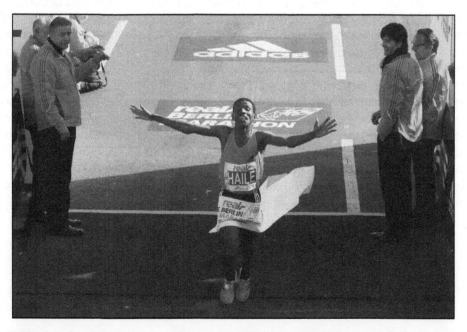

Haile Gebrselassie of Ethiopia sets the world record (2:03:59) at the 2008 Berlin Marathon. During this race, Gebrselassie drank at an estimated rate of 0.89 L/hr. In the 2009 Dubai Marathon, he drank at a rate of 0.83 L/hr, sweated at a rate of 3.6 L/hr, and lost 9.8% of his starting body weight. Yet he won that race in 2:06:08 (Beis, Wright-Whyte, Fudge et al., 2012).

Imago/Icon SMI

in body water content or their brains are less sensitive to a normal increase in ECF osmolality (solute concentration). But either way, the fact that athletes with the greatest levels of weight loss are usually the fastest finishers in endurance events shows that the response of their brains to body water loss has been entirely appropriate, perhaps optimal.

There is no direct evidence that exercise performance is impaired in those who lose weight during exercise, provided they drink to the dictates of thirst and do not become thirsty (Goulet, 2011; Sawka and Noakes, 2007). In fact, evidence that the best marathon runners have a remarkable capacity to resist high levels of fluid loss has been provided in countless races around the world.

Summary

Before the 1960s, endurance athletes often restricted their fluid intake, with no ill effects on health or performance. Although a person could argue that athletes can, equally safely, be advised to drink ad libitum, in the decades after the 1960s, the pendulum swung far to the other end of the spectrum, and all athletes are now advised to drink even before they sense thirst. But for endurance athletes this contradicts the built-in protections clearly offered by the body's thirst mechanism, protections that will serve us well, if we will only let them.

To compound matters, the definition and symptoms of dehydration became muddied. The sports drink industry drew attention exclusively to results of studies that failed to accurately interpret the explanations and consequences of dehydration. Dehydration is simply a reduction in the total body water content. The only symptom of dehydration is thirst, and often it is an overwhelming sense. If at any time a healthy athlete does not sense thirst, the athlete is not dehydrated. Period.

Further, many accomplished endurance athletes are able to successfully compete, even place high and win, with no ill health effects, at significantly higher percentages of dehydration than are currently recommended by leading sports medicine organizations. Could it be that these athletes are simply following their natural inclinations to exercise now and take in fluid later, often along with a post-race or evening meal? And have our efforts to protect athletes actually undone the natural protections offered by our bodies, causing hundreds of athletes to overdrink, leading not to *good* health and performance but to dangerous medical conditions?

CHAPTER 3

Water's Role in Thermoregulation

> . . . whenever one's body temperature rises, even for physiological reasons, we enter into danger and anything that interferes with physiological cooling, or adds to the internal heat load, exacerbates that danger. The wonder is, not that anyone gets hyperpyrexia, but that so few do.
>
> **W.S. Ladell (1957, p. 206)**

The year 1969, my first as a medical student, a rower, and a runner in two short-distance races, was also a pivotal year in the history of the exercise sciences. It was the year after the first summer Olympic Games had been held at altitude (2,200 m) in Mexico City. For the first time, the exercise sciences were challenged to answer two simple questions: Is it safe to compete at that altitude? How long does it take to adapt optimally for competition at altitude?

The 1968 Olympics was also the first time that the former East Germany (German Democratic Republic) competed as a country separate from (West) Germany. Their growing success in Olympic competition and the threat it posed to Western democracies, especially the United States, stimulated an unprecedented interest in the practical application of the sport sciences for achieving superior athletic performances, especially in Olympic competition.

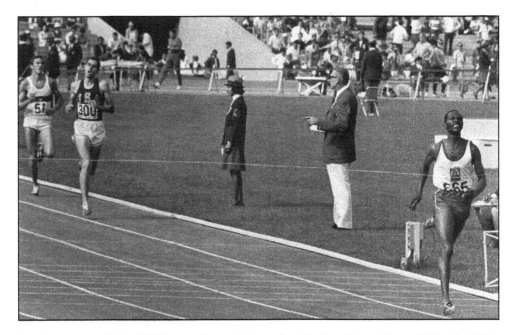

In an iconic moment in the 1968 Olympic Games in Mexico City, Kipchoge Keino of Kenya finishes the 1500m run in a new Olympic record time of 3:34.9, finishing ahead of Jim Ryun of the United States and Bodo Tummler of West Germany. This performance signaled the beginning of the dominance of distance running by East Africans.

AP Photo

Practical experience rather than science would answer both questions. An absence of fatalities showed that it was safe to compete at that altitude. But the dominance of the long-distance running events by athletes from the highlands of East Africa suggested to Sir Roger Bannister that for an optimal adaptation to occur, athletes probably had to live at altitude all their lives.[1]

1 History seems to have proved Dr. Bannister's opinion. The dominance of modern distance running by East African, especially Kenyan, runners, all of whom are born at altitude, suggests that living and training at altitude for a lifetime are beneficial either because these act over the athletic lifetime of each runner or because they have acted over the lifetimes of many generations of each runner's ancestors, producing beneficial biological changes that are now built into each Kenyan runner's DNA. On balance, I suspect that the latter explanation is more probable. However, the mental belief induced by the Kenyans' success over the past 30 years now complements any possible biological advantages that their generations at altitude may have produced.

The year 1969 also produced a scientific publication that would become one of the most influential in this evolving discipline. That the study was completed by two South African scientists, eminent in their discipline, and was published in the local *South African Medical Journal* ensured perhaps that I would be more likely to discover the article in 1970 when I ventured for the first time into the medical library at the University of Cape Town. There I discovered an overpowering personal addiction to published scientific information in biology and medicine.

Not that their article would have been prescribed reading for medical students anywhere in the world, the scientific study of sport and especially marathon running was not something that medical professors either in South Africa or elsewhere would have considered an appropriate choice for young students harboring genuine aspirations for a career in medicine or science.

In their paper that within two decades would become a classic cited frequently by the sports drink industry, Professors Cyril Wyndham and Nic Strydom,[2] then working for the Chamber of Mines in Johannesburg, Transvaal (Gauteng), advanced the theory that marathon runners who fail to drink adequately during exercise risked serious health consequences. Thus ". . . the present practice of marathon runners drinking only small quantities of water is dangerous . . . (so that) . . . the international ruling which forbids the drinking of water in the first 10 miles (16 km) is criminal folly in warm weather" (Wyndham and Strydom, 1969, p. 896). As a result, Wyndham and Strydom advised that marathon runners should drink about 300 ml (10.1 fl oz) every 20 minutes (900 ml per hour) in order to prevent these "dangers." This advice was clearly a revolutionary advance on the conventional wisdom, which held that drinking during exercise is unnecessary, certainly a sign of weakness, and probably detrimental.

Wyndham and Strydom based their conclusion on their finding that runners who drank little during competitive 32 km (19.9 mile) races developed higher body temperatures than did those who drank more and ran slower and who, as a consequence, were less dehydrated at the finish of those races. They concluded that these two observations were causally linked (box 3.1, page 62): that sweat losses during exercise induced a physiological state of dehydration, which, unless prevented by appropriate drinking, caused the body temperature to rise in direct proportion to the extent of underdrinking and hence the level of dehydration that developed during exercise. When the dehydration was severe, the body temperature would become catastrophically elevated, sufficient to cause the potentially fatal medical emergency of heatstroke (figure 3.1).

The authors concluded (incorrectly; see box 3.1, page 62) that the two phenomena were causally related so that the level of dehydration that develops during exercise determines the postexercise body temperature. This finding would become the key evidence supporting

2   When they published their study, Wyndham and Strydom were rightly recognized internationally as among the world's leading thermal physiologists. They had published extensively on all aspects of exercise in the heat and were especially renowned for their studies of heat acclimatization in South African miners. Over a period of 20 years between 1950 and 1970, the practical application of their work reduced the number of fatal heatstroke cases among South African gold miners from values that were unacceptably high to almost zero. Thus it is entirely understandable that their landmark paper titled "The Danger of an Inadequate Water Intake During Marathon Running," published in 1969, should have had a global impact that persists even at the time of this writing. Two of the world's greatest thermal experts had delivered the warning that if they do not drink sufficiently during exercise, marathon runners will die from heatstroke. Only later would we learn that their interpretation was quite wrong.

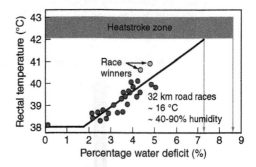

FIGURE 3.1   In a study of runners in two 32 km races in Johannesburg, South Africa, Wyndham and Strydom reported a linear relationship between the degree of weight loss during the race (horizontal x-axis) and the postrace rectal temperature (vertical y-axis). The athlete (arrowed) who won both races lost the most weight and finished with the highest body temperature.

Adapted, by permission, from C.H. Wyndham and N.B. Strydom, 1969, "The danger of an inadequate water intake during marathon running," *South African Medical Journal* 43(July), 893-896.

BOX 3.1   Analyzing Wyndham and Strydom's Conclusion

Why was Wyndham and Strydom's conclusion false that the level of dehydration determines the body temperature during exercise? Figure 3.1 shows an *association* between higher body temperatures and increasing levels of body weight loss in athletes completing 32 km running races. The unwary would naturally assume that the two observations are causally linked so that higher levels of weight loss during exercise are the sole and direct cause of a proportional increase in body temperature according to the physiological explanation seen in figure 3.2.

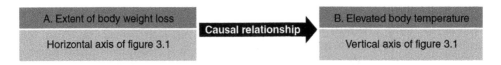

FIGURE 3.2   Physiological model 1, showing a causal link.

If we conclude that A causes B, we then can begin to develop a biological model of how the body works during exercise. Particularly, this model must be able to explain why A causes B. This model then becomes the "truth"—the preconception if you will—which will determine how we interpret any new information relating to prolonged exercise, fluid ingestion, and body temperature. Therefore, the biological model that Wyndham and Strydom developed predicts that the level of dehydration that develops during exercise is the most important determinant of the extent to which the body temperature rises.

But the great challenge for scientists is to be absolutely certain that the two variables A and B are causally linked since there may be many other possible explanations for an apparent relationship. Thus the function of the scientist is to exclude all other possible explanations until only one remains. It is a serious error to assume that the only two variables that one measures in any study must be causally related so that all other possible explanations can be summarily excluded. Wyndham and Strydom failed to consider at least one other obvious explanation for their finding (figure 3.3):

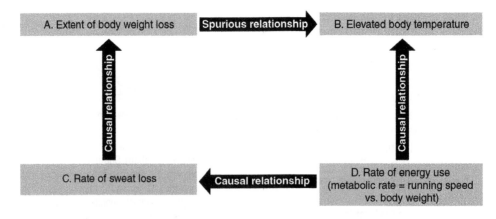

FIGURE 3.3   Physiological model 2, showing the true causal relationships and illuminating the spurious relationship.

In this second model, the rate of energy use (metabolic rate, D) determines both the rate of sweat loss (sweat rate, C), which it does (Greenhaff and Clough, 1989; Saltin and Hermansen, 1966), and the extent to which the body temperature (B) rises during exercise, which it does (Lind, 1963; Nielson, 1938; Nielson and Nielson, 1962; Noakes, Myburgh, et al., 1991). As a result, the metabolic rate, which is a function of the running speed and the runner's body weight, determines both the extent to which the body temperature is elevated during exercise and the sweat rate. This would mean that the relationship between A and B is incidental (spurious), not causal, since both A and B are dependent on a shared third factor, D, the metabolic rate.

The only way to distinguish between physiological models 1 and 2 is to conduct a randomized controlled intervention trial (RCT) in which the effect of changing only one experimental variable at a time is measured. For example, an RCT designed to measure the relative effects of either the metabolic rate or the rate of drinking on the extent to which the body temperature rises during exercise requires two separate experiments. In one, the metabolic rate is uncontrolled and allowed to vary while the drinking rate is held constant; in the other, the amount of fluid drunk during exercise is varied while the metabolic rate is held constant. Only this experimental design can detect relationships that are causal.

Despite their great experience with such trials,[3] Wyndham and Strydom were inexplicably blind to this error, perhaps because they believed their message was too important to await confirmation in a properly conducted RCT. Probably because they had witnessed the frightening consequences of heatstroke in the mining industry, they wished to ensure that the same would not happen in marathon running. But they failed to notice that in the 71 years since the first official marathon footrace had been run in the 1896 Athens Olympic Games, there had been very few cases of heatstroke: The few real cases that occurred were sometimes caused by the injudicious use of performance-enhancing drugs, especially amphetamines.

An RCT conducted by Jonathan Dugas (Dugas, Oosthuizen, et al., 2009) later accurately detected the relationship. Dugas' study included ad libitum drinking, and athletes were allowed to regulate their effort. This study showed that the athletes went slower from the start when told they would

3 Wyndham and Strydom conducted countless properly controlled clinical trials including, for example, some quite exceptional trials of the effects of heat acclimatization on human exercise responses (Wyndham, 1974). They even completed a well-controlled randomized prospective study of the effects of fluid restriction on performance during a prolonged march in which many of the design flaws in their classic study were avoided (Strydom, Wyndham, et al., 1966). The principal error in their prospective study was that they compared ad libitum drinking to not drinking at all during exercise. But the complete avoidance of all drinking is not the current practice of humans during exercise. Their study was therefore an example of one in which the normal response (drinking ad libitum) was compared to the worst possible option (not drinking). This study design is more likely to produce a definitive finding in favor of the chosen intervention—not that dishonesty was Wyndham and Strydom's motive. At the time they completed their studies, the usual behavior was not to drink anything during exercise.

A better design would have been to compare ad libitum drinking with drinking either more or less. Indeed, when they completed one such study, they found that "there was no improvement in body temperature responses, over those observed in men on water ad libitum, when men were forced to drink as much water as they lost in sweat or if they drank hypotonic saline, but it was found to be desirable, from the body metabolism point of view, to add 100 g of sucrose to the water taken at the mid-shift period (Benade, Jansen, et al., 1973)" (Wyndham, 1973, p. 119). As a result, all miners working in wet-bulb temperatures in excess of 29 °C were provided "with at least 3 liters of palatable water per (8 hour) shift" (p. 119).

(continued)

BOX 3.1 **Analyzing Wyndham and Strydom's Conclusion** *(continued)*

not be allowed to drink during the time trial. But their end-rectal temperatures were identical regardless of how much they drank during the trial. This shows that athletes change their performance in order to maintain the same end-rectal temperature. Other RCTs have attempted to properly discern the relationships, but they have been flawed. For example, Montain and Coyle (1992) fixed the work rate and did not compare ad libitum drinking. Therefore, the study did not allow the brain to change the work rate in order to prevent any excessive rise in body temperature. They also did not allow proper cooling with fans to optimize convective cooling.

Unfortunately, Wyndham and Strydom's paper became one of the foundational studies used to justify the dogma that runners must "consume the maximal amount that can be tolerated" (Convertino, Armstrong, et al., 1996, p. i), lest they become dehydrated and so risk their health during exercise. There is an important analogy to the 1944 study by Ladell (Ladell, Waterlow, et al., 1944a; Ladell, Waterlow, et al., 1944b) that led to the conclusion that either salt or water deficiency cause two different forms of heat exhaustion. Since Ladell measured only sodium and water balance in the ill soldiers he studied, he would inevitably conclude that all were suffering from either water deficiency or salt deficiency. Ladell would live long enough to admit his error (Ladell, 1965). Sadly Wyndham and Strydom both died before they could address the damage caused by their error.

Instead, Wyndham and Strydom's study was used to promote the **dehydration myth,** which holds (a) that the extent of dehydration is the most important determinant of the body temperature response during exercise; (b) that levels of dehydration greater than 3% are especially dangerous because they will inevitably lead to heatstroke; and (c) that athletes who collapse after exercise are both dehydrated and hyperthermic and must therefore be treated, without delay, with copious volumes of intravenous fluids (figure 3.4).

But a physiological truth is true only in the confines of the physiological model within which it is interpreted. If the model is wrong, so will be the "truth" that it supports. For this reason, truth is a relative concept. As anthropologist Richard Leakey once wrote, "Absolute truth is like a mirage. It tends to disappear when you approach it" (Leakey and Lewin, 1992, p. xviii).

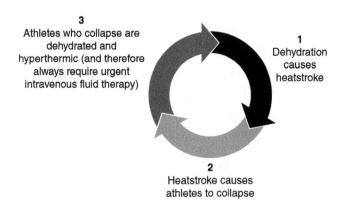

3
Athletes who collapse are dehydrated and hyperthermic (and therefore always require urgent intravenous fluid therapy)

1
Dehydration causes heatstroke

2
Heatstroke causes athletes to collapse

FIGURE 3.4 The circular argument linking post-exercise collapse, dehydration, and the need for intravenous fluid therapy. However, Wyndham and Strydom did not show that dehydration causes post-exercise collapse. The most dehydrated runner in their study was the race winner (figure 3.1, page 61), as is usually the case.

the initial foundational myth that any level of dehydration is dangerous since it elevates the body temperature, increasing the risk that athletes who drink too little during exercise will die of heatstroke.

But any athlete schooled in the 1880 to 1968 idea that drinking during exercise was detrimental would have drawn the exact opposite conclusion: that *the avoidance of drinking* during these races was clearly beneficial because the athlete who won both races was the most dehydrated and had the highest postrace body temperature, presumably because he had drunk sparingly during the race.

Note that there appears to be no relationship between the postrace body temperature and the level of dehydration below a "percentage water deficit" less than about 2.5%. Although they acknowledged this finding, Wyndham and Strydom's original figure did not show this. Instead they truncated the *x*-axis beginning at a "percentage water deficit" of 2% so that the data for runner A in this figure were indicated by an arrow pointing to a "percentage water deficit" of 0%. As a result to the unwary, their figure seemed to suggest that any effect of dehydration on the rectal temperature during exercise begins at a level of dehydration of 0%. This question remains: Why did Wyndham and Strydom choose to present their data in that way rather than in the correct manner (figure 3.1, page 61)?

The point perhaps is that the debate of whether or not it is "safe" to lose some body weight during exercise and, if so, how much, continues unabated. The 2007 position stand of the ACSM (Sawka, Burke, et al., 2007) continues to argue that a body mass loss of up to only 2% is advisable. I, on the other hand, argue that the body will decide itself the safe level of dehydration that it will allow during exercise (Sawka and Noakes, 2007); for some this might be 1% and for others 12% (figure 3.17, page 92). This will be determined by each individual's thirst response, as discussed in chapter 2. Thus, prescribing a one-response-fits-all solution is, in my view, unlikely to be helpful for the majority of athletes.

Early Study Challenges the Wyndham and Strydom Hypothesis

By the time I realized that drinking too much during exercise was dangerous and could likely be fatal, I had just begun my career as an exercise scientist having just completed my medical PhD (MD) degree, studying the effects of exercise on the heart and particularly the factors that determine the maximal functioning of the rat heart. Besides my developing interest in heatstroke and in fluid replacement during exercise, the study of the factors determining fatigue and peak exercise performance in human athletes would become my other consuming passion.

Fortunately, because this new career choice took me from the established research laboratories with the comforting conformity of secure funding streams into a scientific backwater characterized by disinterest and neglect, we initially had neither the equipment nor the money to undertake anything but the most rudimentary research studies. This in turn forced us to study real athletes, not in the laboratory, since we did not have one worthy of the name, but in real-life athletic competitions. The advantage was that these athletes did not expect to be paid for their efforts, and they almost always give a 100% effort. More important, by using simple tools like an accurate (digital) bathroom scale (one of our very first purchases, and which stretched our limited financial resources), a few rectal thermometers (borrowed from the hospital, I suspect), and an army of helpers to record how much athletes reported they drank during competitions, we could begin to address this simple question: What effects does dehydration have on the health and performance of athletes competing in real competitions?

Thus beginning in 1983, we began to collect information on athletes in the more important South African running and canoeing races. Within the first two years, we collected information on 64 individual performances in 42 km (26 mile) races and 48 individual performances in the 56 km (34.8 mile) Two Oceans Marathon, a race that is run in our immediate vicinity. In addition, we had data on 91 individual performances in canoeing races from 30 to 65 km. The goal of this research was as we then wrote: "(i) to determine the rates of water loss, . . . drinking patterns and post-race temperatures of . . . athletes, and (ii) to re-examine the relationship between the degree of exercise-induced dehydration and post-race . . . temperature" (Noakes, Adams, et al., 1988, p. 211). We discovered the following:

- Average rates of fluid intake in the running races varied from 0.43 to 0.62 L/hr. We noted that these values were very similar to rates of 0.13 to 0.59 L/hr reported in the 15 studies that had been reported in the literature at that time (table 4 in Noakes, Adams, et al., 1988).

Thus we concluded that fluid intake of ~500 ml/hr (17 fl oz/hr) "appears to be what athletes involved in prolonged exercise choose" (p. 214) so that "During prolonged exercise in mild . . . conditions, intake of 0.5L/hr will prevent dehydration in the majority . . ." (p. 210). This information would become very important 8 years later when the 1996 ACSM drinking guidelines were introduced, which encouraged athletes to drink "as much as tolerable" or 600 to 1200 ml/hour (20.3 to 40.6 fl oz/hr). Instead, on the basis of these real data we had consistently argued for a decade that rates of 400 to 800 ml/hr (13.5 to 27 fl oz/hr) appeared far more appropriate since this is the range athletes naturally choose. So this 400 to 800 ml/hr range was the one we chose for the guidelines we developed for the International Marathon Medical Directors Association (IMMDA) in 2003. When the ACSM guidelines were revised in 2007, they confirmed that our opinion had been correct since they revised their drinking guidelines from 600 to 1200 ml/hr down to 400 to 800 ml/hr. This was a welcome, albeit overdue, change of position.

- Average sweat rates ranged from 0.7 to 1.3 L/hr (23.7 to 44 fl oz/hr), values that were also similar to those reported by others (table 4 in Noakes Adams, et al., 1988). We noted that only when environmental temperatures were greater than 25 °C (77 °F) were higher sweat rates likely. Only later would I read the study of Nielsen (1938), which showed that both the sweat rate and the rectal temperature during exercise are essentially independent of environmental conditions at air temperatures up to 22 °C (71.6 °F) (figure 3.5).

In 1938 Danish physician and exercise scientist Marius Nielsen published a classic paper that showed the rectal temperature rose during exercise and reached a plateau value after about 50 minutes (Nielsen, 1938) at all exercise intensities except the most extreme (top line of figure 3.5a). This plateau value was determined by the intensity of the exercise (figure 3.5a) and was little affected by the environmental conditions that were studied (figure 3.5b) since the plateau (peak) rectal temperature *at the same exercise intensity* was the same whether the exercise was performed at 11, 16, or 22 °C. Interestingly, this concept that the rectal temperature during exercise is determined by the rate at which the exercise is performed (the exercise intensity) and is "practically independent of environmental temperatures between 5 and 30 °C" (Nielsen and Nielsen, 1962, p. 120) was the accepted teaching in the exercise sciences until the beginning of the 1970s. Thereafter, this accepted concept was exchanged for one in which the level of dehydration was considered to be the most important factor determining the rectal temperature response during exercise. It is my contention that the development of the world's first sports drink by Dr. Cade in 1965 was one of the most important factors driving this change (chapters 5 and 6). Like others at the time, Dr. Cade was convinced that the level of dehydration determines the extent to which the body temperature rises during exercise.

- Postrace body temperatures were only moderately elevated (average values of 38.0 to 39.2 °C in the different races). This, too, was similar to all the information reported in the literature.

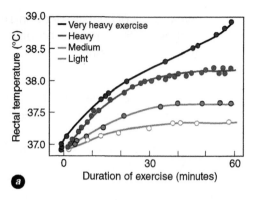

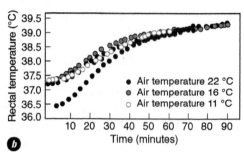

FIGURE 3.5 Rectal temperature at (a) four different exercise intensities and (b) three different air temperatures. Rectal temperature reaches a plateau after 50 minutes, except during the most intense exercise, and was independent of the environmental air temperature up to 22 °C. The dependence of the rise in rectal temperature on the intensity of the exercise is important to our discussion.

From B. Nielsen, 1938, "Die regulation der körpertemperatur bei muskelarbeit," *Skandinavisches Archiv für Physiologie* 79: 195-230. Reprinted by permission of the Scandinavian Physiological Society.

Thus we wrote that although it had been propagated that marked hyperthermia is inevitable during marathon running, the findings of our study did not support this belief. In addition, most of the previous studies reported only moderately elevated rectal temperatures in marathon runners. We noted that the highest postrace rectal temperatures were, without exception, measured in the fastest runners, and we recognized that rectal temperature had been related to running speed in the last part of the race (Maughan, 1985; Maughan, Leiper, et al., 1985).

We also reminded readers that "the highest . . . temperatures and the greatest incidence of heatstroke are found in highly-trained athletes competing in shorter distance events lasting 20-40 min" (Hughson, Staudt, et al., 1983; Noakes, 1982; Robinson, 1963, p. 216)

"These studies . . . suggest . . . running speed is a . . . determinant of rectal temperature during running" (p. 216). It would take nearly 20 years before this prediction would finally be proven beyond doubt (Byrne, Lee, et al., 2006; Lee, Nio, et al., 2010). But I suspect it will take considerably longer before it is accepted that the risk of heatstroke during marathon running is essentially negligible except in those with a genetic predisposition, plus one or more initiating factors other than exercise alone.

■ In contrast to the predictions of the Wyndham and Strydom theory, there was absolutely no relationship between the percentage of weight loss during exercise and the postrace body temperature. We noted that other scientists also did not find any relationship between these variables (Blake and Larrabee, 1903; Maughan, 1985). Accordingly, we concluded that "the level of dehydration plays only a permissive role in determining the rectal temperature during marathon running" (p. 217). Rather, we argued that it is the speed maintained over the last segment of the race, as also found by others (Maughan, 1985; Maughan, Leiper, et al., 1985) that predicts the extent to which the rectal temperature rises during exercise.

Speed ⟶

We concluded that the metabolic rate (running speed multiplied by body weight) is the major determinant of the body temperature during exercise and that the level of dehydration plays only a small (permissive) role. Thus, "Athletes who run slowly during marathon competition could . . . become . . . dehydrated if they did not drink, but would be protected from hyperthermia by . . . low metabolic rates" so that "in cold . . . conditions such runners are at greater risk of hypothermia than of hyperthermia" (p. 217). We also noted this in a statement of some prescience: ". . . it is only those studies which have reported the very high sweat rates during marathon running which have been quoted (American College of Sports Medicine, 1985) to justify the importance of high fluid intakes during running" (p. 216).

Although we had conducted this research between 1983 and 1985, because of a quite demanding teaching load at that time, I submitted the write-up of the paper for publication only in late 1987. By then the ACSM had produced new drinking guidelines for exercise. These were heavily influenced by the Wyndham and Strydom theory that dehydration is the major determinant of the rectal temperature during exercise as well as the risk that heatstroke will develop. Accordingly, these guidelines advised that athletes competing in running races should have access to 300 to 360 ml (10-12 oz) of fluid every 4 km (12-24 min running time), giving a fluid intake of 1.65 L/hr (55.8 fl oz/hr) (fast runners) and 0.83 L/hr (28 fl oz/hr) (slow runners).

Since by then we had reported cases of water intoxication in runners whose rates of fluid intake fell within this range; 9 of 16 hospital admissions at the 1985 90 km Comrades Marathon were due to water intoxication; and 20% of finishers in the 1984 and 1985 226 km Ironman Hawaii Triathlon had EAH (Hiller, O'Toole, et al., 1985), we began to question whether these guidelines might be potentially hazardous, especially if they promoted drinking rates greater than those naturally chosen by athletes. We concluded with this statement: ". . . proposals of the American College of Sports Medicine (1987) in part perpetuates these errors by promoting unrealistically high fluid intakes during exercise and emphasising the risk of hyperthermia during prolonged rather than short, high intensity exercise. Environmental conditions, metabolic rate and individual susceptibility (Jardon, 1982), not dehydration, are the . . . risk factors for hyperthermia during exercise and should be so identified" (p. 218).

We titled the article "The Danger of an Inadequate Water Intake During Prolonged Exercise: A Novel Concept Revisited" (Noakes, Adams, et al., 1988). The paper was accepted and published without serious challenge from the reviewers. It would be the last occasion for a long time in which we would be so fortunate. In 1987, Gatorade formed the Gatorade Sports Science Institute under the direction of Dr. Bob Murray. Thereafter, research that challenged the GSS's position was less likely to be published.

Historical Evidence Against the Wyndham and Strydom Hypothesis

A key understanding in science is that it is not the information that supports a hypothesis that is important. Rather, the hypothesis survives for only as long as there is not a *single* published study with data that refute the predictions of that theory. But as soon as there is a single study that conflicts with that hypothesis, it is time to man the lifeboats because the ship may well be sinking. And the most clever scientists are usually those who are the first to abandon ship; those who stay on board risk going down with the ship. This at least is how science should be conducted according to the Popperian model (Popper, 1959).

So as I became more interested in this topic, I acquainted myself with the literature and asked this question: Is there any evidence in the published literature to show that athletes who do not drink according to these new 1987 ACSM guidelines place themselves at great risk of ill health and perform poorly? Fortunately, because most athletes drank little or nothing during exercise until the 1970s, I expected that there would be plenty of published evidence answering this question.

It follows that if runners drank little before the 1970s, then all must have finished competitive races with marked levels of dehydration and, according to the Wyndham and Strydom hypothesis, very high body temperatures. According to the evolving belief about dehydration, their performances must also have been poor. This theory, often advanced in USARIEM, ACSM, and Gatorade-funded publications, would also predict that the fastest runners would be those able (somehow) to develop the lowest levels of dehydration even if they did not drink during exercise and also to finish with the lowest body temperatures. What I read surprised me.

Body Weight Loss and Body Temperature: 1901 to 1967

Perhaps the first study of body weight loss and body temperatures in marathon runners was undertaken by Blake and Larabee (1903), who studied runners in the 1901, 1902, and 1903 Boston Marathons. The athletes were allowed to "eat or drink what they please during the race" (p. 195). During the races, athletes lost 0.5 to 5.0 kg (1.1-11 lb) and "in general the heaviest men and those who ran fastest lost the greatest amounts" (p. 196). Postrace rectal temperatures ranged from 96.0 to 104.4 °F (35.5-40.2 °C). Interestingly, no athletes gained weight during these races, and the range of body weight losses varied from 2% to 8.5% (figure 3.6, page 70). Two athletes developed hypothermia; it is probable that they became exhausted and walked for the last part of the race.

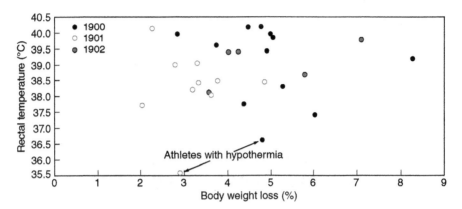

FIGURE 3.6 A plot of the data from the study of Blake and Larabee (1903) shows that there was no clear relationship ($r^2 = 0.058$; $p = 0.2$) between the degree of weight loss in runners in the 1901, 1902, and 1903 Boston Marathon and their postrace rectal temperatures. (The data were plotted on the assumption that the same numbers for data in different tables for weight loss and rectal temperatures referred to the same athletes.).
Data from Blake and Larabee 1903.

Note the wide range in the degree of body weight loss during the race and the postrace rectal temperatures. Note also the absence of any postrace rectal temperatures in excess of 40.5 °C and conversely the presence of hypothermia in two athletes (arrowed).

The authors concluded the article with the statement: "In the entire three years we neither saw nor heard of any serious, persistent after-effects, and it is yet to be proven that even these strenuous contests leave behind them any permanent injury" (p. 206). This would seem to suggest that in the first few years of the 20th century, marathon runners were quite capable of safely completing marathon races without being told exactly how they should conduct themselves, especially that they needed to drink in a manner other than dictated by their bodies.

The next study (Buskirk and Beetham, 1960) was inspired by the finding in one of the classic exercise studies undertaken during World War II in the Nevada Desert that work performance was reduced in the dehydrated individual, whether the work was performed in hot, comfortable, or cool conditions. In some this occurred at weight losses of as little as 2.5%. The question these scientists wished to answer was whether "higher values for dehydration may be necessary to produce . . . failure or a . . . decrement in the well-conditioned athlete." (p. 493). Their research questions were as follows: "What level of dehydration will man undergo during the course of marathon running? How is this level of dehydration related to the thermal response that occurs with running? Can this level of dehydration be considered debilitating to the marathon runner?" The authors also defined dehydration as "body water loss as estimated from the loss in . . . weight" (p. 494).

The authors studied 7 runners in the 1959 Boston Marathon and 10 runners in two 30 km runs. The runners' body weights were measured before and after each run and their core (rectal) temperatures within a few minutes of the completion of each run. Runners were encouraged to drink according to their normal practices during these races and "no attempt was made to curtail drinking during the . . . race" (p. 464).

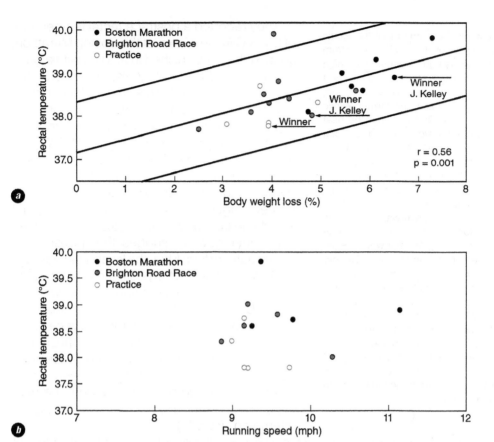

FIGURE 3.7 The study of Buskirk and Beetham (1960) found *(a)* a linear relationship with a positive slope between the percentage of body weight loss and the postrace rectal temperatures in Boston runners in three races, including the 1959 Boston Marathon. In contrast *(b)* there was no relationship between the average running speeds maintained during these races and the postrace rectal temperatures.
Data from Buskirk and Beetham 1960.

The authors found that percentage of body weight loss during the Boston Marathon ranged from 4.8 to 7.4% (average 6.0%), corresponding to an average weight loss per hour, essentially equivalent to the sweat rate, of 1.5 kg/hr (3.3 lb/hr) (figure 3.7). During the shorter runs, the equivalent data were 2.5% to 5.6% (average 4.0%) and 1.3 kg/hr (2.9 lb/hr). The postrace rectal temperatures varied from 38.1 to 39.8 °C (average 38.9 °C) in the Boston Marathon and from 38.1 to 38.5 °C (average 38.3 °C) in the 30 km runs.

The authors noted that the two highest temperatures recorded in these runners (39.8 and 39.9 °C) were substantially lower than values of 41 °C (106 °F) measured in Don Lash[4] after a 3-mile run in an air temperature of 29.5 °C with 65% humidity. They concluded that "significant body heat storage must have occurred [in Lash], and the runners were approaching limiting heat storage capacities. In contrast, this situation did not develop in the marathon runners" (p. 500).

4 I subsequently learned that the iconic U.S. thermal physiologist Sid Robinson from Indiana University had measured very high rectal temperatures in athletes running short distances at very high intensities (Robinson, 1963). Thus, Don Lash, the former 2-mile world-record holder in 1936 when he beat Paavo Nurmi's record, reached a rectal temperature of 39.7 °C when he ran 5 km in 15:00 in cool conditions (16 °C, or 60.8 °F). When he ran 10 km in 31:00 in an air temperature of 30 °C (86 °F), he finished with a rectal temperature of 41.1 °C but without any evidence of distress. Lash was an obvious subject for study since he was a student at Robinson's university. Another world-record holder in the indoor 2 and 3 miles, Gregory Rice from Notre Dame University, also reached a rectal temperature of 41.1 °C when he ran 3 miles in 14:15, also in hot conditions (30.6 °C). By an astonishing coincidence, my copy of the book from which references on this topic come and which I purchased over the Internet was clearly the personal copy of Dr. Robinson since it carries the inscription written with a pen in black ink: Sid Robinson February 26, 1971.

They reported a postrace rectal temperature of 38.9 °C in the winner of the Boston Marathon, John Kelley, who finished in 2:20:05 with a body weight loss of 6%. Kelley also won the 30 km race in 1:44:01, finishing with a rectal temperature of 38.0 °C and a body weight loss of 4.9%. Rectal temperatures for both races and for a 30 km training run were related to %BW loss (figure 3.7a), as had been found by Wyndham and Strydom (figure 3.1, page 61) but were unrelated to the running speeds attained by the runners (figure 3.7b). These findings conflict with those from more recent studies, discussed subsequently, which suggest the opposite.

The authors found that the level of dehydration did indeed influence the postexercise rectal temperature. But they did not believe that dehydration had influenced the runners' performances: "Weight loss in the marathon runners varied from 2.5 to 7.4%, yet a . . . decrement in these men . . . did not occur. Running speed (pace) was maintained essentially constant by each man in all races—there was no let down in pace near the end. . . . In fact, a sprint finish was frequently attempted" (p. 503).

The authors concluded with some speculation of the potential value of dehydration to athletes: ". . . a new level of thermal regulation during work may be established which is . . . partly dependent on the level of dehydration. . . . dehydration of the order of 2 to 3% may . . . prove beneficial . . . if 'warm-up' is regarded as essential for best performance. . . . By incurring a dehydration of this amount, his 'warm-up' time might . . . be reduced [less time to reach a given rectal temperature than when normally hydrated, my addition] while the debilitating effects of dehydration may . . . be minimal or absent at 2 to 3% level in the well-conditioned man" (p. 504).

This study did not produce any evidence to alarm these authors that the levels of dehydration that developed in marathon runners who drank according to their normal practices might pose a threat to either their health or their performances. In contrast, the authors proposed that mild dehydration could aid performance.

Clearly, despite quite marked levels of dehydration that showed a significant relationship to their postrace rectal temperature, these runners did not have profoundly elevated body temperatures in the range found in patients with heatstroke (42 °C, 107.6 °F). Also, these data did not fit the Wyndham and Strydom prediction that a 6% loss in body weight should elevate the body temperature to 41° C (figure 3.1, page 61).

Instead, the authors concluded that postrace rectal temperature suggested successful thermoregulation during the late stages of the race: "Thus, well conditioned men running in a cool environment seem to tolerate a 3 to 7% dehydration rather well" (p. 503). Their data seemingly disprove the theory that athletes who became dehydrated by up to 7% risk their health and must have an impaired exercise performance.

The obvious conclusion from both these early studies is that it is entirely safe for competitors in the Boston Marathon to drink as they wish during the race regardless of how fast they run. But by the time Cynthia Lucero ran the 2002 Boston Marathon, this advice had been substantially changed so that recreational athletes were encouraged to drink at least 1,200 ml/hr (40.6 fl oz) or else their "performance could suffer."

The British physiologist R.H. Fox (1960) was the next to address the thermoregulatory challenges posed by running marathons in the heat. He was concerned that "heat stress may prove to be an important problem at the [1960] Olympic Games in Rome" (p. 310).He calculated that if the race was held at an air temperature of 85 °F (29 °C) in moderate humidity (40-50%) and if athletes ran at 16 km/hr, in order to maintain their body temperatures within a safe range they would need to sweat at rates of 1.5 to 2 L/hr for a total sweat loss of 4.5 L (152 fl oz) during the race. He concluded the article with this question: "What effect will the loss of such a large volume of fluid have on the runner's performance? It is difficult to make any prediction except to say that with the circulation already extended by demands of both metabolism and temperature regulation, the withdrawal of even a relatively small quantity of body fluid would be expected to affect performance adversely" (pp. 311-312).[5]

In fact, the Rome Olympic marathon was won by Ethiopian Abebe Bikila in an Olympic-record and world-record time of 2:15:16.2, which was 8 minutes faster than the previous Olympic record established by Emil Zátopek in the 1952 Helsinki Olympic Games. Just as Zátopek had not drunk during his record-setting performance, neither did Bikila: "The little moustachioed, brown-skinned man is running so lightly that his feet scarcely seem to touch the ground. Most of his competitors have taken some refreshment meanwhile at a snack-bar beside the course which purveys blueberry juice, glucose and similar fortifiers. But Abebe refuses any nourishment. He is used to running, thirsty or not" (Judah, 2008, p. 81).

The next study was performed in England by their most eminent exercise physiologist of the 20th century, Griffiths Pugh. Pugh's status was the result of his work in high-altitude physiology, which was crucial to the success of the 1953 British Everest expedition. Pugh also completed landmark studies of body temperature regulation in English Channel swimmers and the performance of athletes adapting to training at altitude before the 1968 Olympic Games in Mexico City. The study was inspired by Fox's contention that environmental conditions could limit performance during marathon running. The authors believed that neither sweat rates nor

5 This theory is correct only if the circulation determines performance during prolonged exercise. In fact, the circulation is merely a passenger, albeit a rather important one. Instead, exercise performance is regulated by a complex brain control that integrates information from all of the body's organ systems to ensure that all continue to function within their safe functional limits (homeostasis). In this way, the body is protected and does not "fail" catastrophically. The evidence appears to be that the "loss of a large volume of fluid" can be quite well tolerated by some (but probably not all) athletes provided that fluid loss does not threaten their internal homeostasis. It appears that some world-class athletes can achieve exceptional performances even when they lose 7% to 10% of their body weight during competition.

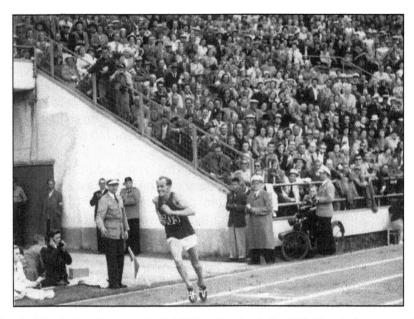

Emil Zátopek of Czechoslovakia enters the Helsinki stadium to win the 1952 Olympic Games marathon in a new Olympic record of 2:23:3. Like Abebe Bikila, winner of the 1960 and 1964 Olympic marathons, both in record times, Zátopek did not drink anything during this race.
AP Photo

body temperatures had previously been measured in marathon runners—clearly they were unaware of the work of Blake and Larabee (1903) and Buskirk and Beetham (1960). So on June 10, 1966, the year in which I completed my high school education, Pugh and his team traveled to a marathon staged by the Witney Road Runners' Club at Witney, near Oxford, England.

For their study, Pugh, Corbett, and colleagues (1967) weighed 75 of the 77 competitors in the race, which was run in temperatures of 22.0 to 23.5 °C (71.6 to 74.3 °F) with a relative humidity of 52% to 58%. In addition, rectal temperatures were measured at the finish line. The method for this measurement was the following: "Competitors were handed rectal thermometers and they retired to a nearby lavatory to insert them. They were asked to insert them to a depth of 8 cm, keep them in place for 5 min, and bring them to the observers to read" (p. 347). Only 47 runners complied with this request.

The 56 runners who completed the race lost an average of 2.85 kg (6.3 lb, 5.2% of starting body weight) during the race with a range of 1.0 to 5.2 kg (figure 3.8a). Average sweat rate during the race was 960 ml/hr (32.5 fl oz/hr), whereas the average rate of fluid intake was 420 ml/hr (14.2 fl oz/hr), again confirming that competitive athletes choose not to drink as much as they sweat when racing.

As in the study of Wyndham and Strydom (figure 3.1, page 61), the winner finished the race with the greatest weight loss and the highest postrace rectal temperature. The mean postrace rectal temperature was 39.0 °C (102.2 °F) ranging from 36.7 to 41.1 °C (figure 3.8b). Seven runners, including three of the first four finishers, had rectal temperatures in excess of 40.0 °C (104 °F); the highest rectal temperature (41.1 °C, 105.98 °F) was measured in the winner. The race

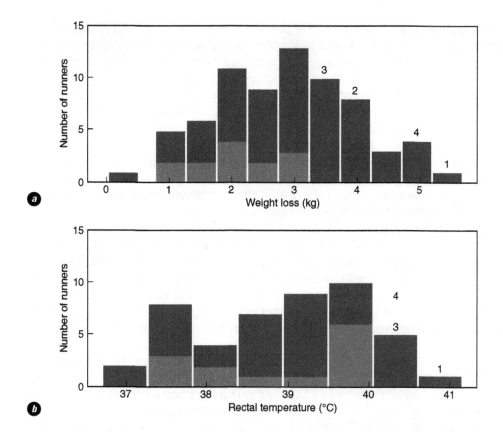

FIGURE 3.8 (a) Marathon runners lost 1.0 to 5.2 kg during a race run in cool conditions in England. The runners who finished in the top positions in the race (numbers 1 to 4) tended to lose the most weight; the winner lost in excess of 5 kg. (b) The postrace rectal temperatures of these runners ranged from 36.7 to 41.1 °C; the top finishers recorded the highest temperatures. The light gray indicates data for nonfinishers. Data from Pugh, Corbett, et al. (1967).

Adapted, by permission, from L.G. Pugh, J.L. Corbett, and R.H. Johnson, 1967, "Rectal temperatures, weight losses, and sweat rates in marathon running," *Journal of Applied Physiology* 23(3): 347-352.

winner also lost the most weight (5.2 kg, equivalent to 6.9% of his body weight) as a result of his very high sweat rate (1.81 L/hr). Indeed, the first four finishers in that race achieved the highest levels of weight loss and the highest postrace rectal temperatures. Interestingly, Wyndham and Strydom had failed to notice the same phenomenon: The person who won the two 32 km races they studied also lost the most weight and had the highest postrace rectal temperatures (arrowed in figure 3.1, page 61).

The authors also reported that four athletes collapsed 30 to 60 minutes after the race with symptoms of faintness, "blacking out," weakness, and nausea with or without vomiting. When they were lying flat, the blood pressures of these athletes were normal. The authors concluded that no cause for collapse could be found in these athletes but that "fluid loss and *muscle vasodilation* [my emphasis] following prolonged exercise are likely factors" (p. 351).[6]

> **6** These athletes were clearly suffering from **EAPH**, the condition that caused such distress to the unacclimatized U.S. soldiers on first exposure to jungle heat in World War II (see chapter 2, page 50).

The authors concluded this: "The present evidence implies that tolerance of a high body temperature is a necessary condition of success in marathon running. . . . Another condition of success seems to be a high tolerance to fluid loss. The winners' weight loss was 5.33 kg corresponding to a fluid loss of 5.1 kg, or 6.7% of his body weight. Dehydration of this degree, especially if rapid, reduces endurance and is a cause of collapse in non athletes. . . . The sweat rate of the winner (1.8L/hr) was compatible with the highest figures reported for heat-acclimatised men exercising under heat stress over similar periods of time" (p. 350).

They also considered the role of solar heat gain by radiation in athletes running in direct sunlight proposing that "when the solar heat load has been avoided by running a marathon before sunrise or after sundown, good times have been recorded in surprisingly severe thermal conditions" (p. 351).

Pugh and his colleagues clearly did not consider it particularly dangerous for marathon runners to drink only 420 ml/hr (14.2 fl oz/hr) during a marathon in which some sweated at up to 1.8 L/hr (60.9 fl oz/hr) and lost up to 6% of their starting body weights, finishing with rectal temperatures as high as 41.1 °C (105.98 °F). Pugh and his colleagues also speculated that a rectal temperature of 41.1 °C might be considered "critical" and higher values might be dangerous. But since they did not measure higher temperatures in ill runners, their conclusion was speculative.

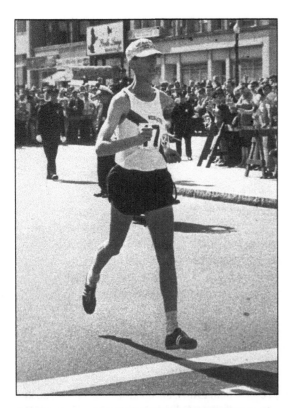

Amby Burfoot crosses the finish line to win the 1968 Boston Marathon in 2:22:17. Burfoot did not drink during the race, losing 4.1 kg, equivalent to 6.5% of his starting body weight.
AP Photo

Thus by 1967 four studies of fluid ingestion and rectal temperatures in marathon runners had all come to essentially the same conclusions:

- Marathon runners drank little, lost a great deal of weight, and finished with high rectal temperatures.
- The fastest runners were always the hottest and the most dehydrated.
- There was no evidence that drinking relatively little and losing up to 6% of body weight during marathon racing was undesirable, dangerous, or impaired running performance.

Body Weight Loss and Body Temperature: 1968 to the 1980s

Ambrose Burfoot, a student from Wesleyan University in Connecticut, won the 1968 Boston Marathon. Running on a hot afternoon, he completed the race in 2:22:17 while losing 4.1 kg (9 lb; 6.5% of starting body weight). Burfoot recalls that, as was the custom of the day, he did not drink anything during that race (see Foreword). In December of that year, Burfoot ran nearly 8 minutes faster in the Fukuoka (Japan) Marathon, again without drinking, missing the U.S. record by 1 second. Burfoot recalls that the Boston race took place on a sunny, warm day, whereas it was much cooler in the Japanese race. Thus, without changing his drinking behavior, Burfoot was able to improve his time by nearly 8 minutes simply by running in a cooler race.

In his professional career, Burfoot would become one of the iconic writers on running and the executive editor of *Runner's World* magazine. He would also be a subject in the first Gatorade-funded study of the effects of fluid ingestion on the rectal temperature response during prolonged exercise in the heat (Costill, Kammer, et al., 1970) (chapter 6). Nearly 40 years after his Boston triumph and the publication of that study in which he was an important participant, Burfoot would begin to question whether the advice that marathon runners should drink "as much as tolerable" was appropriate or whether his choice not to drink in the 1968 Boston Marathon was better.[7]

The year 1968 was one of the most remarkable in the history of the world; *Time* magazine described it thus: "Nineteen sixty eight was a knife blade that severed past from future" (Morrow, 1988; Morrow, 1989, p. 7). The Olympic Games that year mirrored the changes that were overtaking society (Hoffer, 2009).

In the exercise sciences, 1968 would also herald the beginning of the modern applied exercise sciences in which research would increasingly focus on ways to help athletes perform better. In the United States, there was no better example of this modern approach than that adopted by David Costill, PhD, professor emeritus of exercise science at Ball State University in Muncie, Indiana.

Early in his career, Costill became interested in the factors determining success in marathon running. He soon concluded this: "Probably no other single factor poses a greater threat to the marathoner's health than does hyperthermia . . . [so that] any factor that tends to overload the cardiovascular system or reduce sweat evaporation will drastically impair the marathoner's performance and risk overheating" (Costill, 1972, 1027).[8] Of course this is an interesting opinion given that four separate studies of

7 In a 2009 *Runner's World* article, Amby Burfoot concluded that "a modest dehydration is a normal and temporary condition for many marathoners and doesn't lead to any serious medical conditions. Excessive fluid consumption, on the other hand, can prove deadly" (Burfoot, 2009, p. 5). His final piece of advice was such: "6. Drink when you're thirsty. While it's true that your thirst doesn't kick in until you're 1 to 2 percent dehydrated, there's nothing terribly wrong with that. Remember. Your body has an 'exquisitely tuned' water balance mechanism. Use it" (p. 10). Perfect advice from a perfect gentleman.

8 This indicates that Dr. Costill believed in the "catastrophe" model of human exercise physiology (Noakes, St. Clair Gibson, et al., 2005), in which the exercising human continues without control or anticipation of future danger until the body suddenly collapses, catastrophically in this case, with the development of heatstroke. This is a "brainless" model of human physiology since it presumes that the brain will continue to drive the skeletal muscles to the point at which all the heat the muscles produce in pursuit of an exceptional athletic performance is allowed to overwhelm the body's cooling mechanisms, causing death from heatstroke. Hunters with this biological design would never have survived their hunts in extreme heat (chapter 1) and would have disappeared down an evolutionary dead end as indeed occurred to certain of the early hominins including *Australopithecus africanus, Paranthropus robustus, Homo habilis,* and the Neanderthals.

In fact, the brain modifies the exercise behavior "in anticipation" by causing the athlete to exercise more slowly in hot environmental conditions (see note 4 of chapter 6, page 191). This slows the rate of heat production ensuring that serious damage or death does not usually occur, except according to my theory in those with a predisposition, either genetic or transient.

9 This race was run at 24 °C (75.2 °F) with relative humidity of 54% (Costill, 1972), conditions that were typical for marathon races at that time. For example, the 1954 Commonwealth and Empire Games Marathon began at 12:00 noon in mid-August heat (~28 °C, windless with no cloud cover) in Vancouver, Canada, on 7 August, 1954. In that race, the world-record holder, Jim Peters, collapsed ~300 m from the finish and never again ran a competitive race. Although it has been presumed that Peters collapsed because he had developed heatstroke, the evidence to support this diagnosis is not absolutely convincing (Noakes, Mekler, et al., 2008).

The 1964 Yonkers (New York) Marathon was designated as one of two qualifying races to select runners for the 1964 Olympic Games Marathon. That race occurred in midday heat of 33 °C (91.4°F) with humidity and cloudless skies. The winner was Buddy Edelen, who, while living in England, had trained in a tracksuit in the cool specifically so that he would be adapted for racing in the heat. Both Olympic Marathons were won by Ethiopian runners, Abebe Bikila in 1964 and Mamo Walde in 1968. Neither race was run in particularly hot conditions.

marathon runners had each come to the opposite conclusion.

In one of his first field studies, Costill (1972) studied water losses and sweat rates of runners in the 1968 U.S. Olympic Marathon trials.[9] He measured weight losses of 6.1 kg and sweat rates of 1.09 L/m²/hr and noted that "few runners are able to drink more than 300 ml of water" in competitive races. He concluded that "marathoners are physically incapable of consuming sufficient amounts of fluids to keep pace with sweat losses" (p. 1028). As a result, "successful marathon performance is often dictated by one's ability to dissipate excess body heat and to tolerate large body fluid losses" (p. 1029). He did not consider that those are exactly the characteristics that allowed early humans to survive on the dry, hot African savannah. Yet Costill was such an influential scientist that his opinion that overheating was the greatest threat to marathoners would most likely be adopted without question by those who had not read the literature available at that time or who did not yet understand the impact of our biological past.

The next important study was performed at the 1970 Commonwealth Games Marathon, held in Edinburgh, Scotland, on 23 July, 1970. The race took place in mild environmental conditions; the temperature rose from 13.7 to 16.0 °C (56.7 to 60.8 °F) during the race, and humidity was low. The race winner, Ron Hill, a doctor of chemistry, passed the halfway mark in 1:02:35.2, winning in 2:09:28, a new British and Commonwealth Games record, perhaps also the fastest time ever on a circular course that had been correctly measured.

Even though there were five drinking stations on the course, Hill chose not to drink any fluid during the race. As a result, he lost 2.3 kg (5.1 lb) during the race (3.9% of his starting weight of 59.4 kg, corresponding to a sweat rate of 1.06 L/hr). Of 18 out of the 20 runners in the race from whom data were collected, the majority (10) did not drink anything during the race (Muir, Percy-Robb, et al., 1970); three drank 100 ml, two 200 ml, one 600 ml, and two 800 ml. The average weight loss was 3.1 kg (6.8 lb, 5.1% of the average starting body weight of 61.8 kg). The greatest weight loss was 6.4 kg (14.1 lb, 11.7%) in a Kenyan runner who completed the race in 2:22:40 and who drank 800 ml/hr (27 fl oz/hr). If these data are correct, that runner achieved an estimated sweat rate of 2.77 L/hr (93.7 fl oz/hr), one of the highest ever recorded.

The authors were surprised that these runners could undergo such large weight losses. They noted that Jim Alder, who had lost 3.6 kg (5.6% BW) when he won the previous Commonwealth Games Marathon in much hotter conditions in Jamaica (27.2 to 30.0 °C [86 °F] with 75% RH), had finished in second place in 2:12:04, while drinking 100 ml and losing 3.2 kg (5.0%). Thus Alder's weight loss was similar in the hot and cool marathons; the difference was that he ran considerably faster (10 min) in the cooler race but lost a similar amount of weight. Perhaps Alder's performances were regulated to ensure that he could run only fast enough to always incur a ~3% level of dehydration, regardless of the environmental conditions.

The third and fourth runners at Edinburgh, Englishman Donald Fairclouth and New Zealander John Foster, also did not drink during the race, losing 2.3 kg (4.0%) and 3.2 kg (5.1%) while finishing in 2:12:19 and 2:14:14, respectively. The authors were clearly surprised by these findings: "This degree of dehydration, which must have been greatly exceeded by some of the Edinburgh competitors, might be expected to give rise to symptoms and also signs of physiological inefficiency. That it does not do so is indicated by the fact that in Edinburgh few runners took trouble to correct it by drinking during the race. Perhaps their arduous training protects them in some way against the adverse effects of dehydration" (p. 1126). These conclusions were not different from those of Buskirk and Beetham (1960) and Pugh, Corbett, and colleagues (1967).

There followed a series of other studies in which levels of dehydration and rectal temperatures in 32 to 42 km distance runners were studied in smaller groups of subjects (Adams, Fox, et al., 1975; Magazanik, Shapiro, et al., 1974; Maron, Horvath, et al., 1975; Maron, Wagner, et al., 1977; Maughan, 1985; Maughan, Leiper, et al., 1985; Myhre, Hartung, et al., 1982; Myhre, Hartung, et al., 1985; Owen, Kregel, et al., 1986; Wells, Schrader, et al., 1985). Despite the athletes in these studies having varying levels of dehydration, in none of the studies was the postrace rectal temperatures dangerously elevated nor did heat stroke develop. The highest postrace rectal temperature was 41.7 °C (107.06 °F) in an asymptomatic athlete.

A particularly interesting study was the first in which the rectal temperature was measured continuously during a competitive marathon race, the Polytechnic Marathon between Windsor Castle and Chiswick, London, and during two laboratory treadmill runs of ~165 minutes (figure 3.9) (Adams, Fox, et al., 1975), rather than only after a run.

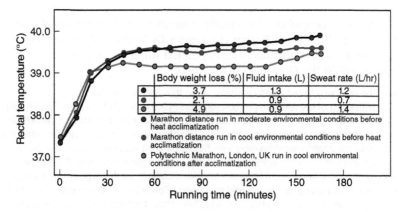

FIGURE 3.9 The first study to measure the rectal temperature response during as opposed to only after a marathon (Polytechnic Marathon, London, UK; Adams, Fox, et al., 1975).

Adapted, by permission, from W.C. Adams, R.H. Fox, A.J. Fry, and I.C. MacDonald, 1975, "Thermoregulation during marathon running in cool, moderate, and hot environments," *Journal of Applied Physiology* 38(6): 1030-1037.

The novel finding was that the rectal temperature rose progressively for the first 30 to 45 minutes and then only slightly thereafter in three runs of 165 minutes, despite the development of a progressive dehydration. The temperature was slightly higher in hotter conditions and was reduced by a period of heat acclimatization. The greatest level of dehydration (4.9%) was reached in the Polytechnic Marathon, which produced the lowest postexercise rectal temperature. Dr. Adams, himself the subject, drank sparingly during all these events, ~350 ml/hr as was the practice of the day. There was no obvious relationship between dehydration and rectal temperature response during those runs.

Dr. Michael Maron reported similar data in a competitive marathon race. Like Dr. Adams, Dr. Maron had to be the subject for his studies. More than 40 years later, Dr. Maron described how he conducted the study on himself (box 3.2) as he ran the Santa Barbara Marathon in California in 1975 (Maron, Wagner, et al., 1977). While the response in Dr. Maron's friend (figure 3.10) was similar to that recorded in Dr. Adams, Dr. Maron's response was quite different in that he reached a much higher temperature (41.8 °C, 107.2 °F), which he sustained for the final 40 minutes of the race without apparent negative consequence, other than the anxiety he caused his colleagues who were measuring his temperature during the race.

Perhaps inspired by Dr. Maron's personal heroics, in 1980, Carol Christensen and R.O. Ruhling reported measuring the rectal temperature of a 38-year-old female runner, Christensen herself, when she completed the Salt Lake City (Pioneer Day) Marathon in 03:55. Her rectal temperature rose from 37.5 °C at the start of the race to 38.9 °C after 20 minutes of running. Her temperature remained between 38.9 and 39.1 °C for most of the race except for a 20-minute period between 60 and 80 minutes as she ran up a 4 km hill, when her rectal temperature rose to 40.0 °C. Forty-five minutes after the race, her rectal temperature returned to 37.5 °C. The authors concluded this: "There was no evidence of either heat stress or decrement

---

BOX 3.2   Maron's Temperature Approaches 42 °C

Forty years after the completion of the study in which he evaluated his rectal temperature response during the 1975 Santa Barbara Marathon, Dr. Michael Maron recalled the details of that experiment and in particular what happened when his core temperature began to approach 42 °C (107.6 °F). He wrote the following:

> I figured the only way to get another runner to do this was to volunteer myself. . . . In our study, a car met up with each of the runners periodically during the race, and the investigators plugged our probes into a Yellow Springs thermometer device to record our temperatures. Unbeknownst to me, at the time my temperature started to climb, Jim Wagner (a wonderful environmental physiologist who completed his postdoctoral training with Sid Robinson) was having serious discussions with the other members of the team about whether they should get me to stop. If it had been a laboratory situation, the guidelines of the time would have dictated that the experiment be stopped. They ultimately decided it was not in the lab and that I was allowing them to peek at an event that would be happening regardless of their presence and that I didn't look too bad for someone who had run 20 miles. They made the correct decision; I would not have stopped. Being good experimentalists, they also never told me that I was hot until after finishing.

Personal communication between Professor Michael Maron and Dr. Chris Byrne, 2007. Reproduced with permission.

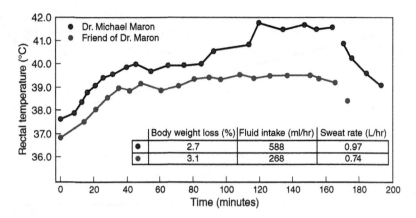

FIGURE 3.10 Two runners show different rectal temperature responses during the 1975 Santa Barbara Marathon.

Adapted, by permission, from M.B. Maron, J.A. Wagner, S.M. Horvath, 1977, "Thermoregulatory responses during competitive marathon running," *Journal of Applied Physiology* 42(6): 909-914.

in performance associated with the high rectal temperature in our woman runner. Although the evidence is scant, it appears that high body temperatures can be maintained by woman marathon runners for considerable lengths of time with no apparent adverse effects" (p. 132). Forty years later, Dr. Christensen recalls that she placed the probe herself and that her temperature was recorded by two graduate students who rode a motor bike and who "periodically came alongside me to take readings—I would slow my pace while they took the reading, but I don't remember having to stop" (personal communication, March 2010).

The study of Dr. Ron Maughan and colleagues (1985) showed that the sweat rate in runners in a cool (12 °C, 53.6 °F) marathon was related to finishing time (figure 3.11a, page 82), whereas the rectal temperature (figure 3.11b) was related to the time to run the second half of the race. Both these findings can be best explained if both sweat rate and rectal temperature are determined by the athlete's metabolic rate as originally taught (Nielsen, 1938) and as argued in box 3.1 (figure 3.3, page 62). The authors noted that none of their subjects had postrace rectal temperatures above 40 °C, and temperatures were below 38 °C in 18 of 59 runners. Their subsequent study (Maughan, Leiper, et al., 1985) showed that the postrace rectal temperature was related to the time required to cover the final 10 km of the race. Runners who slowed down during the final 10 km in this race in cool conditions (exact temperatures not given) became at risk of hypothermia (reduced body temperature), the precise opposite of the dangers proposed by Wyndham and Strydom. One runner who failed to finish was treated in the medical facility for hypothermia (rectal temperature of 33.4 °C). The authors warned that "hypothermia rather than hyperthermia is likely to be a problem among marathon runners competing in races held on days when the wind chill factor is equivalent to an air temperature of less than 12 °C (53.6 °F) and a head wind (speed) greater than 3 m/s (10.8 km/hr)" (pp.193-194).

The final relevant study from this era (Davies and Thompson, 1986) was completed at the Queen's Medical Centre in Nottingham, UK, and published in 1986. For that study, the authors convinced 10 ultramarathon runners who regularly

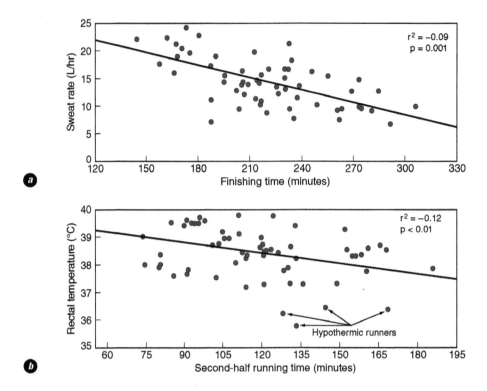

FIGURE 3.11 *(a)* There was a linear relationship with a negative slope between the sweat rate and race finishing time of runners in the 1982 Aberdeen Marathon, whereas *(b)* the postrace rectal temperature was related to the time taken to finish the final 21 km of the race (Maughan, 1985). Four runners finished with rectal temperatures below normal (arrowed).

Reprinted, by permission, from R.J. Maughan, 1985, "Thermoregulation in marathon competition at low ambient temperature," *International Journal of Sports Medicine* 6: 15-19.

trained between 100 and 200 km/week (62 and 124 miles/week) to run for 4 hours on an indoor treadmill while exercising at between 65% and 70% of their maximal capacity. During exercise their metabolic rate, sweat rate, cardiac output, and rectal temperature were measured frequently. Subjects lost an average of 5.5% of their body weight during the 4 hours, losing an average of 3.5 kg (7.7 lb). Their total fluid intake varied from 0 to 1.49 L with an average of only 864 ml (29.2 fl oz), equivalent to 216 ml/hr. Despite these quite high levels of dehydration, the rectal temperature reached an average of only 39.1 °C after 4 hours. There was also no evidence for "cardiovascular strain" since the heart output stayed constant during the exercise. Nor was there any relationship between the amount of fluid ingested and the final rectal temperature. Rather, the rectal temperature was determined by the metabolic rate during exercise as predicted by physiological model 2 (figure 3.3, page 62). The researchers also noted that the "athletes tolerated sweat losses equivalent to ~5.5% body weight without apparent discomfort. Despite this level of dehydration, the athletes ingested very little water (which was freely available) during the exercise" (p. 616).

The authors concluded that despite the low rates of fluid intake during 4 hours leading to quite a high level of dehydration, there was "no evidence of a spiraling increase in the rectal temperature and loss of thermal control during the latter part of exercise" (p. 616). Instead, during the 4 hours of exercise, "the rectal temperature remains within the normal physiological range for exercise and at no point exceeds 39.3 °C" (p. 616).

The authors also noted that the circulating blood (plasma) volume was maintained during exercise despite significant weight loss. This finding has been noted before. Thus "the vascular compartment resisted volume depletion" (Saltin, 1964).[10] This has also been noted by others (Adams, Fox, et al., 1975; Maron, Horvath, et al., 1975; Myhre, Hartung, et al., 1985). This would occur if the loss of sodium in sweat was buffered by movement of sodium from an internal store into the extracellular space.

In summary, the findings of these original studies were remarkably similar and did not provide any evidence to suggest that dehydration was particularly dangerous or that marathon runners were especially likely to develop heatstroke during exercise.

The other famous study of this series is that of Wyndham and Strydom (1969) reviewed earlier in this chapter. Of all these studies, it is the one that would be the most remembered, even though it produced a conclusion that was the converse of all the other related studies reviewed here. That it drew conclusions that (a) are the complete opposite of all the other studies then published and (b) do not fit with our evolutionary biological design has not detracted from its global scientific acceptance and promotion, especially as a cornerstone for the ACSM's drinking guidelines over the past three decades. As covered in chapter 5, heatstroke occurs with extreme rarity in marathon runners—in fact, there are only four such cases that I could trace in the entire scientific literature—but is much more common in athletes involved in short-duration exercise of higher intensity. And as we have learned here, elite marathon runners have produced world-class performances without drinking and without suffering any adverse consequences.

10 This information that the plasma (blood) volume is relatively protected when athletes become dehydrated during exercise would later be forgotten because it conflicted with the theory of human thermoregulatory function during exercise that was developed after Dr. Cade developed Gatorade in 1965. This new model requires that dehydration causes a dramatic reduction in the volume of blood in the center of the body (the central blood volume) that provides the pressure to the blood filling the heart. A reduced pressure driving the blood filling the heart leads to "cardiovascular strain," which prevents an adequate blood flow to the skin, causing heat retention and a rising body temperature. Unless adequate volumes of fluid, especially sports drinks, are ingested during exercise, this heat retention will progress until the athlete collapses from heatstroke. But this model ignores the findings of Costill, Kammer, et al. 1970, reviewed in chapter 6, and the fact that the brain insures that homeostasis is regulated during exercise by modifying both the rate at which heat is produced by the body (by regulating the number of muscle fibers that are recruited in the exercising limbs) and the rate at which heat is lost from the body into the environment (by regulating the rate of sweating).

Testing the Wyndham and Strydom Hypothesis

By 1987, I had clearly decided that it was time to test the Wyndham and Strydom theory that the level of dehydration determines the body temperature response in marathon running. Our research team set out to test the contrasting hypothesis clearly evident in the data of Maughan and his colleagues from Aberdeen that the rate of energy use (metabolic rate) determines both the sweat rate (and thus strongly influences the level of dehydration that develops during exercise) and

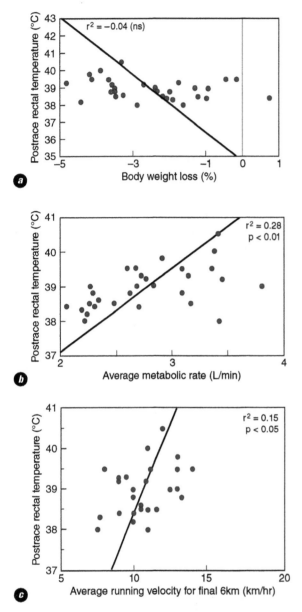

FIGURE 3.12 Our study (Noakes, Myburgh, et al., 1991) of runners in the 1987 Peninsula Marathon showed that there was *(a)* no significant relationship between the postrace rectal temperature and the percentage of weight loss (level of dehydration) during the race. Instead, the postrace rectal temperature was related to measures of rates of heat production (metabolic rate) during the race, including *(b)* the average metabolic rate and *(c)* the running velocity for the final 6 km of the race. Note that differences in the average metabolic rate explained 28% and the average running velocity 15% of the variation in the postrace rectal temperatures in these runners.

Adapted, by permission, from T.D. Noakes, K.H. Myburgh, P.J. du Plessis, et al., 1991, "Metabolic rate, not percent dehydration, predicts rectal temperature in marathon runners," *Medicine & Science in Sports & Exercise* 23(4): 443-449.

the postrace rectal temperature in marathon runners.

Accordingly, we weighed 30 runners before and after the 1987 Peninsula 42 km (26 mile) Marathon in Cape Town and also measured their rectal temperatures within minutes of their completing the race (Noakes, Myburgh, et al., 1991). We also recorded their running speeds over various sections of the course. Then beginning a week after the race, the athletes came to our laboratory where we measured their rates of energy use (metabolic rate) at the range of speeds each had achieved in the race. This allowed us to predict their average metabolic rates during the full 42 km distance, during the first and second halves, and also during the final 6 km of the race.

The results of the study showed that the runners lost an average of 2 kg (4.4 lb; range: –3.3 to +0.6kg) during the race, their average post-race rectal temperature was 38.9 °C (range 38.0 to 40.5 °C), and their average rate of fluid intake during the race was what they had been advised before the race—600 ml/hr (20.3 fl oz/hr; range 0.4 to 0.7 L/hr). Their average estimated sweat rate was 1.0 L/hr (33.8 fl oz/hr; range: 0.5 to 1.7 L/hr). These data were essentially identical to those reported in other published studies of marathon runners.

We found no relationship between the level of dehydration and the postrace rectal temperature (figure 3.12*a*), whereas there was a significant relationship between the postrace rectal temperature and the average metabolic rate (figure 3.12*b*) and running velocity (figure 3.12*c*) for the final 6 km.

There was also a significant relationship between sweat rate and both the average metabolic rate for the entire race (figure 3.13*a*) and for the final 6 km of the race (figure 3.13*b*). The average metabolic rate during the race could explain 17%, and the average metabolic rate during the final 6 km 15% of the variation in the average sweat rates of these runners during the race. Average metabolic rate during the race was also significantly related to the product of the average running velocity during the race and the starting body weight (figure 3.14, page 86). Average running velocity could explain 15%, and the body mass 27%, of the variation in the average metabolic rates in these runners.

This indicates that average running velocity and body mass can be used as a proxy for metabolic rate and hence the rate of heat production during marathon races. This finding also supports the general prediction that the athletes who run the fastest will have the highest metabolic rates during marathon running and, as a result, the highest sweat rates and postrace rectal temperatures. If they do not drink more than other athletes, they will also finish with the greatest levels of weight loss and hence the highest levels of dehydration. As a result, it will appear as if dehydration could explain these findings according to the logic shown in figure 3.2

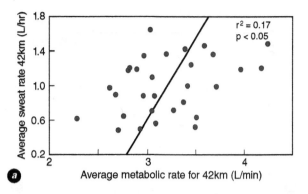

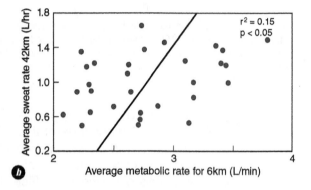

FIGURE 3.13 A linear relationship with a positive slope was present between the sweat rate and the average metabolic rate for *(a)* the entire race and *(b)* for the final 6 km, indicating that the sweat rate during the race was related to measures of the rate of heat production (metabolic rate) as predicted by physiological model 2 presented in figure 3.3 (1987 Peninsula Marathon, Cape Town, South Africa).

Adapted, by permission, from T.D. Noakes, K.H. Myburgh, P.J. du Plessis, et al., 1991, "Metabolic rate, not percent dehydration, predicts rectal temperature in marathon runners," *Medicine & Science in Sports & Exercise* 23(4): 443-449.

(page 62), whereas the dependence of both sweat rate and rectal temperature on the metabolic rate (figure 3.3, page 62) provides a more convincing explanation. According to this interpretation, the apparent relationship between postrace rectal temperature and level of dehydration reported by Wyndham and Strydom (figure 3.1, page 61) might be better explained by the faster running speed of those who became the most dehydrated and who also developed the highest postrace rectal temperatures (because they were running the fastest). In this way, the relationship between the level of dehydration and the postrace rectal temperature is spurious since both are dependent on the metabolic rate (figure 3.3).

Accordingly, we concluded that the level of dehydration in the runners in this 42 km standard marathon was unrelated to the postrace rectal temperature and that this finding was similar to the majority of other studies of marathon runners. Hence, the level of dehydration cannot be the most important factor determining the rectal temperature during marathon running. As a result, dehydration cannot be a factor determining whether or not heatstroke will develop in marathon runners.

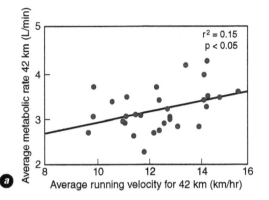
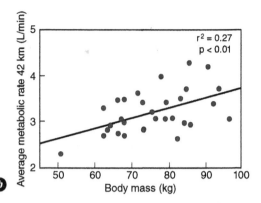

FIGURE 3.14 Average metabolic rate during the 42 km race was related to the athlete's *(a)* average running velocity and *(b)* the athlete's body mass (1987 Peninsula Marathon, Cape Town, South Africa).

Adapted, by permission, from T.D. Noakes, K.H. Myburgh, P.J. du Plessis, et al., 1991, "Metabolic rate, not percent dehydration, predicts rectal temperature in marathon runners," *Medicine & Science in Sports & Exercise* 23(4): 443-449.

We acknowledged that although dehydration does affect the body temperature during exercise, the magnitude of this effect might be smaller than other influences. At the time I did not yet appreciate that this elevation might in any case be regulated as part of our biological design to ensure that exercise continues safely (while heat is lost in the most efficient ways) without the risk of a catastrophic failure such as the development of heatstroke.[11]

We speculated that the effect of dehydration on rectal temperature may be relatively small such that it may not be quantifiable in cross-sectional studies. We wrote, "Thus the argument is not that dehydration does not influence the rectal temperature response during exercise. Rather, it is that other factors may be the more important determinants of that response" (Noakes, Myburgh, et al., 1991, p. 447).

Obviously we wanted to argue that the rate of energy use (metabolic rate or equally the rate of heat production) was likely to be that factor since there was

11 Shortly after the beginning of exercise, it is as if the athlete's brain calculates the "hotness" of the environment and, on the basis of that calculation, chooses an exercise intensity that is appropriate for the duration of exercise that the brain has also already decided it wishes to perform. We do not yet know exactly how the brain makes this calculation since it would require the measurement of all the variables that contribute to the environmental heat load, including air temperature, humidity, radiant heat load, and wind speed. Probably the brain monitors continuously the rate at which the body is storing heat. It then adjusts the exercise intensity that it will allow to ensure that, regardless of the environmental conditions, the rate of heat gain will not cause the rectal temperature to rise above the critical value of about 42 °C before the planned exercise bout terminates. As a result, when it is hot and humid and therefore more difficult for the body to lose heat to the environment, humans will naturally choose to exercise at a lower intensity than when it is cooler (Marino, 2004) but will likely end with final rectal temperatures that may be identical regardless of the environmental conditions (Tucker, Rauch, et al., 2004).

In this way, the brain ensures that the rate at which the body accumulates heat will not produce a rectal temperature in excess of 42 °C before the intended exercise bout is due to end.

already a large body of published evidence showing that the metabolic rate is the principal determinant of the rectal temperature during exercise. Indeed Wyndham and his colleagues (Wyndham, Strydom, et al., 1970) had themselves provided clear evidence for this relationship (figure 3.15). They overlooked the existence of this relationship when they compiled their paper.

Since we had found a significant relationship between both the metabolic rate and the running velocity during the final 6 km of the race, we concluded: "These data would seem to confirm that it is only the running velocity or metabolic rate during the preceding 30 to 100 min which determines the post-exercise rectal temperature" (pp. 447-448).

We also found that the average sweat rate was also related to the average metabolic rate during the full 42 km race and suggested that Wyndham and Strydom's finding that dehydration predicted the postexercise rectal temperature might perhaps be explained "by the co-dependence of sweat rate (and therefore percent dehydration) and rectal temperature on metabolic rate in their particular study." This is the basis of the argument presented in box 3.1 (figure 3.3, page 62).

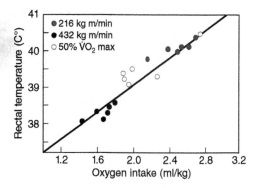

FIGURE 3.15 Research in Professor Wyndham's laboratory (Wyndham, Strydom, et al., 1970) clearly showed a very close relationship between the exercising metabolic rate, measured as the oxygen intake, and the rectal temperature during exercise. Note that the differently shaded dots in this figure relate to different work rates in different experiments.

Adapted, by permission, from C.H. Wyndham, N.B. Strydom, A.J. Van Rensburg, A.J.S. Benade, and A.J. Heyns, 1970, "Relation between VO₂max and body temperature in hot humid air conditions," *Journal of Applied Physiology* 29(1): 45-50.

The range of the rectal temperatures in our study (38.0 to 40.5 °C) was essentially identical to that in Wyndham and Strydom's study (38.3 to 40.9 °C) and indeed in the study of Pugh and colleagues (36.7 to 41.1 °C). But since our runners had been instructed to drink 600 ml/hr during the race, a rate that was considerably more than the average rates achieved by the runners in the studies of Pugh and colleagues (0.42 L/hr) and Wyndham and Strydom (~0.2 L/hr) and they finished the race somewhat less dehydrated (2.5%) than the runners in the two other studies (5.3% and ~4.0%), we were able to conclude that "dehydration alone was not the most important factor determining the rectal temperature in their runners" (p. 448).

We noted this: "This study again confirms that profound dehydration-induced hyperthermia is not a common feature of modern-day marathon races, at least in the recreational runners who comprise the vast majority of competitors. Rates of fluid intake (±0.6 L/hr) and sweat loss (±1.0 L/hr) were similar to those previously reported (Noakes, Adams, et al., 1988) and were lower than values which are usually quoted (American College of Sports Medicine, 1985). *This again confirms that high rates of fluid intake are not required for the prevention of significant dehydration in recreational marathon runners*" [my emphasis] (p. 448).

This later conclusion had little impact; 6 years after the publication of this paper, the ACSM produced their 1996 drinking guidelines, which stressed the need for runners to "consume the maximal amount that can be tolerated" (Convertino,

Armstrong, et al., 1996, p. i) to optimize their performances and to prevent the allegedly dangerous consequences of dehydration.

We concluded, "The most important practical point of this finding is that the risk of heat injury is greatest in those runners who maintain the highest metabolic rates during competition. Even the maintenance of optimum hydration may not negate that risk in that particular group of athletes" (Noakes, Myburgh, et al., 1991, p. 448).

In retrospect, it is surprising that the implications of this paper and the one describing the first cases of water intoxication (Noakes, Goodwin, et al., 1985), both published in the official scientific publication of the ACSM, *Medicine and Science in Sports and Exercise* (MSSE), were not evident when the ACSM released its drinking guidelines. In subsequent years, we found it increasingly difficult to have our papers on fluid balance and exercise published, especially in scientific publications originating in the United States. The anonymous reviewers of our submissions would repeatedly inform us that our papers were flawed since they did not conform to what everyone else knew to be "true." The possibility that this topic might be the victim of "abnormal science" was considered only by the editors of the *British Journal of Sports Medicine* and by Dr. Winne Meeuwisse, editor of the *Clinical Journal of Sports Medicine*, published in Canada.

Only after the publication of the study by Chris Byrne and colleagues (Byrne, Lee, et al., 2006), reviewed subsequently, and the revision of the ACSM guidelines in 2007 so that they essentially mirrored our 2003 guidelines (Noakes, 2003a), did this hardline resistance lessen somewhat, but not completely.[12]

By the end of 1991, our group had published the classic paper on water intoxication (Noakes, Goodwin, et al., 1985); a paper establishing the real rates at which athletes drink during competition (Noakes, Adams, et al., 1988); a paper showing that metabolic rate, not the level of dehydration, determines the rectal temperature response during exercise (Noakes, Myburgh, et al., 1991); and a fourth paper reviewed in chapter 9, confirming that EAH and EAHE are caused solely by overdrinking and to which the development of a sodium deficit plays no part (Irving, Noakes, Buck, et al., 1991).

When combined, these studies should have been sufficient for formulating safe drinking guidelines for competitive athletes as I finally did in 2003, using only this information (Noakes, 2003a). But a 16-year period of "abnormal science" lay ahead before that truth could emerge.

12 My letter (Noakes, 2007c) to that journal stressing the importance of the paper by Dr. Chris Byrne and his colleagues had to be modified at the editor's request before it was finally published. What I had written, the original title, "Study Findings Challenge Core Components of ACSM Drinking Guidelines," was not acceptable. But the title "Study Findings Challenge Core Components of a Current Model of Thermoregulation" was found to be more acceptable. The focus then became a criticism of the thermoregulatory model of exercise developed by the GSSI and in which the level of dehydration is considered the most important determinant of the body temperature during prolonged exercise. The editor of the journal at that time was Andrew Young, PhD, who is employed by the USARIEM, the same organization that employs Michael Sawka, Samuel Cheuvront, and Scott Montain, all of whom have provided much of the opinion that is used by the ACSM and the U.S. military in the formulation of their various position stands over the years.

Identification of the Dehydration Myth

On the basis of these studies, by the early 1990s I had concluded that a myth had developed in the exercise sciences, the dehydration myth, fostered mainly by the incorrect interpretation of the Wyndham and Strydom paper. In 1990, I wrote a paper titled "The Dehydration Myth and Carbohydrate Replacement During Prolonged Exercise" (Noakes, 1990) for a short-lived journal, *Cycling Science*, edited and published by my friend Chester Kyle, whose knowledge of cycling aerodynamics was legendary and who was responsible for revolutionary changes in bicycle designs in the 1980s (Kyle, 1984; Kyle, 1988). In the short history of the journal, readers selected this paper as the most interesting. Unfortunately, the paper's impact was restricted only to the readers of that journal.

The article began thus: "The belief is widespread that dehydration occurs inevitably in all athletes during prolonged exercise; that dehydration is the most important cause of impaired performance during prolonged exercise; and that dehydration is the essential ingredient causing collapse and heatstroke in endurance athletes, especially marathon runners and triathletes. As a result, both the scientific and lay literature is replete with articles stressing that the prevention of dehydration is the single most important factor influencing performance and risk of collapse during prolonged exercise" (p. 23).

I then reviewed the published evidence showing that (a) the sickest athletes at greatest risk of dying during and after prolonged endurance exercise are those who have drunk the most and so have developed EAHE and (b) that there is no evidence linking either postexercise collapse or heatstroke to dehydration. The focus of the article became carbohydrate ingestion, because evidence was beginning to accumulate that compared to the ingestion of water alone, the ingestion of carbohydrate delayed fatigue and improved performance during exercise lasting more than 2 hours, and especially during the last quarter of this type of prolonged exercise.

Five years later, I again addressed this question (Noakes, 1995). Because the article was intended for sport physicians who treat athletes at endurance events, the focus was more on whether or not dehydration is a proven cause of ill health in endurance athletes.

The article presented the evidence that athletes collapse after exercise not because they are dehydrated and hot (hyperthermic), but because they have exercise-associated postural hypotension (EAPH) in which their bodies are unable to regulate the blood pressure immediately on cessation of prolonged exercise, especially in the heat. Since we had discovered serendipitously that the best method for treating patients with EAPH was simply to lay them down with their feet and pelvis elevated above the level of the heart, we proposed that this form of treatment "has essentially removed the need for intravenous fluid therapy from the management of the vast majority of athletes who collapse *after* completing marathon and ultramarathon races" (Noakes, 1995, p. 126). We reiterated the suggestion that athletes who collapse *after* exercise should not simply be treated with intravenous fluids on the assumption that they are dehydrated. Rather, "like all patients, the collapsed athlete first deserves a rational diagnosis before initiation of the most appropriate therapy for the specific diagnosis (Noakes, 1988a).

There is no evidence that, if the diagnosis is not readily apparent, withholding therapy for a few minutes will have any detrimental consequences" (p. 127). Had this advice been understood and adopted some time in the following 7 years, some fatal cases of EAHE need never have occurred.

The article also included one other important statement related to what I believed should be included in drinking guidelines: ". . . athletes can safely be encouraged to maintain low levels of dehydration by drinking 'enough but not too much' during exercise. *But they should be warned that very high rates of fluid ingestion* (1.5 L/hr) sustained for many hours can lead to hyponatremia with a potentially fatal outcome" (Noakes, 1993, p. 127).

Studies of the Dehydration Myth at the South African Ironman Triathlons

When the inaugural 2000 and 2001 South African Ironman Triathlons were held in Cape Town, I was appointed the race medical director by my friend Gerhardt Mynhardt, who was the race organizer. As a consequence, we were able to test many of these ideas in the field. By this time I had learned from the example of my New Zealand colleague and collaborator, Dr. Dale Speedy, that it is possible to study fluid balance in large numbers (hundreds) of Ironman triathletes, provided one adopts the correct methods. This was a revelation to me, because in all our previous studies we had usually restricted ourselves to the studies of tens, not hundreds, of athletes.

Accordingly, at both the 2000 and 2001 South African Ironman races, we employed a large team of collaborators to measure the body weights and blood sodium concentrations of about 300 entrants before and after they had completed either race (Sharwood, Collins, et al., 2002; Sharwood, Collins, et al., 2004). In addition, in an attempt to identify the cause, we studied those who collapsed. We also measured postrace rectal temperatures in all those who would consent to the personal indignity. In 2000, 157 athletes consented, and in 2001, 337 consented.[13]

13 One of the reasons, in my view, why the dehydration myth has been sustained for so long is the natural reluctance of most researchers and clinicians to measure rectal temperatures in large numbers of collapsed and noncollapsed athletes after endurance events. As soon as it is shown that the range of rectal temperatures in the control group of noncollapsed athletes is exactly the same as it is in collapsed athletes, then it is clear that the cause of the collapse cannot be hyperthermia. If one believes that dehydration causes collapse by raising the body temperature to unsafe levels (according to the Wyndham and Strydom hypothesis), then one can only conclude that collapsed athletes cannot be significantly dehydrated since they are not abnormally hot.

From the 2000 race we learned that whereas the postrace blood sodium concentration was significantly but inversely related to percentage of body weight loss during the race (as found in all the previous studies) so that those who lost the most weight during the race had the highest postrace blood sodium concentrations (and those who gained weight had lower blood sodium concentrations), there was no relationship between the absolute body weight loss (in kg or L) during the race and either the postrace rectal temperature (figure 3.16a) or the total performance time in the race (figure 3.16b). This seemed to confirm the conclusion that the level of dehydration was unrelated to either the

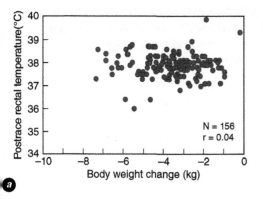
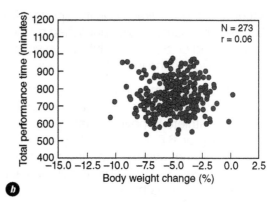

FIGURE 3.16 Studies at the 2000 South African Ironman Triathlon showed that there was no significant relationship between the degree of weight loss during this race and either *(a)* the postrace rectal temperature or *(b)* the overall performance time.

Reprinted, by permission, from K. Sharwood, M. Collins, J. Goedecke, G. Wilson, and T. Noakes, 2002, "Weight changes, sodium levels, and performance in the South African Ironman Triathlon," *Clinical Journal of Sport Medicine* 12(6): 391-399.

postrace rectal temperature or the performance time. When we analyzed the data from both the 2000 and 2001 races, it was clear that higher levels of weight loss were associated with superior performance, but again there was no relationship between weight loss and postrace body temperature.

In our study (Sharwood, Collins, et al., 2002), we could again confidently conclude the following: "There was no evidence that in this study, more severe levels of weight loss or dehydration were related to either higher body temperatures or impaired performance" (p. 391) so that "we conclude that a conservative drinking policy can be advocated for those Ironman Triathlons that are held in the moderate environmental conditions similar to those present in this race, without risking the health of the triathletes" (p. 398).

After the 2001 race, we decided to combine the results from both races for our next publication (Sharwood, Collins, et al., 2004). Since the findings from the combined data were even more conclusive, we chose to send our manuscript to *Medicine & Science in Sports & Exercise (MSSE)*, the official sports medicine and science journal of the Gatorade-funded ACSM. By this time, the ACSM had published its 1996 guidelines, which were firmly grounded on the dehydration myth.

We stated the hypothesis under study (Sharwood, Collins et al. 2004): "Our hypothesis was that there is no increased risk of medical complication associated with high levels of weight loss during an ultraendurance competitive event performed out of doors in a moderate environment. Thus the specific aim of the study was to answer the questions: Is a weight loss of 7% or more incapacitating, and are such high levels of weight loss associated with a higher prevalence of diagnosable medical conditions?" (p. 719).

This article was not accepted for publication in MSSE, perhaps because its findings were incompatible with the dehydration myth on which the 1996 ACSM drinking guidelines were based. Instead, the article was subsequently accepted by the *British Journal of Sports Medicine*, which is perhaps less at risk of a potential conflict of interest since it has only ever published one set of (industry-funded) drinking guidelines (Maughan, Goodburn, et al., 1993) and now has no financial dependence, either directly or indirectly, on the sports drink industry either in North America or in Europe. The journal is also published by the *British Medical Journal*, which takes a strong stand on conflicts of interest in scientific research and publication.

Following are the important findings of this study:

- Blood sodium concentrations were highest in the triathletes who lost the most weight. The only athlete requiring treatment for EAHE was also the only athlete to have gained a significant amount of weight during the race (3 kg, or 6.6 lb). He had ignored our prerace admonition that triathletes should not overdrink during the race. He had also outwitted our attempts to prevent EAHE by limiting fluid availability during the cycling and running legs of the triathlon.

- There was a very weak relationship between the percentage of body weight loss and the postrace rectal temperature. But it was in the wrong direction because the triathletes who lost the most weight had the lowest postrace rectal temperatures (figure 3.17), the opposite of the prediction of the Wyndham and Strydom theory.

- There was a significant relationship between the total performance time and the percentage of change in body weight so that the fastest finishers lost the most amount of weight during the race and vice versa (see figure 2.4a, page 55). Three years later we were able to confirm this relationship in finishers in the 2004 New Zealand Ironman Triathlon (see figure 2.4b on page 55).

These findings conflict with the popular theory that a weight loss of more than 2% during exercise will produce a 20% to 55% reduction in performance (Craig and Cummings, 1966) (figure 3.18, page 94). Were this correct, some of these triathletes could have finished this race in less than 6:45 if they had just drunk more. But this would have produced the world's fastest Ironman triathlon times by more than an hour. If only these athletes had known beforehand that just by drinking a little more they could have finished so much sooner and so would have established incredible new world records

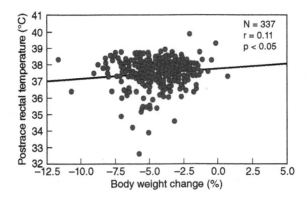

FIGURE 3.17 Our study of competitors in the 2000 and 2001 South African Ironman Triathlons found that if there was any relationship between body weight loss and the postrace rectal temperature, it was in the wrong direction so that those who lost the most weight had the lowest postrace rectal temperatures. This finding must be spurious.

Reproduced from *British Journal of Sports Medicine*, K.A. Sharwood, M. Collins, J.H. Goedecke, G. Wilson, and T. Noakes, 38(6), 718-724, 38, with permission from BMJ Publishing Group Ltd.

that would remain unmatched until some other triathletes had discovered their incredible secret!

▪ The level of dehydration was unrelated to either the incidence or nature of the medical diagnoses in athletes requiring medical care after the race.

▪ Experienced clinicians were unable accurately to predict the level of dehydration in these triathletes on the basis of the signs that are used to determine the extent of dehydration in clinical medicine. These signs include the presence of sunken eyes, a decreased skin turgor, and the inability to spit.[14]

▪ Blood pressures measured in the supine (lying faceup) position were not different in those who had lost little, some, or a great deal of weight during the race. We concluded that "resting cardiovascular function in the supine position does not appear to be abnormally compromised even in athletes who have lost significant amounts of weight during prolonged exercise" (Sharwood, Collins et al. 2004, p. 722).

> **14**   This study was incomplete and not entirely conclusive. It stimulated a much more thorough and definitive study directed by our New Zealand colleagues (McGarvey, Thompson, et al., 2010). Their conclusions were, however, identical: "The five parameters (decreased skin turgor, sensation of thirst, sunken eyes, inability to spit and dry mucous membranes) tested in this study did not precisely identify runners with total weight loss >3% at the end of a marathon" (p. 716).

The novel conclusion of this study was that a weight loss greater than 7% was "apparently without penalty" (p. 722) for some athletes who completed the race in less than 9 hours, even though their weight loss exceeded 7%. This finding also conflicted with the popular theory that a weight loss greater than 2.5% causes a linear impairment in exercise performance from 20% to 55% or even as much as 125% (see box 3.3 and figure 3.18, page 94)!

Instead, we found that the weight change during the race could predict only 5% of the variation of performance during the race, leaving 95% to be explained by other factors. As a result, "we can thus conclude that high levels of weight loss have, at least, a marginal effect on total performance time" (p. 723). We proposed that "the doctrine that 'weight loss during exercise must be less than 2% (Convertino, Armstrong, et al., 1996)' needs to be properly evaluated in prospective trials lasting longer than a few minutes" (p. 723).[15]

> **15**   I can only presume that I added this as a challenge to an anonymous reviewer who, on reviewing our first submission of this paper to MSSE, had written in capital letters the following: "THERE IS NO QUESTION THAT DEHYDRATION (WATER LOSS INCURRED DURING EXERCISE) IN EXCESS OF 2% BODY WEIGHT IMPAIRS ENDURANCE EXERCISE PERFORMANCE." At that time the ACSM drinking guidelines were still based on the industry-favored "zero % dehydration rule," which encouraged athletes to ensure that they did not lose any weight during exercise by drinking "as much as tolerable." The 2007 ACSM drinking guidelines changed this to the "2% dehydration rule," which stipulated that athletes should drink enough to ensure that they did not become dehydrated by more than 2% during exercise.
>
> My belief is that these recommendations are still too prescriptive because it could encourage dehydration-resistant athletes, able to perform optimally even when dehydrated by more than 2%, to overdrink during exercise and so underperform. Nor is there any evidence that a weight loss of more than 2% will affect the health of those who drink sufficiently to prevent the development of thirst during exercise.

BOX 3.3 Predictions of Performance Impairment

Dr. Michael Sawka, from the United States Army Research Institute of Environmental Medicine (USARIEM), who was first author of the *2007 ACSM Position Stand on Exercise and Fluid Replacement* (Sawka, Burke, et al., 2007), has consistently argued that weight loss during exercise is undesirable because it increases the risk for heat illness and impairs exercise performance. To prove the latter, in one article (Sawka, Montain, et al., 2001), he produced a figure including the work of Craig and Cummings (1966) and of Pichan, Gauttam, and colleagues (1988), which apparently measured reductions in exercise capacity of 20% to 50% at levels of dehydration of 2% to 4%. Appropriately extrapolated as I have done in figure 3.18, these data predict that athletes who finish races with weight losses of 6% to 10% as measured in many Ironman triathletes (figure 3.17, page 92) could expect their performances to be impaired by 55% to 75% (lower arrows) or 100% to 120% (upper arrows), respectively.

These extrapolations show that laboratory studies assessing the impact of certain interventions on athletic performance can produce results that have absolutely no relevance to the real athletic world. Many scientists in this discipline believe that only laboratory research is real science, so they choose not to study athletes participating in real athletic competitions. When studies of competitive athletes produce results at variance with those measured in the laboratory, some scientists either dismiss the athletic studies as misleading (Cheuvront, Carter, et al., 2003) or attempt to explain why athletic studies only confirm what has already been found in the laboratory (Cheuvront, Kenefick, et al., 2007) when the opposite is true.

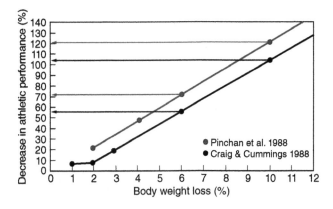

FIGURE 3.18 Data extrapolated from the papers of Craig and Cummings (1966) and Pichan, Gauttam, et al. (1988). If believed, the data predict that athletes who finish races with body weight losses of 6% to 10% could expect their performances to be impaired by 55% to 75% (lower arrows) or 100% to 120% (upper arrows).

Data from Craig and Cummings 1966; Pichan, Gauttam, Tomar, et al., 1988.

Finally we concluded this: "Large changes in body weight during a triathlon were not associated with a greater prevalence of medical complications or higher rectal temperatures, but were associated with higher serum sodium concentrations" (Sharwood, Collins, et al. 2004, p. 718) so that "there is no logical basis to encourage high rates of fluid intake especially to reduce the risk of heat illness in Ironman triathletes competing in relatively mild environmental conditions" (p. 723). There was surprisingly little response to this article.

The next paper of interest (Cheu-vront, Carter, et al., 2003) came from the U.S. Army Research Institute of Environmental Medicine (USARIEM). It analyzed 24 studies of marathon runners in which data were reported for both weight loss and running speed during these races. They found a linear relationship with a positive slope between these two variables so that the most dehydrated runners ran the fastest (figure 3.19). This is the opposite of what is found in laboratory studies (figure 3.18) but matches exactly what has always been found in competitive athletics. The authors concluded this: "The positive correlation in this figure should not be wrongly interpreted as support for the ergogenic effect of dehydration." The authors then attempted unsuccessfully to explain why the findings

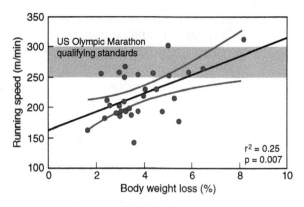

FIGURE 3.19 A linear relation with a positive slope between the level of postrace body weight loss and 42 km marathon running speed was reported by Cheuvront et al. (Cheuvront, Carter, et al., 2003) from USARIEM. The data used for this analysis came from 24 studies of marathon runners, all of which show that the fastest finishers in marathon races are inevitably the most dehydrated. According to this study, 25% of the athletes' performances could be explained by the extent to which they lost weight during these marathons.

Reprinted, by permission, from S.N. Cheuvront, R. Carter III, and M.N. Sawka, 2003, "Fluid balance and endurance exercise performance," *Current Sports Medicine Reports* 2(4): 202-208.

cannot be real: "The physiologic paradox of high performance when markedly dehydrated may also have several simpler explanations" (p. 204), while concluding, "but the question of how competitive runners perform so well when dehydrated remains" (p. 204). Rather than effectively addressing this paradox and the implications it might hold for the advice given to athletes, the authors merely restated their apparent bias: "Dehydration by anything over 2% of body weight significantly degrades endurance exercise performance, especially in hot environments" (p. 206). As a result, "To minimize the adverse consequences of body water deficits on endurance exercise performance, it is recommended that fluid intake be sufficient to minimize dehydration to less than 2% of body weight loss. This can usually be achieved with fluid intakes of under 1 L · h^{-1}" (p. 202). The abstract to the article carries no reference to the paradoxical finding that these conclusions do not appear to be valid for marathon runners. The senior author of this paper, Michael Sawka, is the first author of the *2007 ACSM Position Stand on Exercise and Fluid Replacement*. Those guidelines also advise that exercisers should drink enough to prevent a >2% weight loss during exercise. This position was steadfastly defended by Dr. Sawka in our debate published in 2007 (Sawka and Noakes, 2007).

The Evidence Mounts

In recent years, the evidence disproving Wyndham and Strydom's hypothesis has continued to accumulate. A series of studies was performed by the Defence Medical and Environmental Research Institute of the Republic of Singapore (Byrne, Lee, et al., 2006; Lee, Nio, et al., 2010). For these studies, Jason Lee and colleagues measured body weight loss, intestinal temperature recorded continuously with an ingested telemetric thermometer, and racing performance in competitors in the 2003 and 2007 Singapore Bay Run and Army Half-Marathon (21 km, or 13 miles), which was run in hot (26 °C-30.6 °C, or 78.8 °F-87.1 °F), humid (75-90%) conditions. There were a number of unexpected findings.

First, some athletes reached very high intestinal temperatures (41.3 and 41.7 °C) even though they were completely without symptoms (asymptomatic). This shows that some humans can reach these high temperatures without risk to their health (as had already been proven by Dr. Maron in his study on himself, figure 3.10, page 81). Furthermore, rectal temperatures lower than these values cannot be assumed to explain the symptoms in athletes who collapse after exercise. Rather, other possible causes, such as EAPH, need to be excluded before the condition can be ascribed purely to an elevated body temperature.

Second, there was no relationship between the postrace intestinal temperature and the percentage of body weight loss during either race, in keeping with the findings from all our studies (figures 3.17 and 2.4, pages 92 and 55). Third, there was no relationship between the total amount of fluid that the athletes ingested during the race and either their postrace intestinal temperatures or their average running speeds during either race. Fourth, there was also no relationship between the 21 km finishing time and the percentage of weight loss during either race. However there was a significant relationship between the postrace intestinal temperature and the running speed during the race.

From the data of the 2003 race, the authors concluded that "dehydration was not a major determinant of the core body temperature during 2 hr of self-paced outdoor running in the heat" (Byrne, Lee, et al., 2006, p. 744). Rather, "It seems timely to reaffirm that the major determinant of the core body temperature during running is relative exercise intensity" (p. 744). From the similar data of the 2007 race, they wrote, "In conclusion, our study findings suggest that hyperthermia, defined by a body core temperature greater than 39.5 °C, is common in trained individuals undertaking outdoor distance running in environmental heat, without evidence for fatigue or heat illness. Running velocity was the main significant predictor variable for the change in core body temperature at 21 km. . . . Fluid volumes ingested during competitive races have no detectable effect on any of the variables relating to core body temperature or performance" (Lee, Nio, et al., 2010, p. 897).

These authors have undertaken an even more ambitious study (J.K. Lee, personal communication) in which they monitored the intestinal temperatures and, with GPS, the running speeds of 19 competitors, 12 male and 7 female, in the 2008 Standard Charter Singapore Marathon. Then, as we had in our 1991 paper (Noakes, Myburgh, et al., 1991), they also measured the oxygen consumption of these athletes at a range of running speeds so that they were able to predict the metabolic rates and hence rates of heat production of these athletes during the various stages of the race.

These authors found that the average body weight loss during the race was 2.3 kg (3.9%); men lost more weight (2.8 kg; 4.3%) than women (1.5 kg; 3.3%). Mean fluid intake during the race was 2.0 L for men and 1.7 L for women. Half the runners reached intestinal temperatures in excess of 38.5 °C, but none exceeded

40 °C. As is usual, the race winner lost the most weight (7.0%). Again, there was no relationship between the percentage of weight loss during the race and the postrace intestinal temperature. Running velocity (and metabolic rate) during the race but not the degree of weight loss (dehydration) most accurately predicted the intestinal temperature during exercise (figure 3.20). It was rewarding to see that our less sophisticated study in 1991 had produced the correct conclusions and that metabolic rate, not percentage of dehydration, is indeed the more important determinant of the body temperature during exercise.

Our groups have combined forces to measure the same variables in runners competing in the 56 km Two Oceans Marathon in Cape Town and in the 90 km Comrades Marathon between Durban and Pietermaritzburg, South Africa. The collected data from all these studies provide a key piece of information that is perhaps the single best piece of evidence that disproves the dehydration myth. The data show that the postexercise intestinal temperature is lower the longer the distance run and so is highest

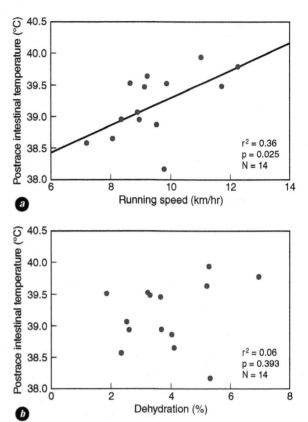

FIGURE 3.20 The study of Lee and colleagues (personal communication) at the 2008 Standard Charter Singapore Marathon has established that (a) the running speed but not (b) the degree of weight loss is related to the postrace intestinal temperature in runners during a 42 km marathon.

Data from Lee, Nio, Lim, et al., 2010.

after the 21 km race (figure 3.21a, page 98) and lowest after the 89 km Comrades Marathon. This is because the average running speed falls with running distance (figure 3.21b), whereas the level of dehydration is relatively unaffected by distance run and was not greater in 89 km runners than in those racing only 21 km (figure 3.21c). This suggests that the thirst mechanism is acting appropriately at all running distances. Postrace intestinal temperature was paradoxically weakly related to the level of dehydration so that those who lost the most weight had the lowest postrace temperatures (figure 3.21d) but was more strongly related to the running speed (figure 3.21e). The authors naturally believe that they will find even higher temperatures in races of 5 to 10 km as perhaps already shown by Robinson in his study of Don Lash running 3 miles (4.8 km) (see note 4, page 72). A study by Ely, Ely, and colleagues (2009) found average rectal temperatures greater than 40 °C after an 8 km race, confirming this prediction. The published evidence shows that heatstroke becomes increasingly less common the longer the duration of exercise.

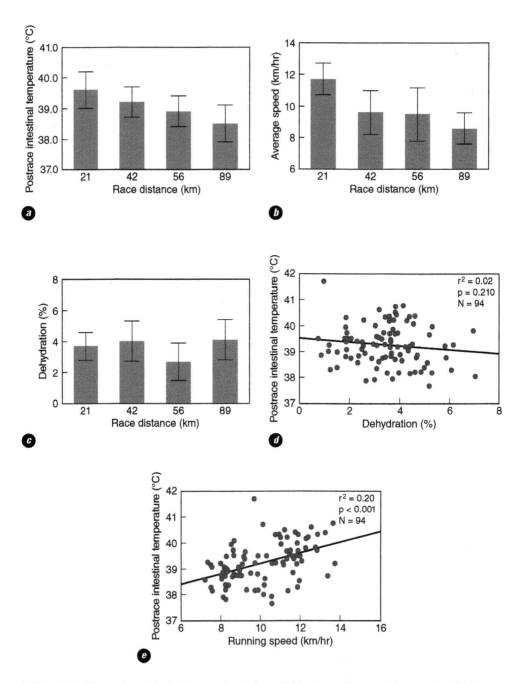

FIGURE 3.21 The postrace intestinal temperature is lower *(a)* the longer the race distance as *(b)* athletes run slower. The degree of weight loss is *(c)* quite similar at all running distances, but *(d)* there is only a weak relationship between the degree of weight loss and the postrace intestinal temperature in the 94 athletes who were studied in these four races. Instead, *(e)* running speed is a significant predictor of the postrace intestinal temperature (Byrne, 2007; Byrne, Lee, et al., 2006) (Lee, Nio, et al., 2010).

Data from Byrne 2007; Byrne, Lee, Chew, et al., 2006; Lee, Nio, Lim, et al., 2010.

The authors concluded that how fast a person runs, not how much that person drinks, determines the extent to which body temperature rises during exercise. This has been known since 1938 (figure 3.5, page 67). But sometimes it takes 70 years for a truth to be rediscovered, especially if there are reasons some might not wish this fact to be widely known.

Another study that confirms that prolonged exercise does not pose a major threat to human thermoregulatory capacity was performed by a group from Western Australia at the 2004 Ironman Western Australia (Laursen, Suriano, et al., 2006). During the race, the intestinal temperatures were measured in 10 well-trained athletes who completed the race in a mean time of 10 hours and 11 minutes with average swim, cycle, and run times of 58:00; 5:14:00, and 3:59:00, respectively. Seven of the athletes finished in less than 10 hours, indicating that they were superior athletes. Despite their relatively fast overall finishing times, the athletes performed each individual event at quite low intensities relative to their capacities. Thus, their average cycling speed was 34 km/hr and their average running pace was 10.6 km/hr (5:40/km). In contrast, the world-record holder in the 42 km marathon runs almost twice as fast (20.5 km/hr; 2:56/km). Since the metabolic rate determines the body temperature during exercise, it was perhaps not surprising that the intestinal temperatures of these triathletes averaged ~38 °C throughout the entire race even as the athletes became progressively more dehydrated, so that they finished with an average weight loss of 2.3 kg (3.0%). The highest temperatures were measured immediately after the swim and were 38.5 °C. The highest individual intestinal temperature (40.5 °C) was measured in the fastest swimmer, who finished 8th overall in the swim in a time of ~49 minutes. Like us, the authors could not find any relationship between the intestinal temperature during exercise and the level of dehydration that developed during the race. The authors concluded that despite a body weight loss of ~3%, intestinal temperatures were elevated only about 1° C above prerace resting values, hardly evidence for serious thermoregulatory strain despite 10 hours of exercise that temporarily exhausted the athletes.

The authors assumed that since this was the first modern study in which core body temperature was measured in an event lasting more than 3 hours, they would not find any difficulty publishing the article in a leading U.S. scientific journal devoted to the exercise sciences. But they presumed wrong: The article was returned with comments from peer reviewers who concluded that these data must be false because they conflict with what is known to be "true." The article finally found a home in the *British Journal of Sports Medicine*.

Dr. Wei-Fong Kao and his colleagues from the Veterans General Hospital in Taipei, Taiwan (Kao, Shyu, et al., 2008), measured body weight changes continuously during 12- and 24-hour races in Taipei in 2003. They showed that in both races, body weights fell progressively for the first 8 hours of these races before stabilizing for the remainder of the race. The point of stabilization was a ~3% weight loss in the 12-hour race and a ~4% weight loss in the 24-hour race (figure 3.22, page 100). This stabilization of weight loss is most interesting. In a review published in 1993 (Noakes, 1993) I noticed that there was a "remarkable

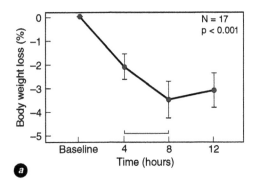 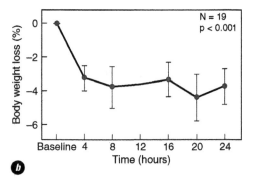

FIGURE 3.22 Weight loss during the *(a)* 12-hour and *(b)* 24-hour 2003 Soochow University International Ultra-marathon races stabilized after the first 8 hours of each race at either 3% or 4% depending on the race duration. This suggests that this degree of weight loss could be regulated and may represent the loss of metabolic fuel and a water reserve that does not require immediate replacement during exercise (Kao, Shyu, et al., 2008).

Reprinted, by permission, from W-F Kao, C-L Shyu, X-W Yang, et al., 2008, "Athletic performance and serial weight changes during 12- and 24-hour ultra-marathons," *Clinical Journal of Sport Medicine* 18(2): 155-158.

constancy of the weight loss (2-3 kg) experienced by athletes during prolonged exercise. This appears to be relatively independent of the type or duration of the activity. *It is as if the total weight loss during exercise is a regulated variable* [my emphasis]" (p. 309).

But more interestingly, Kao and his colleagues (2008) showed a strong linear relationship with a negative slope between distance run in the 24-hour race and the percentage of body weight loss during the race (figure 3.23) so that the athlete who lost the most weight (~7%) covered the second-greatest distance (~260 km). The race winner ran a little farther (~275 km), even though his weight loss of ~4.2% greatly exceeded the ACSM cutoff of 2% at which exercise performance begins to be "seriously degraded" according to their publications (Convertino, Armstrong, et al., 1996; Sawka, Burke, et al., 2007; Sawka and Noakes, 2007). This is not a new finding, having been reported previously by many others (figures 3.1, 3.7, and 3.17, pages 61, 71, and 92). By contrast, the athlete who drank the most so that his weight increased by ~1.7% could manage only 150 km. Similarly, five of the six athletes who ran the farthest in the 12-hour race lost more than 3% of their body weight during the race.

Kao and his colleagues concluded that "greater weight loss is associated with better performance in the 24-hour race" so that "these findings, if conclusively confirmed, have important practical implications with regard to hydration recommendations" (p. 158).

Of the 11 best performers in that race, only 1 lost less than 2% of body weight during the race, whereas 7 lost more than 4% body weight. This conflicts with the popular theory advanced in many USARIEM, ACSM, and Gatorade publications that any weight loss greater than 2% is associated with a substantially impaired exercise performance. Scientists who advise those organizations will argue that the most dehydrated athletes in these studies would have performed even better had they just drunk more and lost less weight. But if they truly believe this, they should attempt to disprove this hypothesis in prospective studies performed under field conditions. Until the results of such studies are known, we are allowed to conclude that weight loss during exercise is a relatively poor predictor of performance and that if there is any link, it is between greater levels of weight loss and better performances.

Subsequent studies continue to fit the alternate theory that better performance usually occurs in those who lose the most weight during competition. These include our study of EAH in the 2004 New Zealand Ironman Triathlon, which again showed a linear relationship between the degree of weight loss and finishing time in triathletes in that race (figure 2.4b, page 55); a study of adventure racers (Clark, Barker, et al., 2005), which found that those who had the darkest urine after the race performed the best; and another of professional cyclists in two multiday cycling tours in Australia and France (Ebert, Martin, et al., 2007). As in the studies of runners, there was a significant relationship between the cyclists' degrees of weight loss and their finishing positions so that the cyclists who finished in the highest positions were more dehydrated than those who finished in lower positions. Interestingly, cyclists drank more than runners (up to 1.3 L/hr, 44 fl oz/hr) and finished with lesser degrees of dehydration. Average levels of dehydration in different races ranged from 1.2% to 3.5%.

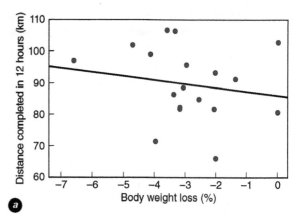

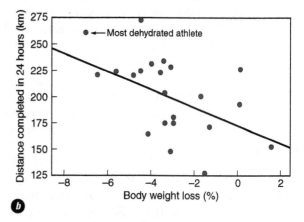

FIGURE 3.23 A linear relationship with a negative slope between the degree of weight loss during (a) 12-hour and (b) 24-hour Soochow University International Ultramarathon races. The athlete who lost the most weight in the 24-hour ultramarathon (arrowed, bottom) covered the second greatest distance (Kao, Shyu, et al., 2008).

Reprinted, by permission, from W-F Kao, C-L Shyu, X-W Yang, et al., 2008, "Athletic performance and serial weight changes during 12- and 24-hour ultra-marathons," *Clinical Journal of Sport Medicine* 18(2): 155-158.

A study of runners in the 2008 Rio Del Lago 100-mile (161 km) Endurance Run in California also found that the degree of weight loss during the race was significantly related to race finishing time so that runners who lost the most weight finished in the shortest time. The race winner lost 6% of his body weight during the race. During this race, the runners studied lost 5.6% to 6.6% of their body mass and 4.6% to 6.3% of their total body water (Lebus, Casazza, et al., 2010).

More recent studies from a group of French scientists continue to confirm these findings. They showed that the fastest runner they studied in the 7-day 230 km (142.9 mile) Marathon of the Sands in the Sahara Desert lost more than 9% of his body weight during the race but finished 6th of 650 competitors (Zouhal, Groussard, et al., 2009). In a study of 643 runners in the 2009 Mont Saint-Michael

Marathon in France (Zouhal, Groussard, et al., 2011), the authors found a significant linear relationship with a negative slope between the degree of weight loss during the race and the finishing time. As a result, athletes who finished the race in less than 3 hours lost an average of 3.1% body weight, those finishing in between 3 and 4 hours lost 2.5% body weight, and those taking longer than 4 hours lost only 1.8% body weight.

So the clear evidence from all studies is that the faster athletes run, the higher their body temperatures will be and in general the greater their levels of dehydration will be. The dependence of the rectal temperature on the running speed maintained during the race was most clearly shown by the studies of Byrne and colleagues (figure 3.21e, page 98). During the course of our collaborative studies, we frequently discussed the need to undertake a study of body temperatures during very short-duration exercise such as a 5 km running race so that we could again show that (a) the highest body temperatures are reached during exercise of short duration of high intensity (and not during prolonged exercise of lower intensity in which athletes are more likely to become dehydrated) and (b) very high body temperatures can be safely sustained since the brain will regulate the athlete's pace to ensure that a catastrophic elevation in body temperature does not occur (Tucker, Marle, et al., 2006; Tucker, Rauch, et al., 2004). Scientists from the USARIEM were the first to undertake that study.

USARIEM scientists including Drs. Cheuvront and Montain studied intestinal temperatures during 8 km time trials conducted in hot and cool conditions (Ely, Ely, et al., 2009). In exactly half of 24 individual trials, athletes reached rectal temperatures in excess of 40 °C. There was no evidence that these temperatures impaired running performance. This study is especially important because it originates from USARIEM and is coauthored by Dr. Scott Montain. In 1992, Montain published a study that concluded that athletes should drink 1.2 L/hr, which is essentially as much as is tolerable, because this drinking approach lowered the body temperature by about 0.2° C compared to drinking substantially less (0.7 L/hr), more in line with ad libitum drinking. This logic then steered the 1996 American College of Sports Medicine to advise that athletes should be encouraged to drink either 1.2 L/hr or "as much as tolerable" during all forms of exercise because this approach would produce the lowest body temperatures during exercise—the implication of which is that the lower the temperature, the better the performance.

Yet in Montain and colleagues' 1992 study, the final rectal temperatures were always lower than 40 °C, even when subjects did not drink at all during 2 hours of vigorous exercise in moderately severe heat. Had this new study been completed before 1992, it would have forced a quite different interpretation of the 1992 paper on which the 1996 ACSM drinking guidelines—the guidelines that were to have such a profound effect on runners' drinking behaviors—were based. If the goal of drinking is to maintain a safe rectal temperature and if a temperature of even 40 °C does not impair running performance, then the 1992 study could have been interpreted as evidence that athletes do not need to drink at all during 2 hours of vigorous exercise in moderately severe heat. In that case, the *1996 ACSM Position Stand on Heat and Cold Illnesses during Distance Running* would have been quite different. In turn, the global epidemic of EAH and EAHE might never have occurred. And this book would not have been written.

Summary

It seems that the speculative conclusions we drew in our 1988 paper, which state that (a) dehydration has little effect on the body temperature response during marathon running and (b) high rates of fluid ingestion are not necessarily beneficial for better performance, have been vindicated by the (few) relevant studies that have been performed in the following 20 years. Confirmation that dehydration in those who drink ad libitum has little effect on athletic performance, as I had argued in my debate with Michael Sawka (Sawka and Noakes, 2007), has now been confirmed in a meta-analysis of all the relevant studies. On the basis of those studies, Professor Eric Goulet has concluded that "This meta-analysis . . . [has] shown that drinking to the dictate of thirst significantly improves time trial (TT) performance compared with a rate of drinking below thirst sensation . . . [so] that drinking sufficiently to satisfy thirst will provide a . . . performance advantage 98% and 62% of the time compared with a rate of drinking below and above thirst . . . , respectively. . . . (T)his meta-analysis [also] showed that an exercise-induced dehydration (EID) level of 2.2% BW was not associated with a decrease in TT performance compared with euhydration. . . . The findings of this meta-analysis support the theory . . . developed by Noakes (Sawka and Noakes, 2007) . . . that it is not the effect of EID . . . that is responsible for the decrement in exercise performance (EP), but rather the fact of not drinking to the satisfaction of thirst, and contradict and abolish the old and much-believed dogma stating that during prolonged exercise it is of capital importance to drink ahead of thirst, otherwise it is . . . too late, and EP has already started to decrease" (Goulet, 2011, p. 7).

Thus, "The results of the present meta-analysis are in sharp contradiction with the message that has been conveyed by the scientific literature for . . . a long time (Cheuvront, Carter, et al., 2003; Sawka, Burke, et al., 2007) and indicate that, under real-world . . . conditions, EID does not alter EP in a statistical as well as a practical manner in trained cyclists, compared with the maintenance of euhydration" (p. 6).

Instead Dr. Goulet concluded: "this meta-analysis showed for the first time that drinking according to the dictates of thirst will maximize EP" (p. 7).

Clearly, these findings have practical implications for fluid replacement guidelines during exercise. But it remains to be seen when these definitive findings will be properly acknowledged so that appropriate drinking guidelines for exercise can be adopted universally. Perhaps this book will help by providing the untarnished scientific truth.

CHAPTER 4

Salt Balance in the Body

It ain't easy to do nothing, now that society is telling everyone that the body is fundamentally flawed and about to self-destruct. People expect perfect health. It's a brand-spanking-new Madison Avenue expectation. It's our job to tell them that imperfect health is and always has been perfect health.

The Fat Man, medical resident in
***The House of God* (Shem, 2003, p. 193)**

Humans evolved as hot, sweaty, long-distance hunters able to outlast all other mammals when running in a hot, arid environment—the African savannah—in which salt was in short supply. Most of the Earth's salt exists in our planet's oceans. The only rich source of salt on the savannah was in the bodies of other animals.

Once our ancestors became accomplished hunters, able to outrun fleet-footed antelope, the problem of an inadequate salt supply was essentially solved since animal flesh has a much higher salt content than do plants. In addition, the blood, urine, and gastrointestinal contents of mammals are another rich source of sodium. Modern !Xo hunters, for example, collect the stomach and intestinal fluids of the antelope they hunt (Liebenberg, 1990). The higher salt intake that resulted from the capture of large mammals would have allowed an increase in the total body water content and hence in body size.

As part of this development, humans must have evolved a capacity (a) to delay drinking in order to hunt successfully as well as (b) a great capacity to minimize urinary water production through secretion of the hormone arginine vasopressin (AVP), also known as vasopressin, argipressin, or antidiuretic hormone (ADH), and commonly denoted as AVP/ADH. As a result, daily urine production can be safely reduced to 500 ml and daily water requirement to a minimum of ~2 L in humans resting in cool conditions. The presence of salt in sweat does not immediately make sense any more than does a high sweat rate in mammals living in relatively arid conditions where both water and salt are in short supply. The explanation for the high sweat rates is now apparent—it is the essential adaptation that makes persistent hunting possible in the midday heat. But why should humans waste a precious commodity, salt, in sweat? I argue that the presence of salt in human sweat could be an important adaptation for delaying thirst by slowing the rate at which the serum sodium concentration and osmolality rise in response to water loss from sweating.

To maximize the value of this novel source of salt, that is, animal bodies, human hunters forced to sweat when hunting for long hours in the heat would have benefitted from two other adaptations. First would be an ability to regulate the amount of salt lost in sweat (and urine) so that these losses matched exactly the habitual sodium intakes (over weeks or months). Second would be the ability to store sodium in an internal store that could be filled in times of plenty and slowly depleted over a period of weeks or months when dietary salt was scarce.

The first evidence that humans began to increase their salt intakes from sources other than meat comes from the discovery of salt works at Lake Xiechi in Shanxi, China, dated to about 6000 BCE. The original value of salt came with the accidental discovery that salt immersion can preserve meat over winter. By about 2800 BCE, the Egyptians were using salt to preserve fish, which they then sold to the Phoenicians in exchange for glass and dyes.

The coastal areas abutting the North Sea, including England, Holland, and Scandinavia were rich in salt as the peat exposed at low tide was impregnated with salt. The extraction and sale of that salt were the initial sources of wealth for those nations as it was for the city of Venice. Inland salt harvesting in Europe developed in the three central Austrian cities of Salzburg ("salt city"), Hallstat ("salt town"), and Hallein ("salt work"), all of which lie on the river Salzach ("salt water"). The rise in the level of the world's oceans between CE 300 and 1000 prevented the extraction of salt from peat, producing Britain's first economic recession. The retreat of the oceans re-exposed the peat after CE 1000, restored the salt industry, and attracted invaders. Thus the centers of salt production in England and France fell under the control of invading Norsemen and Arabs.

The availability of salt influenced the nature of the political systems introduced into different countries in the first century of this millennium. The ample supplies of salt along the shores of the Mediterranean and the North Sea were associated with freer, more democratic societies. In contrast, the scanty salt reserves in salt-poor countries were monopolized by rulers and priests who stored the salt under heavy guard and controlled its release to manipulate their salt-addicted populations. Thus, "Where salt was plentiful, the society tended to be free, independent and democratic, where it was scarce, he who controlled the salt, controlled the people" (Bloch, 1963, p. 95).

Salt availability also influenced the outcome of military conflicts. A salt short-age became a critical factor for the conduct of the U.S. Civil War since the main source of salt production for the Confederate forces was in the North and was lost early in the conflict. A key tactic of the Union forces was to limit salt entry into the Southern states. Salt provision to the Confederate states produced a thriving black market but this did not help, and a lack of adequate salt for the Confeder-ate troops was considered a major factor determining the outcome of that war (Lonn, 1965; Meneely, Tucker, et al., 1953).

This rich history attests to the importance of salt in the development of the modern world, and the salt trade that became the first great global industry after 6000 BCE has ensured that we are exposed daily to a lavish salt intake to such an extent that many now believe that our habitually too-high dietary sodium intake is an important cause of certain diseases, most especially high blood pressure. Thus in just the past 5,000 years, the human diet has evolved from one in which salt was present in small amounts to one in which salt is a cheap, freely available commodity that is present in excess of human dietary needs even in poor com-munities. In addition, humans (and other mammals) have an overpowering drive to ingest salt when a salt deficiency develops.

So it is an astonishing achievement of the sports drink industry that it has convinced us of the exact opposite—that modern human athletes lack biological controls to ensure that they ingest enough salt and so are at risk of developing a syndrome of salt deficiency even when eating a diet that is stuffed with salt.

Despite an average daily salt intake in the United States of ~10 to 15 g, which greatly exceeds the minimum expected daily requirement of perhaps 3 g in habitual exercisers, the myth has developed that all U.S. athletes are at risk of becoming salt deficient especially when they run marathons or compete in ultradistance events like the Ironman Hawaii Triathlon or the Western States 100-mile race. This is especially so in those who are "salty sweaters." It is held that such salt deficiency is then the cause of EAH and EAHE, heat illness, and muscle cramps. Since this theory would seem to be highly implausible (even if humans were not potent salt conservers), it raises another question: How could this improbable theory ever have gained any credence whatsoever especially in an apparently scientifically sophisticated nation such as the United States and among endurance athletes like distance runners and Ironman triathletes, many of whom might consider themselves highly educated and too sophisticated to believe an unsubstantiated dogma?

Blood Sodium Concentration and Osmolality

Let's start with an understanding of how blood sodium concentration is regulated. About 60% of the human body is made up of water distributed into two predominant compartments—the intracellular fluid compartment (within the cells, ICF) and the extracellular fluid compartment (outside the cells, ECF). The ECF includes the interstitial fluid compartment (between the cells, ISF) and the fluid contained in the vascular space, also known as the plasma volume (PV).

More of this fluid is contained inside rather than outside the cells: In a 70 kg (154 lb) human with a total body water content of 42 L, about 28 L are found inside the cells in the ICF, and the remaining 14 L are outside the cells in the ECF, including the ISF and PV (figure 4.1).

The circulating blood volume of about 5 L comprises 3 L of fluid that is part of the ECF; this is the plasma volume. The circulating red blood cells float in this fluid. The remaining 2 L of the blood volume comprises the fluid inside the red blood cells and is therefore a part of the ICF volume.

The ISF facilitates the transfer of fluid and other biological chemicals between the bloodstream and the cells. Water travels freely across the membranes that divide the intracellular and extracellular compartments. Its movement across these membranes is directed by the osmotic pull exerted on either side of these dividing membranes. The extent of this osmotic pull is determined by any difference in the number of molecules contained within the separated compartments. As a result, the osmotic pull—the osmolality—of the extracellular and intracellular compartments is always the same; if a difference develops in the concentrations of the molecules on either side of these water-permeable membranes, water simply crosses the membrane in either direction until the osmolality inside and outside the cells is the same (even though the concentration of the molecules on either side of the membrane has not changed).

The major determinant of the osmolality of the ECF is the number of sodium ions (Na^+) it contains. These ions contribute about 50% of the osmolality of the ECF. Similarly, the major determinant of the osmolality of the ICF is the other major body electrolyte, potassium (K^+).

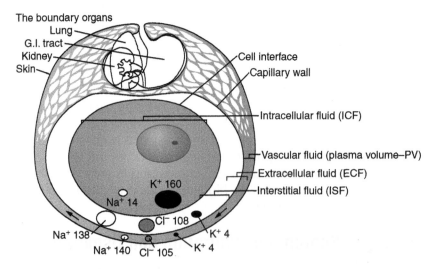

FIGURE 4.1 Distribution of water in the human body. The most important constituents of each of the fluid compartments are shown; the size of the circle depicting each constituent represents the absolute concentration of each, and the number gives the concentration in millimoles per liter (mmol/L, often denoted as mM, but in this publication, mmol/L is used). The boundary organs that influence whole body fluid balance—the kidneys, gastrointestinal tract, and the lungs—are also shown. The relative size of the compartments is depicted by the volume that each fills on this diagram so that the ICF contains about 28 L in a 70 kg human, whereas the ECF (ISF and PV) together total about 14 L.

Adapted from *Of water, salt, and life: An atlas of fluid and electrolyte balance in health and disease*, 1956 (Milwaukee: Lakeside Laboratories), plate 1.

The body regulates its osmolality principally by controlling the amount of sodium and potassium that it contains, specifically the Na^+ content of the ECF and the K^+ content of the ICF.[1] As a result, the volume of the ECF is regulated by how many Na^+ ions it contains, whereas the volume of the ICF is determined largely by the number of K^+ ions present within the cells.

The body is designed to regulate the osmolality of the ECF and especially the ICF within a narrow range. In the extracellular space, the sodium chloride (NaCl) concentration is always between 135 and 145 mmol/L, and this is regulated by the number of molecules of sodium in the ECF, which in turn determines the amount of fluid that can be accommodated in the ECF. Similarly, if the osmolality of the ICF either rises too high or drops too low, the cells either shrink or swell beyond the range at which they function optimally. Brain cells have an added complexity: When they swell, the pressure within the rigid skull bones increases. If this pressure increases too much in those with EAHE, death results from the suppression of key brain functions, including those regulating breathing and the beating of the heart. At the time of this writing, 12 athletes or soldiers are known to have died in this way. All deaths would probably have been prevented if the pressure inside the skull had been rapidly reduced with the use of hypertonic (3-5%) saline solutions administered intravenously. It follows that the volumes of the ECF and the ICF compartments are regulated by controlling the number of osmolality-producing molecules contained in either compartment, most especially sodium in the ECF and potassium in the ICF.

The typical Western diet contains about 10 g of salt per day (Institute of Medicine of the National Academies, 2005). But obligatory salt losses in sweat and urine even in an athlete exercising 120 minutes a day 7 days a week are only about 2 to 3 g per day, as we confirmed in the elite athletes we studied in Kenya (Fudge, Easton, et al., 2008; Fudge, Pitsiladis, et al., 2007). Thus, many Western athletes running even 2 hours a day will have a daily positive sodium balance of as much as 8 g and must rid their bodies of that excess each day by excreting the sodium in either sweat or urine.

One consequence of excreting that excess sodium in sweat is the salty sweater, whose sweat contains a high sodium concentration. Some of this excess may be stored in the exchangeable, osmotically inactive sodium stores within the cells (see note 1).

Excess sodium can also be excreted by the kidneys through inhibition of the secretion of the hormone aldosterone by the adrenal glands. Aldosterone acts to increase sodium reabsorption by the kidneys and sweat glands (figure 4.2, page 110), thus raising blood osmolality. To achieve this effect, aldosterone causes an increased excretion of potassium by the body. A rising blood osmolality will in turn switch on production of AVP/ADH in the brain; this hormone increases water reabsorption by the kidneys. As a result, the volume of the ECF will increase until

1 This is a simplified explanation. The osmolality of the body is determined by the total amount of *exchangeable* sodium and potassium in the body. In particular, the amount of exchangeable sodium in the body exceeds the total amount present in the ECF by some margin. This extra amount is believed to exist in an osmotically inactive form within certain cells, such as bone and skin. This sodium store is continuously exchanging (osmotically inactive) sodium (Na) within the cells with osmotically active sodium (Na^+) in the ECF. This exchange process may be an important determinant of whether those who overdrink during exercise and who have SIADH also develop EAH or EAHE.

the normal osmolality is restored. In contrast, inhibition of aldosterone secretion increases sodium losses in urine and sweat.

Another cause of increased sodium loss from the body occurs when the blood volume rises. This causes secretion of the hormone atrial natriuretic peptide (ANP) by the atrial chamber of the heart (in response to stretching of the atrium). This hormone acts on the kidney to increase sodium excretion. Patients with EAH and EAHE excrete sodium at paradoxically high concentrations in the urine. This increased sodium excretion in the urine (natriuresis) in the presence of a low blood sodium concentration is paradoxical and is probably due to the combined effects of AVP (Kawai, Baba, et al., 2001) and ANP (Kamoi, Ebe, et al., 1990; Kawai, Baba, et al., 2001), and perhaps brain swelling causing the condition known as

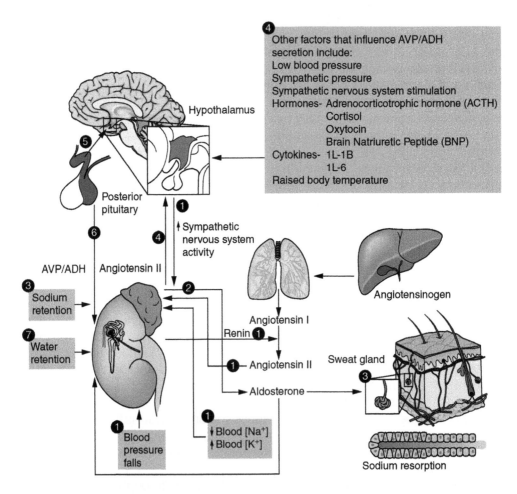

FIGURE 4.2 The complex mechanisms regulating the sodium content of the body. In response to many stimuli, including (1) increased renin release from the kidney (which converts angiotensin I to angiotensin II), a falling blood sodium concentration, rising blood potassium or angiotensin II concentrations, reduced blood pressure, or a variety of stresses including anxiety, (2) aldosterone production by the adrenal cortex is increased. Aldosterone acts on the (3) kidneys and sweat glands to increase sodium reabsorption in exchange for the excretion of potassium. (4) Angiotensin and a number of other factors act (5) on the hypothalamus to increase (6) AVP/ADH secretion from the posterior pituitary gland. Increased blood AVP/ADH concentrations act (7) on the kidneys to increase water retention.

cerebral salt wasting (CSW). The mechanisms by which conditions of the brain cause CSW are still unknown.

Potassium losses from the body are small because potassium is an intracellular electrolyte present in low concentrations in the blood perfusing the kidneys and sweat glands and is therefore in low concentrations in urine and sweat. Control of potassium excretion is via aldosterone, which increases potassium excretion in exchange for sodium reabsorption by the kidneys (figure 4.2).

Some years ago it was suggested that potassium losses are large in exercising humans (Knochel, 1974) and could cause potassium deficiency leading to heatstroke.[2] But many subsequent studies have shown that this idea, like the theory of sodium deficiency in endurance athletes, is a myth (box 4.1). There is no risk that potassium deficiency will occur in healthy human athletes because dietary potassium intake always exceeds urinary and sweat losses (Costill, 1977; Costill, Cote, et al., 1975; Costill, Cote, et al., 1982).

2 This is yet another example of the catastrophe model of human physiology. According to this model, normal physiological processes, in this case the secretion of potassium in the urine and sweat in exercising humans, occurs without control until a catastrophic physiological failure occurs, leading to death. But if humans were designed this way, we would not have survived our dangerous evolutionary past. The point is that our evolution provided us with exquisite homeostatic controls to ensure that our daily urinary and sweat potassium losses exactly balance our daily dietary potassium intakes. The same applies for sodium.

BOX 4.1 The Mystery of Sodium Stores

The major determinant of the volume of fluid in the ECF is the amount of sodium chloride (NaCl) that it contains. There is usually enough NaCl in the 14 L of the ECF to ensure that the NaCl concentration is 140 mmol/L. If all the sodium in the body is contained in the ECF, then this should equal 1,960 mmol, which is 140 mmol multiplied by 14 L. Since 1,000 mmol of sodium weighs 23 g (1,000 mmol of sodium chloride weighs 58 g), the total amount of sodium present in the ECF is 45 g. Sodium exists in small amounts in the ICF, but this amount is negligible compared to the sodium found in the ECF.

One of the great uncertainties of physiology is that, were there only 1,960 mmol of sodium (45 g) in the human body, we would be unable to function because the osmolality of the body (a measure of the concentration of the molecules dissolved in all bodily fluids) would be less than the measured value of ~300 milliosmols per liter (mOsmol/L). This has led to the theory that the actual amount of sodium stored in the human body is much greater, closer to 3,000 mmol in a 70 kg human (Edelman, Leibman, et al., 1958). Exactly where that sodium is stored is the greater mystery. Although the possibility that the body has this additional sodium store was actively researched in the 1950s, there has been much less interest in the past 5 decades. This mystery has important implications since it could mean that this sodium acts as a reserve that can be mobilized when sodium is lost from the body, for example during exercise, or stored when subjects eat a high-sodium diet.

Perhaps the important point is there is still enough uncertainty about the complexity of human sodium metabolism that we should be wary of adopting dogmatic positions, especially about the existence of a condition of sodium deficiency in humans. What is known is that during exercise, both water and sodium are lost in sweat. But sweat has a low NaCl concentration, usually between about 20 and 40 mmol/L in persons eating the

(continued)

BOX 4.1 **The Mystery of Sodium Stores** *(continued)*

---

high sodium diet prevalent in developed nations; much lower sweat NaCl concentrations (down to 1 mmol/L) are found in those ingesting low-sodium diets. As a result, sweating removes relatively more water than salt from the body, causing the blood NaCl concentration to increase, since there is relatively less NaCl in sweat than in the bodily fluid (plasma or blood) from which sweat originates.

The crucial point is that the volume of fluid in the extracellular space is tightly regulated to ensure that the NaCl concentration is always between 135 and 145 mmol/L; thus in a healthy person the NaCl concentration is the variable that is protected or regulated (Hew-Butler, Verbalis, et al., 2006), *not the volume of fluid in the extracellular space,* nor indeed the athlete's body weight. This means that the ECF volume will be sacrificed, if necessary, in order to protect the NaCl concentration. It follows that if the NaCl concentration is suddenly reduced within hours as occurs in EAH and EAHE, then the primary abnormality has to be in the (abnormal) regulation of the volume of the ECF, which has been allowed to expand in excess of the total amount of NaCl that it contains.

EAH and EAHE cannot be due exclusively to a loss of NaCl; if that were the case, the volume of the ECF would simply be adjusted (reduced) to ensure that the NaCl concentration remained within the normal range until enough NaCl had been ingested to correct the deficit. This is a remarkably effective mechanism because simply reducing the ECF volume by 1 L (figure 9.12*b*, page 277) reduces by 140 mmol (3.2 g) the amount of sodium needed to maintain the blood sodium concentration (at 140 mmol/L). This is the amount of sodium present in 3 to 7 L of the sweat of an acclimatized human athlete eating a moderately high-salt diet.

One of the persistent claims of the sports drink industry has been that EAH and EAHE are caused by large and uncorrected NaCl losses in the sweat of salty sweaters so that this condition can be prevented only by ingesting NaCl-containing sports drink, even though the NaCl content of such drinks is in the homeopathic range (~20 mmol/L) compared to the blood sodium concentration (140 mmol/L).

This advice is simply wrong. Had it been acknowledged after 1985 that EAH and EAHE are preventable diseases caused by abnormalities in the regulation of the body water content and are not due to sodium deficiency, lives could have been saved.

The sports drink industry has staked its claims on the principles of salt deficiency, proclaiming that the sodium consumed in a person's general diet is not enough and that sodium supplementation, via electrolyte-containing sports drinks, can prevent muscle cramps, heat illness, and sodium deficiency during long-duration exercise. These claims ignore the body's exquisite regulations of sodium concentration and a wealth of research on the subject.

Salt Deficiency and Muscle Cramps

K. Neville Moss, professor of coal mining at Birmingham University (UK), was one of the first to undertake relevant studies of "heat" cramps in 1923 (Moss, 1923). He studied miners working underground and showed that their hourly sweat rates during a 5½-hour shift ranged from 400 to 1,450 ml/hr, whereas average fluid intake rates were reportedly 730 to 1,775 ml/hr. He also noted that heat-acclimatized miners sweated more than did unacclimatized miners and that the average sweat sodium chloride concentration was 0.224% (39 mmol/L) but that this "great loss of chloride by sweating is evidently related to the extra quantity of salt in the diet of the miners working in hot mines" (p. 193). He also noted that manual laborers in India "can lose 10 lbs (4.5 kg) in five hours without any apparent symptoms, though this represents 10% of his total body weight. . . . He could doubtlessly lose more before he commenced to suffer badly" (p. 194).

Together with three iconic British physiologists, Professor J.S. Haldane, his son J.B.S. Haldane, and Professor A.V. Hill, Moss then set out to study miners in Lancashire who developed muscle cramps during activity. Haldane "suggested that cramp may depend upon excessive losses of chloride by sweating" (p. 196). As a result, the excited trio of Haldane Jr., Hill, and Moss went to a "deep coal face at Pendleton Colliery and examined the urine. A sample of urine obtained at the end of the shift from one of the colliers who was subject to cramp was found to be practically free from chloride,[3] though very little urine was passed. It gave only the slightest cloudiness with silver nitrate, though only 5cc were secreted during 4½ hours. This phenomenon, which is never met with under normal conditions, and hardly ever at any time, made it quite clear that there was excessive shortage of chlorides in the blood" (p. 196). Moss understood that sweating alone would not produce this effect because sweat contains a lower (sodium) chloride content than does blood so that "sweating by itself would tend to concentrate the chloride in the blood plasma" (p. 196). But Moss was aware of a publication showing that animals forced to ingest large volumes of water developed "water poisoning" (Rowntree, 1923) in which they developed "twitching of the muscles, passing on into convulsions" (p. 196). Thus he concluded that "Miner's cramp, and with it the symptoms of fatigue . . . must thus apparently be attributed to water poisoning" (p. 196).

Moss' solution was to provide miners with salt drinks made by the addition of 10 grams of NaCl to a gallon (3.79 L) of water. This solution had a sodium chloride concentration of 45 mmol/L (0.26%), which is approximately 3 times the concentration of Gatorade. Four of seven miners treated with this solution felt they benefitted, but one felt worse. "Curing" only four of seven subjects is not a meaningful effect.

Thus was born the theory that muscle cramping is due to a sodium deficit caused by excessive sodium losses in sweat, the forerunner of the salty sweater myth, and is compounded by an excessive water intake. According to a theory first proposed in 1929 that excessive and unregulated sodium losses in sweat cause a sodium deficit which in turn causes muscle cramping—a theory that would continue to be promoted by the scientists advising GSSI and ACSM as recently as 2007—Hancock, Whitehouse, and Haldane explained how a sodium deficit that develops during exercise causes this to happen: "It is clear that if a man is sweating, and at the same time replacing the fluid lost by

3 Prior to about the 1950s it was not possible to measure the concentration of sodium in biological samples. But since the chloride ion concentration in biological samples varies with charges in the sodium concentrations, the chloride ion concentrations can be used as a surrogate measure of the sodium concentration. Thus, before they were able to measure sodium concentrations in biological samples, scientists used the chloride concentration as a surrogate indicator of body sodium content and hence the adequacy of the body sodium stores.

Testing the urine for its chloride concentration also became the method for determining whether a patient was sodium deficient. During my medical training, this test—known as the Fantus test—was the standard laboratory method for determining the presence or absence of sodium deficiency. But today we are encouraged to believe that it is unnecessary to study the urine if one wishes to detect sodium deficiency or the adequacy of sodium balance. Instead, it is argued that the presence of abnormally high concentrations of sodium in the sweat indicates the presence of a sodium deficiency—truly a remarkable distortion.

drinking ordinary water, there will be a tendency, since much chloride may be lost in the sweat, for the percentage of chloride in the blood-plasma and whole body to fall, with corresponding tendency for what is at present usually called the 'osmotic pressure' of the blood-plasma to fall. This tendency is, however, ordinarily met to a large extent by the action of the kidneys, which excrete the excess of water while retaining chloride which would otherwise be excreted. During hard muscular work, however, the kidneys are thrown out of action . . . this being doubtless due to the blood-supply being diverted from the kidneys to the muscles and skin. The body is thus left defenseless against the effects of loss of chloride, with the result that unless a good reserve of chloride is available the acute symptoms [of muscle cramping] described by Moss may be produced" (Hancock, Whitehouse, et al., 1929a, p. 43).

According to this theory, miner's cramps developed when "warnings against drinking too much water have been disregarded" (Moss, 1923, p. 198). But in later decades, studies of fluid balance in some patients with heat cramps failed to show that all were overhydrated, because most either lost weight during exercise or gained weight during recovery, indicating that they had lost some body water at the time the cramps developed (Noakes, 1992). However, urine output was high, indicating that severe dehydration was not a likely etiological factor (because dehydration reduces urine production).

Professor Haldane was an enthusiastic supporter of the accuracy of his theory now considered "proven" by Dr. Moss' analysis of a single urine sample in one miner who did not have cramps at the time the sample was taken: "Now a man who is both sweating and working hard, and is at the same time drinking water to relieve his thirst, is losing chloride rapidly in his sweat and at the same time replacing the sweat, which contains about a quarter per cent of sodium chloride, by practically pure water.[4] The kidneys at the same time are out of action, so cannot deal with the excess diffusion pressure of water. The result is an acute rise in the diffusion pressure of water or fall in the 'osmotic pressure'; and violent attacks of cramp are symptomatic of this" (Haldane, 1928, pp. 609-610). He continued, "Perhaps few persons realize how much sweat, and therefore how much chloride, a man who is thoroughly acclimatized to heat may lose in a short time" (p. 610).[5] Thus he concluded that the cause of heat cramp is "acute poisoning by water" (p. 609).

Prevention was based on the approach first proposed by Moss: Haldane suggested ingesting more sodium by eating red herrings and highly salted bacon or adding salt to their water or tea. That this advice crossed the Atlantic and reached the United States by the 1930s is shown by a publication on muscle cramps written by

---

4   This is the explanation provided by Drs. Hiller and Laird for the EAH and EAHE that they detected in the Ironman Hawaii triathletes after 1983.

5   In another publication, Haldane reported that one man lost 18 pounds (8 kg) of sweat in the course of a shift, and this sweat contained about an ounce (28 g) of salt—twice what the average man consumed in all forms per day. Twenty-eight grams of sodium chloride equates to 483 mmoles in 8 L of sweat at a sweat sodium (chloride) concentration of 60 mmol/L. This high concentration indicates that these miners were indeed eating diets with very high salt contents. In fact, Haldane reported that "the salt loss was instinctively made up above ground by means of bacon, kippers, salted beer, and the like" (Brockbank, 1929, p. 65).

Dr. John H. Talbot of the Harvard Fatigue Laboratory (Talbott, 1935). There, Talbot concluded this: "This lowering of the sodium and chloride in the serum,[6] from loss in the sweat without adequate replacement is considered to be the principal causative mechanism in the production of heat cramps"[7] (p. 359) so that "in the condition under discussion there is a loss of salt and water from the body with a replacement principally of water. If this major process is continued irrespective of the secondary processes, there will be a lowering of the sodium and chloride concentration below normal. When the critical level for sodium and chloride is reached in the working subject, muscle cramps will occur" (pp. 359-360). As a result, prevention of the condition was relatively simple: Ingest more sodium.

Other studies also claimed that salt ingestion prevented these cramps, suggesting that the condition is due to sodium deficiency or "water intoxication" or both (Brockbank, 1929; Derrick, 1934; Glover, 1931; Ladell, 1949; Oswald, 1925; Talbott and Michelsen, 1933), but the reported data do not provide any convincing evidence that muscle cramping during exercise is caused by salt deficiency. Perhaps as a consequence of this, the U.S. military was advising its soldiers to ingest 0.5% to 1.0% sodium chloride solutions "under all conditions conducive to undue chloride losses" (McCord, 1931).

6 Talbot actually measured the osmolality of blood in subjects with muscle cramps and found that it was not reduced in 10 of 13 subjects he treated. Thus, "the lowering of the concentration of certain electrolytes in the serum from loss in the sweat is associated with a concomitant increase in other constituents so that the osmotic pressure is maintained" (Talbott, 1935, p. 359). But this is anomalous because he also reported that both blood sodium and chloride concentrations were reduced. Since the blood sodium concentration is the principal determinant of the blood osmolality, this finding is improbable. This means that there was likely an error in Talbot's measurements of either the blood sodium concentrations or of blood osmolality. If his blood sodium measurements were incorrect, his theory that muscle cramps are due to sodium deficiency is undermined.

7 This advice sounds suspiciously similar to that offered by the GSSI and its scientific spokespersons for the prevention of EAH and muscle cramps in the 1990s (chapter 9) suggesting that knowledge on this topic has not advanced much in nearly 100 years.

More than 85 years later, the GSSI and its scientists continue to evoke this explanation for both EAH and muscle cramping even though it cannot be correct because (a) athletes who develop muscle cramps do not have low blood sodium concentrations so that a sodium deficiency cannot cause the condition (Maughan, 1986; Schwellnus, 2007; Schwellnus, 2009; Schwellnus, Drew et al., 2011; Schwellnus, Nicol, et al., 2004; Sulzer, Schwellnus, et al., 2005); (b) conversely, people with EAH and EAHE do not complain of muscle cramping even though they can develop large increases in blood enzyme concentrations (Bruso, Hoffman, et al., 2010; Ellis, Cuthill, et al., 2009) compatible with severely impaired muscle cell function; (c) as is proven in chapter 9, EAH is not caused by sodium deficiency; and (d) EAH cannot occur only as a result of overdrinking water. Rather, there must also be abnormal fluid retention as a result of syndrome of inappropriate antidiuretic hormone hypersecretion (SIADH) or related phenomena.

In summary, the theory that muscle cramping is due to the development of a sodium deficit during exercise is based on the measurement of a single urine sample in a healthy miner working at the Pendleton Colliery, Lancashire, in the early 1920s and who did not have cramps at the time the measurement was made. Such is the power of dogma (box 4.2, page 116).

BOX 4.2   Dogma of Muscle Cramping

That muscle cramps are caused by salt deficiency is a historical dogma based on a single urine sample and sustained for more than 80 years in the absence of definitive evidence. "Cramps are almost an inevitable consequence of a low concentration of sodium in the extracellular fluid, and have always been associated with hard work in the heat (Moss, 1923; Talbott, 1935). . . . These cramps start locally and may spread to the whole muscle and to adjacent muscle groups, but are promptly relieved by intravenous hypertonic saline (Ladell, 1949)" (Ladell, 1957, p. 193). Thus spoke W.S.S. Ladell, MD, PhD, at the 21 February, 1957, meeting of the Royal Society of Tropical Medicine and Hygiene held in London, England. At the time, Ladell was stationed in Lagos, Nigeria, at the Hot Climate Physiological Research Unit. The audience could only infer from his statement that hard work in the heat induced large sodium losses in sweat and that such losses then caused the "concentration of sodium in the extracellular fluid" (of which blood is a part) to fall substantially. According to this explanation, losses of salt in sweat must always cause the blood sodium concentrations to fall, leading to EAH as currently understood. But, in fact, neither Moss (1923) nor Talbott (1935) ever showed that their miners with muscle cramps had water intoxication or as we currently understand the condition, EAH. The sole evidence for an altered sodium metabolism in this condition was that single urine sample collected from the miner in the Pendleton Colliery in 1923. Recall also that muscle cramping is a disease of antiquity, whereas EAH was first described in 1981. Nor has it ever been shown that EAH is associated with muscle cramps as the principal symptom (even though the integrity of the muscle cells is clearly affected as shown by the substantial leakage of enzymes from the interior of the cells into the blood stream (Bruso, Hoffman, et al., 2010; Ellis, Cuthill, et al., 2009). Rather, the main symptom of EAH is an altered level of consciousness.

This failure of proof has led to the adoption 50 years later of a circular logic favored by many scientists with attachments to the sports drink industry (figure 4.3): The presence of muscle cramping indicates that there is a sodium deficiency since muscle cramps are always caused by a sodium deficiency. (We "know" this to be "true" because it was proven by Moss in 1923). If the blood sodium concentration is normal in people with muscle cramps (as historically proven), then this must be because a true sodium deficiency can occur, for example in muscle, even though a sodium deficiency cannot exist in the ECF (since the blood sodium concentration is normal). Thus, exercise-associated muscle cramping (EAMC) is a special case of sodium deficiency in which a normal blood sodium concentration fails to expose the presence of a true sodium deficiency inside the muscle cells. Hence, modern scientists have discovered a novel disease not previously described: *sodium-deficiency muscle cramping in the presence of a normal blood sodium concentration.*[8]

It is inconceivable that there could be a deficit located only in the intracellular sodium store with an intact extracellular sodium store. This would require either a failure of inward movement of sodium from the ECF into the ICF or, alternatively, a failure of regulation of the normal processes by which sodium is pumped from the ICF into the ECF. Since the latter is an energy-requiring process, failure of that process always leads to the accumulation of sodium in the ICF, not in the ECF. The promotion of physiological myths leads ultimately to their exposure as wishful thinking dressed up in the guise of truth. Even so, the concept became established that salt deficiency could occur in those who exercised vigorously and sweated profusely for prolonged periods in extremely hot conditions

8   Sodium "deficiency" might occur without loss of sodium from the body if osmotically active sodium was osmotically inactivated and stored in an intracellular site. But this would still cause the blood sodium concentration to fall (figure 9.15, page 288).

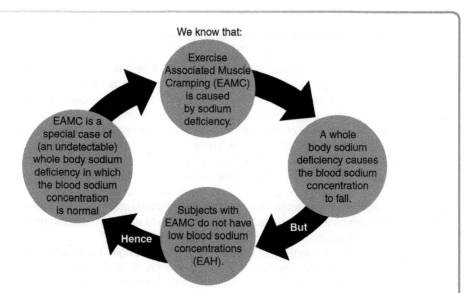

We know that:

Exercise Associated Muscle Cramping (EAMC) is caused by sodium deficiency.

A whole body sodium deficiency causes the blood sodium concentration to fall.

But

Subjects with EAMC do not have low blood sodium concentrations (EAH).

Hence

EAMC is a special case of (an undetectable) whole body sodium deficiency in which the blood sodium concentration is normal

FIGURE 4.3 The circular argument that has been necessary for sustaining the myth that a whole body sodium deficit causes EAMC. The finding that athletes with EAMC have normal blood sodium concentrations indicates that they do not have a sodium deficit in the largest body sodium store, the ECF.

while drinking only water. This salt deficiency caused a condition known as heat cramps. Since EAH had not been described at that time, scientists like Ladell missed the obvious conclusion of their theory: Muscle cramps must be a complication of EAH since they occur when a state of advanced sodium deficiency has developed, causing the blood sodium concentration also to fall. But people suffering from EAH do not complain of muscle cramps.

It turns out that not much has changed in the past 85 years. In July 2008 the ACSM (and therefore Gatorade-funded) journal *Current Sports Medicine Reports* published a series of articles on sodium in athletes. Prominent in the journal was an article by Michael Bergeron, PhD, titled "Muscle Cramps During Exercise: Is It Fatigue or Is It Electrolyte Deficit?" (Bergeron, 2008). Dr. Bergeron has conducted many Gatorade-funded studies and serves on the GSSI. Bergeron argued that there are "two distinct and dissimilar general categories of exercise-associated muscle cramps" (p. S50). The first, according to Bergeron, is due to overuse or overconditioning; the second is due to "extensive sweating and a consequent significant whole-body exchangeable sodium deficit," which "can lead to more widespread muscle cramping, even when there is minimal or no muscle overload and fatigue" (p. S50).

For his explanation of muscle cramping caused by muscle overload and fatigue, Dr. Bergeron refers to the motor neuron control theory of muscle cramping, the theory that has been developed by my colleague, Professor Martin Schwellnus, and is discussed subsequently. Bergeron expends relatively little effort on this theory, preferring rather to focus on the more traditional "electrolyte deficit" theory of muscle cramping.

Bergeron begins by quoting his own work and that of other Gatorade-funded scientists showing that "Whether during a single race, match, game, or training session or consequent to multiple game or repeated-day exercise bouts, a sizeable whole-body exchangeable sodium deficit develops when sweat sodium and chloride losses measurably exceed salt (Bergeron, 1996; Bergeron, 2003; Stofan, Zachwieja, et al., 2005) intake" (p. S51). The only problem is that in none of these studies was whole-body sodium balance measured. Thus,

(continued)

BOX 4.2 **Dogma of Muscle Cramping** *(continued)*

---

the basis for his subsequent discussion that explains *how* this "whole-body exchangeable sodium deficit" develops is trite. But ultimately Dr. Bergeron is faced with the problem of how to explain the presence of a "whole-body exchangeable sodium deficit" when the blood sodium concentration is normal (figure 4.3). He is unable to provide a single reference in which the presence of this sodium deficit has been shown to exist in a subject with a normal blood sodium concentration and muscle cramping. Dr. Bergeron concludes that "maintenance of hydration and sodium balance is the proven effective prevention strategy for averting exertional heat cramps in athletes and workers during training, competition, and other physical activities" (p. S53). Unfortunately, he does not cite a randomized, controlled clinical trial showing that athletes who maintain their "hydration and sodium balance" develop fewer muscle cramps than do those who fail especially to maintain "sodium balance" during training and competition.

As shown in box 4.4 (page 125), it takes more than a single 1.8-hour tennis match and the excretion of ~160 mmol of sodium in sweat (Bergeron, 1996; Bergeron, 2003) to develop such deficits, if indeed it is ever possible to develop such deficits given the nature of the controls that humans have developed to maintain sodium balance (figure 4.1, page 108).

Causes of Exercise-Associated Muscle Cramping (EAMC)

The theory that large sodium losses in sweat causes heat or muscle cramps originated in England in the 1920s and was soon adopted by David Dill in the United States. The original evidence on which this theory is based was that single urine sample taken by the Haldanes on the miner in the Pendelton Colliery. It is surprising that there is still no good evidence that sodium deficiency plays any role in causing muscle cramping. The person most responsible for pointing out this fact is my colleague Professor Martin Schwellnus (Schwellnus, 2007; Schwellnus, Derman, et al., 1997; Schwellnus, Drew, et al., 2008).

9 In the end, Schwellnus chose not to include his paper in *Current Reports in Sports Medicine,* choosing rather an independent, peer-reviewed journal, the *British Journal of Sports Medicine.*

In a paper presented at the Gatorade-sponsored 2007 Vail Conference on Sodium Balance and Exercise, Schwellnus (2009) presented the following observations and arguments:[9]

- Muscle cramping can occur in individuals exercising in cool conditions and even extreme cold water in the case of swimmers. There is no evidence that the body temperatures of subjects with muscle cramping are any higher than those of control subjects performing the same exercise, nor does passive heating cause muscle cramping. Thus the term *heat cramps* is a misnomer.
- Not a single published scientific paper shows that blood electrolyte concentrations, including the sodium concentration, are abnormal at the time subjects develop EAMC. In contrast, four separate studies have established that athletes with EAMC have normal blood sodium concentrations (Drew, 2006; Maughan, 1986; Schwellnus, Nicol, et al., 2004; Sulzer, Schwellnus,

et al., 2005). Thus, Schwellnus (2009) concludes that "the available evidence to date does not support the hypothesis that electrolyte depletion or dehydration causes EAMC—therefore an alternate hypothesis . . . has to be considered" (p. 404).

■ There is not a single published scientific paper showing that athletes with EAMC are more dehydrated than controls without the condition. Instead, four separate studies (Drew, 2006; Maughan, 1986; Schwellnus, Nicol, et al., 2004; Sulzer, Schwellnus, et al., 2005) show that athletes with EAMC are no more dehydrated than control subjects who complete the same exercise bouts without developing EAMC.

■ The sole evidence that salty sweating causes EAMC comes from case reports of 23 subjects from three separate studies authored either by Dr. Bergeron (1996; 2003) or originating from the GSSI (Stofan, Zachwieja, et al., 2005). In most of these reports, there were no adequate control groups, and in none were either sweat sodium concentrations or total body sodium stores measured at the time that EAMC developed. In addition, in one study the daily salt intake of crampers was higher than that of noncrampers. In addition, sweat sodium concentrations were high in crampers (53 mmol/L) (Horswill, Stofan, et al., 2009), indicating that subjects were in positive sodium balance, the opposite of the authors' conclusion.

■ There is no sweat sodium concentration that defines a salty sweater. However, the sweat sodium concentrations in the three cited studies were either normal or low when compared to values reported in other studies of subjects who did not develop EAMC.

■ When cramping occurs in people with medical conditions causing hyponatremia, the cramps occur at rest and are generalized, affecting multiple muscles. In contrast, EAMC typically affects only muscle groups that are involved in the repetitive contractions associated with that specific activity. It is not clear how a generalized sodium deficiency can cause cramping that is localized exclusively to the muscles used in the activity.

■ Recovery from EAMC occurs with rest and passive stretching. In addition, stretching is known to prevent one form of cramping, those that occur during sleep—nocturnal cramps (Daniell, 1979). It is not clear how these findings can be explained simply on the basis of an unreplaced sodium deficit.

Since the theory of sodium deficit and dehydration does not explain the development of EAMC, Schwellnus has been instrumental in developing an alternative "altered neuromuscular control" hypothesis for the cause of EAMC. This theory was first published in 1997 (Schwellnus, Derman, et al., 1997), shortly after the 1996 ACSM position stand had just been released. That position stand includes this statement: "Electrolytes (primarily NaCl) should be added to the fluid replacement solution to . . . reduce the probability for development of hyponatremia" (Convertino, Armstrong, et al., 1996, p. iv). Eleven years later, the 2007 position stand (Armstrong, Casa, et al. 2007) includes these statements: "Sweat Na^+ losses that are replaced with hypotonic fluid has been proposed as the primary cause of EAMC" (p. 564) and "EAMC responds well to rest, prolonged stretch with the muscle groups at full length, and oral NaCl ingestion in fluids or foods (i.e., 1/8-1/4 teaspoon of table salt added to 300-500 ml of fluids or sports drink") (p. 564).

This neuromuscular control theory of EAMC suggests that muscle cramping occurs when reflexes that normally inhibit the actions of a "cramp generator" (Khan and Burne, 2007) (situated somewhere in the nervous system, probably in the spinal cord) become quiescent. As a result, the activity of the generator is unchecked, causing muscle cramping. Muscle fatigue, in particular, increases the activity of the generator and reduces inhibitory reflexes (Hutton and Nelson, 1986; Nelson and Hutton, 1985).

The first study suggesting that the motor activity in cramps was originating in the central nervous system was reported in 1957 (Norris, Gasteiger, et al., 1957). Other studies have shown that it is possible to produce muscle cramping by stimulation of the muscle at a specific threshold frequency (Minetto, Botter, et al., 2008; Stone, Edwards, et al., 2003) and conversely that stimulation of the Achilles tendon inhibits the muscle cramp (Khan and Burne, 2007). More recently a magical effect of ingestion of pickle juice has been reported (box 4.3). In contrast, the ingestion of Gatorade was associated with a higher incidence of postexercise experimentally induced muscle cramping (69%) than was the incidence (54%) when the same subjects ingested nothing during the experiments (Jung, Bishop, et al., 2005). The authors concluded this: "It would appear that hydration or electrolyte supplementation did not influence the incidence of cramps" (p. 74). The GSSI and its scientists have not adopted this information in their publications. All these studies favor the theory that "altered neuromuscular control during fatiguing muscular exercise is the principal mechanism in the etiology of acute EAMC" (Schwellnus, 2009, p. 407).

BOX 4.3   Pickle Juice and Electrically Induced Muscle Cramping

Intrigued by the reports of athletic trainers that cramps can be reversed by the ingestion of pickle juice (an acidic brine), Kevin Miller and colleagues from North Dakota State University (Miller, Mack, et al., 2010b) designed an experiment to evaluate this observation. They showed that ingestion of pickle juice immediately reduced the duration of electrically induced muscle cramping in subjects who had exercised sufficiently to lose 3% of their body weight and 145 mmol of sodium. Thus 75 ml of pickle juice ingested at the onset of an electrically induced muscle cramp reduced the duration of the cramp by 49 seconds compared to the duration of cramps that occurred without ingestion of pickle juice or when only water was ingested.

Because the effect occurred within about 90 seconds of ingestion of pickle juice, it could not have been due to changes in blood sodium concentrations or the reversal of dehydration since the fluid would still have been retained in the stomach at that time. A subsequent study showed that the ingestion of an effective volume of pickle juice does not change blood sodium concentrations (Miller, Mack, et al., 2009). The authors speculated that drinking pickle juice, with its high acid content, may stimulate a reflex in the back of the throat, and this in turn triggers a reflex that lessens or stops the cramp. This finding supports Schwellnus' neuromuscular theory of how muscle cramps are caused.

A separate study from the United States found that nonfatiguing exercise that caused a 3% loss in body weight did not alter the strength of the electrical stimulus needed for inducing muscle cramping. The authors concluded that "cramps may be more associated with neuromuscular fatigue than dehydration/electrolyte losses" (Miller, Mack, et al., 2010a, p. 2056).

More recently, Schwellnus and colleagues have completed the first prospective study of the factors that identify those at risk of developing EAMC (Schwellnus, Drew, et al., 2011). Forty-four of a cohort of 210 athletes competing in the South African Ironman Triathlon developed EAMC during the race. There was no difference in body weight changes or blood sodium concentrations between those who did and did not develop EAMC. Instead, triathletes who developed EAMC had faster overall times and a higher prevalence of previous EAMC. The authors concluded that there were two factors that predicted risk of EAMC—a history and a faster finishing time—suggesting that those who exercise at a higher intensity are at greater risk. The study again showed that dehydration and altered serum electrolyte concentrations are unrelated to EAMC.

Salt Deficiency and Heat Illness

As with the idea that sodium deficiency can cause muscle cramps, a myth has developed that sodium deficiency can cause heat illness. My search suggests that Dr. Ladell was one of the first scientists who attempted to determine whether humans could become salt deficient during exposure to the heat. At the time, Ladell was a young, recently certified medical doctor serving with the British Army in North Africa during World War II. In time, Ladell would become a highly regarded thermal physiologist. In his studies in the British Army, Ladell attempted to measure sodium and fluid balance in the soldiers he was treating for heat exhaustion.[10] He concluded that some were salt deficient (heat exhaustion type I—salt deficiency) (Ladell, Waterlow, et al., 1944b) and some were water deficient (heat exhaustion type II—water deficiency) (Ladell, Waterlow, et al., 1944a). These conditions then became part of the accepted classification of the heat illnesses, and the terms are still in use today. The diagnosis of salt deficiency was made on the basis of the *absence* of chloride in the urine using the Fantus test (Marriott, 1947, p. 289). More recently the condition has been diagnosed on the basis of excessive amounts of sodium in urine and sweat, an unfortunate distortion.

But the problem with this classification is that the sodium chloride content of the body regulates its water content as described earlier in this chapter. As a result, at least acutely (i.e., over a period less than 48 hours), a pure salt deficiency will produce essentially the same consequences as a pure water deficit with the exception that the blood sodium concentration is more likely to be normal in

10   There is the ongoing problem of exactly what constitutes the heat illnesses and especially heat exhaustion. As described subsequently, Ladell and colleagues described the symptoms and signs that they considered to be diagnostic of heat exhaustion. The symptoms were all related to a reduction of blood pressure on standing. Thus, the condition he was describing is exercise-associated postural hypotension (EAPH), which is caused by abnormalities in the regulation of blood pressure immediately on the termination of exercise and which has nothing to do with sodium deficiency, or dehydration for that matter.

a pure salt deficit. In both cases the total body water content will be reduced and the body will attempt to maintain the blood sodium concentration within the normal range that does not cause brain damage. The physiological differences between the two conditions are described in table 4.1.

This theoretical exercise shows that the predominant feature of a pure sodium deficit is circulatory failure, not muscle cramping. It also shows that the body can potentially adapt to a low sodium intake but not to an absence of water. By reducing sodium losses in the urine especially but also in the sweat and by mobilizing Na^+ from the internal exchangeable sodium stores, the body should theoretically be able to adapt to a low salt intake for prolonged periods (weeks or months perhaps) until the exchangeable sodium reserves are depleted. While this occurs, the TBW could theoretically be protected, the blood sodium concentration would be within the normal range, and the only measurable change would be a reduction in the amount of osmotically inactive Na in the internal body stores. Ultimately when these reserves are depleted, the athlete would present with a reduction in TBW and a low blood pressure, similar to the condition known as Addison's disease, which occurs in people who (among other abnormalities) are unable to secrete aldosterone usually because of damage to the adrenal gland. In contrast, a true pure water deficit will produce incapacitation within 2 to 3 days as a result of overwhelming thirst, hypotension, and ultimately kidney failure.

TABLE 4.1   Physiological Responses to Either Pure Water or Pure Sodium Deficits

	Pure water deficit	Pure sodium deficit
Blood sodium concentration	Increased.	Normal.
Extent of reduction in TBW	In proportion to the extent of the water deficit.	In proportion to the extent of the sodium deficit.
Site of fluid loss	All fluid compartments.	Predominantly from the ECF.
Mechanism of control	1. Increased sodium and water retention by the kidneys (as a result of increased AVP/ADH) and renin/aldosterone secretion. 2. Removal of Na^+ from the ECF with storage as osmotically inactive Na in the internal body stores.	1. Increased sodium retention by the kidneys as a result of increased renin/aldosterone secretion. 2. Initially water excretion to maintain a normal blood sodium concentration. Later water retention leads to hyponatremia. 3. Mobilization of osmotically inactive Na to Na^+ in the ECF.
Diagnosis	Pure dehydration with sodium and water retention leading to varying levels of hypernatremia. Low urine volume. Marked thirst. Unimpaired cardiovascular function until the dehydration becomes severe (>15-20% BW loss).	Volume depletion (of the ECF) leading progressively to apathy and hypotension (electrolyte shock) (Nadal, Pedersen, et al., 1941); and ultimately hyponatremia after 2-3 days (box 4.4, page 125). Urine volume in proportion to intake. Absence of thirst.

Data from Mange, Matsuura, Cizman, et al., 1997; Marriott 1947; Spital 2007.

Ladell began his research when he was posted to Shaiba in Southern Iraq from May to October 1943. The daily temperatures during that period were in excess of 38 °C (100.4 °F) for 4 consecutive months; for 3 weeks during that period daily temperatures were in excess of 46 °C (114.8 °F). Relative humidity was generally lower than 15%. The soldiers needed to drink about 7.5 L each day to stay in fluid balance or about three times as much as those living in more temperate environments. They were also encouraged to take in ~30 g of sodium chloride per day. If we assume that subjects lost 6.5 L of sweat and 1 L of urine per day and if urine sodium losses were minimal due to activation of sodium-conserving mechanisms, this would require their sweat sodium chloride concentrations to be 4.6 g/L or 79 mmol/L. This value is about twice that measured in modern athletes who are in sodium balance (Costill, 1977). Since such high values are measured only in subjects eating a sodium-rich diet, the conclusion must be that Ladell's subjects (a) were eating a high-sodium diet (as they were) and (b) could not have been sodium deficient.

Ladell's problem was that he began his research with the strong belief that sodium deficiency is likely to be the most important factor causing heat illness in the British Army in Iraq. Why else would he have brought with him from England the instruments that would allow him to measure blood and urine sodium concentrations in these soldiers? He could, after all, have brought equipment to measure any number of other variables. But he chose to study salt. Since salt was his passion, his natural bias would be to presume that whatever he observed was definitely caused by what he was measuring, specifically blood and urine sodium concentrations. How could it be otherwise?[11]

Ladell measured daily sweat losses (~7 L) during the hottest periods and also sweat sodium concentrations. From this he calculated that subjects were losing 15 to 25 g of sodium chloride per day. But chloride was always present in the subjects' urine, indicating that no one was sodium deficient. Thus the conditions he described were not due to sodium deficiency. This is further proven by the high sweat sodium concentrations that he measured in many subjects (figure 4.4, page 124). Since the sweat sodium concentration can be reduced to below 10 mmol/L in those ingesting little sodium, the presence of such high sweat sodium concentrations in his subjects proves that they were not truly sodium deficient. Rather, these data prove only that his subjects were suffering from a condition of excessive sodium intake producing a physiological state of high salt losses during sweating (excretion), or salt wasting, the opposite of Ladell's conclusion. To diagnose a state of true salt deficiency, Ladell needed to show that these soldiers were excreting essentially no salt (chloride) in either their sweat or their urine.

But Ladell failed to show that any of his subjects were sodium deficient. Yet he (and many others since) believed that he distinguished two types of heat exhaustion, the features of which he was the first to describe, and which he considered to be due to either water or salt deficiency. It is not clear how he distinguished

11 A real challenge for scientists is that they tend to believe that whatever they measure as part of their research must also be the sole explanation for what they discover. Thus, Ladell would be inclined to believe that the "disease" he was studying—heat exhaustion—was caused exclusively by what he was measuring, specifically sodium and water balance. Such reductionism ignores the fact that humans are complex organisms so that simple explanations of causation are never likely to be the complete truth.

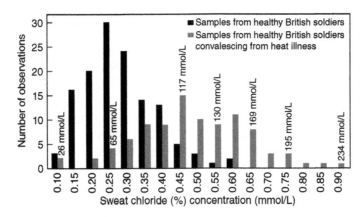

FIGURE 4.4 Sweat chloride concentrations in subjects with heat illness studied by Ladell, Waterlow, et al., 1944b. The very high values in excess of 140 mmol/L are biologically impossible since the blood chloride concentration (from which the sweat is derived) is seldom higher than this value. Thus Dr. Ladell's analytical methods must have produced inaccurate results in a number of subjects. According to these results, most of these soldiers have cystic fibrosis, which is not possible because that disease precludes military service.

Adapted from *The Lancet*, vol. 244, W.S. Ladell, J.C. Waterlow, and M.F. Hudson, "Desert climate: Physiological and clinical observations," 491-497, copyright 1944, with permission from Elsevier.

between the two conditions. Table 4.1 suggests that the only way to distinguish between the two conditions would be to measure the blood sodium concentration, the rates of water excretion by the kidneys, blood AVP/ADH concentrations, and changes in the size of the internal exchangeable sodium stores. But Ladell measured none of these variables. Instead, because of his training as a doctor, he focused on the key symptoms the soldiers reported:

"The effect of standing was dramatic. The pulse became progressively more difficult to feel and more rapid. The blood pressure fell, and often could not be taken because the sounds were inaudible. The patient became increasingly pale, began to sweat profusely, to yawn and to complain of dizziness. He was obviously on the verge of syncope after standing for only one or two minutes" (Ladell, Waterlow, et al., 1944b, p. 495).

But people with true sodium deficiencies have low blood pressures when lying down, not just when standing (table 4.1). Instead, Ladell is describing the classic features of postural hypotension, which is caused by abnormalities in the regulation of cardiovascular function, in particular an abnormally low arteriolar vascular resistance resulting from inadequate activation of the sympathetic nervous system or excessive activation of the parasympathetic nervous system. Since this condition occurs most commonly after exercise in people who are neither significantly salt nor water deficient, it cannot be due to either or both of these abnormalities. Instead, the problem resides within the regulation of the blood pressure by the sympathetic and parasympathetic nervous systems. Thus, whether or not these subjects were sodium or water deficient, the cause of their illness was the development of postural hypotension as a result of inappropriate regulation of their peripheral vascular resistance.

The relevance of these studies to sport is difficult to understand because it is not clear whether the British soldiers who presented with "heat illness" had been active or simply living in hot conditions for prolonged periods. In addition, subjects were ingesting 25 g of salt per day so that predictably the sweat of most contained significant amounts of chloride (figure 4.4), the opposite of what happens in true sodium deficiency.

Some years later Ladell (1965) confessed to his errors: "It is apparent from what has been written above that it is impossible to predict what the electrolyte needs may be. *The controls are so good, however, that balance can be achieved at any level of intake over a wide range* [my emphasis]. Both the salt-starved but sweating Indonesian and the salt-replete sedentary American executive are taking exactly as much salt as will keep them in balance. Before this was realized high salt intakes, up to 40 g/day, were sometimes recommended for men in the troops, *probably contributed to rather than prevented their breakdown in the heat* [my emphasis]. Regrettably this tendency to 'oversalt' is not yet dead" (Ladell, 1957, p. 247). Presumably, as long as there are salt supplements and salt-containing sports drinks to be sold, this tendency to oversalt will not disappear in the immediate future (Moss, 2010).

As we shall see, humans can decrease their sweat sodium concentrations to almost zero when they must survive on a low-sodium diet, so the presence of high sweat sodium concentrations confirms the absence of a sodium deficiency. Despite this, it has become part of the literature that salt deficiency is an important cause of heat cramps and heat exhaustion (Armstrong, 2003; Pandolf and Burr, 2010).

The relevant question is *not* whether some military personnel exposed to extreme heat for months on end may fall ill and appear to improve when they are allowed to recover while ingesting salt and water. The important question is whether modern recreational athletes—in the course of a single tennis match or when competing in a 42 km marathon, the 90 km Comrades Marathon, the 160 km Western States Race, or the 226 km Ironman Hawaii Triathlon—are ever at risk of becoming salt deficient, given that the modern diet contains so much salt and that humans have an extraordinary capacity to conserve sodium (box 4.4).

BOX 4.4 Experimental Sodium Deficiency

In the early 1930s, R.A. McCance, assistant physician in charge of biochemical research at King's College Hospital, London, set out to determine if he could induce a state of sodium deficiency in humans. He wished to study the features of a disease caused by a pure sodium chloride deficiency without the associated water deficit that typically accompanies sodium chloride deficiency in patients with persistent vomiting or diarrhea.

McCance realized that mammals that do not sweat can exist on a very low sodium intake;[12] thus, the most appropriate species for study would be sweaty humans. To produce a state of chronic sodium deficiency, he decided to expose a group of subjects to a very low-salt diet for a prolonged period while they were forced to sweat profusely, at least once a day. Accordingly, he recruited four subjects whose names are recorded for posterity: Dr. McCance himself; P.M. Edwards, a female medical student from King's College Hospital; and R.B. Niven and D. Whitteridge, two male medical students from Oxford.

12 The common fruit fly, drosophila, can probably exist without any salt intake. Plants contain very little salt because they do not have extracellular fluid (where sodium is the most important electrolyte). Thus, salt may be important for humans but it is certainly not a crucial ingredient for many other living creatures.

(continued)

BOX 4.4 **Experimental Sodium Deficiency** *(continued)*

To ensure that they ate a low-salt diet, Mrs. McCance kindly allowed the two male subjects to live at the McCance household with her husband while she fed them a salt-free diet comprising "salt-free 'casein' bread, synthetic sodium chloride-free milk, salt-free butter, thrice boiled vegetables, jam, fruit, home-made salt-free shortbread and coffee" (McCance, 1936a, p. 823). To increase salt losses from the body, subjects lay in a radiant heat bath set at a temperature of 100 °F (38 °C) for 2 hours a day. This caused a sweat loss of 2 to 3 L. As a result, subjects lost about 1 kg of weight per day, or about 2 to 3 g sodium chloride.

Generally it took "about a week" (equivalent to a sweat loss of 14-21 L) to make the subjects "seriously deficient" (McCance, 1936a, p. 823), by which time the total loss of sodium chloride varied from 23 to 27 grams (390-460 mmol). McCance did not attempt to explain the origins of this sodium.

The subjects were then maintained in that state for 3 to 4 days. Common symptoms that they developed included general lethargy and mild cramps. McCance noted that the cramps were not of the severe, localized type previously described in miners but were "widespread, frequent, not very painful, and generally controllable" (McCance, 1936b, p. 250).

Initially the body weight loss tracked the sodium loss, but after the first 2 to 4 days the sodium loss continued, whereas body weight stabilized (figure 4.5a). During this time average blood sodium concentrations dropped by 14 mmol/L, from 155 to 137 mmol/L (McCance, 1937). Urine sodium losses dropped steeply from ~3 g/day on day 1 to 0.3 g or less thereafter. By the end of the experiment, urinary sodium losses had fallen to 10 mg/day.[13]

The findings in figure 4.5 can be explained if the initial response to human salt deficiency is a contraction of the ECF volume with maintenance of a normal or elevated blood sodium concentration. Thereafter the falling ECF volume produces a volume signal to increase AVP/ADH secretion with protection of the ECF volume despite an increasing sodium deficit. During this period, hyponatremia develops[14] as a result of increased water retention resulting from this increased AVP/ADH secretion, causing an increase in the ECF volume out of proportion to its sodium content.

McCance did not measure what happened to the sweat sodium concentrations during this time. Probably he assumed (incorrectly) that sweat sodium concentrations are not subject to change even as the body becomes progressively more sodium deficient.

13 McCance did not ask himself what biological mechanism produced this outcome. Had he asked that question, he might have been the person to discover the action of the adrenal cortical hormone aldosterone. Instead, Jerome Conn would be the first to do this less than 10 years later. In science, it is always important to ask the right questions.

14 Hyponatremia should be prevented by the mobilization of the osmotically inactive sodium stores according to the predictions of table 4.1, page 122. That this does not occur is surprising and indicates that our knowledge of why hyponatremia develops is still incomplete.

During recovery, subjects ate "highly salted foods such as anchovies and bacon" (McCance, 1936a, p. 823). "We ate the bacon out of the frying pan to avoid losing any of its salt, and then, to make assurance doubly sure, we washed out the pan with a little hot water and drank the washings." (p. 823). To correct the original deficit they needed to ingest the same amount of salt lost during the experiment (~20 g). Recovery was rapid as soon as >20 g of salt had been ingested. This usually occurred overnight with a regain of all the lost weight.

Interestingly, of the four subjects in Dr. McCance's original study, Miss Edwards, who did not live with the McCance family, failed to develop a sodium deficiency and her data were not included (McCance, 1937). I suspect that cooking her own food proved too much of a temptation for Miss Edwards and she was unable to re-create Mrs. McCance's salt-free cooking. Others have found it extremely difficult to generate a salt deficiency in free-living humans.

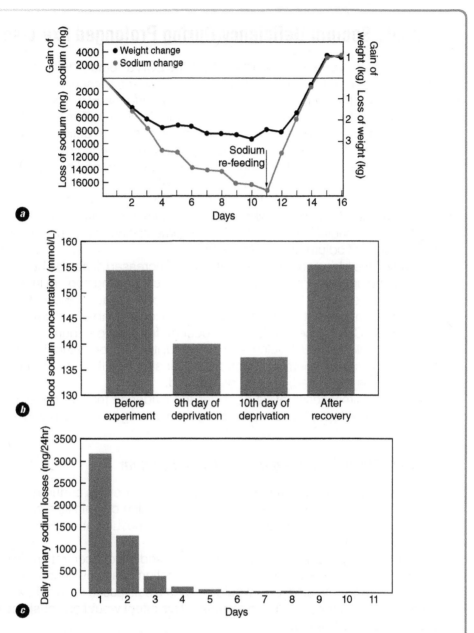

FIGURE 4.5 (a) Weight changes in a subject in the study of McCance et al. (1936b) who developed a progressive sodium deficit as a result of heavy daily sodium losses induced by sweating while ingesting very little dietary sodium. Sodium refeeding occurred on the 11th day of the experiment. (b) Blood sodium concentrations in the South African medical student R.B. Niven during the 15-day experiment. (c) Changes in daily urinary sodium losses in Dr. R.A. McCance showing an almost complete disappearance of sodium in his urine by the 5th day of the experiment.

Data from McCance 1936b.

Probably the most important conclusion of this study is that because we live in an environment in which salt is ubiquitous, cheap, freely available, and highly desirable, a sodium deficit is extremely difficult, perhaps impossible, to generate in free-living humans. Only under the most artificial laboratory conditions can such a deficit be produced.

Acute Sodium Deficiency During Prolonged Exercise

Because sodium is present predominantly in the ECF, a sodium deficiency can be diagnosed by a reduction in the total amount of sodium present in the ECF. This requires that both the ECF sodium concentration *and* the ECF volume be measured concurrently. Since it is difficult to measure the ECF volume, and because this measurement is seldom made, the diagnosis of sodium deficiency is usually made simply on the basis of the blood (ECF) sodium concentration. But this is illogical since the blood sodium concentration may be reduced because the ECF volume is increased (as occurs in EAH and EAHE). Unless the ECF volume is known, it cannot be established whether the body sodium content is increased, normal, or reduced in subjects whose blood sodium concentrations are reduced. All that can be concluded is that the ECF volume is increased out of proportion to the amount of sodium present in the ECF.

Similarly, if the blood sodium concentration is increased, it can be because the total body sodium content has increased (in those ingesting sodium in excess of bodily requirements and those who have an impaired capacity to lose the excess in urine or sweat or to store the excess in the exchangeable sodium stores) or because the ECF volume has fallen as occurs, for example, during prolonged exercise. But unless the ECF volume is measured, it cannot be determined whether an increased blood sodium concentration indicates that the total body sodium concentration is increased, normal, or reduced.

Given these limitations, let us consider the evidence that we currently have for "sodium deficiency" in athletes based on changes in the blood sodium concentrations.

Endurance Athletes Drinking Not at All or Ad Libitum

Before the early 1980s, athletes drank little during competitive endurance events. Usually they drank water or a cola drink, both of which contain little sodium. For example, the sodium content of Coca-Cola is ~7 mmol/L or about 60% less than that present in Gatorade.

Thus an analysis of published studies of blood sodium concentrations in endurance athletes in that era would provide an indication of any evidence for sodium deficiency in these athletes. This would happen if salt losses in sweat exceeded the amount of salt ingested during exercise. This effect would obviously be most apparent in salty sweaters.

Table 4.2 shows that only 1 (out of 30) of those studies contained some athletes whose blood sodium concentrations were low both before and after the race. Those data appear to be erroneous.[15] Every other study at the time reported exactly the same finding: *Blood sodium concentrations* always *rose during exercise.* In fact, blood sodium concentrations were not reduced in even one of the subjects in the other studies reviewed in the table. Since these athletes had all lost sodium in their sweat and urine during those races, their total body sodium contents must have been reduced after the race compared to their prerace values. But since humans are designed to regulate their blood sodium concentrations and the sodium content of the ECF regulates the ECF volume, so the sweating-induced reduction in ECF sodium content must cause a reduction in ECF volume, thereby maintaining near-normal blood sodium concentrations in these athletes.

TABLE 4.2   Serum Sodium Concentrations [Na⁺], Body Weight Loss (%), and Volumes of Fluid Ingested in Athletes Involved in Endurance Events

Race distance	Mean ± SD prerace plasma or serum [Na⁺] (mmol/L)	Mean ± SD postrace plasma or serum [Na⁺] (mmol/L)	Mean % BW loss	Mean volume of fluid ingested during race (ml)	n	Range of postrace plasma or serum [Na⁺] (mmol/L)	Reference
42 km R	141	156	5.1	ND	10	ND	Beckner and Winsor, 1954
85 km S	144 ± 3	152 ± 1	~5.0	2000	6	150-153	Astrand and Saltin, 1964
42 km R	ND	143 ± 3	~4.9	520	4	139-147	Pugh, Corbett, et al., 1967
42 km R	139 ± 2	145 ± 1	ND	ND	8	144-147	Rose, Carroll, et al., 1970
90 km R	136±4	137 ± 4	ND	ND	33	130-142 (prerace range 126-151)	Dancaster and Whereat, 1971
42 km R	146 ± 2	143 ± 3	ND	ND	14	ND	Viru and Korge, 1971
90 km S	142	141	2.6	2370	41	135-147	Refsum, Tveit, et al., 1973
42 km R	143 ± 1	148 ± 1	5.4	Ad libitum	5	ND	Riley, Pyke, et al., 1975
42 km R	141 ± 1	141 ± 1	4.3	520	6	ND	Maron, Horvath, et al., 1975
160 km R	144 ± 1	140 ± 3	3.1	ND	13	135-145	Noakes and Carter, 1976
42 km R	146 ± 2	148 ± 2	3.3	1590	9	145-150	Kavanagh and Shephard, 1977
42 km R	139 ± 3	142 ± 1	2.9	1361	18	138-146	Cohen and Zimmerman, 1978
500 km R in 20 days	141± 1	139± 1	~2.0	Ad libitum	10	ND	Wade, Dressend-orfer, et al., 1981
90 km R	139 ± 4	146 ± 1	ND	ND	40	ND	McKechnie, Leary, et al., 1982
42 km R	140 ± 2	146 ± 2	2.9	ND	90	ND	Whiting, Maughan, et al., 1984
80 km C	ND	140 ± 1	1.1	3200	5	ND	Noakes, Nathan, et al., 1985

(continued)

TABLE 4.2 Serum Sodium Concentrations [Na⁺], Body Weight Loss (%), and Volumes of Fluid Ingested in Athletes Involved in Endurance Events *(continued)*

Race distance	Mean ± SD prerace plasma or serum [Na⁺] (mmol/L)	Mean ± SD postrace plasma or serum [Na⁺] (mmol/L)	Mean % BW loss	Mean volume of fluid ingested during race (ml)	n	Range of postrace plasma or serum [Na⁺] (mmol/L)	Reference
32 km R	135 ± 3	142 ± 3	5.0	1200	10	ND	Wells, Schrader, et al., 1985
42 km R	142 ± 1	140 ± 1	2.4	Ad libitum	6	ND	Irving, Noakes, et al., 1986a
2 hr tread-mill R	139	144	ND	1200	5x4	ND	Owen, Kregel, et al., 1986
2 hour C	140	145	3.1%	0	6	ND	Nielsen, Sjogaard, et al., 1986
42 km R	139 ± 1	142 ± 1	2.5	Ad libitum	45	ND	Nelson, Ellis, et al., 1989
42 km R	144	149	4.9	Nil	16	ND	Rocker, Kirsch, et al., 1989
24 hr R	140 ± 1	138 ± 1	3.1 ± 1.55	ND	9	ND	Fellmann, Bedu, et al., 1989
186 km T	142 ± 4	143 ± 5	ND	Ad libitum	101	131-149	Noakes, Norman, et al., 1990
56 km R	136 ± 1	137 ± 2	2.7	Ad libitum	8	ND	Irving, Noakes, et al., 1990
42 km R	~144	146 ± 1 (G) 145 ± 1 (½G) 144 ± 1 (W)	4.2 4.0 4.5	2200 1200 1200	7 7 7	ND	Cade, Packer, et al., 1992
40 km R	141 ± 1	144 ± 1	3.9	1947	8	ND	Millard-Stafford, Sparling, et al., 1995
100 km R	142 ± 7	161 ± 7	4.6	3250	7	152-170 (?)	Rama, Ibanez, et al., 1994
42 km R	144 ± 2	147 ± 2	3.1	1464	6	ND	Pastene, Germain, et al., 1996
1600 km in 11 days or longer	138 ± 2	141 ± 2	ND	Ad libitum	9	ND	Fallon, Sivyer, et al., 1999

Data are mean (±SD) or range.
R = running; S = cross-country skiing; T = triathlon; C = sea canoe/kayak; G = Gatorade; ½G = half-strength Gatorade; W = water; ND = no data; (?) = data appear to be improbable.

The point is that there was no suggestion during this period that athletes were salt deficient and needed to ingest sodium during exercise to ensure that their (elevated) blood sodium concentrations did not fall. Rather, there was some interest in the concept that sodium ingestion might maintain the ECF volume and therefore enhance performance by preventing "cardiovascular strain." But studies by our group (Sanders, Noakes, et al., 1999; Sanders, Noakes, et al., 2001) and others failed to show that this effect could be achieved without the ingestion of salt from drinks that were so concentrated that they were unpalatable.

It was only after we had described the first cases of EAH and EAHE that quite suddenly the need to increase sodium intake during exercise was promoted in order to prevent this novel disease, which began to be marketed as one of sodium deficiency, not fluid excess.

15 The exception was the study of Comrades Marathon runners conducted by Dancaster and Whereat (1971). In their paper published in the *South African Medical Journal* (SAMJ), Dancaster and Whereat also measured blood sodium concentrations before and after the race. Surprisingly, before the race, they apparently found that 51% of the 35 runners they studied had blood sodium concentrations equal to or below 136 mmol/L, indicating a significant incidence of *prerace* hyponatremia. The lowest prerace value was 126 mmol/L with another value of 130 mmol/L. Such values are impossible in healthy asymptomatic athletes preparing to begin a 90 km ultramarathon footrace. We have since measured thousands of blood sodium concentrations in athletes before ultraendurance events and have yet to find one such low blood value *before* exercise. The only reasonable explanation is that either sample storage or the method of measuring blood sodium concentrations produced seriously erroneous readings in these runners.

Sodium Chloride Balance During Repeated Days of Exercise

Several research studies have been conducted since World War I to determine the amount of sodium especially soldiers need to ingest to stay in sodium balance when exercising daily in the heat. These studies have been conducted by some of the most eminent scientists in the history of the exercise sciences.

Beginning in 1933, Dr. David Dill, founder of the Harvard Fatigue Laboratory, undertook a series of studies to evaluate "sodium economy" in subjects exercising in the heat (Daly and Dill, 1937; Dill, Jones, et al., 1933). Sodium balance was compared in the same subjects when living next to the sea in La Jolla, California, and in Boulder City in the Nevada Desert, while eating the same diet. Dill, Jones, and colleagues (1933) concluded that as long as some sodium (or chloride) was present in the urine, "the serum (sodium) chloride level remains within the normal range" (p. 764). They were perhaps the first to report that sweat sodium concentrations fell with exposure to heat (heat acclimatization) and that values as low as 5 mmol/L were present in some subjects. Thus, high sweat sodium concentrations "are not maintained in profuse and continued sweating" (p. 765). Instead, as the result of adaptation to the heat, the concentration of salt in sweat decreases after the first days in a hot environment so that "if there has been an opportunity for acclimatization, the product of the sweat glands is so dilute that 10 litres per day may be secreted without the necessity of an abnormal salt intake" (p. 766).

In 1943, Taylor, Henschel, and colleagues reported a study in which they evaluated the ability of subjects to acclimatize to heat when they exercised for prolonged periods each day in extreme heat (dry bulb temperature 49 °C; wet bulb temperature 29 °C) so that they sweated 5 to 8 L while ingesting 6, 13, or 30 grams of sodium chloride per day. They concluded that "men sweating 5 to 8 liters in the tropics will not require more than 15-17 grams of NaCl a day (p. 448). . . . An increase in salt intake above this level (17 g per day) results in increased loss of salt and water in the urine with no apparent advantage" (p. 450). Sodium chloride losses in urine and sweat sodium fell on the low-salt diet.

The study also evaluated the role of salt intake in the development of heat exhaustion. Whereas only 1 of 39 men on a moderate intake of sodium chloride (13 g) developed heat exhaustion, 5 of 20 men on the low salt intake (6 g) developed vomiting, nausea, and weakness suggestive of the development of postural hypotension. But rectal temperatures in cases of heat exhaustion ranged from only 37.3 to 39.8 °C, indicating that none was suffering from a true heat illness.

The authors concluded the following: "Heat exhaustion appears to be circulatory failure or impending circulatory failure during activity. The subject cannot perform continuous physical work, indeed he may faint while attempting it, but if he ceases physical activity and lies down the capacity of his cardiovascular system is adequate to meet the requirements of resting metabolism" (p. 449).[16] The authors also noted than no subject developed heat cramps so that "these observations serve to emphasize that no one factor accounts for the development of true heat cramps (Dill, Bock, et al., 1936). . . . it is clear that NaCl loss per se and the resulting reduction of plasma chlorides[17] will not necessarily result in heat cramps but will lead in many cases to heat exhaustion" (p. 449).

The conclusion seems to be that a sodium deficit causes a reduction in body water content, which increases the probability that postural hypotension will develop. One possibility might be that a progressive sodium deficit that develops in those who are unable to reduce their daily sodium chloride losses to less than their intakes predisposes such people to the development of postural hypotension during and after exercise. The development of postural hypotension is related to the action of the sympathetic nervous system and the inability to increase the peripheral vascular resistance when the cardiac output falls either during or after exercise (chapter 2). Thus, the development of a sodium deficit during heat acclimatization in those ingesting too little salt might be related to an unrecognized influence of sodium chloride on the activity of the sympathetic nervous system. To my knowledge, this possibility has not been considered.

The following year (1944), Dr. Jerome Conn (box 4.5) and Margaret W. Johnston established that acclimatized men working in heat (29 °C, 85% RH) and sweating at 4 to 9 L per day were able to maintain sodium balance on a daily salt intake of 5 g/day because they reduced their urine sodium losses immediately after their dietary sodium intake was reduced. One to two days later there was a reduction in sweat sodium concentrations. The authors concluded that "an

16 In fact, the principal function of the cardiovascular system is to maintain a blood pressure that is sufficient for sustaining the erect position. The condition described here is exercise-associated postural hypotension (EAPH), which has essentially nothing to do with dehydration and sodium deficiency.

17 This is a surprising conclusion because the authors seem ignorant of the fact that humans are designed to homeostatically regulate their milieu intérieur. Simply because chloride is lost in sweat does not mean that the blood sodium concentration must fall. Rather, the body is designed to ensure that any such reduction is the exception, not the rule, and occurs under only the most bizarre circumstances.

BOX 4.5 Hormonal Basis for Sodium Conservation

As an unexpected consequence of the Japanese air attack on the U.S. Navy battleships anchored at Pearl Harbor on December 7, 1941, Jerome Conn, MD, discovered the hormonal basis for sodium conservation by the kidneys and sweat glands during heat acclimatization. At the time, Conn was professor of internal medicine at the University of Michigan at Ann Arbor. Conn's area of expertise was endocrinology—the study of the body hormones and the diseases caused by either their excess or deficiency.

The entry of the United States into World War II that resulted from that attack soon occasioned a visit by members of the U.S. Armed Services to Conn's laboratory (Conn, 1962). They wished to know whether Conn would be prepared to study the processes of human acclimatization to heat. The U.S. Armed Forces were aware that in a war with Japan their troops would be exposed to hot, humid conditions in the battle to capture the Pacific Islands before Japan could itself be attacked.

For reasons best known to him, Conn decided to study sodium and water balance in conscientious objectors undergoing an extended period of heat acclimatization. He began by studying subjects exercising in heat (32 °C, 80-90% RH) who lost 5 to 7 L of sweat per day while ingesting 14 g of salt each day (Conn, 1949a; Conn, 1962). He observed that the sweat sodium chloride concentration (figure 4.6, page 134) fell from about 3 g/L (52 mmol/L) in the unacclimatized state to about 1 g/L (17 mmol/L) by the 10th day (arrow A in figure 4.6), a savings of 10 to 14 grams of salt daily. Urinary salt secretion fell immediately after the training in the heat began (arrow B) but increased (arrow C) once the sweat sodium chloride concentration had reduced (arrow A) so that sweat sodium chloride losses had been reduced. Note that the sum of the daily sweat (~1 g/day) and urine salt losses (~12 g/day) exactly matched the level of sodium chloride intake (14 g/day) during the first 40 days of the experiment.

Figure 4.6 also shows the effect of a sudden reduction in the sodium chloride intake from 14 g/day to 3 g/day on day 50 (arrow D). The immediate effect is a reduction in the urinary sodium losses to <0.5 g/day by day 54 (arrow E). Again, the reduction in sweat sodium concentrations after day 50 occurs more slowly (arrow F) than the reduction in urinary sodium losses. And again, the sum of the urinary and sweat salt losses matched the greatly reduced dietary intake from days 51 to 54. Increasing the daily salt intake to 8 g/day on day 65 was followed by an abrupt increase in urinary salt losses (arrow G), which was followed only about 12 days later by an increase in daily sweat salt losses (arrow H). Conn reports that in some subjects, sweat sodium chloride concentrations as low as 1 mmol/L were achieved. These subjects were able to remain in positive sodium balance even when ingesting only 3 g/day of salt while sweating up to 7 L/day.

Because he was a complete scientist, Conn also measured urinary nitrogen excretion each day of the experiment. He noticed that urinary nitrogen excretion rose progressively (arrows I and K) when the daily salt intake was reduced, indicating a period of negative nitrogen balance. This state reverted to normal (arrows J and L) sometime after daily sweat salt losses had reached their lowest values.

Conn's genius was to conclude that all these effects must be due to the secretion of a hormone that (a) modifies sodium chloride losses in urine and sweat and (b) produces a negative nitrogen balance. Since he knew that hormones secreted by the cortex of the adrenal gland produce both these effects, originally he termed the unknown substance desoxycorticosterone-like adrenal steroid (DLAS). In 1952 the hormone was isolated for the first time and soon became known as aldosterone.

In a subsequent study (Conn, 1962), Conn measured changes in urinary and sweat sodium chloride excretion in response to progressive reductions in daily dietary salt intakes (figure 4.7, page 134). As already established in figure 4.6, the amount of salt lost in sweat and urine adjusted immediately to match the daily salt intake.

(continued)

BOX 4.5 **Hormonal Basis for Sodium Conservation** *(continued)*

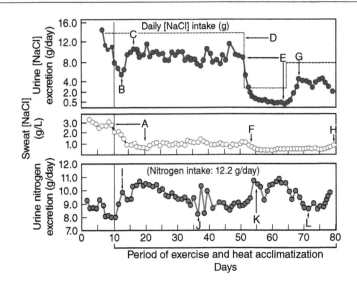

FIGURE 4.6 Changes in *(top)* daily urinary sodium chloride excretion, *(middle)* sweat sodium chloride concentrations, and *(bottom)* urinary nitrogen excretion in response to exercise in the heat in subjects who ingested 14 g/day of salt on days 10 to 50 of the experiment and then 3 g/day from days 51 to 65. Note that urinary sodium chloride excretion fell within hours of the change in dietary sodium intake with a reduction in sweat sodium concentrations following 1 to 2 days later.

Adapted from *Advances in Internal Medicine*, vol. 3, J.W. Conn, "The mechanism of acclimatization to heat," 373-393, copyright 1949.

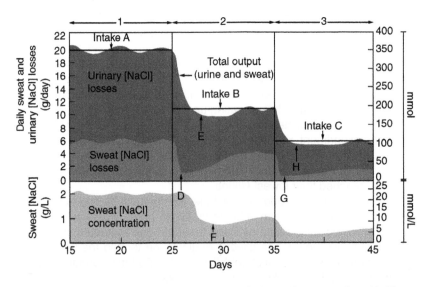

FIGURE 4.7 Changes in daily sodium chloride losses in sweat and urine and in sweat sodium chloride concentrations in response to three levels of daily sodium intake (1: 20g/day; 2: 11g/day; 3: 6 g/day).

Adapted, by permission, from J.W. Conn, 1962, "Some clinical and climatological aspects of aldosteronism in man," *Transactions of the American Clinical and Climatological Association* 74: 61-91.

In the first part of the experiment from days 15 to 25 (section 1), the daily sodium chloride intake was ~20 g/day (arrow A) with urinary and sweat sodium chloride losses of ~6 and ~14 g/day. After day 25, the daily sodium chloride intake was reduced to ~11 g/day (section 2, arrow B). This was followed immediately by a reduction in urinary sodium chloride losses to ~1 g/day already on day 26 (arrow D) and a more gradual reduction in the sweat sodium chloride losses (arrow E) as the result of a reduction in the sweat sodium chloride concentration that was minimized only by day 30 (arrow F).

The same response occurred when the daily sodium chloride intake was reduced further to 6 g/day (section 3, arrow C). Once again, within about 2 days, daily sodium chloride losses in sweat (arrow G) and urine (arrow H) were reduced until they exactly matched the intake.

While there was a wide variation in these responses, most subjects could adapt to a daily salt intake as low as 6 g/day and some to yet lower intakes even when they exercised sufficiently to expend up to 17 megajoules (MJ) of energy each day, requiring total sweat losses of up to 9 L (Conn and Johnston, 1944). Some were able to achieve sodium balance even when ingesting only 1.9 g/day (Conn, 1949a). Conn concluded that the critical factors determining successful adaptation to heat were the speed at which the salt content of sweat losses could be reduced and the extent to which those could be decreased (Conn, 1962). Thus, "The metabolism of early acclimatization to heat was characterized by intense salt-saving activities of both the kidneys and the sweat glands" (p. 64). As a result, "probably the most sequential mechanism that we observed, was the ability of the acclimatized man to maneuver himself into a state of positive sodium balance" (p. 64). This would be a natural consequence of a mammal that evolved in a salt-deficient environment.

Conn next concluded that this response must be hormonally based and was likely due to a hormone secreted by the adrenal cortex. As a result he decided to inject desoxycorticosterone acetate (DCA), an analog of the adrenal cortical hormone desoxycorticosterone, into an unacclimatized subject undergoing the early phase of heat acclimatization. To his great joy, the hormone produced an immediate and dramatic reduction in urine and sweat sodium chloride excretion (figure 4.8, page 136) associated with an increase in body weight. Thus this hormone was able to replicate the fall in urine and sweat sodium concentrations induced by heat acclimatization. The increase in body weight would be due to an increased body water content secondary to sodium and water retention.

Conn concluded that the main determinant of successful acclimatization to heat was the ability to secrete a "salt-saving steroid" (analogous to DCA) from the adrenal cortex. In time, it would become clear that the adrenal cortical hormone involved in this mechanism is aldosterone, not corticosterone. Thus "when one considers that the aldosterone-sweat gland system can reduce [salt] losses from the skin by as much as 95%, we must conclude that all forms of temperature regulation in hot climates would fail were it not for the activity of this [aldosterone—sweat gland] system in maintaining the volume of the extracellular fluid" (p. 67).

In a subsequent experiment (Conn, 1949a), Conn administered DCA for 7 days to a fully acclimatized man who was working and living in the heat chamber that was used for their experiments. The results were similar to those in the previous experiment on an unacclimatized subject: The DCA produced the expected results suggestive of further heat acclimatization (even though no additional heat acclimatization had occurred).

On removal of DCA treatment, the subject developed the classic symptoms of the unacclimatized man on first exposure to heat: postural hypotension, a sharp increase in rectal temperature, muscular weakness, cardiovascular strain shown as an increase in heart

(continued)

BOX 4.5 **Hormonal Basis for Sodium Conservation** *(continued)*

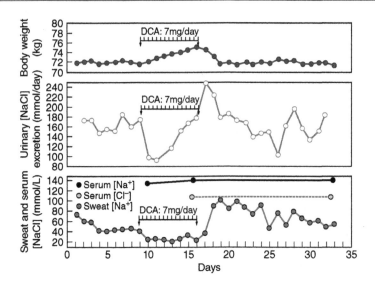

FIGURE 4.8   Injection of desoxycorticosterone acetate (DCA) into subject DB from days 9 to 16 produced *(top)* a progressive increase in body weight with *(middle)* an immediate reduction in urinary sodium chloride excretion followed by *(bottom)* a more gradual reduction in sweat sodium chloride concentrations. Blood (serum) sodium concentrations were unchanged during the experiment. These changes, which reversed immediately when the DCA injections were terminated, were the same as those produced by a period of natural acclimatization to heat. In the original drawing, Conn reported urinary NaCl excretion in the units of g/day. I have corrected this to mmol/day because daily urinary NaCl excretions of ~180 g/day are impossible in humans.

Adapted, by permission, from J.W. Conn, 1962, "Some clinical and climatological aspects of aldosteronism in man," *Transactions of the American Clinical and Climatological Association* 74: 61-91.

rate, and the inability to complete the usual exercise bouts in the heat. Body weight fell as sweat sodium chloride losses increased dramatically. These are the features of the condition known as Addison's disease, discussed subsequently.

Conn concluded that the administration of DCA had inhibited the natural production of DLAS (aldosterone) by the adrenal gland. As a result, when DCA was removed from the previously acclimatized subject, he was temporarily without any natural DLAS, the production of which had been suppressed by the DCA and which needed time for its production to again reach normal levels. Consequently, the subject was again unacclimatized to heat for a period of about 5 days while the production of DLAS again returned to normal.

Conn concluded the following as the process of heat acclimatization: "The ability of the sweat glands to decrease the loss of salt from the skin to less than 5 per cent of the original loss, when necessary, makes it possible for the acclimatizing man receiving an average intake of sodium chloride to maneuver himself into a period of positive sodium balance with which he can now gradually increase his extracellular fluid volume" (Conn, 1962, p. 71). "It thus seems reasonable to believe that one of the *major functions* of aldosterone[18] is its indispensable place in bringing about the cutaneous, renal and cardiovascular adjustments which are necessary for man's survival in hot climates" (p. 72). It was "possible to explain the *results* of acclimatization to heat almost wholly on the basis of increased production of aldosterone." This conclusion implies that the postural hypotension that occurs on first exposure to heat is not due to "cardiovascular strain" as much as it is due to a failure of an aldosterone-dependent sodium conservation with expansion of the ECF volume.

Subsequently, Ladell and Shephard (1962) showed that the injection of spironolactone, a chemical that antagonizes the action of aldosterone, increased sweat sodium chloride concentrations, further confirming the role of aldosterone in the regulation of sweat sodium concentrations. Finally, Conn (1949a) showed

18 Aldosterone was isolated, identified, and synthesized between 1952 and 1954 (Conn, 1962; Simpson, Tait, et al., 1952; Williams and Williams, 2003).

that ACTH, the pituitary hormone that causes release of the adrenocortical hormones, including aldosterone, from the adrenal cortex, also decreased urinary and sweat sodium chloride concentrations. He concluded this: "Under the conditions of our experiments, the need for the conservation of body salt constitutes the stimulus which 'fires' the mechanism and which realizes the level of activity of the pituitary-adrenal axis" (p. 391).

In April 1954, Conn was confronted with a patient with a complex disturbance in electrolyte metabolism. Conn concluded that all the abnormalities could be explained by the hypersecretion of aldosterone, termed primary hyperaldosteronism (Conn, 1955). It became apparent that the source was an aldosterone-secreting tumor of the adrenal cortex, an aldosteronoma. Surgical removal of the tumor cured the condition by causing a large excretion of urinary water and sodium. Sweat sodium concentrations rose from 9 mmol/L to 45 mmol/L by the 8th postoperative day. Interestingly, muscle sodium concentrations were increased and potassium concentrations reduced.

In honor of its discoverer, the condition is now known as Conn's syndrome. The opposite condition is known as Addison's disease. In this condition, a failure of adequate aldosterone secretion causes very high sweat sodium concentrations in excess of 60 mmol/L, which Conn considered to be the upper range of normal (Hsu, Lee, et al., 1997). Indeed, some patients with Addison's disease can have sweat sodium concentrations as high as 110 mmol/L (Conn, 1949b). This is the condition of salty sweating.

Subsequently in 1960, Conn's research team confirmed that aldosterone secretion increases in response to a period of heat acclimatization (Streeten, Conn, et al., 1960). They termed this condition secondary aldosteronism. They next showed that patients with primary hyperaldosteronism (Conn's syndrome) may have a reduced capacity to transfer sodium into the exchangeable sodium stores, especially in the bone (Streeten, Rapoport, et al., 1963). When they subsequently treated rats with aldosterone or DCA, there was a reduced uptake of sodium from blood to bone, whereas the aldosterone antagonist, spironolactone, increased sodium uptake by bone (Rovner, Streeten, et al., 1963).

On the basis of these studies, Rovner and colleagues concluded that aldosterone may play a role "in regulating the transfer of electrolytes between bone and extracellular fluid" (p. 938). If correct, aldosterone would act to mobilize sodium from the osmotically inactive exchangeable sodium stores, increasing the blood sodium concentration. This effect of aldosterone could explain why 70% of athletes who gain weight during exercise do not necessarily develop EAH or EAHE. In contrast, the absence of this action would exacerbate the drop in blood sodium concentrations in those who overdrink.

Sadly, not everyone wishes to remember the meaning of Dr. Conn's work.

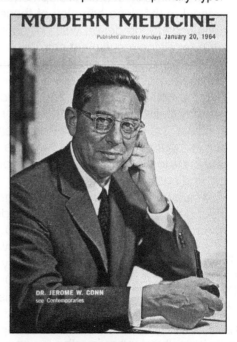

American endocrinologist Jerome Conn.
Courtesy of the National Library of Medicine

average diet, containing 10-15 grams of NaCl, provides sufficient protection in acclimatized men to make the use of salt supplements unnecessary" (p. 933). Thus, "under conditions of large sweat volume and average intake the sweat glands are very efficient in salt conservation" (p. 136).

Beginning also in the late 1940s, Dr. Sid Robinson of the University of Indiana conducted a series of studies of sodium balance and heat acclimatization that would confirm many of Conn's findings. They established the following:

- Sweat sodium losses are determined by the level of daily salt intake in the diet. This has since been confirmed (Costa, Calloway, et al., 1969).
- Sweat sodium concentrations fall during a period of heat acclimatization especially when the daily sodium chloride intake is low. When the daily salt intake was increased, sweat and urine losses increased.
- Sweat (sodium) chloride concentrations may be as low as 15 mmol/L.
- In response to a low-salt diet and daily exercise in the heat, the kidneys begin to reduce their salt output within 1 to 2 hours, whereas salt excretion in sweat begins to fall only after 8 to 24 hours and requires several days to achieve a maximum effect (Robinson, Nicholas, et al., 1955). They also noted that intermittent exposure to exercise and heat produced a more rapid response.
- The administration of DCA produced lower sweat and urine sodium concentrations but increased blood sodium concentrations (perhaps as the result of mobilization of sodium from the exchangeable stores).

The classic studies of U.S. soldiers in the desert conducted by Adolph (1947) also failed to detect the development of salt deficiency. Since chloride was always present in the urine samples of these soldiers, the authors concluded that salt deficiency in the desert was not common since "less than 5% of desert troops were receiving insufficient salt" (p. 106). Indeed Adolph noted that "a few men may accumulate considerable crusts of salt on the skin during a single day's exposure. Such individuals consistently show from day to day more salt on the skin than others do, and *they characteristically eat excessive quantities of salt* [my emphasis]. Large intakes of salt may give rise to high concentrations of salt in sweat" (p. 106).[19] They also observed that "in the man partially depleted of salt its concentration in this sweat is also reduced. Sweat, like urine, therefore responds to the call for conservation of salt" (p. 108). This observation anticipated the findings of Dr. Conn.

A study by Weiner and van Heyningen (1952) reported very high sweat (sodium) chloride concentrations and concluded that those exercising in the heat for 4 hours a day would need to ingest 20 to 24 g of salt daily. But their data actually showed that subjects were able to adapt to a daily sodium chloride intake of 10 g.

Dr. Malhotra and colleagues from the Indian Ministry of Defence studied groups of Indian soldiers while they walked 11 km in 2 hours in temperatures of about 35 °C dry bulb and 30 °C wet bulb when they ingested 16.2, 11.2, 8.7, 6.2, or 3.1 g of salt per day (1960). Only subjects

19 The presence of salt crusting on the skin or in clothing indicates a high rate of salt loss in sweat. This in turn indicates that the athlete's dietary salt intake is high. Athletes with salt crusting should be advised to reduce their dietary salt intakes, not to increase the intakes, because they are eating too much, not too little.

ingesting 3.1 g/day developed signs and symptoms of sodium deficiency. These included headache, giddiness, lassitude, weakness, a disinclination to do any physical or mental work, and a fall in the blood chloride concentration.

Predictably (as in figures 4.6 and 4.7, page 134), urine and sweat sodium losses exactly matched salt intakes equal to or greater than 6.2 g as a result of constant urinary sodium losses at all intakes (figure 4.9) but with increasing sweat sodium losses with increasing intakes. The authors extrapolated their data to predict that subjects who exercised for 8 hours a day in even hotter conditions (43 °C dry bulb) might need to ingest up to 15 g salt per day. But this extrapolation ignores the findings of Conn and colleagues who showed that most humans can readily adapt to sodium intakes as low as 6 g/day even when exercising for many hours a day in heat.

A series of studies in Israel have led to the conclusion that it is impossible to develop a state of sodium deficiency in free-living individuals who have access to as much salt as their taste dictates. Yoram Epstein and Ezra Sohar (1985) evaluated 10 soldiers who covered 27 km/day daily in the desert for 24 consecutive days and whose sweat rates ranged from 5 to 10 L/day. Their mean daily sodium intake was 264 mmol and their mean daily urinary sodium loss was 176 mmol. The presence of so much sodium in the urine convinced the authors that these subjects were not sodium deficient: "Since the kidneys reabsorb almost all sodium when sodium depletion occurs, it is obvious that during the whole march, despite heavy sweating, sodium was always present in abundance" (p. 130). Another study in the hottest area of Israel found that people involved in strenuous physical work and who sweated several liters per day had a mean urinary sodium excretion of 156 mmol per day when eating their normal diets. When their diets were supplemented with an additional 180 mmol/day of sodium, mean daily urinary sodium output rose to 446 mmol, confirming that the diet contained an excess of sodium. A further study of agricultural workers whose daily sodium chloride intake

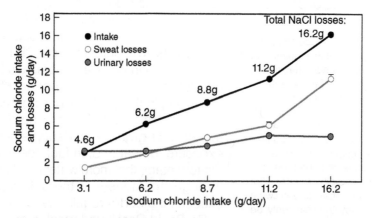

FIGURE 4.9 There was a progressive increase in the amount of salt lost in urine and sweat each day in subjects ingesting increasing amounts of dietary sodium chloride while exercising vigorously for 2 hours in extreme heat. Thus, salty sweating in this experiment occurred as the result of an increased daily sodium chloride intake. Total losses in urine and sweat (numbers above line for daily salt intake) exactly matched salt intakes except at an intake of 3.1 g, at which a negative sodium balance developed in these subjects because they continued to lose salt in excess in urine. This response is unusual.

Data from Malhotra 1960.

was very low (34 mmol, or 2 g, per day) found that their sweat sodium concentrations were also very low (17 mmol/L), indicating the presence of an appropriate response to a habitual low sodium intake. The authors also noted that there are several people (Morse and McGill, 1937) who live on low sodium intakes of 45 to 90 mmol/day "with no ill effects" (p. 130)

As a result of these studies, Epstein and Sohar (1985) have concluded with admirable directness: "It seems that in the so-called 'salt deficiency heat exhaustion' we may be dealing with yet another case of 'christening by conjecture' (Asher, 1951). A syndrome which is alleged to be due to pure salt deficiency, as the name suggests, should fulfill the following criteria: (a) it should be shown by direct and accurate measurement that the amount of sodium lost in the sweat (and urine, my addition) exceeds the amount of salt in the diet; (b) typical signs and symptoms should appear after sodium depletion has reached a critical level; (c) sodium deficiency should be proved by laboratory methods; and (d) recovery should be brought about by administration of sodium chloride alone. Such a syndrome has never been proven to exist and is disproved by the findings cited above. Nor has sodium depletion due to salt loss in the sweat ever been observed in the extensive 20 years of field experience of the Environmental Unit at the Heller Institute at Tel-Hashomer" (p. 131). As a result, "intake of salt tablets during profuse sweating is not only unnecessary but may be harmful. Instances of nausea and vomiting after intake of salt tablets have been observed. . . . This point emerges clearly on examining the consequences of sea-water drinking. Sea-water is not suitable to quench thirst since its salt concentration is twice the maximum urinary salt concentration. Consequently, the body must use its dearly needed water to excrete the salt ingested with the sea water" (p. 130-131).*

In 1973 Wyndham, Strydom, and colleagues (1973) reported their study in which they evaluated South African miners during an 8-day heat acclimatization program when they exercised for 4 hours in a dry bulb temperature of 33.3 °C and a wet bulb temperature of 31.7 °C. Miners did not lose more than 15 g of sodium chloride per day (range of 9 to 14 g/day) and did not benefit from the ingestion of supplementary salt tablets. The authors wrote, "Put in simple language, man generally increases his intake of salt to the required 15 g per day[20] when he is working in the heat, and losing that amount of salt in his sweat. There is no advantage, therefore in giving a salt supplement during exposure to heat and, in fact, there may be a disadvantage that more water must be passed through the kidneys if the salt supplement exceeds the bodily requirement" (p. 1779).

Dr. David Costill undertook a study funded by Johnson and Johnson to determine whether the ingestion of water or that company's prototypical electrolyte-containing sports drink,

20 This explanation is, of course, the reverse. Sodium losses match intakes, not the converse. These miners were habituated to a daily salt intake of 15 g. Had the authors studied others who were habituated to much lower intakes, they would have come to a different conclusion, specifically that the level of the habitual sodium chloride intake determines the amount of salt lost in urine and sweat.

This error would continue to be promoted as part of the myth of the salty sweater. That myth holds that high rates of salt loss in sweat cause sodium deficiency that can only be prevented by ingesting ever-large amounts of dietary salt. Instead, excessive amounts of salt in sweat indicate the presence of too much salt in the diet.

*Reprinted from Y. Epstein and E. Sohar, 1985, "Fluid balance in hot climates: Sweating, water intake, and prevention of dehydration," *Public Health Reviews* 13: 115-137, by permission of Professor Epstein.

Brake Time Thirst Quencher, could offset the electrolyte losses incurred during five bouts of exercise on consecutive days in heat (37-38 °C, 55-65% RH) (Costill, Cote, et al., 1975). The goal of the exercise was to produce a 3% body weight loss (~2.1 kg) in subjects ingesting fluid ad libitum during exercise. Generally it required about 1.5 to 2.5 hours to achieve this degree of weight loss.[21]

There were two critical findings in that study. First, whether or not they ingested the sports drink during exercise, subjects remained in positive sodium (and potassium and chloride) balance for the duration of the experiment. Second, the only effects of the sports drink were to increase the total sodium ingested each day (figure 4.10*a*) and as a consequence the urinary sodium losses (figure 4.10*b*). Sweat sodium losses were unchanged.[22] The data indicate that subjects were habitually ingesting a diet with a very high sodium content (225 mmol, or ~13 g, per day). The sports drink added a further 25 to 75 mmol to this excess.

As a result, Dr Costill's group showed that the ingestion of Brake Time Thirst Quencher was an expensive method of increasing the amount of sodium excreted in the urine, a predictable response in athletes whose diets already contain a large sodium excess.

21 This finding shows how long it takes to lose substantial amounts of weight during exercise in athletes who either do not drink or who drink according to the dictates of thirst during exercise. In my opinion research showing that it may take 1 to 2 hours for athletes to become dehydrated by 3% was unwelcome news to the sports drink industry. So, that interest must have been pleased when the ACSM adopted the zero % dehydration rule in 1996. If subjects were encouraged to drink only in activities likely to produce dehydration levels in excess of 3%, then only those exercising for more than an hour would need to drink. Since relatively few humans exercise for this duration, the market size for sports drinks would be much smaller. The zero % dehydration rule would, however, ensure that everyone who exercises, regardless of duration, would need to drink. The ACSM finally revised its guidelines away from the zero % dehydration rule in 2007, tacit acknowledgment that my guidelines (Noakes, 2003c) were more appropriate.

22 This is because there was no risk of sodium deficit developing. The studies of Conn discussed earlier show that urinary sodium losses are first decreased before there is a fall in sweat sodium concentrations. Hence, only when there is a risk that sodium deficiency will occur (because sodium intake does not match losses) will the sweat sodium concentrations also fall.

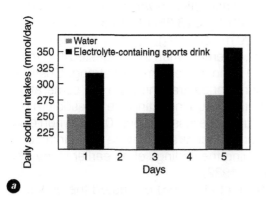

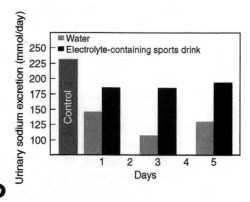

FIGURE 4.10 *(a)* Daily sodium intakes in subjects drinking either water or a sodium-containing sports drink (Brake Time Thirst Quencher) during prolonged exercise in the heat. *(b)* Urinary sodium excretion on days 1, 3, and 5 of this experiment when either water or the sports drink was ingested. Note that all the extra sodium ingested in the sports drink appears in the urine and that daily urinary sodium losses are very high when the sports drink is ingested.
Data from Costill, Coté, Miller, et al., 1975.

In the control condition, the urine contained a sodium excess of 225 mmol/24 hr (5 g/24 hr), whereas the sweat sodium losses were only ~80 mmol per exercise bout. As a result, on the days that subjects exercised, they accurately reduced their urinary sodium excretion by ~80 mmol (figure 4.10b). Since their sodium intakes exceeded their maximum requirements by ~225 mmol/day, they could have exercised each day for almost three times as long as they did (i.e., for up to 7.5 hours a day) while remaining in sodium balance. And if they had chosen to exercise more, they would simply have eaten more salt during the time that they were not exercising, or activate their sodium-conserving mechanisms that evolved to reduce the amount of sodium excreted in their urine and sweat.

This classic study shows that humans ingest far too much salt daily and would need to exercise for 7.5 hours a day to ensure that the ~13 g excess is secreted in sweat (as opposed to secreted in urine).

In later studies, Costill's group showed that muscle sodium and chloride concentrations measured from muscle biopsy samples remained normal even when they exercised sufficiently in extreme heat (39.5 °C, 25% RH) to lower their body weights by 5.8% (Costill, Cote, et al., 1976). Again this degree of weight loss was not easily achieved but required up to 4.5 hours of exercise. A subsequent study (Costill, Cote, et al., 1981) reported similar findings after exercise lasting 2 hours, although sodium losses were proportionately smaller.

Numerous other studies have confirmed this biological law that humans regulate their total body sodium stores exquisitely accurately despite any acute or chronic changes that may occur in the rates of either sodium intake or sodium losses (Reinhardt and Seeliger, 2000). Included among the scientists who undertook this research was Lawrence Armstrong, PhD, who was the senior author of the 1996 and 2007 ACSM position stands and who would later propose that EAH and EAHE can be due to the development of an acute sodium deficiency within a few hours of exercise. In a set of three publications that were initiated while he was a doctoral student in Dr. Costill's laboratory at Ball State University in Muncie, Indiana, which continued while he was employed by the USARIEM, Armstrong established the following:

During 8 consecutive days of heat acclimatization in which they exercised for 90 minutes a day in uncomfortable heat (40.1 °C, 23.5% RH, limited convection), subjects ingesting a low-sodium diet (100 mmol, or 6 g, sodium/day) developed a negative sodium balance of 230 mmol, whereas when they ingested 400 mmol sodium (24 g) per day they gained 900 mmol of sodium (Armstrong, Costill, et al., 1987). But blood and muscle sodium concentrations were the same at the end of the experiment, in part because the group ingesting the low-sodium diet lost 0.7 kg due to a reduction in ECF volume; the loss was only 0.2 kg when extra sodium was ingested. Muscle potassium concentrations were also unaffected (Armstrong, Costill, et al., 1985), confirming the findings of an earlier study also by Dr. Costill's group (Costill, Cote, et al., 1982).

A second study (Armstrong, Hubbard, et al., 1993) evaluated the effects of an even lower sodium intake (68 mmol, or 4g, per day) during 10 days of heat acclimatization (Robinson, Nicholas, et al., 1955) in which subjects exercised for 30 minutes each hour for 8 hours a day for 17.5 consecutive days in the same severe environmental conditions (41 °C, 21% RH). Subjects walked 22.4 km per day up a gradient of 5% at a speed of 5.6 km/hr. This study was completed in collaboration with scientists from the USARIEM. The study was designed to determine whether the U.S. Dietary Guidelines that humans should ingest less than 104 mmol (6 g) of sodium per day could apply also to those exercising daily in hot conditions.

After 17 days of the experiment, there were no "cases of heat exhaustion, heat syncope, heat cramps, or heatstroke" (p. 214), even though subjects drank only water during exercise. Nor did any subject develop EAH; instead blood sodium concentrations remained in the normal range for the duration of the experiment. The reason was that subjects reduced their urinary sodium concentrations to ~5 to 10 mmol when ingesting little sodium. Instead, the major complaint of the subjects was "numerous foot blisters and minor orthopedic injuries" (p. 214).

At the end of the experiment, most subjects were in neutral or positive sodium balance. Thus, despite losing 60 L of sweat during the 17 days of the experiment, "no subject exhibited the symptoms of salt-depletion heat exhaustion (e.g., vertigo, hypotension, tachycardia, vomiting)" (p. 219).

The authors concluded that their findings were "in agreement with the results of Johnson et al. (Johnson, Pitts, et al., 1944) who concluded that "a well-balanced diet and a regimen of hourly water consumption adequately maintained performance and resulted in normal fluid-electrolyte measurements during strenuous physical activity (5 hr/day) in a hot environment" (p. 219).[23]

Dr. Armstrong and his group (Armstrong, Hubbard, Szlyk, et al., 1985) also completed a study in which subjects walked on a treadmill for 30 minutes every hour for 6 hours in uncomfortable heat (40.6 °C) while they drank fluids at different temperatures. Fluid intake was greatest when water at the lowest temperature (6 °C) was ingested and was twice as great as the fluid intake from a hot solution (46 °C). Sweat sodium losses during the experiment ranged from 70 to 250 mmol and were paradoxically lowest in subjects when they drank the least and lost the most weight.[24] The authors concluded that "K+ (potassium) depletion may be more of a problem than Na+ depletion during extended heat and exercise exposure because food may be supplemented readily with sodium chloride" (p. 769). This conclusion conflicts somewhat with Armstrong's subsequent statements on the importance of ingesting sodium during exercise (see chapter 9).

23 I find it difficult to understand how Dr. Armstrong was able to reconcile these findings with his subsequent statements to the effect that EAH is due to sodium deficiency that can be produced within a few hours of exercise. In these experiments he had been completely unable to induce a state of sodium deficiency even in subjects exercising daily for 4 hours while ingesting a sodium-restricted diet. Instead, he has chosen to support the USARIEM model of how EAH develops (figure 9.12, page 277), even though his own studies clearly establish that humans are designed to conserve sodium.

24 The point is that despite losing the most sodium, subjects maintained their blood osmolalities (and hence blood sodium concentrations since the blood sodium concentration is the most important determinant of the blood osmolality), whereas those who lost the least weight showed the largest increases in blood osmolality. This should have alerted Dr. Armstrong to the possibility that the blood sodium concentration is not determined by sodium losses during exercise but by associated changes in body water content. Since blood osmolalities stayed within the normal range in all these experiments, there were no cases of EAH.

The next study (Armstrong, Costill, et al., 1985) evaluated sodium and potassium losses during acclimatization in subjects who walked at 5.6 km/hr on a treadmill at a grade of 6% for 90 minutes in the same hot conditions (40.6 °C, 24% RH) for 8 days when they ingested either 399 (24 g) or 98 (6 g) mmol sodium per day. The authors wished to determine whether potassium deficiency might occur under these conditions. However, body potassium stores increased even on the low-sodium diet. Thus they concluded that the findings did not support their "previous claim that dietary sodium levels affect K^+ balance" (p. 391).

In a reverse experiment, Konikoff, Shoenfeld, and colleagues (1986) from Tel Aviv University increased the salt intake of heat-acclimatized subjects exercising under controlled laboratory conditions by 10 g/day. When evaluated during exercise, there was no measurable cardiovascular or thermoregulatory benefit of this increased salt intake. Instead, the additional sodium predictably appeared in the urine. The authors concluded that "acclimatized people living in a hot dry climate need no supplementary salt to their daily dietary intake while engaging in physical exercise or sport activities up to two hours a day. Salt loading under such conditions has no beneficial effects and, on the contrary, it may even be hazardous" (p. 300).

Allsopp, Sutherland, and colleagues (1998) pointed out that sodium conservation by the kidneys does not require that a sodium deficit must first be present. Rather, sodium conservation can occur *before* the deficit occurs; that is, it occurs "in anticipation" specifically to ensure that a sodium deficit does not occur. Thus, the mechanisms that produce sodium conservation when the sodium intake is reduced, including the increased production of aldosterone, are more complex than is usually considered.

Fudge and Easton (2008) studied a group of 14 elite Kenyan endurance athletes over a 5-day period while they were preparing for the 2005 IAAF Athletics World Championships. Daily fluid and sodium balance was measured as these athletes drank fluids ad libitum. They chose not to drink during exercise. Daily sodium intake was 3.2 g, which exactly matched total daily sodium losses of 3.2 g (urine 2.3 g, sweat 0.9 g); daily water intake was 3.8 L, most of which came from milky tea and water. Sweat sodium concentrations were 37 mmol/L. The high rates of urinary sodium losses indicate that these athletes could easily have adapted to a daily sodium intake of about 1 g/day, but the ease of availability of salt and their taste habituation ensured that they chose to ingest more salt each day than they required.

Summary

Evidence simply does not exist that recreational or professional athletes competing in long-duration events will inevitably develop a state of salt deficiency or dehydration. By adjusting fluid volume, the human body regulates osmolality within a narrow range: The NaCl concentration of the ECF is always 135 to 145 mmol/L. It is impossible for healthy humans, whether nonexercising or exercising, to become salt deficient when they have free access to dietary salt. Since our bodies are designed by our evolutionary history to defend against a sodium deficiency even when ingesting only a fraction of the sodium present in the modern Western diet, as shown by the research presented in this chapter, sodium deficiency is an unproven and highly improbable cause of exercise-associated muscle cramps or heat illness.

Humans have an advanced capacity to conserve sodium and can safely exist on a sodium intake of as little as 3 g/day even when exercising vigorously in the heat on a daily basis. Humans always lose weight and increase their blood sodium concentrations (table 4.2, page 129) when they exercise. To suggest that the body cannot sustain long-term exercise in the heat without ingesting supplemental sodium ignores not only our biological design but also reams of research proving otherwise.

CHAPTER 5

Emergence of the Sports Drink Industry

I never thought about the commercial market. The financial success of this stuff really surprised us. I am proud that Gatorade was based on research into what the body loses in exercise. The other sports drinks were created by marketing companies.

**Dr. Robert Cade,
inventor of Gatorade
("James Robert Cade," 2007)**

The previous chapters present a foundation of the truth about the thirst mechanism, thermoregulation of the human body, and sodium balance during exercise. If you have run the journey with me, you have learned the following truths:

- Scientists subscribe to either a catastrophe model of exercise physiology, in which the brain does not exert control over physiological systems, or more likely a homeostatic control or survival model, in which the human body has developed biological controls to preserve function and survival.
- Dehydration is simply a reduction in the total body water content. The only symptom of dehydration is thirst, which becomes increasingly persistent and impossible to ignore as the level of fluid loss persists. If at any time a healthy athlete does not sense thirst, the athlete is not dehydrated.

■ Leading sports medicine organizations advise athletes to drink even before they sense thirst. But this ignores the built-in controls provided by the body's thirst mechanisms. These mechanisms have evolved over hundreds of millions of years to ensure that all the creatures on Earth are able to regulate their body water contents accurately without being told when and how much they need to drink.

■ Dehydration in those who drink ad libitum (at one's own discretion) has no proven detrimental effect on athletic performance. In fact, drinking ad libitum during exercise will improve time-trial performance more than drinking either less or more than the volumes directed by the thirst mechanism.

■ The human body regulates osmolality within a narrow range; the sodium chloride concentration of the extracellular fluid is always 135 to 145 mmol/L.

■ In almost every circumstance in health, it is the blood sodium chloride concentration that is regulated. It is not the volume of fluid in the extracellular space nor the athlete's body weight that is regulated.

■ Blood sodium concentrations always stay the same or rise during all forms of exercise in those who drink according to the dictates of thirst.

■ Neither muscle cramps nor heat illnesses are caused by sodium deficiency.

So it is with great interest that we turn our attention to the sports drink industry, whose remarkable commercial success would be achieved despite these truths.

Gatorade is a sports drink that was developed by Dr. Robert Cade, MD, at the University of Florida in 1965. In 1967 the company Stokely-Van Camp purchased the brand, selling it to Quaker Oats in 1983 that, in turn, sold Gatorade to PepsiCo in 2000.

In 2008 and 2009 two scientific papers reporting research funded by PepsiCo through their Gatorade Sports Science Institute (GSSI) confirmed what we had already established nearly 2 decades earlier: Exercise-Associated Hyponatremia (EAH) is caused by abnormal fluid retention in those who have been encouraged to overdrink during exercise. These studies confirmed that abnormal sweat sodium chloride losses play no role in the development of EAH.

Dr. Cade's Concoction

In 1965, Robert Cade (box 5.1) was assistant professor in the renal division in the College of Medicine at the University of Florida, an institution known more for the quality of its football players than for its marathon and ultramarathon runners. In that year, Cade developed Gatorade, the world's first drink specifically designed and marketed for ingestion during exercise. Gatorade would become the world's most successful, most iconic, and (according to its marketing department) most scientifically researched sports drink: "Gatorade is the most thoroughly researched beverage in the world, and the only sports drink with more than 40 years of science to back up its claims that it works, hydrating athletes, replenishing electrolytes and providing fuel for working muscles" (Hein, 2009).[1]

1 Despite all of this research, the composition of Gatorade has changed very little in 40 years. Perhaps it would be more correct to state that Gatorade is the sports drink whose effects on the human body during exercise have been the most thoroughly studied.

BOX 5.1   The Gentlemanly Inventor of Gatorade

Robert Cade graduated with a medical degree from the University of Texas Southwestern Medical School at Dallas. He completed his residency in internal medicine at Parkland Memorial Hospital, a hospital that received international focus on 22 November, 1963, when President John F. Kennedy was admitted there after his fatal shooting in Dealey Plaza, Dallas. In 1961 Dr. Cade joined the renal division of the department of medicine at the University of Florida. He was promoted to professor in 1971 and served as division chief from 1971 to 1978. His noncurricular interests ranged from playing the violin to reading and writing poetry, growing roses, and restoring and showing antique Studebaker cars (Nordlie, 2004).

During his career as professor of medicine and physiology at the University of Florida, Dr. Cade conducted research on a variety of medical conditions treated in the division of nephrology, hypertension, and renal transplantation. Besides designing the world's first commercially marketed sports drink, Gatorade, in 1965, Dr. Cade developed a theory for a possible link between autism and schizophrenia and dietary milk and grain intake (Nordlie, 2004). His hypothesis was that an inability to break down casein in milk and gliadin in wheat leads to the secretion of morphine-like substances, which cause damaging proteins to accumulate in the brain. These abnormal proteins cause the transmission of false brain signals that explain the features of these diseases. He proposed that a diet free of gluten, casein, milk, and grain products would help about 80% of patients with autism, Down's syndrome, and schizophrenia. This idea remains popular but unproven.

Dr. Cade, who died on 27 November, 2007, at age 80, was known for his generosity and ability as a researcher, clinician, educator, and humanitarian. He was also described as a maverick and an ennobler: "He ennobled the school, ennobled himself, ennobled the University, and contributed warmth and kindness and decency in a collegial fashion" (Nordlie, 2004, p. 2). His generosity included his donation of the J. Robert Cade, MD, Professorship of Nephrology Fund. He was described as gentle, creative, and inspiring—a "gem of a man." The basis for Dr. Cade's philanthropy was "God has blessed me in all kinds of ways—including a big income. In the book of Deuteronomy God tells the Israelites a man should give as he is blessed. I think I am duty bound to do as He suggests" ("Dr. Robert Cade," 1990, p. 2).

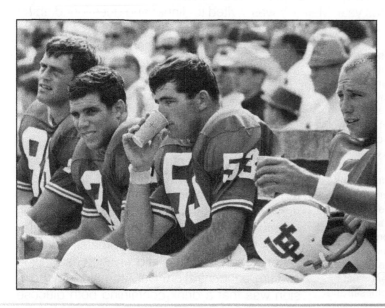

Kim Helton, a football player for the University of Florida Gators in 1965, drinking the ancestral Gatorade solution during a game.
AP Photo

Several versions exist of the story of how Gatorade was invented, including those involving the University of Florida's football players or coaches being concerned about athletes not urinating enough; athletes being nauseated, sluggish, or hospitalized after playing in the Florida heat; and the flagging second-half performance of the team.

In his book *First in Thirst,* Darren Rovell (2005) presents a rather complete version of the story and the one that will probably become the authentic version. Rovell writes that in August 1965, Dewayne Douglas, assistant coach of the Gators freshman football team, shared lunch with Dr. Dana Shires, who at that time was working as a fellow with Dr. Cade in the renal division. Douglas reputedly stated that 25 players from this freshman football team had been admitted to the hospital infirmary the previous weekend because of heat exhaustion and dehydration. He "pleaded with Shires to come up with something to negate the strain that the brutal summer heat had inflicted upon his players" (p. 10). Douglas also apparently reported that "players who drank too much water would get stomach cramps while players who put too much salt in their bodies would often experience leg cramps" (p. 10). According to Rovell, Shires informed Cade of the discussion and the two set about developing the solution.

Rovell describes that "Cade and others *knew* [my emphasis] that replacing fluids would be a true advantage for the team, as the team's loss of fluids led to dehydration, serious salt depletion, and in some cases severe heatstroke" (p. 11).[2]

Although Cade and Shires knew something about sweating, they reportedly sent another of Cade's fellows, Alex DeQuesada, a Cuban who had arrived at the university just one month earlier, to the medical library with $5 in his pocket. "In just two hours, DeQuesada returned with almost everything that had ever been written about this topic" (Rovell, 2005, p. 12). The key paper that DeQuesada uncovered had been presented by Dr. Sidney Malawer at the American Society for Clinical Investigation, two months earlier (Malawer, Ewton, et al., 1965). By supreme coincidence, Malawer had worked as a medical resident at the University of Florida the previous year. Malawer was invited to dinner and questioned about his research in which he had passed a tube into the small intestine of 18 men and measured the rate at which fluid was absorbed across the intestinal wall from solutions infused into the intestine and that differed in their glucose and sodium concentrations.

These studies showed that the addition of glucose at increasing concentrations increased the rate at which both sodium and water were absorbed by the intestine from a salt-containing solution. Maximal water absorption was achieved from the most concentrated glucose solution.[3] Increasing the glucose concentration of the drink had a much greater effect on water absorption than did an increase in the sodium concentration. But the natural conclusion was that a drink containing both glucose and sodium would be especially valuable for

2 The defining function of science, in my opinion, is to disprove, not to prove, hypotheses. No scientist can ever be certain that he or she has completed the definitive experiment to prove a theory that some more sophisticated future experiment might yet disprove. So the best a scientist can do is to keep testing her hypotheses in an attempt to disprove them. With each "disproof" the original hypothesis is modified and so slightly improved. If further experiments are unable to disprove it, this does not mean the theory is true; the theory simply survives for another round of experimentation. So a true scientist does not presume to know that his theory is correct. Claude Bernard warned that "the results of an experiment must be noted by a mind stripped of hypotheses and preconceived ideas" (Bernard, 1957, p. 24).

athletes requiring instantaneous rehydration. But this conclusion, which appears so obviously correct, may not necessarily be true for the reason that all the sodium needed for optimizing fluid absorption can be provided by secretions from the pancreas into the small bowel (figure 2.1, page 42) and so does not have to be in the original solution that is ingested.

Convinced by this information that their drink needed to include glucose and salt, Cade and Shires next needed permission to test the effects of their concoction on human athletes. The coach of the varsity football team, Ray Graves, gave consent for the University of Florida freshman team to be studied, but he drew the line at allowing his varsity players to be studied. Cade and his team began by studying weight, blood, and urine changes during practice in two players each afternoon in September 1965.

3 Medawar and his colleagues did not study the effect of varying the sodium concentration of the solutions they tested; they varied only the glucose concentration and maintained the sodium concentration constant at 140 mmol/L. Thus, it is not clear why Dr. Cade decided to include sodium only at quite low concentrations in the ancestral Gatorade formulation. But, in fact, it does not matter because all solutions have the same sodium content once they enter the small bowel regardless of how much sodium was present in the ingested solution. This is because the secretions of the pancreas enter the small bowel through the bile duct (figure 2.1, page 42).

The passage of time has ensured that the results of those tests have become ever more definitive: Rovell (2005) writes that they showed that two 240-plus-pound (110 kg) subjects lost about 25% of their total body sodium stores—"an amount that could have been lethally dangerous" (p. 16). Subjects also became dehydrated, which "can cause headaches, dizziness and muscle cramps, with heatstroke being the most extreme result" (p. 17). Cade recalls the results rather more vividly: "The results were eye-opening. The players' electrolytes were completely out of balance, their blood sugar was low and their total blood volume was low. The impact on the body of this upheaval in chemistry was profound. 'Each of these conditions, by itself, would to some extent incapacitate a player' Cade says in his oral history. 'Put them all together and you can have real problems'" (Kays and Phillips-Han, 2003, p. 2).

On the basis of their physiological hunch that the players needed water, salt, and glucose, Cade and Shires developed the prototypical drink. Initially it tasted "like toilet bowl cleaner" ("Gatorade Celebrates 35 Years," 2002, p. 1) but the addition of lemon juice on the advice of Mrs. Cade made the solution at least drinkable. By October 1965, the drink was ready for field testing.

So on 1 October, 1965, the freshman team lined up against the varsity B team in a traditional game known as the Toilet Bowl. Because of their experience and superior size—about 10 kg per man—the varsity B team usually prevailed. During this match, the freshmen would receive the new solution, whereas the varsity B team would drink water

By the end of the first half, the freshman team "had been beaten pretty badly" and were trailing 13-0. But then the freshmen were "given the solution and by the second half, had given the B team a real run for their money. . . . They scored touchdown after touchdown and didn't give up a point the rest of the way" (Rovell, 2005, p. 19). Coach Graves was so impressed by this turnabout that he asked Cade to supply the varsity team with the drink for the game the following day against "heavily favored" (p. 21) Louisiana State, who were ranked the fifth best college football team in the nation at that time.

So Cade and his team "worked through the night, scavenging the labs for the ingredients and hand-squeezing lemons." (Kays and Phillips-Han, 2003, p. 1). Dr. Cade recalls, "We all met in the lab that night and realized we only had one bottle of glucose, and we needed at least 20. We started calling drug stores, supply houses and pharmacies, and we couldn't find any. We were in a dark funk about this when Sgt. Douglas walked in, the very same Douglas who coached the freshman team. In his afterhours coach Dewayne Douglas worked as chief of hospital security. We told him about our dilemma. A big smile crossed his face. Being a security officer, he had a key to every lab in both the hospital and the medical school, so we went around and borrowed enough glucose to make the stuff" ("When Wife Game Him Lemons," 2004, pp. 1-2). Within a few hours 100 L of the solution were prepared, poured into two 50 L vats, and stored overnight in the hospital's walk-in freezer.

Before the game, Dr. Cade filled hundreds of Dixie cups and placed them near the players, who had not been informed of the nature of the experiment of which they were unwittingly a part. The result of the match played the previous day was the only evidence that Dr. Cade had for the value of his product. Yet as he handed his solution to the bemused players, he apparently told them, "This is a glucose and electrolyte mixture. If you drink it during the game, you'll be stronger and feel better in the third and fourth quarters" (Rovell, 2005, p. 22).[4]

The University of Florida Gators came from behind to win 14-7, and the legend was born. But the role that the solution actually played on that day cannot be known and was probably small "since not many players partook of the drink during its surprise introduction on the sidelines that day" (Rovell, 2005, p. 22). In addition, the effect could have been due to a powerful placebo effect, since the Louisiana State players had not been informed they were part of the experiment and were therefore not a proper control group. Without a proper control group it is not possible to draw any definitive conclusions. Dr. Jim Free, who coined the name for this novel solution—Gatorade—would later say, "If we had lost, you probably never would have heard of Gatorade again" (p. 22).

Influenced by the outcome of this uncontrolled experiment and assured by Dr. Cade and his colleagues that Gatorade was better than water "since it travelled through the stomach fast enough that they could drink more of it and wouldn't get bloated" (Rovell, 2005, p. 23), coach Graves ordered the drink to be on the sidelines both for practices and games for his varsity team for the entire 1965 season.

After the Gators ended the 1965 season with a respectable 7-4 record, Dr. Cade began to wonder how he might be able to commercialize his product. He suggested a price of $5 per gallon to Graves, who politely refused: The 1966 Gators would have to perform without Gatorade.

4 The Gators probably began the experiment with a different expectation than did the Louisiana State players who may or may not have been drinking water (or Coca-Cola or whatever) and who thought that they were simply playing a football match without knowing that they were participating in an experiment that would determine the future of the global sports drink industry in the 20th century. Had they known this, they might have played a little harder in the fourth quarter and so obviated the need to write this book.

Studies in our laboratory have found that subjects told they were receiving a carbohydrate solution when they were actually drinking water performed 2% better than when told truthfully that they were drinking only water (Clark, Hopkins, et al., 2000). Others have reported this effect (Nassif, Ferreira, et al., 2008). This is a measure of the power of the placebo.

But on the first day of the 1966 season, 7 Gators were treated for "heat illness"; the following day it was 17. Graves called Dr. Cade and told him that "he needed Gatorade at whatever cost for both games and practices" (Rovell, 2005, p. 26). So Dr. Cade informed him that the cost would now be $10 a gallon. One result, it is claimed, was that over the next 5 years only one player (not using Gatorade) was hospitalized for the treatment of "heat illness" (Kays and Phillips-Han, 2003, p. 1)

The Gators completed the 1966 season with an 8-2 record and were considered the best football team ever to wear the Gator uniform. Their particular strength was their ability to be the stronger team in the second half. Since Dr. Cade had promised that Gatorade would produce this effect, his faith in his product was apparently vindicated. Rovell, on the other hand, reports that the Gators were fortunate to have Steve O. Spurrier (SOS) as their quarterback. Spurrier would win the 1966 Heisman Trophy, awarded to the best collegiate football player in the United States, in part because of his ability to secure late victories—hence his nickname, SOS. His center, All-American Bill Carr, concluded, "I think Gatorade gave us a physiological and psychological edge and then Steve just made things happen. He had such a great ability to manage the clock and he had us all believing every time we stepped out there" (Rovell, 2005, p. 27).

Spurrier's faith did not include any belief in a special Gatorade effect: "I don't have any answer for whether the Gatorade helped us be a better second-half team or not. We drank it, but whether it helped us in the second-half, who knows" (Rovell, 2005, p. 28).[5]

Rovell records that one of the team's two losses during the 1966 season may have been self-inflicted. Having won the first seven games of the season, the Gators traveled to Jacksonville, Florida, to play the University of Georgia Bulldogs at a neutral venue. Dr. Cade wished to see what would happen if the Gators were Gatoradeless.[6] He reportedly trashed the Gatorade cartons, or stored them overnight on a truck in Gainesville. Without their Gatorade, the Gators lost 26-10, going scoreless in the second half. In an interview after a season-ending loss to the University of Miami, coach Graves mentioned how beneficial the sports drink had been to his team. The story was carried on November 30, 1966, by the Associated Press and United Press International: "A liquid solution that tastes like a mint and works like a miracle may be one of the factors behind the success of the University of Florida football team this year" (p. 33). The article was titled "Florida's Pause That Refreshes: 'Nip of Gatorade'" (p. 33).

To explain why the Florida team had improved from their 7-4 win-loss record in the 1965 season, for a part of which they had used Gatorade, Dr. Cade theorized, "This year is a different solution. It's been modified . . . we've added a couple of

[5] Spurrier reportedly drank Coca-Cola, not Gatorade, during these games (Rovell, 2005). SOS Spurrier went on to play 10 seasons as a professional player in the National Football League and has enjoyed a successful coaching career at his alma mater and with other teams. His son, Steve Jr., would become an assistant football coach at the University of Oklahoma.

[6] Although this was a true intervention trial, which could have tested whether two variables were causally related (i.e., drinking Gatorade directly caused a football team to win its matches), the study results could still have been explained by another variable that was not adequately controlled in the study. Thus, the sudden absence of what they had been expecting (the presence of the ancestral Gatorade solution on the sidelines in their matches) could have exerted a negative psychological effect on the players.

other electrolytes" (Rovell, 2005, p. 34). This is a classic example of reductionist logic. Dr. Cade's presumption is that the explanation for the success of a college football team can be reduced to a single variable, in this case to the presence of additional electrolytes in their sports drink. In reality, the factors determining success in professional team sports are so complex that they defy the analysis and control of all but a very few coaching geniuses. In fact, the Gatorade formula changed little from 1965 to 1966. The players on the 1966 varsity team were different; indeed, they are remembered as being extraordinarily talented and included the Heisman Trophy winner Steve Spurrier in perhaps the team's most important position, quarterback.

Their successful season saw the Gators invited to the Orange Bowl, played on 1 January, 1967. There, coach Graves' team outplayed the Georgia Tech team coached by Bobby Dodds, under whom Graves had served his coaching apprenticeship from 1947 to 1959. The Gators scored 20 of their winning 27 points in the second half; Georgia Tech scored 6 points in each half. After the game, Dodds told Graves, "We didn't have Gatorade, that made the difference" (Rovell, 2005, p. 35). But Spurrier was less convinced: "We drank Coca-Cola at half-time at the games because that is what they gave us" (p. 36).

Gatorade Goes National

Having in this way "proved" its efficacy on the football field, the further story of Gatorade has much to do with its commercialization. In March 1967, Dr. Dana Shires, on behalf of Dr. Cade, entered into discussions with the Indianapolis-based company Stokely-Van Camp to market the product nationally. On 16 May, 1967, the two parties reached an agreement. The first challenge was to improve the palatability of the drink. Technicians at the company increased the sugar content by 2% "and determined that this didn't have much effect on the speed of absorption of the liquid" (Rovell, 2005, p. 47).[7]

7 This statement cannot be true because the technicians at Stokely-Van Camp would have had to perform research on humans to prove this theory. And this research could be undertaken only in a medical institution. Only many years later would the GSSI fund research to investigate the factors that regulate the rate of fluid absorption by the intestine.

The second challenge was to increase the national profile of the new product. With the support of the marketing division of Stokely-Van Camp, Gatorade rapidly spread throughout U.S. collegiate sport in 1967. Collegiate football standouts Notre Dame and Purdue started using the product in the 1967 season, and the NFL signed a contract the same year to make Gatorade the official drink of the NFL. During that time, the Gators became known as the second-half team: Since they began using Gatorade, they outscored their opponents by 379-221 in the second half compared to 290-204 in the first half. By 1969, Gatorade was widely used throughout all U.S. sports; in Dr. Cade's words, "Our stuff was on its way" (Kays and Phillips-Han, 2003, p. 2).

Gatorade crossed the gulf dividing college from professional football with the help of the Kansas City Chiefs. "Back in the late 1960s, several of the Chiefs' star players suffered from dehydration in the hot and humid Missouri heat." Hall of Fame linebacker and center E.J. Holub, known as the toughest player in the NFL, reported, "In the pre-season I passed out in the huddle, and coach Stram knew

8 Not so. Athletes do not pass out (lose consciousness) because of exercise-induced dehydration (see chapter 2). They may feel dizzy and develop low blood pressure when standing after exercise, the condition known as exercise-associated postural hypotension (EAPH). But this condition is not caused by dehydration. Rather, it is due to a delayed recovery of blood vessel control (vasoconstriction) necessary for the regulation of blood pressure after exercise.

Any athlete who loses consciousness before, during, or after exercise has a potentially serious medical condition, often of the heart, that needs to be investigated urgently by a cardiologist before the athlete is allowed to return to sport. If E.J. Holub did in fact pass out, he should have been seen by a cardiologist.

it was from dehydration" (Rovell, 2005, p. 63)*.[8] Concerned, coach Stram spoke with his friend, University of Florida coach Ray Graves, in search of a solution.

"Coach Graves told coach Stram about a relatively new concoction, Gatorade, which helped replenish and rehydrate his college football players, improving their performance. Coach Stram received a few cases of Gatorade, which he and trainer Wayne Rudy introduced to the team, and the rest is history. The Chiefs noticed dramatic improvements in their energy levels and performance, and went on to become the champions of Super Bowl IV during this time" ("Gatorade Returns to 'Origins,'", 2003).

In a January 2004 interview with a reporter from the University of Texas Southwestern Medical Center at Dallas before an award from the University of Florida for his "discovery" of Gatorade, Dr. Cade confirmed that, in his mind, he developed Gatorade in response to University of Florida freshman football team coach Dewayne Douglas' inquiry of why football players did not go to the rest room during or after a game during which they frequently lost 12 to 18 pounds as a result of "sweating under the scorching Florida sun. . . . Dr. Cade couldn't find any research on the subject, so he did his own" ("When Wife Gave Him Lemons," 2004, p.1). The findings of those studies are reviewed subsequently.

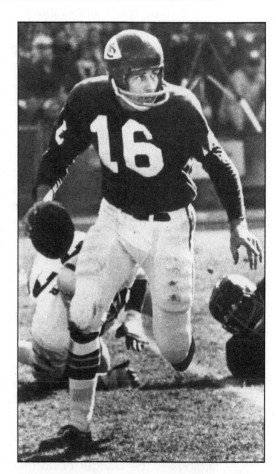

Quarterback Len Dawson of the Super Bowl champions, the Kansas City Chiefs, in 1969. The Chiefs were the first NFL team to use Gatorade.
AP Photo

The sudden and unprecedented growth in sales of Gatorade is especially impressive because all the great achievements in sports from antiquity until about 1970 were achieved by athletes who were encouraged to drink little or preferably nothing during both training and competition. Recorded sales of Gatorade before

1982 are not traceable. Starting in 1982, sales grew steadily, with cumulative annual sales up to 2005 of at least $18 billion.

The success of Gatorade naturally spurred the production of competing sports drinks. Some of the notable offerings include the following:

- Accelerade, produced by PacificHealth Laboratories and launched in 2003, is the first sports drink to include both carbohydrate and protein, together with the usual electrolytes, sodium and potassium. The manufacturers claim that the protein improves performance and speeds recovery more effectively than do sports drinks that contain only carbohydrate.

- Powerade, launched in 1988 by Coca-Cola as the official sports drink of the Olympic Games, has a composition very similar to Gatorade but with less sodium and more carbohydrate. By 2010, Powerade had achieved 22% of the sports drink market compared to the 77% share of Gatorade.

- Energade was introduced into South Africa by Cadbury Schweppes in 1993 and soon became the dominant brand. The composition is similar to the Gatorade formulation.

- Lucozade Sport is the leading European sports drink produced by Glaxo-SmithKline. It is the official sports drink of the London Marathon, the Lawn Tennis Association of the United Kingdom, and the FA Premier League. The drink contains 6% carbohydrate, a "trace" of sodium, and a variety of vitamins.

- Isostar was developed in Switzerland in 1977 and introduced into the European market in the 1980s. It has a higher carbohydrate content (9%) than other sports drinks and includes a greater range of electrolytes: sodium, potassium, magnesium, phosphorus, and calcium.

Dehydration and Heatstroke

A crucial element of the folklore that has propped up the "science of hydration" over the past several decades is the myth that dehydration causes heatstroke. Dr. Cade's preconceived belief, evident in all his writings, was that the only way to prevent heatstroke during exercise is to drink plenty of fluids. He was not alone in this belief. In particular, the 1969 study of Wyndham and Strydom influenced, for 40 years, scientists' beliefs on dehydration during exercise.

Wyndham and Strydom's misleadingly titled article that described their findings—"The Danger of an Inadequate Water Intake During Marathon Running"—launched a novel "science of hydration," which incorrectly proved the need for the revolutionary change in drinking behaviors that occurred thereafter. But in describing such "danger," Wyndham and Strydom committed a series of scientific errors (box 3.1, page 62), the most important of which was to allow their prejudice to determine their conclusions.

Wyndham and Strydom's study promoted the concept that dehydration during exercise was dangerous. Consequently, they opened the field to a host of studies, many funded by the fledgling sports drink industry (Gisolfi, 1996), of which the scientific goal may have been to establish the value of drinking during exercise but which, I argue, have primarily served a commercial purpose. I first discussed Wyndham and Strydom's research in chapter 3. Wyndham and Strydom's study became the intellectual foundation for the erroneous "foundation myth," which holds that dehydration is the single most important factor determining the rise in rectal temperature during exercise and hence the risk that heatstroke or other medical "dangers" will develop during prolonged exercise, especially in the heat.

Recall that these scientists believed they had shown that an increased level of dehydration directly leads to an increased rectal temperature. Rectal temperature beyond 42 °C can lead to heatstroke. Therefore, the myth was born that dehydration leads to heatstroke. In addition to concerns over heatstroke in American football players, scientists began to assume that the danger of heatstroke was of utmost concern for marathoners.

If it is true that underdrinking does indeed cause heatstroke, then there must have been a considerable number of cases of heatstroke during that period before 1975 when athletes were advised to avoid drinking, and an absence of cases after the introduction of frequent drinking stations in marathons beginning in the 1980s. To provide some scientific evidence to address this question, I searched the published literature for reported cases of heatstroke during exercise and compiled a summary of all the cases that I could trace in appendix C. The list will not be absolutely complete and might be missing some cases published in more obscure or non-English-language medical journals and perhaps some military case series that I was unable to trace. But my goal was not to provide a definitive list of every single reported case. Rather, I wished to collect all the information I could (nothing that I traced has been excluded) in an attempt to answer four questions:

1. How many cases of heatstroke have been described in marathon runners?

2. Is heatstroke more prevalent during more prolonged exercise when "dangerous dehydration" is more likely to occur than during short-duration exercise lasting less than, say, 60 minutes and in which significant dehydration does not occur?

3. What is the published evidence showing that subjects with exercise-induced heatstroke are more dehydrated than control subjects involved in the same physical activities but who did not develop heatstroke?

4. Are there factors other than dehydration that predispose a person to heatstroke during exercise? Why, for example, does heatstroke occur in only one or some of many athletes exercising at the same time in the same conditions, and why does it occur quite often in cool conditions?

1. How many cases of heatstroke have been described in marathon runners?

This was the easiest to answer. In the entire published scientific record to which I have access, I could trace only six published reports of heatstroke in marathon runners, two of which we had ourselves described (Noakes, Mekler, et al., 2008; Rae, Knobel, et al., 2008) and another two of which may or may not actually have had heatstroke. Furthermore, in one of these cases, that of Jim Peters in the 1954 Vancouver Commonwealth and Empire Games Marathon (Rae, Knobel, et al., 2008), whose case is usually considered the iconic example of heatstroke in a marathon runner who failed to drink adequately during exercise, the diagnosis was not absolutely certain. Although Peters was reportedly unconscious for at least 2 hours after the Vancouver Empire Games Marathon, his body temperature was only 39 °C when measured about an hour after he first collapsed. He also recovered without requiring active cooling. Without active cooling, people who have true heatstroke usually die. We concluded that he had developed abnormal brain function (encephalopathy) that was not necessarily due solely to an elevated body temperature. In addition to these few cases, there were three cases of heatstroke in professional cyclists involved in exercise lasting a few hours.

By contrast, one single race, the 1988 11 km Falmouth Road Race, produced nine cases of heatstroke in a single year (Brodeur, Dennett, et al., 1989), and I personally treated four cases of heatstroke in a single 12 km National Cross-Country Championship race in Cape Town in 1981. Thus, it is clear that marathon running does not pose as great a threat of heatstroke as do running events of much shorter distance. Indirect evidence to support this conclusion is a report from the 1980 Melbourne Marathon (Kretsch, Grogan, et al., 1984). The study reported that only about 50% of a sample of 5,423 runners drank anything during the race. Despite this low rate of fluid intake, "there were no cases of heat exhaustion, heat stroke, or problems caused by asthma, cardiac disease or renal failure" (p. 812). Instead, the article lists a litany of running injuries that affected the athletes' ability to complete the race.

William Roberts, medical director of the Twin Cities Marathon, was in attendance at the race for 24 years from 1982 (Roberts, 2000) before he encountered the first case of heatstroke in that race in 2005 (Roberts, 2006). During that time, probably at least 150,000 athletes completed the race without developing heatstroke (Roberts, 2000). If the average finishing time for all those runners was 4.5 hours, then the incidence of heatstroke in that marathon was 1 case per 600,000 marathon running hours. This confirms my experience that the number of athletes seeking medical care at the end of marathon races was extremely low in the 1980s and only began to increase after athletes were told that they should drink more during exercise.

Given the millions of marathon performances in the past century, the fact that the scientific literature includes only six described cases of heatstroke in marathon runners indicates that the condition must occur extremely rarely in this group of athletes. Obviously many cases go unreported; I myself have not reported all the cases of heatstroke that I have treated in marathon runners over the years. But the absence of such reports *increases*, not decreases, the likelihood that articles describing such cases will be reported in the medical literature. Rarity increases the probability that journal editors will publish case reports.

The overriding conclusion must be that these data do not support the statements of some of the scientists working with the sports drink industry to the effect that "the greatest threat to health and well-being during prolonged exercise, especially when performed in heat, is dehydration. If this heat is not dissipated, it will lead to hyperthermia and the potential to suffer a fatal heat stroke" (Gisolfi, 1996, S159) and "Hypohydrated persons who exercise in the heat will incur significant adverse consequences. . . . If strenuous exercise is performed in hypohydrated persons, the medical consequences can be devastating" (Sawka and Montain, 2000, p. 564S).

2. Is heatstroke more prevalent during more prolonged exercise when "dangerous dehydration" is more likely to occur?

This, too, was easy to answer. I was able to trace the reports of 1,939 cases of heatstroke in the literature from 1941 to 2008 in running or other forms of exercise. Of these cases, the majority (1,536 cases) were reported in the militaries of various nations with far fewer numbers in football (predominantly U.S. gridiron) (153 cases) and running (137 cases). The only other large number of cases was reported from the South African gold mines (97 cases).

The exercise duration measured as distance run was reported in all but two of the cases of heatstroke in those runners or military personnel who developed heatstroke while running. Table 5.1 lists the frequency (%) of the distances that athletes had run before they developed heatstroke.

Eighty-nine percent of all cases occurred in those who ran less than 20 km; 44% occurred at distances less than 10 km. Remarkably, 10% of subjects developed heatstroke even though they had run less than 5 km. The clear observation is that heatstroke is more likely to occur in those running less than 20 km. Since such a large number of athletes now run marathons each year in different locations around the world, the small number of heatstroke cases in marathon runners cannot be because fewer people run marathons than they do shorter distances.

Similarly, the frequency of reported distances that military personnel had *marched* before they developed heatstroke mirrors that found with the runners: Even when marching rather than running, and hence expending less energy than if they were running, the majority of cases (51%) occurred before the subject had marched even 10 km, and 75% occurred in soldiers who had marched less than 20 km. Thus heatstroke is more likely to occur in exercise of short duration, in which dehydration cannot be a factor (Epstein, Moran, et al., 1999). Yet the most recent ACSM position stand on exertional heat illness specifically states that the "greatest risk for heat stroke occurs . . . in strenuous exercise that lasts longer than I h(our)" (Armstrong, Casa, et al., 2007, p. 558). I suspect the draftees of

TABLE 5.1 Frequency (%) of Reported Distance That 137 Subjects (Runners or Military Personnel) Had Run Before Developing Heatstroke

Distance run (km)	Number of cases	% of all cases
0-5	14	10
5-10	47	34
10-20	61	45
20-40	8	6
42 or greater	5	4
No data	2	1
Total	137	100

9 To put this risk in perspective, consider this rough estimate: Let us assume that there are 250,000 marathoners in the United States, each of whom runs two, four-hour marathons a year for a total running exposure of 2 million exercise hours. If there are two fatal cases of EAHE per year in U.S. marathon runners, then the rate of fatal EAHE is one per one million hours of marathon competition. Next let us assume that there are twice as many football players who train 10 hours a week for 18 weeks per year, giving a total of 90 million hours of training each year. If two football players die each year from heat stroke, then the relative risk of heatstroke is 1 per 45 million exercise hours in football players, which is 45-fold lower than the annual risk of death from EAHE in marathon runners.

The reason why American football is so safe is because it does not greatly tax the human thermoregulatory capacity designed for more severe demands. When training in severe environmental conditions (34 °C, 37-45% RH), the core temperatures of football players are 38 °C to 39 °C, similar to values measured in distance runners training for about 50 minutes in the same environmental conditions (Fowkes, Godek, et al., 2004). The core temperatures of the football players fell during rest periods between plays so that players "seem to dissipate heat adequately during rest periods" (p. 2451).

No relationship was found between the football players' weight loss during practice (level of dehydration) and their postpractice core body temperatures (Godek, Bartolozzi, et al., 2006), further evidence against the dehydration myth. Some 138 kg NFL linemen lost up to 8 L of sweat during approximately 3 hours of daily practice (2.4 L/hr), but were able to drink fluid at rates of up to 2 L/hr without apparently experiencing intestinal fullness (Fowkes Godek, Bartolozzi, et al., 2008). Much smaller (60-70 kg) runners develop symptoms when they ingest fluid at rates in excess of 800 ml/hr for more than about an hour.

the ACSM document followed the historic logic: Heatstroke is caused by dehydration (figure 3.1, page 61) and thus must be more likely to occur when the exercise exceeds 1 hour (since it is not possible for "significant" dehydration to occur in the first hour of exercise). Had they evaluated the published record, they might have come to an opposite conclusion.

American football has been played at U.S. colleges since 1869 and professionally since the 1890s (the Ohio League). From what we can tell, for the 96 years before Dr. Cade experienced his epiphanous moment, administrators, coaches, and players in U.S. football had not considered it prudent to drink fluids in order to prevent heat exhaustion or dehydration. In fact, the incidence of heatstroke in American football players is surprisingly low, reportedly either 21 deaths from 1995 to 2001 (3 per year) (Bergeron, McKeag, et al., 2005) or 31 deaths from 1995 to 2010 (2 per year) (2010).[9] This is relatively easily explained. First, the activity is intermittent, allowing the body to cool between bouts of exercise. Second, the structure of the game limits the duration for which a team must either attack or defend. As a result, a set of offensive or defensive plays seldom lasts more than about 10 minutes. In addition, players are frequently substituted and may not play every down in such a sequence.

Heatstroke occurs much more frequently in exercise of short duration compared to exercise of long duration. On the basis of this evidence, the dehydration that develops normally during exercise lasting less than 60 minutes cannot be a significant contributor to heatstroke. Rather, one might (facetiously) argue the opposite: It is the *absence* of dehydration that is the more likely predictor of heatstroke risk, since most cases occur in exercise in which high levels of dehydration cannot occur.

3. What evidence is there that heatstroke is caused by dehydration?

Since most cases of heatstroke occur within 60 minutes of the start of exercise, significant or "dangerous dehydration," a term favored by some scientists working with the sports drink industry, could not have been a factor, since such dehydration requires at least 3 hours to develop in those who must also refuse to drink anything during that time.

A number of large-scale studies of cases of heatstroke have failed to provide any evidence that dehydration occurs frequently in patients with exercise-induced heatstroke. A study of 157 cases of fatal heatstroke in U.S. soldiers training during World War II found that dehydration was a probable factor in only 6 cases, whereas there was a tendency toward overhydration ("hydremia") in the majority (Malamud, Haymaker, et al., 1946; Schickele, 1947). Another large study found that 6% to 16% of soldiers with heatstroke were dehydrated (Carter, Cheuvront, et al., 2005). A similar proportion (16%) of Israeli soldiers with heatstroke were considered to be dehydrated (Epstein, Moran, et al., 1999). Many other studies have not found that dehydration occurs frequently in exercise-associated heatstroke (Aarseth, Eide, et al., 1986; Al-Harthi, Sharaf El-Deane, et al., 1989; Austin and Berry, 1956; Beller and Boyd, 1975; Ferris, Blankenhorn, et al., 1938; Henderson, Simon, et al., 1986; O'Donnell, 1975; Seraj, Channa, et al., 1991).

Yet somehow the authors of the 2007 ACSM position stand interpreted these and related data as evidence that dehydration is a risk factor for heatstroke.

An outspoken voice on this topic is Dr. A.M.W. Porter, who wrote the following (2000): "In the context of collapses from heat injury in present-day army training in the UK, however, water discipline and intake are largely irrelevant. To say this is to invite rebuttal, *but to dehydrate an individual to the point when sweating ceases is almost impossible* [my emphasis]. . . . British soldiers in training who collapse and die from heat illness have not had time to become severely dehydrated, and the insistence on water discipline suggests that they are unlikely to be in any way meaningfully dehydrated. . . . Drinking will not itself solve the imbalance between the large metabolic heat load and the impeded evaporated heat loss. The pre-occupation of medical officers and instructors with water intake is a dangerous distraction from the real issue" (p. 570).

It appears that the initial fascination with dehydration as a cause of heatstroke arose from the belief that (a) heatstroke developed after a cessation of sweating and (b) dehydration, caused by either water or sodium loss or both, caused a cessation of sweating as a result of "fatigue" of the sweat glands (Schwartz and Itoh, 1956). Thus, the explanation of how heatstroke develops was quite simple: Excessive dehydration causes a cessation of sweating and prevents heat loss. As a result, heat accumulates progressively until heatstroke develops.

The problem arose when it became apparent already in the early 1960s that dehydration does not decrease the sweat rate to any important degree. As a consequence, it became necessary to develop an alternative model of how heatstroke could develop in those who were still sweating profusely when they collapsed. "Its [dehydration's] deleterious action is in impairing the proper function of the cardio-vascular system, which is unable to dissipate the heat accumulated in the internal organs and muscles, due to decreased blood and cellular fluid volume. Since dehydration is present in many cases of heat stroke, the importance and the means of its prevention should be clearly explained to all concerned" (Gilat, Shibolet, et al., 1963, p. 210). This appears to explain the origins of the cardiovascular model of thermoregulation during exercise (CMTE), which is based on the theory that dehydration is the factor that initiates the condition. One way in which this theory has evolved in the past 60 years is shown in figure 5.1 (page 162).

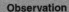

Observation

Dehydration occurs in cases of heat stroke.

Intellectual model

Dehydration due to unreplaced water or sodium
losses causes heat stroke.

Proposed mechanism

Dehydration causes the termination of sweating.
As a result the dehydrated human is unable to
lose heat during exercise. Instead heat accumulates
progressively until heat stroke develops.

Inconvenient finding

Dehydration does not cause
any impairment of sweating.

Proposed new mechanism

Dehydration causes heat accumulation because of a failure of
cardiovascular function—The Cardiovascular Model of Thermoregulation
during Exercise (CMTE). As a result the cardiovascular system is
unable to adequately transport heat from the muscles to the skin. Instead heat
accumulates "in the internal organs and muscles" and heat stroke develops.

Inconvenient finding

There is no published scientific evidence that shows
dehydration or impaired heart function as necessary or even
common features of heat stroke.

Solution

Suppress this inconvenient truth. Instead promote
dehydration as a novel disease of exercise.

FIGURE 5.1 Intellectual steps leading to the development of the cardiovascular model of thermoregulation during exercise (CMTE).

The problem is that there is now no evidence that dehydration plays any role in the causation of heatstroke. Thus, the entire basis for this intellectual model is flawed and needs to be replaced with fact. The key problem, in my view, is that the error in the original theoretical model led to the idea that it is primarily a failure in the rate of heat loss that causes heatstroke. But the alternative possibility is that heatstroke is caused by a massively excessive endogenous heat production (within the body) that indeed overwhelms the normally more-than-adequate heat-losing mechanisms (Rae, Knobel, et al., 2008). This model, which better explains most of the observations described here, has the disadvantage that it was not the original explanation, nor has it yet been embraced by a majority of those exercise scientists with the greatest influence in the discipline.

A review of all the cases of heatstroke does not provide any convincing evidence that dehydration occurs even as frequently as might be expected, given that all were involved in exercise that must produce some weight loss. Thus, the conclusion that dehydration is a risk factor for heatstroke, as repeatedly proposed in the ACSM position stands, is simply untrue.

4. Are there factors other than dehydration that predispose a person to heatstroke during exercise?

Why, for example, does heatstroke occur to only one or some of many athletes exercising at the same time in the same conditions? And why does it often occur in cool conditions? I found several pieces of evidence that contradict earlier explanations for how heatstroke develops.

First, the incidence of heatstroke is most common in exercise of short duration, for example, races of less than 21 km, which are usually completed within an hour (by those at risk of developing heatstroke) and in which high levels of "dangerous dehydration" simply cannot occur. The same would apply to American football and other sports of short duration and frequent rest breaks.

Second, no study has ever shown that athletes with heatstroke are more dehydrated than those control subjects who complete the same activities but without developing heatstroke. The importance of this missing evidence cannot be ignored forever.

Third, subjects who develop heatstroke either at rest or during exercise are inevitably sweating profusely and do not show any evidence for heart failure (Ferris, Blankenhorn, et al., 1938; O'Donnell and Clowes, 1972) at the time they collapse. The point is that if subjects with heatstroke are sweating appropriately and have normal heart function (apart from a low blood pressure) when they collapse, then the cause of their collapse cannot be a failure of heat loss. Instead, it must be because *they are generating heat too rapidly* for it to be lost into the environment. This is either because the environment is too hot to absorb that heat or because the subjects are generating heat at an abnormally rapid rate.

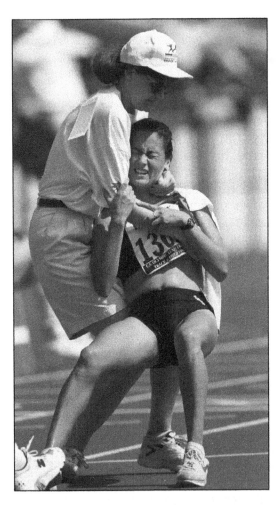

An athlete collapses during the U.S. Olympic 10 km walk trials in Atlanta, June 1996. Cases of heat stroke typically occur in short-distance races (less than 15km) in which dehydration cannot be a factor.

AP Photo/Rick Bowmer

Fourth, many cases of heatstroke occur in environmental conditions that are too cool to seriously challenge the extraordinary human heat-losing capacity. Several clinicians have made this point repeatedly (Bartley, 1977; Epstein, Moran, et al., 1999; Kark, Burr, et al., 1996; Molnar, 1947; Schickele, 1947; Schrier, Henderson, et al., 1967). For example, a study of exertional heat illness in the U.S. Marine Corps reported that "Most of the cases occurred during the cooler early morning hours when recruits performed strenuous exercise" (Kark, Burr, et al., 1996, p. 354).

The fifth piece of evidence that contradicts other explanations for heatstroke is that if the exercise alone was the factor causing subjects with heatstroke to overheat, then they should begin to cool immediately after they stop exercising. Instead, without proper cooling, patients with heatstroke will inevitably die. Thus, the question becomes this: Is this excessive heat production (Yu, Lu, et al., 1997) the cause or simply the consequence of the heatstroke?

The traditional explanation is that an inability to lose heat adequately during exercise in the heat causes heat retention, which becomes toxic to the body cells when the temperature exceeds about 41 °C. Sometimes long-held logical assumptions conceal an opposite truth. In this case, the opposite truth would be that heatstroke is caused not by abnormalities in the heat-dissipating mechanisms but by a state of abnormal heat production—what we have called *excessive endogenous* (within the body) *heat production* (Rae, Knobel, et al., 2008)—which produces heat so rapidly that the heat-dissipating mechanisms of the body are overwhelmed. This is the only possible explanation for the large number of cases of heatstroke that occur in cool conditions, or in athletes exercising at a low intensity, or in those who have been physically active for only a short time, or in those who require to be actively cooled for many hours after they collapse, or in those who show a secondary rise in body temperature after they were initially cooled (figure 5.2).

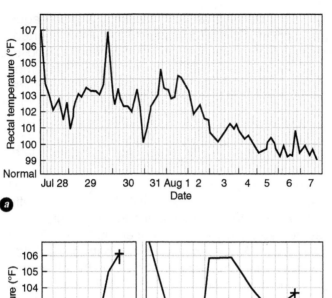

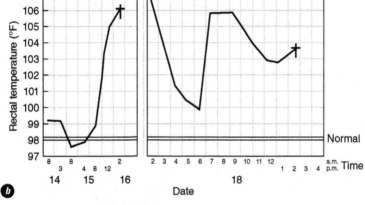

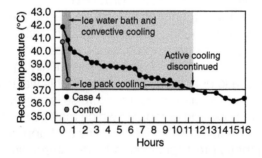

FIGURE 5.2 *(a)* Rectal temperature response over 11 days in a U.S. soldier who was hospitalized and treated for heatstroke on day 1. *(b)* Rectal temperature in 2 U.S. soldiers who died following effective initial treatment for heatstroke (Malamud, Haymaker, et al., 1946). *(c)* Temperatures in two athletes treated for hyperthermia after the 56 km Two Oceans Marathon in Cape Town, South Africa (Rae, Knobel, et al., 2008). † = deceased.

(a, b) Reprinted, by permission, from N. Malamud, W. Haymaker, and R.P. Custer, 1946, "Heat stroke: A clinico-pathologic study of 125 fatal cases," *Military Surgeon* 97: 397-449. © Military Medicine: International Journal of AMSUS. *(c)* Reprinted, by permission, from D.E. Rae, G.J. Knobel, T. Mann, et al., 2008, "Heatstroke during endurance exercise: Is there evidence for excessive endothermy?" *Medicine & Science in Sports & Exercise* 40(7): 1193-1204.

Although they did not identify it as such, Malamud and colleagues (1946) provided evidence in support of this theory (figure 5.2a). They reported cases of fatal heatstroke in which subjects initially responded to cooling but whose temperatures subsequently rose despite continued cooling: "Initially high temperatures were often reduced by ice packs and other cooling measures, sometimes to subnormal levels, but as a rule there was a secondary rise and, in cases of long duration, several rises . . . [these] subsequent fluctuations suggest a persistent disturbance in thermoregulation" (p. 401). The only explanation for the cases shown in figure 5.2 is the persistence into recovery of an abnormal state of excessive endogenous heat production.

In two soldiers, a secondary rise in rectal temperature preceded a fatal outcome (figure 5.2b). Their rectal temperatures were initially reduced by effective cooling but rose inexorably within a few hours, leading to a fatal outcome.

In two athletes treated for hyperthermia after the 56 km Two Oceans Marathon in Cape Town, South Africa, immersion in a bath of ice-cold water rapidly reduced one athlete's rectal temperature, whereas in the other athlete, the fall in rectal temperature was much slower (figure 5.2c). That athlete with heatstroke required 11 hours of continuous cooling before his rectal temperature stabilized in the normal range.

These cases can be explained only if their heatstroke was due not to a failure of their heat-losing mechanisms as is the usual explanation, but because of an abnormal state of heat production (excessive endogenous heat production) that (a) overwhelms their normal heat-losing mechanisms causing heatstroke to occur and (b) continues for hours or days after their initial collapse from heatstroke. In addition, these cases prove that not all cases of fatal heatstroke can be prevented by early and effective cooling. Rather, heatstroke is a complex disease with varying degrees of severity, some mild and some that will produce a fatal outcome regardless of the quality of medical care provided.

If some or perhaps the majority of heatstroke cases are due to this abnormal state of excessive endogenous heat production, rather than to a failure of heat-dissipating mechanisms caused by cardiovascular failure—the commonly accepted explanation—then the condition is essentially incidental to exercise since it must be a genetic or acquired condition that is waiting to occur as soon as a toxic combination of factors is present. Exercise is only one factor in this toxic combination. Other factors, one or more of which may be necessary in combination to cause heatstroke to occur so infrequently and apparently randomly as it does, are likely a genetic predisposition, an intercurrent viral or bacterial infection (Carter, III, Cheuvront, et al., 2007; Wyndham, 1965), or chemical agents, including specific drugs (Vassallo and Delaney, 1989) such as ephedra, cocaine, or amphetamines or drugs that interfere with sweating, such as atropine, propantheline, or scopolamine.

There may also be a brain component to the initiation of the excessive endogenous heat production. German scientists (Kochs, Hoffman, et al., 1990) have shown alterations in brain function in pigs with malignant hyperthermia. These changes occur before the onset of the metabolic disturbances that indicate the onset of hyperthermia. Changes may occur well in advance of the changes in skeletal muscle that induce the catastrophic rise in body temperature.

It is a common observation that the abnormalities in brain function in people with heatstroke are out of proportion to the degree to which the body temperature is raised since higher temperatures in fever are not associated with the same degree of brain dysfunction. In addition, body temperatures of up to 42 °C can be safely induced in awake humans without any serious alterations in brain function (Pettigrew, Galt, et al., 1974). Marathon runners can also achieve such high temperatures without adverse effects or even the awareness that they are so hot (figure 3.8, page 75; box 2.2, page 49). Perhaps the brain also plays a role in the initiation of heatstroke in human athletes.

Summary of Findings on Dehydration and Heatstroke

There is no published scientific evidence to support the hypothesis that heatstroke is caused by dehydration and that it can be prevented by drinking as much as tolerable during exercise. Rather, the evidence is that heatstroke is a complex and often fatal medical condition that occurs infrequently during prolonged exercise probably because the exercise intensity is below some critical rate necessary to activate the condition. In contrast the risk increases in exercise of short duration in which the exercise intensity is high and in which, coincidentally, the rate of heat production is also high.

Since heatstroke strikes only a few individuals among tens of thousands of athletes competing in the same events or to few among millions of American football players, common factors experienced by all the athletes in those same activities cannot be the cause of heatstroke in the affected few. Rather, there must be individual factors unique to the affected few that explain why only they are afflicted. Shibolet, Coll, and colleagues (1967) made this point already in 1967: "The factor of individual susceptibility is brought out by the fact that usually only one of a group fell victim to heatstroke, and when more than one was claimed, these occurred after variable durations of exertion and varied in severity or affliction" (p. 544).

My interpretation is that, just as is the case with EAH and EAHE, heatstroke must occur when several factors occur simultaneously. First, there must be an individual susceptibility, for example an underlying muscle disorder related to but usually distinct from that causing the medical condition known as malignant hyperthermia (Hopkins and Wappler, 2007). Then there must also be an initiating factor—perhaps a latent bacterial or viral infection or a chemical agent such as amphetamines or cocaine known to be associated with heatstroke. Then there must be exercise, usually of a moderately high intensity. The environment plays a part since the hotter and more humid the environment, the more quickly the body temperature will rise above 41 °C producing the characteristic features of heatstroke if the brain fails to slow the athlete down soon enough as it should. According to this explanation, dehydration need play no part in the production of heatstroke. Rather, an abnormality in skeletal muscle is activated, perhaps when the temperature rises above some critical value, inducing explosive endogenous heat production and muscle cell breakdown with release of toxic chemicals that have widespread deleterious effects on multiple organs. Alternatively, heatstroke might result from abnormalities in the regulation of body temperature by antagonists acting on the vanilloid receptor TRPV1 in peripheral tissues (Gavva, 2008).

Finally, the finding that heatstroke occurs so infrequently in marathon runners raises this question: Why has the myth developed that marathon runners are the group at highest risk for the development of heatstroke, whereas it is 5 to 15 km runners who are at the greatest risk? The tragedy is that the wrong treatment (fluid ingestion at high rates) for a rare condition (heatstroke in marathon runners) that is not even caused by the condition (dehydration) for which the treatment is prescribed would produce a novel, sometimes fatal disease (EAHE) in those who were at absolutely no risk for that rare condition (heatstroke) because they were running at a very low intensity often in cool to cold environmental conditions. Heatstroke can occur in cool environmental conditions, but we have shown that fluid ingestion has little to do with preventing it. Had this myth not taken hold, there would have been no need for this book.

Dr. Cade's Original Studies

Dr. Cade's writings indicate that he shared the belief of Wyndham and Strydom that dehydration reduces heat loss by sweating, often referred to as sweat gland fatigue, causing heat retention and leading inevitably to heatstroke. A feature of the Gatorade phenomenon is that the product launched the sports drink industry even though the evidence for any beneficial effect was initially limited to the purely observational evidence that its use turned the University of Florida football team into the leading U.S. college football team in 1966. Among many other possibilities, the success of the 1966 Gators could have been due to the play of its Heisman Trophy-winning quarterback, who apparently did not drink much Gatorade.

While Dr. Cade did undertake some studies of the Gator football players, those studies were first published in 1971 and 1972, long after the product had already achieved the initial breakthrough that ensured its future success. It is likely that the scientific papers describing the results of those experiments would never have been published but for the legal battle between Dr. Cade and the University of Florida over the university's rights to a share of the royalties for a product developed by its staff on its campus and that conveniently used its football team for marketing and promotion (box 5.2).

Dr. Cade's First Gatorade Study

"Changes in body fluid composition and volume during vigorous exercise by athletes."

Authors: J.R. Cade, H.J. Free, A.M. de Quesada, D.L. Shires, and L. Roby. Department of medicine, University of Florida Medical School. Published in *Journal of Sports Medicine and Physical Fitness,* Volume II, pp. 172-178, 1971.

The focus of this study was to evaluate the effects of the loss of "large amounts of water and salt as sweat, and, as sweat is a hypotonic solution, this should produce electrolyte concentration disturbances as well as marked volume depletion" (Cade, Free, et al., 1971, p. 172). Accordingly "the study was designed to elucidate the changes in composition and volume of body fluids in athletes who exercise in a warm and humid environment" (p. 172). The authors also suggested

BOX 5.2   Legal Battles Over Gatorade Royalties

Few scientists ever enjoy the good fortune of a discovery that produces a massive financial return. Dr. Cade's discovery was perhaps more of a product development than of a true scientific discovery; yet it brought a financial windfall for which no one was prepared. Dr. Cade would write in 1968, "Sometimes I'm sorry I ever invented the thing. If Gatorade didn't get any publicity or make any money, no one would care about it. . . . My lawyers tell me that if the drink is successful, I can expect to get sued two or three times a year from now on" (Rovell, 2005, p. 67). The legal battles for the Gatorade royalties actually fueled the science behind the dehydration myth and a novel science of hydration.

Dr. Cade sold his idea and the name, Gatorade, to Stokely-Van Camp in exchange for royalties payable to the Gatorade Trust. Those royalties were then distributed to 46 trustees in proportion to the size of their shareholding. Since the University of Florida was not an original shareholder in the Gatorade Trust, it was not eligible for any of these royalties.

But believing that the Gatorade brand achieved credibility through its association with its developer who was an employee of the university, and the association of the product with its successful football teams, the University of Florida initiated legal action against Dr. Cade, the Gatorade Trust, and Stokely-Van Camp in July 1971. In a judgment delivered in July 1972, the University of Florida was granted 20% of the royalties to Gatorade retroactively and for the life of the product. In addition, Dr. Cade was refused permission to patent the chemical composition of Gatorade. However, he and Stokely-Van Camp were given the right to retain the brand name, Gatorade, on condition that Dr. Cade described the chemical composition of his product in a scientific publication.

The last legal requirement would explain two questions that puzzled me as I reviewed the two original Gatorade publications discussed subsequently.

First, why were these papers first published 5 years after they had been completed? Either paper could have been written up within a few months and published, at worst, within a year of their completion. Second, why were the papers published in a relatively obscure scientific journal? The journal that Dr. Cade and his colleagues selected for their first two Gatorade publications was the *Journal of Sports Medicine and Physical Fitness.* This journal is published by the Italian company Minerva Medica, which specializes in publishing medical journals for Italian doctors. This begs a question: If the science behind this novel product was so extraordinary, why did the authors choose to publish their findings in such a modest scientific journal?

My conclusion is that the first two Gatorade papers published in 1971 and 1972 were written because they had to be written. Without them and, in particular, their disclosure of the chemical composition of the original Gatorade formulation, the legal case between the University of Florida and Dr. Cade and his associates would not have been concluded to the mutual satisfaction of all parties. That the legal decision was eminently fair has been vindicated. By 2005 the University of Florida had earned about $100 million from Gatorade royalties and the Gatorade Trust about $400 million. As the principal shareholder in the Gatorade Trust, Dr. Cade would also have been remunerated handsomely.

With the publication of Dr. Cade's articles in 1971 and 1972, following in the steps of Wyndham and Strydom's study, the dehydration myth was born. This myth contends that the dehydration that develops during exercise will lead to death unless it is prevented by the act of ingesting fluid at rates that prevent any weight loss during exercise.

It was not Dr. Cade's doing alone that caused his dogma to become the international mantra of sport during the 1990s and beyond. That required the support of a group of scientists who shared his convictions.

that these changes might occur, "in varying degree, among a wide segment of the population" (p. 172).

The subjects for the study were the 10 University of Florida freshmen football players who were studied at the start of the 1965 college football season. A pair of players was studied each day for 5 days during the first week of September until data were available for all 10. Although the year was not stated in the publication, Rovell's book indicates that this study must have been completed in 1965 before Gatorade began to be used regularly by the University of Florida varsity football team. Subjects were studied before and after a "vigorous two hour practice session in the late afternoon" (Cade, Free, et al., 1971, p. 172). There is no record of the environmental conditions at the time of the experiment.

During exercise, the players lost 2.7 kg (2.9% body weight), somewhat less than the water deficits of 4% to 6% incurred by the winning marathon runners studied in the 1960s. Of this volume, 2 L came from the ECF and 0.3 L from the blood (or plasma) volume. The concentration of sodium in the sweat was less than what was present in the blood; thus, the players were sweating the equivalent of a dilute solution of blood. As a result, "… plasma sodium concentrations increased in all subjects as a result of severe sweating" (Cade, Free, et al., 1971, p. 174). This despite their calculations that subjects lost 34 to 370 mmol of sodium (0.78-8.5 g since 1 mmol of sodium = .0229 g).

Since the authors did not measure the rectal temperatures of their players—Rovell (2005) records that none would consent to this indignity—the authors were unable to determine whether or not these players had actually become excessively hot because they did not drink during exercise.[10] Indeed, their paper contains no reference to the appearance of any symptoms of heat illness in any player during the experiment. To link their findings to documented cases of heat illness, the authors quoted evidence from other studies that had no relevance to their own study and findings. They quoted a study in which (a) a 10% to 32% reduction in plasma volume was measured in subjects who collapsed during "fever therapy" and (b) elevated serum sodium concentration (indicating the presence of dehydration) was found in some subjects with heatstroke (Baxter and Teschan, 1958).

Without finding any evidence for heat illness or establishing any link between sweating, fluid loss, and heat illness in their players, Cade and colleagues (1971) concluded that "the few reported observations of volume and compositional change in patients with heatstroke differ from our findings only in degree. That loss of volume adversely affects the ability of the body to dissipate heat (Sargent, 1962) seems quite likely, and may, indeed, be of major importance in the genesis of heatstroke" (p. 176).

10 Ultimately U.S. football players did consent to have their body temperatures measured, but not with the use of a rectal thermometer. Rather, the development of an ingestible pill that transmitted the (intestinal) body temperature to a receiver outside the body was used. Using this technique, studies of the Pittsburgh Steelers NFL football team, among others, have found that professional football players do not become particularly hot during football training. In fact, they stay quite cool (Fowkes, Godek, et al., 2004). In addition, drinking does not alter the extent to which their temperatures rise during football practices. The main factors determining their body temperatures appear to be their metabolic rates during play and the length of the rest periods between plays. The intermittent nature of American football means that the average metabolic rate sustained by players is quite low even if players exert themselves vigorously during each play. When conditions are excessively hot, the best advice is to allow the players longer rest periods to cool down after each set of downs.

The focus of science must be to evaluate causation rather than to speculate why such causation, unproven by one's studies, *must* exist. This is especially relevant if one's study finds no evidence of the primary illness for which one is seeking a cause—in this case heat illness—in any of the 10 University of Florida freshmen football players who were studied (box 5.3). Just as Wyndham and Strydom's study had found no evidence for any "dangers" of drinking sparingly during 2 or more hours of vigorous exercise, nor had Dr. Cade's original study found any evidence that the mild levels of dehydration in these football players was dangerous.

Cade and colleagues (1971) continued with their remonstration, questioning "salt ingestion without adequate water intake," given that sweat is a hypotonic solution. "Indeed, ingestion of salt without water during exercise, a practice common among athletes, would aggravate the basic physiologic disturbance" (p. 176).

In their concluding paragraphs, the authors stated, "Our studies demonstrate that large amounts of salt and water are lost during exercise. . . . The ideal

BOX 5.3 Heatstroke in Subjects Participating in Research Studies

Dr. Cade's finding that the subjects who did not ingest any fluid during exercise did not develop heatstroke despite becoming dehydrated poses this question: What happens to athletes who participate in research studies in which they are not allowed to drink either anything or as much as they might wish during prolonged exercise? Are they at risk of developing heat illness and heatstroke? If so, is it safe to allow such studies? Or should such studies be banned by university research committees charged with ensuring the safety of human subjects participating in studies in which they must exercise in the heat? If the descriptions of the dangers of not drinking during exercise are real, then this is an important ethical question.

I traced 39 studies of fluid ingestion during exercise that included a control trial in which subjects either did not ingest any fluid or whose fluid intake was restricted so that they drank less than their thirst dictated. In total, there were at least 459 individual performances by subjects who either did not drink at all or whose fluid intake during exercise was restricted.

The conclusion is that in none of these studies did a single athlete develop heatstroke despite the severe environmental conditions in which some of the trials were conducted. For example, subjects in the study of Sawka, Young, and colleagues (1992) began exercise in 49 °C (120.2 °F) heat when they were already dehydrated by 8%; yet none developed heatstroke and all terminated exercise with "heat exhaustion" with body temperatures below 40 °C. This suggests that the term "heat exhaustion" applies to a condition that the brain uses to ensure that the athlete stops exercising before her body temperature reaches the heatstroke range.

While the body temperatures at the termination of exercise were predictably higher when no fluid was ingested, the increase was small and in very few cases did rectal temperatures exceed 40 °C in those who did not ingest any fluid during exercise. In only 4 studies (Brown, 1947a; Brown, 1947b; Mudambo, Leese, et al., 1997; Sawka, Young, et al., 1992; Strydom, 1975) was it noted that some subjects developed unpleasant symptoms when they did not ingest fluid during exercise. In none of the laboratory trials of athletes were there any reports of heat illness or heat exhaustion when subjects did not drink at all during exercise.

replacement fluid for an exercising athlete who is vigorously perspiring, then, is a hypotonic salt solution to which glucose has been added. Such a solution has been in use at the University of Florida for the past three years and has significantly decreased the incidence of heat related illness." (p. 177).

Summary of Dr. Cade's First Study This is the study that, according to Dr. Cade's memory 40 years later, produced results that were "eye-opening. The players' electrolytes were completely out of balance, their blood sugars were low and their total blood volume was low. The impact on the body of this upheaval in chemistry was profound. Each of these conditions, by itself, would to some extent incapacitate a player" (Kays and Phillips-Han, 2003, p. 2). From this description one would wonder how it was possible for humans ever to have survived any form of exercise in the heat and certainly not 6 hours of sustained running with minimal fluid ingestion in extreme heat.

The authors were correct in their conclusion that exercise causes a loss of salt and water from the body. But whether or not such losses are "large," as they stated, is not a question for science. Rather, this is a value judgment that exists beyond the realm of science. In fact, the losses they measured were not as large as those measured in winning marathon runners or other ultraendurance athletes, for example those completing the 90 km (56 mile) Comrades Marathon.[11] Nor was there any evidence that the water losses approached the 8 kg (18 lb) that Dr. Cade would later claim. In fact, they were a rather modest ~3 kg, again substantially less than losses reported in runners who completed marathon and ultramarathon races without becoming incapacitated since they generally won those races.

11 Dr. Cade did not actually measure the salt losses in these football players. Rather, he estimated these losses on the basis of changes in body water content and blood sodium concentrations. We measured salt losses of 150 to 200 mmol (8-13 g) in athletes completing ultramarathon races with and without EAH or EAHE (Irving, Noakes, et al., 1991).

These water and sodium losses caused the blood sodium concentration to rise, as is always found in those who do not drink to excess during prolonged exercise. Only later would the GSSI develop the argument that large sodium losses will cause the blood sodium concentration to fall, causing EAH unless a sodium-containing sports drink is ingested during prolonged exercise.

Dr. Cade's study was not designed to determine whether or not their solution was ideal because they included no measure of efficacy. Nor did the study include any data to support their claim that use of their solution has significantly decreased the incidence of heat-related illness. Nor did they indicate in what population at the University of Florida this effect had been observed.

This study provided not a single shred of evidence to support their conclusions. Yet this study would assist in the creation of a novel model of human temperature regulation, subsequently adopted by Gatorade and the GSSI, which holds that dehydration is the most important determinant of the body temperature response to exercise so that, unless prevented, dehydration will lead to death from heat illness or heatstroke.

Dr. Cade's Second Gatorade Study

"Effect of fluid, electrolyte, and glucose replacement during exercise on performance, body temperature, rate of sweat loss, and compositional changes of extracellular fluid."

Authors: R. Cade, G. Spooner, E. Schlein, M. Pickering, R. Dean. Department of medicine, University of Florida Medical School. Published in the *Journal of Sports Medicine and Physical Fitness*, Volume 12, pp. 150-156, 1972.

This paper clearly establishes that by 1972, Dr. Cade and colleagues had developed an intellectual model of the relationship between sweating during exercise and heat illness (figure 5.3) that mirrored what Wyndham and Strydom developed (figure 3.1, page 61). In this model (A) high rates of sweating during exercise in (B) those who drink at low rates (C) cause dehydration (true), which (D) directly causes heat illness, leading ultimately to heatstroke (untrue). Thus the only way to (F and G) optimize health, safety, and performance during exercise is to (E) ingest fluid, glucose, and electrolytes at high rates. This explanation would form the basis for the 1996 ACSM position stand, which promoted the idea that athletes need to drink "the maximal amount that can be tolerated" during exercise in order to prevent heatstroke that develops as the result of "cardiovascular strain" in those who become dehydrated during exercise.

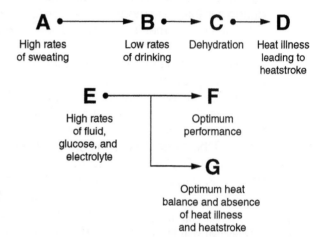

FIGURE 5.3 Dr. Cade's model of thermoregulation during exercise.
Adapted from Cade, Free, De Quesada, Shires, Roby 1971; Cade, Spooner, Schlein, Pickering, Dean 1972.

Gatorade, the GSSI, the ACSM—in their 2007 position stands (Armstrong, Casa, et al., 2007; Sawka, Burke, et al., 2007)—and the scientists undertaking research for Gatorade are still promoting Dr. Cade's interpretation 38 years later, despite an absence of conclusive evidence supporting this revolutionary theory.

To evaluate this hypothesis, Cade and colleagues evaluated the effects of three different drinking options on the time to run 7 miles (11.2 km) in which walking and running were interspersed so that subjects ran a total of 5.25 miles (8.45 km) and walked 1.75 miles (2.82 km). Subjects, not always the same, completed one or more of three different trials in which they drank the following:

1. Nothing.
2. A dilute (0.1%) sodium chloride drink flavored with citric acid and lemon juice, drunk ad libitum (according to the dictates of thirst). (This solution was erroneously called water on one of the tables in the paper.)
3. The original Gatorade solution containing sodium (Na^+) 17 mmol/L, potassium (K^+) 3.5 mmol/L, phosphate (PO^{4-}) 6 mmol/L, chloride (Cl^-) 12 mmol/L,

and 3% glucose, also flavored with citric acid and lemon juice. This solution differs somewhat from the present Gatorade solution of Na^+ 20 mmol/L (464 mg/L), K^+ 3.3 mmol/L (127 mg/L), Cl^- 11.2 mmol/L (392 mg/L), and 6% (5.9g/L) carbohydrate. The reasons the new Gatorade formulation has a higher glucose content is described by Rovell (2005).[12] This solution was also drunk ad libitum.

A total of six subjects were involved in two separate trials. In the first trial, four subjects completed all their three 7-mile runs in a single week while ingesting one of the three solutions in random order. These four subjects then repeated the same three experiments, each week for another two weeks until each had run three times drinking each of the three different solutions for a total of nine experimental runs. Blood sodium and glucose concentrations as well as performance were measured for the full 7 miles and for the final 800 m. Environmental conditions during this trial were moderately warm (27.6-28.9 °C, 37-42% RH). Conditions were substantially warmer in the second set of experiments (32.2-34.4 °C, 40-48% RH).

The authors' first finding was that the blood sodium concentrations rose in all groups during exercise. However, the rise was greatest when the runners did not drink during the trial (figure 5.4). This response conflicts with the theory, subsequently developed, that the failure to drink electrolyte-containing solutions like Gatorade during exercise causes a fall in serum sodium concentrations leading to EAH and EAHE. Rather, drinking dilute sodium-containing fluids substantially reduced the extent to which serum sodium concentrations *rose* during exercise (figure 5.4). These findings were in line with all the evidence available at that time (table 4.2, page 129), which showed that not drinking at all, and therefore incurring the largest sodium deficit, *always* caused the blood sodium concentration to rise during exercise. The identical response was observed by Barr, Costill, and colleagues (1991) (figure 9.14, page 281).

Overall running performance and performance during the final 800 m were significantly superior when the carbohydrate electrolyte drink was ingested compared to drinking either nothing or the saline solution. Ingesting the carbohydrate and electrolyte solution reduced the 7-mile run and walk time from about 82 to 83 minutes in the placebo and saline trials to about 78.5 minutes with the Gatorade solution. This improvement reflects an enhancement in running performance of about 3%. This is compatible with the view that, in exercise of this duration, it is the glucose in the drink, rather than the fluid, that enhances the exercise performance. In only 1 of the 24 runs did an athlete run slower when ingesting the ancestral Gatorade solution than when ingesting either water or saline.

In the second group of experiments, conducted in much hotter conditions, the subjects were asked

12 The original Gatorade solution was sweetened with the artificial sweetener calcium cyclamate. By 1968, there was growing concern that cyclamates might be hazardous for health; by November 1969 the U.S. Secretary for Health and Human Services had declared cyclamates unsafe for human use, and by 1 January, 1970, all soft drinks with cyclamates were removed from the U.S. market. To improve its taste, the manufacturer of Gatorade increased its carbohydrate content from 3% to 6% when the cyclamates were removed. More recently, high-fructose corn syrup was used to sweeten the product, although as of 2011 the sweetness has been provided by dextrose and sucrose. There is growing concern of the possible causative role fructose (present also in sucrose) plays in the development of obesity, diabetes, and perhaps heart disease (Johnson, Perez-Pozo, Sautin, et al., 2009).

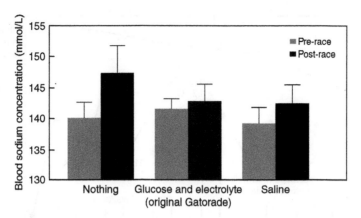

FIGURE 5.4 Blood sodium concentrations during a 7-mile run and walk in subjects who drank either nothing (left), the original Gatorade solution (middle), or a saline solution (right).
Data from Cade, Spooner, Schlein, Pickering, Dean 1972.

to run and walk as far as they could for up to 7 miles. Under these conditions, somewhat surprisingly, no runner completed more than 6.5 miles when drinking nothing, and only three finished the full 7 miles when drinking the 0.1% sodium drink. But all completed 7 miles when drinking the ancestral Gatorade solution. Thirty performances were completed by five subjects, but the design was unbalanced since one subject completed nine trials, three subjects completed six each, and one subject completed only three trials.

In these experiments, rectal temperatures were measured as were body weight changes, in order to calculate sweat rates. Rectal temperatures rose more rapidly in the group ingesting either nothing or saline. But because so few runs were completed in the heat, it was not possible to evaluate the statistical significance of this finding.

Finally in a single subject, it was noted that his rectal temperature rose progressively during exercise and that his skin temperature was higher during running than when walking except in the final five interval runs when this pattern was reversed (220-yard walks, numbers 11,13, and 15) (figure 5.5, page 176).

Dr. Cade and colleagues concluded that the lower skin temperatures in the final five runs indicated the following: "The abrupt reversal in the pattern of skin temperature change was due, we think, to poor perfusion of the skin during running as blood was shunted away from skin and to working muscle. . . . Decrease in perfusion of the skin as a result of volume depletion resulting from severe sweating and shunting of blood to muscles during running is in effect a failure of the heat dissipating mechanism and accounts for the marked rise in rectal temperature which occurred during the last three miles of the run" (p. 153-154). To emphasize their point, the authors also wrote that "the subject's skin became pale when he ran and quite flushed during each 220 yard walk" (p. 153).

In fact, this conclusion is the opposite of the true finding: The rectal temperature rose less than half as high in the final 4 miles as it did in the first 3 miles (figure 5.5, page 176). This, despite the possibility that the athlete might have run faster in the final 800 m, since he knew his performance was being monitored

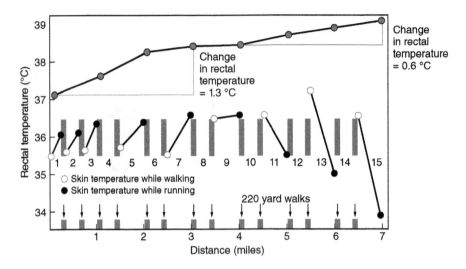

FIGURE 5.5 The rectal and skin temperature response in a single subject in the study of Cade, Spooner, and colleagues, 1972.

Reprinted by permission of Edizioni Minerva Medica from: *J Sports Med Phys Fitness*, 1972 Sep; 12(3): 150-156.

during that section of the race and he was near the end of the event, making a finishing spurt highly probable. The lower skin temperatures in this athlete might have occurred if he ran faster during these runs and so generated an increased convective cooling. Alternatively, the cloud cover might have increased after run 8, reducing the amount of radiant heat to which the runner was exposed. The fall in skin temperature as the subject walked in the 11th, 13th, and 15th intervals of this trial did not indicate the presence of "thermoregulatory failure." Rather, this athlete's thermoregulatory function was superior during the final 4 miles of this run because his core temperature rose less than it did in the first 3 miles, and he terminated exercise with a core body temperature of only 39 °C, well below the tolerable human limit of about 42 °C.

Another unexpected finding was that the average sweat rate was substantially greater when subjects did not drink during the trials (30.3 ml/min/1.73m²) than when they drank either the sodium drink (27.1 ml/min/1.73m²) or the ancestral Gatorade solution (19.7 ml/min/1.73m²). This is the opposite of the popular dogma, advanced in the 1990s, that dehydration caused by not drinking during exercise *reduces* the sweat rate and hence predisposes an athlete to heatstroke by *reducing* the capacity for heat loss from the body. Neither assertion is true.

To explain this unexpected finding, Cade and colleagues proposed that "the greater rate of sweating (when ingesting either nothing or saline) is a result of higher body temperature which is in turn due to less effective perfusion of the skin and the attendant inability to dissipate heat" (p. 155).

While it is correct that the higher body temperature will cause a higher sweat rate (since sweating is probably driven by the rate of heat storage as reflected by the rectal temperature), the higher sweat rate should cool the body more effectively, thus lowering the temperature. The only way to maintain a higher body temperature in the face of an increased sweat rate is to maintain a higher rate of heat production, usually shown as a faster running speed (which did not happen in this study). Either the measurements are in error, or some extraneous factor caused this unusual finding in this experiment. But the authors clearly interpreted this as evidence that by preventing dehydration, the ingestion of fluid allowed greater skin perfusion and superior heat loss. As a result, it was not necessary to sweat as much. This finding fitted their model of thermal regulation (figure 5.3).

The authors also noted that performance was much worse in the heat, suggesting that "heat stress is of major importance in limiting endurance exercise capacity" (p. 155), an extraordinarily important albeit not a novel observation.[13]

Cade and colleagues also proposed that the ability of the ancestral Gatorade solution to slow the rise in body temperature "more strikingly" than did either not drinking or drinking the saline solution "surely recommends the use of such solutions to decrease the likelihood of heat stroke when exercise is performed in a hot climate" (p. 155).

13 The crucial point is that athletes run slower in the heat *from the onset of the exercise bout.* They do not wait to overheat before they slow down. Thus, the response is behavioral and occurs in anticipation (Marino, 2004; Marino, Lambert, et al., 2004; Tucker, Marle, et al., 2006; Tucker, Rauch, et al., 2004) with the aim of ensuring that the body matches its rates of heat production and heat loss from the start of exercise so that heatstroke does not occur.

Summary of Dr. Cade's Second Study   The most important finding of this study was that a 3% glucose solution improved running performance in the heat. The study did not show that it was dangerous not to drink during exercise. As in all the previous studies, there were no cases of heatstroke or heat illness in subjects running in hot conditions, even when they did not drink. The highest body temperature reached by any athlete was only 39.4 °C. The authors reported that running performance was impaired in the heat, but they failed to observe that there was no difference in the final body temperatures in subjects who did or did not complete the full 7-mile run. This is compatible with the theory that the human brain will usually ensure that the athlete slows down or stops running long before the body temperature reaches a dangerous level.

Dr. Cade's Third Gatorade Study

"Marathon running: Physiological and chemical changes accompanying late-race functional deterioration."

Authors: R. Cade, D. Packer, C. Zauner, D. Kaufmann, J. Peterson, D. Mars, M. Privette, N. Hommen, M.J. Fregly, and J. Rogers. Departments of medicine and physiology, and the Center for Physical and Motor Fitness, University of Florida at Gainesville. Published in the *European Journal of Applied Physiology,* Volume 65, pp. 485-491, 1992.

It would be another 20 years before Dr. Cade would complete another study of the effects of fluid ingestion during exercise (Cade R., Packer D. et al., 1992). By then, his conflicts with his university had been resolved and his product had become even more iconic as well as highly profitable. Yet he was apparently still keen to study his "hyperthermia/volume reduction hypothesis" (p. 485) to determine "how vascular volume depletion and its consequent hyperthermia develop and how they and hypoglycemia relate to late-race impairments of performance and specifically to the severe impairment known to runners as 'hitting the wall'" (p. 485).

In this study, three groups of seven runners, each matched for a variety of relevant physiological variables, were studied when they ran a 42 km marathon while drinking either water, Gatorade (glucose 280 mmol/L [5%], sodium 21 mmol/L), or half-strength Gatorade ad libitum. Runners were studied before the race, at 14 and 29 km, and immediately after completion of the race. Race temperatures ranged from 16 to 22.5 °C. Humidity fell from 80% to 60% during the race, and the wind speed varied from 0 to 7 km/hr.

The hypothesis under evaluation was that the late-race deterioration in marathon performance, sometimes known as "hitting the wall," is due to dehydration, which causes a reduction in plasma volume, leading to "cardiovascular strain," impaired skin blood flow, and ultimately heatstroke, according to Dr. Cade's model of thermoregulation during exercise (figure 5.3, page 173).

Their first finding was that the group drinking Gatorade drank significantly more (~2.1 L vs. ~1.3 L) than did the groups drinking either water or half-strength Gatorade. Sweat rate was also higher in the Gatorade group; as a result, the extent of the fluid deficits was similar in all three groups: ~2.8 L (equal to ~2.8 kg). Rectal temperatures during the race were not different between groups (~38-39 °C) and were well below values measured in athletes with heatstroke.[14] However, the rate at which the rectal temperature rose was slightly slower in the runners ingesting Gatorade.

Blood sodium concentrations were best maintained in the group ingesting water and rose the most in the group ingesting Gatorade (figure 5.6a). Total sodium losses

14 That these runners' body temperatures did not reach values measured in cases of heatstroke is to be expected if the human body regulates its physiological functions to ensure that all remain in (homeostatic) balance. This is achieved also by changes in behavior. The fact that athletes "hit the wall" and start to run more slowly can be better understood as a behavioral change that the brain enforces when it perceives that homeostasis cannot be maintained and organ damage prevented if the same behavior (running speed) is maintained for the expected duration of the activity—in this case, running 42 km.

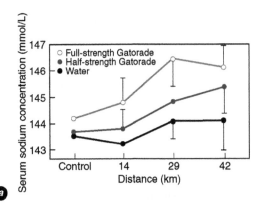

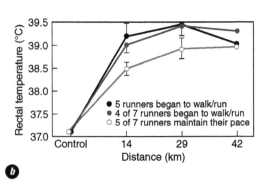

FIGURE 5.6 *(a)* Blood sodium concentrations in three matched groups of 7 runners ingesting either water, Gatorade, or half-strength Gatorade during a 42 km marathon. *(b)* Rectal temperatures in the same three groups during the marathon race.

With kind permission from Springer Science+Business Media: *European Journal of Applied Physiology and Occupational Physiology*, "Marathon running: Physiological and chemical changes accompanying late-race functional deterioration," 65(6), 1992, 485-491, R. Cade, D. Packer, C. Zauner, et al., figure 4, © Springer-Verlag 1992.

averaged about 400 mmol (9.2 g) and were not different between groups. Ingestion of Gatorade replaced only 42 mmol of that loss compared to 0 mmol in the group ingesting water. Plasma volume fell by about 12% in the group ingesting water but by only 8% in the Gatorade group. The reduction in the group ingesting half-strength Gatorade fell between these values (~10% reduction).

Blood glucose concentrations were maintained only in the group ingesting Gatorade, falling in the other two groups. Running time was 3:08 in the Gatorade group versus 3:17 to 3:21 in the water and half-strength Gatorade groups. Only 2 of the 7 athletes (29%) drinking Gatorade ran slower than they had predicted, whereas a much greater proportion (10 of 14, or 71%) of athletes drinking either water or half-strength Gatorade ran slower than they had predicted.

Cade and colleagues concluded this: "The data suggest that poor performance late in the race was due either to exhaustion of carbohydrate stores or to marked reduction of blood volume with its consequent elevation of body temperature, or both. The data also suggest that ingestion of a glucose/electrolyte solution in adequate amounts can either ameliorate or prevent both the energy substrate depletion and the thermal consequences of prolonged vigorous exercise" (p. 491). But this conclusion is not possible since the study did not include a control group that did not drink during the marathon and whose response would have demonstrated "the thermal consequences of prolonged vigorous exercise," whatever those might be.

The study also showed that drinking Gatorade was not the most effective way to reduce the body temperature. Rather, it was to stop running and to start walking as occurred in a number of athletes ingesting water. Once those athletes started walking after 29 km, their rectal temperatures fell sharply (figure 5.6*b*). Paradoxically, according to these data, by allowing athletes to run faster, the provision of fluid and energy *increased* the body temperature during exercise. These findings confirm the importance of running speed as the key determinant of the body temperature during exercise.

The fact that 11 of the 21 runners started walking even when their body temperatures were well below those that cause heatstroke again suggests the protective action of the brain.[15] Finally, the rectal temperatures were precisely within the range reported in all the other studies reviewed in chapter 3.

15 Probably the best example of the phenomenon in which the brain causes the athlete literally to stop in her tracks in order to prevent the development of heatstroke occurred to Englishwoman Paula Radcliffe in the 2004 Athens Olympic Games Marathon for women.

My theory, based on our studies, is that when the environmental conditions exceed about 35 °C with humidity in excess of ~30%, it becomes increasingly unlikely that a runner generating as much heat as Radcliffe (because of her fast running speed) will be able to lose all that excess heat into the environment—not because she was unable to transfer that heat to the environment by increased sweating and blood flow to the skin, but rather because the environment was unable to absorb that heat as rapidly as she was producing it. As a result, Radcliffe would have retained heat as she ran. Ultimately at 36 km, her body temperature likely reached ~42 °C and her brain decided that that was far enough and so it called a stop to her forward progress. Radcliffe reported that she felt as if she could not put one foot in front of the other—a human example of hyperthermic paralysis.

If Dr. Cade's model is correct, then Paula Radcliffe could have won that race if she had simply drunk more during the race. But that is nonsensical. Paula Radcliffe could have finished that race only if (a) she had run slower, (b) if the race had been held in slightly cooler and especially less humid conditions, or (c) if, like the winner of the race (40 kg Japanese runner Mizuki Noguchi), she had been lighter by about 12 kg.

Summary of Dr. Cade's Third Study   The clear finding of Dr. Cade's final study was that the ingestion of Gatorade improved the performance of a group of marathon runners. This appears an incontrovertible finding. However, the method of action was not established since two variables—blood glucose concentrations and plasma volume—were different between the groups ingesting Gatorade, half-strength Gatorade, or water. Determining which of these two effects improved the marathon running performance of the group ingesting Gatorade was not possible since the experimental design did not allow this distinction.

Rather, the authors postulate that this effect was due to the prevention of "the marked reduction of blood volume with its *consequent* [my emphasis] elevation of body temperature" (p. 491). This is entirely dependent on their belief that dehydration causes an elevation of body temperature into the range that impairs performance, a necessary conclusion from the erroneous Wyndham and Strydom interpretation.

But the conclusion is not warranted since there were no differences in rectal temperatures at the finish in the groups who drank either Gatorade or water even though the plasma volume was 4% higher in those who drank Gatorade, despite similar levels of total weight loss (dehydration) in both groups. According to the authors' hypothesis, the group who drank only water should have been hotter at the race finish since they had the greater reduction in plasma volume. But they were not. This finding was therefore not compatible with their conclusion that the maintenance of a higher plasma volume during marathon running improves heat loss (by preventing "cardiovascular strain"), thereby maintaining a lower body temperature.

The most logical explanation is that the rectal temperatures in the water and half-strength Gatorade groups fell from 29 to 42 km because they slowed down, in part because they were developing a progressive reduction in their blood glucose concentrations (hypoglycemia). It is now known that besides the prevention of hypoglycemia, glucose ingestion aids performance during running by lowering the perception of effort at any running speed (Burgess, Robertson, et al., 1991), thereby allowing a faster running speed at the same level of psychic effort. That this effect is due to a central brain effect is also now properly recognized (Gant, Stinear, et al., 2010). The greater metabolic rate engendered by a faster running speed explained the higher body temperatures as described in box 3.1 (page 62).

To elevate the body temperature enough (>42 °C) so that there is a real risk that heatstroke will develop, the athlete must continue to run extremely fast for a short time (20-60 min). This requires superior athletic ability, high levels of fitness, inordinate effort, determination, commitment, and willpower. Only the very fittest, most determined athletes need apply. Even then, heatstroke is likely to occur only in athletes with a genetic predisposition when some other external factor is also acting, be it (among many other possibilities that have yet to be properly studied) an intercurrent viral illness, or the ingestion of either a thermogenic agent like ephedrine or a drug like the amphetamines that interfere with the action of the normal brain controls.

Summary

Dr. Cade's invention of Gatorade changed the world of hydration during exercise for decades to come. Despite the thoroughly upstanding and honorable gentleman that Dr. Cade proved to be throughout his life, he unfortunately followed the example of two highly skilled scientists, Wyndham and Strydom, erroneously identifying dehydration as the singular cause of heatstroke. This would have consequences that he could not have foreseen.

In the first three classic Gatorade studies undertaken by Dr. Cade and his colleagues, a total of 40 subjects were studied:

- 10 freshman football players (Cade, Free, et al., 1971) "during a vigorous two hour practice session in the late afternoon" when they did not ingest any fluid (p. 172).
- 9 athletes as they ran 7 miles in cool or hot conditions when they either drank nothing or an electrolyte-containing solution or an ancestral Gatorade solution. This group completed a total of 66 individual runs.
- 21 runners who completed a marathon drinking either water, or half- or full-strength Gatorade.

Thus there were a total of 97 individual athletic performances. In 22 of these performances, subjects did not drink anything during exercise. An objective assessment of these studies allows the following conclusions:

1. Glucose ingestion improves running performance in races of 7 miles and 42 km.
2. American football players can safely practice for 2 hours in the heat without ingesting fluid.
3. Athletes can safely run 7 miles in moderate heat without drinking.
4. Rectal temperatures did not reach dangerous levels even in those who did not drink in any of these experiments.
5. No athlete developed heat illness, heat cramps, or other medical conditions even when they did not drink. Thus these conditions are not caused exclusively by dehydration in those who do not drink during exercise.
6. Sweat rates during exercise were modest (~1 L/hr).
7. Athletes lost substantial amounts of sodium in their sweat. Yet their blood sodium concentrations *rose*. Thus, athletes do not need to ingest sodium-containing sports drinks to prevent the development of EAH during exercise.

But these would not be the conclusions adopted by the GSSI as it began to market Gatorade as "the most thoroughly researched beverage in the world, and the only sports drink with more than 40 years of science to back up its claims that it works, hydrating athletes, replenishing electrolytes and providing fuel for working muscles" (Hein, 2009, p. 1).

CHAPTER 6

The Shaky Science of Hydration

After you finish the race you should start drinking water as soon as possible. Find the bottled water that is for finishers and drink a full bottle within the first few minutes of finishing. Continue to drink water and sports drink at a rate of about 22 oz per hour.

Hydration advice for runners in the 2005 Dallas Marathon, 20 years after it was first suggested that this advice is likely to cause EAHE in slow runners with SIADH

The main finding of the three studies performed by Dr. Cade and his colleagues reviewed in chapter 5 was that glucose ingestion improved exercise performance. This finding has since been confirmed repeatedly in the past 40 years and is no longer in doubt.[1] This beneficial effect occurs even in exercise of quite short duration (30-60 min) when it is not likely due to a replenishment of depleted carbohydrate stores in the body or the reversal of a low blood glucose concentration.

1 Recall that at this time everyone believed that adequate fluid ingestion was essential for maximizing performance during prolonged exercise and that carbohydrate ingestion was of no value. There was no scientific proof that carbohydrate ingestion improved performance, so most scientists, following David Costill's lead, discounted the possibility that carbohydrate ingestion improved performance. At the sports medicine conference that preceded the 1984 American Medical Joggers Association 80 km ultramarathon in Chicago, Bruce Fordyce established a United States All-Comers 50-mile record of 4:50:51. In response to Fordyce's question to Dr. Costill, Dr. Costill said that carbohydrate ingestion during exercise was more likely to impair than to improve his performance. But Bruce did not agree, informing Dr. Costill, as he told me later, "I am unable to run my best in races of 80 km unless I ingest a high-carbohydrate drink during the race." Only in 1986 would the first irrefutable evidence be presented to confirm what Bruce had discovered for himself—that carbohydrate ingestion during prolonged exercise improves performance.

This suggests the ingested carbohydrate probably acts via the brain,[2] reducing the sensations of effort. We have recently shown that the rate at which the sensations of effort increase during exercise accurately predicts the duration of exercise that the athlete will willingly sustain (Crewe, Tucker, et al., 2008); others have confirmed this finding (Eston, Faulkner, et al., 2007; Eston, Lambrick, et al., 2008). Thus, the reduction in the sensations of effort when carbohydrate is ingested indicates that the athlete will be able to continue exercising either at a higher intensity for the same duration or at the same intensity but for longer. Probably this is because the brain calculates that if carbohydrate is to be provided regularly during exercise, then it is safe to exercise either harder or for longer.

But this really is a side issue. The most important conclusion from those studies must be that they failed to prove that the ingestion of Gatorade during exercise produced the result for which it had originally been formulated by Dr. Cade, specifically to prevent heat illness and heatstroke. Since no subject in any of these studies developed a heat illness even when they did not drink anything during exercise, the experimental design could not determine whether or not the ingestion of Gatorade protected against these conditions.

In this chapter, we look at the continuation of research on sports drinks, specifically the studies that were funded by Gatorade, which influenced the drinking guidelines that were subsequently published by leading sport science organizations.

2 Dr. Asker Jeukendrup and colleagues, who receive funding from GlaxoSmithKline (the manufacturers of Lucozade Sport, the major competitor for Gatorade in Europe), have shown that ingested carbohydrate drinks produce performance effects that do not occur when the same amount of carbohydrate is injected directly into the bloodstream (Carter, Jeukendrup, Jones, 2004). More surprisingly, these studies show that simply swishing a carbohydrate drink in the mouth without swallowing it enhances exercise performance (Carter, Jeukendrup, Mann, et al., 2004).

I interpret this to mean that receptors perhaps in the mouth inform the brain that the athlete is ingesting carbohydrate-containing solutions so that the brain can allow an enhanced exercise performance. A more recent study from this group has identified the brain centers involved in this response (Chambers, Bridge, et al., 2009).

Three Core Gatorade-Funded Studies

If you wish to develop a medicine to cure or prevent an illness, then it is perhaps important to study patients with the illness or who have a predisposition for developing that illness when exposed to the causative agents. Alternatively, it is rather important that the illness you are trying to prevent actually exist and be caused by the mechanism you are studying.

Instead, scientists determined to prove the beneficial effects of fluid ingestion during exercise have developed surrogate measures that they believe identify conditions that will lead to heat illness or heatstroke should the exercise continue for sufficiently long. Such surrogate measures might be an elevated rectal temperature during exercise, which is taken as evidence that heat illness or heatstroke is about to occur, or a falling blood sodium concentration, which is interpreted as evidence that EAH or EAHE will develop if the experiment is continued for 4 to 5 hours, the usual exercise duration required for producing EAH and EAHE.

With two exceptions (Speedy, Noakes, et al., 2001; Stachenfeld and Taylor, 2009), instead of studying athletes who are known to be predisposed to developing heat illness, heatstroke, or EAH/EAHE during exercise, scientists have used surrogate measures in healthy subjects, *at no proven risk for developing any of these specific condition,* to draw conclusions about the probability that the ingestion of a sports drink will prevent the development of these conditions in those (few) individuals who are really predisposed to developing these conditions during exercise. Were sports drinks such as Gatorade registered as therapeutic medicines, then the regulatory authorities would have ensured that those experiments were conducted appropriately before any such medical claims were made.

This error, which began with the studies directed by Dr. Cade (chapter 5), was perpetuated in the very first independent industry-funded study, which was conducted by a highly regarded scientist, Dr. David Costill. This would be the first of three studies from which the myth that humans can exercise safely only if they drink "as much as tolerable" would develop. And from the dissemination of this myth, athletes began to overdrink during exercise.

First Gatorade-Funded Study

"Fluid ingestion during distance running."

Authors: D.L. Costill, W.F. Kammer, and A. Fisher. Published in *Archives of Environmental Health*, Volume 21, pp. 520-525, 1970.

For this first industry-funded study in an independent laboratory, Costill and colleagues (Costill, Kammer, et al., 1970) evaluated four experienced marathon runners who ran at 70% of their maximum oxygen consumption ($\dot{V}O_2$max) for 2 hours in moderate environmental conditions (24.8-25.6 °C, 49-55% RH) while ingesting nothing, or 100 ml water, or 100 ml of the ancestral Gatorade solution with a glucose concentration of 4.4% every 5 minutes for the first 100 minutes of a 120-minute run (rate of intake 1,000 ml/hr). The air velocity produced by the laboratory fans "cooling" the runners during the trials was 5.7 km/hr, considerably less than these runners' usual racing speeds of 18 to 19 km/hr. Those small laboratory fans would also not have caused the constant movement of all the air surrounding the athlete as occurs either during outdoor exercise or during laboratory exercise in a properly constructed wind tunnel (Saunders, Dugas, et al., 2005) (box 6.1, page 186).

BOX 6.1   **Convective Cooling in Laboratory Exercise Testing**

After he had won his fifth Tour de France, the Belgian cyclist Eddy Merckx, considered the greatest and most successful professional cyclist of all time, was invited to demonstrate his exceptional endurance capabilities in a French exercise laboratory (Morrison, 1997). Since Merckx found no difficulty cycling for up to six hours daily at a high intensity during the Tour, it was assumed that he would be able quite easily to cycle at the same pace for just a few hours in the laboratory. So "he began with élan, only to quit, tired, drenched in sweat and bitterly disappointed after an hour. What the lab bike did not provide was the 25-mile-an-hour head wind Eddy took with him everywhere he pedaled. Air drag was his chief adversary, for he had to push aside masses of air to reach speed, but his main ally, too, because that draft alone cooled him as energy income required. No head wind, no cooling, no sustained performance" (p. 150).

With two notable exceptions (Mora-Rodriguez, Del Coso, et al., 2007; Saunders, Dugas, et al., 2005), most laboratory studies of fluid ingestion during exercise, including the original Gatorade-funded studies, have failed to provide adequate convective cooling in the form of large fans that generate wind speeds appropriate for the speed that athletes exercising at that intensity would generate if they were exercising outdoors.

When we were designing the Sports Science Institute of South Africa, I was determined that we should develop a state-of-the-art environmental chamber for the study of exercise in the heat. But I was also determined that we would not fall into the trap exposed by these experiments on Eddy Merckx in which the laboratory where the studies were conducted was unable to match the convective cooling that Merckx would naturally experience when he cycled outdoors in the Tour de France. Thus, we designed a chamber in which four massive fans, each with a diameter of 1.2 m, circulated air around a chamber specially designed to ensure uniform air movement throughout the entire chamber at a preset air velocity appropriate for the work rate at which the athlete was exercising. We (Saunders, Dugas, et al., 2005) wished to determine what the effect was of four different wind velocities (0, 10, 33, and 50 km/hr) on performance and physiological changes when cyclists exercised at a fixed work rate in the environmental conditions (33 °C, 59% RH) studied by Drs. Montain and Coyle (Montain and Coyle, 1992) in their influential study reviewed subsequently in this chapter.

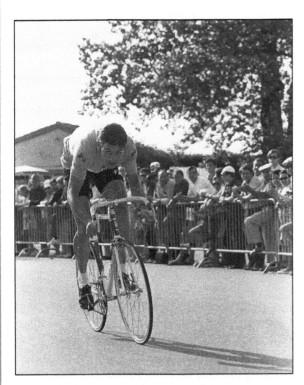

Eddy Merckx racing in the 1970 Tour de France. The athlete who exercises outdoors generates a facing wind speed equal to the speed of progression (presuming there is no tailwind).

AP Photo

First, we found, exactly as Eddy Merckx had discovered, that without any circulating wind subjects stopped after about 60 minutes of cycling. But exercise time increased progressively as the wind speed increased so that the same subjects were able to exercise at the same intensity for more than 2 hours at the highest wind speed of 50 km/hr (figure 6.1a).

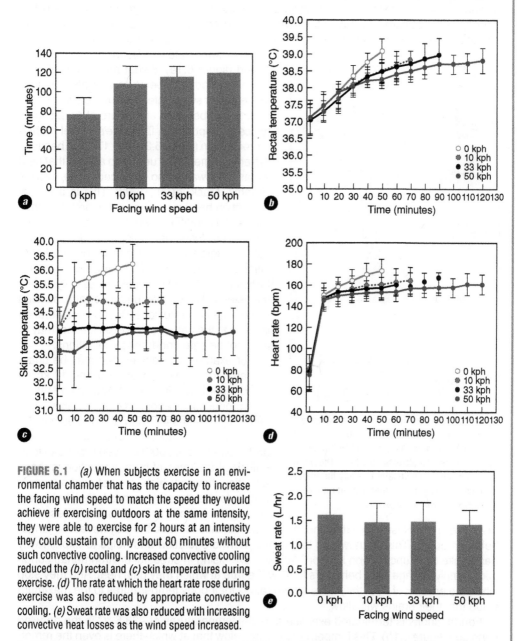

FIGURE 6.1 *(a)* When subjects exercise in an environmental chamber that has the capacity to increase the facing wind speed to match the speed they would achieve if exercising outdoors at the same intensity, they were able to exercise for 2 hours at an intensity they could sustain for only about 80 minutes without such convective cooling. Increased convective cooling reduced the *(b)* rectal and *(c)* skin temperatures during exercise. *(d)* The rate at which the heart rate rose during exercise was also reduced by appropriate convective cooling. *(e)* Sweat rate was also reduced with increasing convective heat losses as the wind speed increased.

(a, e) Data from Saunders, Dugas, Tucker, et al., 2005. *(b-d)* From A.G. Saunders, J.P. Dugas, R. Tucker, M.I. Lambert, and T.D. Noakes, 2005, "The effects of different air velocities on heat storage and body temperature in humans cycling in a hot, humid environment," *Acta Physiologica Scandinavica* 183(3): 241-255. © 2005 Scandinavian Physiological Society. Adapted by permission of John Wiley and Sons.

(continued)

BOX 6.1 Convective Cooling in Laboratory Exercise Testing *(continued)*

Second, increasing wind speed dramatically reduced the rate at which the body stored heat. The skin and rectal temperatures (figure 6.1*b* and *c*) fell to progressively lower values as wind speed increased. One result was that heart rate was also reduced (figure 6.1*d*); hence, so-called cardiovascular strain was reduced simply by ensuring that the laboratory conditions more closely resembled those occurring naturally during exercise outdoors.

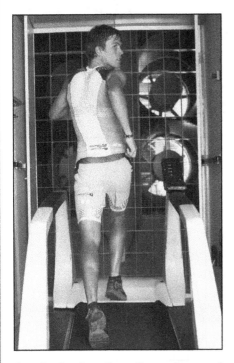

Ryan Sandes, Cape Town ultramarathoner and winner of all 28 stages of the 4 Desert Races, training in the environmental chamber at the Sport Science Institute of South Africa. The chamber is designed specifically to study the effects of convective cooling on human performance.

Shawn Benjamin, www.arkimages.com

Third, sweat rate also fell with increasing wind speed (figure 6.1*e*). Sweat rates were highest when the body temperature was also highest; these higher sweat rates were unable to cool the athlete, not because of a failure of sweating as typically proposed in Dr. Cade's model of thermoregulation (figure 5.3, page 173) but because the environment was unable to absorb that heat as fast as it was being produced by the cyclists (Adams, Mack, et al., 1992). This is a critical distinction because it shows that both the environmental conditions *and* the rate at which heat is being produced determine whether or not it is safe to exercise in specific environmental conditions (Brotherhood, 2008). Yet this is usually forgotten, and blanket guidelines usually dictate that exercise is "unsafe" under certain specified environmental conditions. But no consideration is given to the nature of the exercise that may or may not be safe under those conditions.[3]

For example, conditions that may be unacceptable for running races of 5 and 10 km at world-record pace in which the sustained rate of heat production is about as high as can be sustained by humans for 15 to 30 minutes may be perfectly safe for activities like tennis (Morante and Brotherhood, 2008) or even American football since the rates of heat production in those activities, however high, are not continuous. At least in tennis, the players modify their behaviors so that the hotter the conditions, the less they play—each point lasts a shorter time than in cool conditions—and the players rest for longer between points. This is known as behavioral thermoregulation and helps to explain why heatstroke is so uncommon in sport. Athletes exercising in stressful environmental conditions simply change their behaviors to slow the rate at which they gain heat. And they stop when the amount of heat they have stored raises their body temperatures to the maximum value that their brains will allow.

Fourth, subjects terminated exercise at rectal temperatures of ~38.5 °C in the no-wind condition (figure 6.1*b*). This temperature is well below that at which there is even the remotest risk that heatstroke will develop. This confirms the action of a brain control mechanism, the goal of which is to ensure that the brain does not (usually) try to kill itself by allowing the muscles to continue producing heat faster than the body can lose it.

3 A fundamental misunderstanding that has helped to perpetuate overdrinking in both competitive athletes and hikers is that heatstroke is caused exclusively by environmental conditions, specifically by the hot and humid conditions in which exercise-related heatstroke sometimes occurs. This ignores the obvious biological reality that heatstroke cannot occur in healthy people in these environmental conditions if they do not exercise (and generate a significant heat load). Thus, it is the rate at which metabolic heat is being produced that will always be the most important factor determining the risk of developing heatstroke. The effect of severe environmental conditions is to reduce humans' capacity to lose heat.

But provided athletes produce less heat (by exercising at a lower intensity) so that the heat they produce can still be lost even in severe environmental conditions, then there can be no risk that heatstroke will develop. The probability that heatstroke will develop in any environment must be related primarily to the rate at which the athlete is producing heat. The much slower rate of heat production when walking or hiking slowly in hot conditions will place the walker or hiker at a much lower risk of developing heatstroke than would very fast running (since the lower rate of heat production when walking or hiking slowly will be more easily absorbed by the environment, however hot and humid). Thus, the reason heatstroke is so uncommon in Grand Canyon hikers is quite easy to explain even if it is intriguing (chapter 10, page 322).

Finally, we compared the physiological effects of drinking to replace either 58% (ad libitum) or 80% ("drinking to stay ahead of thirst") of the weight the subjects lost when they cycled in these conditions but into an appropriate facing wind speed of 33 km/hr. Compared to ad libitum drinking, there was no measurable benefit of drinking to stay ahead of thirst.

The relevance of these findings to the interpretation of the findings of the classic Gatorade-funded studies is discussed as each is reviewed.

The four runners in Dr. Costill's study were unusually good: best marathon times of 2:14:28, 2:21:48, 2:33:36, and 2:48:09. The fastest runner was Amby Burfoot, winner of the 1968 Boston Marathon and later the editor of *Runner's World* magazine. This study provided a novel experience for Burfoot since he was not accustomed to drinking during running—he had won the 1968 Boston Marathon even though he had not drunk anything during the race.

The study found that, beginning after 70 minutes of exercise, the runners' rectal temperatures rose significantly more when they did not ingest any fluid (figure 6.2). After 120 minutes of exercise, the terminal rectal temperatures were 39.4 °C (±0.9) in those who did not drink, 38.7 °C (±0.7) in those drinking water, and 38.6 °C (±0.8) in those drinking Gatorade.

Surprisingly, sweat rates were the same in all trials. The authors (Costill, Kammer, et al., 1970a) noted that "each runner's skin was sufficiently wetted by sweating to permit maximal evaporation in all test conditions" (p. 523). Hence, their rate

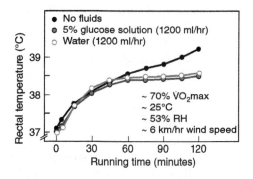

FIGURE 6.2 The rectal temperature response during 2 hours of laboratory exercise in subjects when they drank either nothing, water, or the ancestral Gatorade solution.

Reproduced with permission of The Taylor & Francis Group, from *Archives of Environmental Health*, "Fluid ingestion during distance running," D.L. Costill, W.F. Kammer, and K. Fisher, 21(4), 1970, 520-525. Permission conveyed through Copyright Clearance Center, Inc.

of sweating was not affected by their dehydration when they did not drink during exercise. Since sweating is the major mechanism determining heat loss during exercise in humans, it follows that dehydration had not altered the capacity of these runners to lose the body heat they were producing in these experiments. Thus, the higher rectal temperature in the no-drinking trial was not caused by an impaired sweating capacity.

The failure to drink did not cause the elevation in body temperature by reducing sweating consequent to a reduction in skin blood flow, as proposed in Dr. Cade's original model of thermoregulation during exercise (figure 5.3, page 173). This is an important finding because it cannot be explained by his model, which predicts that dehydration adversely effects thermoregulation during exercise by causing "cardiovascular strain," reducing both skin blood flow and the sweat rate and leading ultimately to heatstroke.

To explain this paradox—namely, that dehydration causes an elevation of body temperature without affecting the capacity of the body to lose heat by sweating—the authors came to the conclusion that the ingested fluid had probably cooled the body. But this is improbable because the amount of heat lost in this way is trivial and a number of other explanations are perhaps more likely.

The authors did make another critical observation that has conveniently been overlooked by subsequent researchers. The experienced marathon runners in this study had great difficulty drinking 100 ml every 5 minutes during exercise (1,200 ml/hr): "All of the runners experienced extreme sensations of fullness during the final five or six feedings [after 75 min of exercise; my addition]. At the end of 100 minutes of running and feeding, it became apparent that further attempts to ingest fluids would have been intolerable" (Costill, Kammer, et al., 1970a, p. 522).

In fact, the researchers passed a tube into their subjects' stomachs to determine how much of the ingested fluid had actually passed from the stomach into the intestine. An average of 340 ml was still present in the stomach at the end of the exercise bout even though the runners had not drunk for the last 25 minutes of the trial. Such a large volume of residual fluid in the stomach would easily explain the runners' increasing discomfort after 75 minutes of running at their best marathon pace.

But this finding has been largely ignored by those who used this study to encourage athletes to drink at even higher rates of at least 1.2 L/hr or even up to 1.8 L/hr during exercise—or even "the maximal amount that can be tolerated" (Convertino, Armstrong, et al., 1996, p. i).

This carefully conducted study established that drinking during exercise lowers the rectal temperature in the second hour of exercise when compared to not drinking anything. However, there was no difference in the rectal temperature response to the ingestion of either water or Gatorade.

The second important finding was that the rectal temperature response to exercise was not influenced by fluid ingestion during the first hour of exercise (figure 6.2). Thus, one might conclude that there may be no physiological reason to drink during exercise lasting less than 60 minutes other than to alleviate thirst.

The third relevant finding was that when they did not drink, the runners did not develop heat illness, heatstroke, muscle cramps, or EAH/EAHE; nor were their temperatures abnormally high. Even when the subjects drank nothing during exercise, they completed 2 hours of quite demanding exercise with average rectal temperatures just above 39 °C and without any apparent adverse effects, as is always found.[4] Water drinking reduced the final rectal temperature by about 0.7 °C (figure 6.2). This finding is consistent with all the studies reported previously or indeed since.

The fourth finding was that each of these well-trained runners was unable to drink at rates of 1,200 ml/hr for more than about 80 minutes when exercising at a reasonable intensity. After that time, they developed disabling gastrointestinal symptoms caused by retention of fluid in the stomach and upper gastrointestinal tract. The development of gastrointestinal symptoms is one factor limiting the extent to which some athletes can replace their fluid losses during exercise. This is predictably due to two factors: (a) the rate at which the stomach is able to release the fluid into the upper intestine, known as the rate of gastric emptying, and (b) the rate at which the intestine is able to absorb that fluid. My conclusion, based on advising some athletes who have developed progressive intestinal fullness and vomiting during prolonged exercise, is that the maximum rates of intestinal fluid absorption in these symptomatic athletes may be 400 ml/hr or even lower.

There are two additional provisos that influence the interpretation of the findings of this study. First, subjects exercised at a fixed, unvarying work rate that was set by the researchers. But this is not how athletes exercise in real life. Rather, they set their own paces, which vary during the event and are set initially on the prior knowledge of either how far or for how long each athlete expects to exercise. This pace is set by the brain. This method of testing does not allow the athlete's brain to alter the behavior if, for example, it wishes to slow the rate of heat accumulation during exercise in the heat. This type of exercise is therefore "brainless" (Noakes, 2008).

Second, the athletes were tested in the laboratory without appropriate convective air movement. This air movement aids cooling by increasing the rate at which cooler air moving over the skin removes body heat by convective cooling (box 6.1, page 186). When Costill (1972) plotted the data from this laboratory study against his data measured in real marathons, he showed (although he probably did not realize it at the time) that the relationship between sweat rate and running speed for his laboratory studies was displaced upward. This indicates that when running at the same speed, subjects sweated more in the laboratory than when running outdoors. This would have resulted from inadequate convective cooling in the laboratory trials. This study found:

■ Costill studied runners in the Boston Marathon and the 1967 U.S. Olympic Marathon Trials held in Alamosa, New Mexico, and he compared the data to the laboratory trial, reported in figure 6.2 (page 189).

■ There was a linear relationship with a positive slope between the measured sweat rate (L/m²/hr) and the estimated energy expenditure (Kcal/min) for all three conditions.

4 The terminal rectal temperatures achieved in all the laboratory studies reviewed in this chapter are much lower than those present in marathon runners competing outdoors. Probably this is the result of the higher environmental heat load, especially that imposed by radiant heat during outdoor exercise or the ability of athletes to run at a higher intensity for longer when competing outdoors rather than in the confines of the laboratory.

- The sweat rate and energy expenditure relationship was very similar for both outdoor marathons in which there was proper convective cooling.
- The sweat rates were about 100 ml/m²/hr higher at racing speeds during the laboratory trial than during the outdoor marathon races due to the inadequate convective cooling in the laboratory.

In summary, this study, conducted in inappropriate environmental conditions with inadequate convective cooling, would in time be interpreted as evidence that a failure to drink during exercise at a fixed work rate caused the body temperature to be (slightly) increased. According to the theory that any elevation of body temperature during exercise is pathological and indicates that heatstroke will be the inevitable consequence, this finding would be grasped by the drinking activists as clear evidence for the dangers of dehydration during exercise.

The contrary evidence that (a) no athlete developed any evidence for heat illness when they did not drink, and conversely that (b) when drinking as much as tolerable, at rates of 1000 ml/hr, these athletes developed disabling gastrointestinal symptoms that would be ignored by these same scientists. Dr. Costill was one of the first to promote the importance of fluid ingestion during exercise, yet he never allowed any external influences, however attractive, to modify his conclusions that athletes can ingest fluid only at relatively slow rates during exercise and that they do not need to ingest any additional electrolytes (box 6.2). Indeed, his opinion was clearly that sports drinks are overrated.

Second Gatorade-Funded Study

"Thermal effects of prolonged exercise in the heat."

Authors: C.V. Gisolfi and J.R. Copping. Published in *Medicine and Science in Sports and Exercise*, Volume 6, pp. 108-113, 1974.

The second Gatorade-funded study further entrenched the novel science of hydration. It was led by Carl Gisolfi, PhD, who would also achieve iconic status in the exercise sciences in the United States, in part, through his association with the Gatorade brand. His contribution to the marketing of the brand is acknowledged by the annual Gatorade-sponsored Carl Gisolfi Tutorial Lecture and the Carl Gisolfi Fun Run at the Annual Congress of the ACSM.

In this study, Drs. Carl Gisolfi and J.R. Copping (1974) studied six athletes, including themselves, running for 1.5 to 2.5 hours at 75% $\dot{V}O_2$max in hot conditions (33.5 °C, 38% RH). Although athletes ran 12.8 to 14.4 km/hr, the air velocity of the fans used to "cool" the runners was only 2.2 km/hr, and even less effective than those used in David Costill's original study. Subjects drank either warm water, cold water, or nothing. The rate of fluid ingestion chosen for the study was 600 ml/hr since "this was approximately what marathon runners ingested if they drank during competition"[5] (p. 109). This was a study of voluntary drinking, that

5 This is an interesting observation because it fits precisely with what we found in our study of marathon runners and canoeists in the early 1980s (Noakes, Adams, et al., 1988a) (chapter 3)—that they typically drank 400 to 600 ml/hr. Yet when the revised guidelines of the ACSM were published in 1996, they advocated that endurance athletes should drink at least twice as much—up to 1,200 ml/hr (chapter 7).

BOX 6.2 David Costill's Integrity Upheld

Dr. David Costill prized and maintained his intellectual independence. Many years after it had been completed, Dr. Costill described the circumstances that led to his iconic study of the effects of fluid ingestion on thermoregulation in marathon runners. It was the first industry-funded study of the effects of a sports drink on thermoregulation during prolonged exercise. An interview with *New York Times* science editor Gina Kolata (2001) produced the following report:

> Arriving at Ball State, Dr. Costill learned that there was little money to study sports, so he decided to seek some. Gatorade had just come onto the market, he said, so he wrote to the company and suggested a study on dehydration among marathon runners. A company doctor called him back. "He said, 'I'm really excited by your idea but there is one problem: You asked for $800,'" Dr. Costill recalled. "I said, 'Oh, gee.' Then he said, 'You ought to add another zero to that'" (Kolata, 2001, p. 2).
>
> Astonished, Dr. Costill did, and used the money to buy laboratory equipment. That was the beginning of a long career in which he pursued every avenue to scrounge money for research in a field that had never been lavishly financed. At the same time, he avoided making deals or giving endorsements.
>
> The study (Costill, Kammer, et al., 1970) did not show that Gatorade was any better than water for dehydration. But it did change marathon rules by documenting that runners were in dire need of fluids (Kolata, 2001).

In fact, the reporter herself was influenced by her own interpretation.[6] The study did not show that runners were in "dire" need of fluids. In fact, it showed that they coped quite well even if they did not drink at all during 2 hours of vigorous exercise in moderately hot conditions (figure 6.2, page 189).

While accepting such research funding, Costill retained a fierce, lifelong independence from any real or imagined commercial pressure. Later he would write this in his popular book on running physiology: "A number of 'sports drinks' containing carbohydrates are currently on the market, grossing more than $100 million each year. Unfortunately many of the claims used to sell these drinks are based on misinterpreted and often inaccurate information. Electrolytes, for example, have long been touted as important ingredients in sports drinks. But research shows that such claims are unfounded. A single meal adequately replaces the electrolytes lost during exercise. The body needs water to bring its concentration of the electrolytes back into balance. . . . Our studies during the marathon and exercise bouts lasting up to six hours suggest that electrolytes are not an essential ingredient for sports drinks" (Costill, 1986, pp. 75-76).

Dr. Costill was clearly never going to be the leading scientific cheerleader for the sports drink industry, which must have caused the industry some distress because it meant they had wasted that extra "zero" they suggested he add to his very first budget application.

6 This conclusion is incorrect and reflects the bias of author Gina Kolata. Because she herself is an athlete and author of a book that seeks the "truth about exercise and health" (Kolata, 2003), her error provides additional proof of the extent to which the dehydration myth (chapter 3) has pervaded the consciousness even of educated and otherwise rational North American athletes. This interpretation implies that if marathon runners do not drink enough, the results will be "dire." But there is still no evidence to show that marathon runners are in dire need of fluids.

is, drinking ad libitum, or according to the dictates of thirst. Subjects sweated at an average rate of ~1550 ml/hr so that when drinking ad libitum, they replaced only 39% of the fluid they lost in sweat.

The principal finding of the study was that subjects who did not ingest fluid developed higher rectal temperatures, but only after 90 minutes of exercise (figure 6.3a). As in the study of Costill, Kammer, and colleagues (1970), sweat rates were the same in all conditions. The failure to ingest fluids during exercise did not impair heat loss by sweating. Rather, some other (more complex) mechanism must have caused the higher postexercise rectal temperatures of those who did not drink during the trial.

Similarly, as in the study of Buskirk and Beetham (1960) and Wyndham and Strydom (1969), there was a linear relationship between the percentage of weight loss during exercise and the postexercise rectal temperature in each subject (figure 6.3b); the group data were not reported. However, terminal rectal temperatures were again well below 40 °C in those subjects who did not ingest any fluid during exercise. Even when those athletes ran without drinking at a fixed running speed in these severe environmental conditions with totally inadequate convective cooling (box 6.1, page 186), there was again no evidence that they were at risk of developing heatstroke. Nor did any report any symptoms of dehydration. Furthermore, drinking reduced the final rectal temperature by only about 1.0 °C (figure 6.3a).

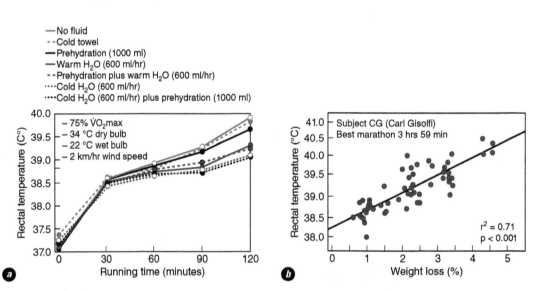

FIGURE 6.3 (a) The ingestion of fluid reduced the rectal temperature response during 2 hours of exercise. This effect was not due to differences in sweat rates, which were the same in all conditions. (b) The relationship between rectal temperature and percentage of weight loss in subject CG (Carl Gisolfi), who had run a 3:59 marathon. Similar findings were reported in two other subjects, although they were somewhat faster marathon runners than Dr. Gisolfi, with best marathon times of 2:36 and 2:44.

Reprinted, by permission, from C.V. Gisolfi and J.R. Copping, 1974, "Thermal effects of prolonged treadmill exercise in the heat," *Medicine & Science in Sports & Exercise* 6(2): 108-113.

This study showed that when drinking ad libitum, at a rate of 600 ml/hr, but sweating at rates of ~1550 ml/hr, athletes of recreational ability finished with rectal temperatures ~1.0 °C lower than when they did not drink at all during exercise in hot, humid conditions with inadequate convective cooling. The temperature-raising effect of not drinking was not due to a failure of sweating because sweat rates were the same under all conditions as also found by Costill and colleagues (1970). No athletes developed medical complications as a result of not drinking during exercise. Finally, the convective cooling of the athletes did not match what naturally occurs when subjects exercise outdoors.

One valid conclusion from this study might have been that athletes can exercise safely for 2 hours in hot, humid, almost wind-still conditions without developing heatstroke or any of the other so-called heat-related illnesses. But this was not what Dr. Gisolfi concluded either then or at any time during the rest of his life. Rather, he would spend the final 3 decades of his life promoting a quite different interpretation. For example, in an article published as a companion to the first ACSM drinking guidelines of 1975, Dr. Gisolfi advised that athletes should drink "200-300 ml of a glucose-electrolyte solution every 15 to 20 minutes (600-1200 ml/ hr)" to prevent "symptomatic dehydration." This, despite the complete absence of any scientific study to determine whether such high rates of fluid ingestion were either helpful or harmful. When the new ACSM guidelines were produced in 1996, they advocated exactly this range of drinking rates. By that time, Dr. Gisolfi was also chairman of the GSSI advisory board.

Third Gatorade-Funded Study

"Influence of graded dehydration on hyperthermia and cardiovascular drift during exercise."

Authors: S.J. Montain and E.F. Coyle. Published in *Journal of Applied Physiology,* Volume 73, pp. 1340-1350, 1992.

While study continued on fluid intake during exercise, researchers—especially Dr. Costill, along with his PhD students Edward Coyle and Carl Foster—were engaging in research on the effects of glucose intake on gastric emptying and exercise performance. In fact, once Dr. Coyle was at the University of Texas at Austin, he and his colleagues conducted a series of studies on the subject. A landmark study of theirs established that carbohydrate ingestion during exercise increased time to fatigue by 33% (approximately 1 hour) in subjects cycling at a fixed work rate at a moderately high exercise intensity (Coyle, Coggan, et al., 1986). Subsequently they showed that the provision of glucose at the point of exhaustion could reverse fatigue (Coggan and Coyle, 1987), a finding first reported in 1939 (Christensen and Hansen, 1939) but that had subsequently been forgotten.

These studies were crucial for many reasons, not least because they finally established that performance during prolonged exercise lasting 3 or more hours cannot be optimized without carbohydrate ingestion (in athletes who are

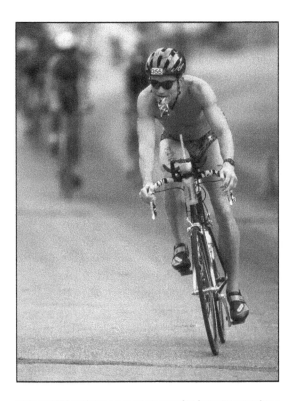

Before 1986 athletes were encouraged to ingest water alone during exercise to optimize performance and prevent heat stroke. A study of cyclists in 1986 by Dr. Edward Coyle at the University of Texas at Austin established for the first time that carbohydrate ingestion during prolonged exercise improved performance.

© Human Kinetics

7 The novel idea that excessive carbohydrate consumption, especially of sucrose and fructose, may contribute to the development of obesity, diabetes, and heart disease in predisposed individuals (Johnson, Perez-Pozo, et al., 2009) forms part of the reevaluation of the value of high-carbohydrate diets not only in the general population (Taubes, 2007; Taubes, 2011), but also in athletes (Cordain and Friel, 2005). It is reasonable to propose, but is yet untested, that athletes who are habitually adapted to a high-fat, high-protein, low-carbohydrate diet may not benefit from carbohydrate ingestion during exercise to the same extent as do those athletes who follow the traditional high-carbohydrate athletic diet.

adapted to the traditional high-carbohydrate athletic diet).[7] The studies also confirmed Dr. Cade's original but unrecognized finding 14 years earlier (Cade, Packer, et al., 1992) and provided the scientific support for the value of sports drinks that contain carbohydrate in quite high concentrations. Thus, the study legitimized the sports drink industry. It was perhaps a natural consequence that the sports drink industry should begin to consider Dr. Coyle a highly attractive scientist and one whom they invited to all 12 of their sponsored symposia from 1987 to 1998.

Dr. Coyle's next contribution (Montain and Coyle, 1992) would, together with the studies of Costill and colleagues (1970) and Gisolfi and Copping (1974), form a trilogy of studies that would develop the faux science that humans can exercise safely only if they drink as much as tolerable. In their industry-funded investigation, Montain and Coyle (1992) studied well-trained cyclists who cycled for 2 hours in hot conditions (33 °C; 50% RH) at 62% to 67% $\dot{V}O_2$max, equivalent to an average power output of 206 (±14) watts (W). The air velocity of the fans cooling the cyclists was only 8.6 km/hr, whereas the predicted cycling velocity at that work rate would have been 35.6 km/hr (Saunders, Dugas, et al., 2005). The wind speed provided for cooling the cyclists should have been ~36 km/hr, not 8.6 km/hr. The laboratory fans would also not have caused all the air in contact with the cyclists' bodies to be in constant motion at a rate equivalent to their speed of forward motion as occurs in outdoor exercise. Thus, the experimental conditions did not produce realistic rates of convective cooling. Graded dehydration was produced by having the athletes drink fluid at four different rates during exercise: 0, 291, 712, or 1190 ml/hr.

The authors reported that graded levels of dehydration produced a graded effect on heat retention[8] during exercise (figure 6.4a, page 198). Postexercise rectal temperatures were highest in those who drank nothing (39.1 ± 0.1°C) and lowest (38.4 ± 0.1 °C) in those who drank 1.2 L/hr (figure 6.4b). However, the difference between those drinking 712 ml/hr and those drinking 1190 ml/hr was trivial (0.2 °C: 38.6 vs. 38.4 °C) and could not be of any biological significance. Indeed, the difference between those who drank the most and those who drank the least was 0.7 °C, somewhat less than the prediction from the data of Wyndham and Strydom. According to Wyndham and Strydom's predictions, the difference in rectal temperature between those dehydrated by 1% and those dehydrated by 4% should have been closer to 2 °C (figure 3.1, page 61). In addition, there was no effect of any level of fluid ingestion on the rectal temperature responses during the first 60 minutes of exercise (figure 6.4a). Regardless of how much fluid was ingested, the final rectal temperatures were always at least 3 °C lower than values measured in athletes with heatstroke.

8 A higher temperature (as found in the groups that did not drink in the studies depicted in figures 6.2 and 6.3, pages 189 and 194) does not mean that the thermoregulatory system has failed so that, in these authors' words, there is abnormal "heat retention." Although the body temperature is higher when no fluid is ingested during exercise, that higher temperature continues to be regulated but at a slightly higher temperature. Thus, a new homeostasis state is reached but at a higher temperature. This is shown by the fact that the temperature of these athletes did not spiral out of control and rapidly reach 42 °C as it would have if there had been a thermoregulatory failure. Instead, the body temperature is either held stable at that higher temperature or continues to rise gradually but does not reach values in excess of 42 °C before exercise terminates.

In effect, the scientists had designed an experiment in which any weakness in human thermoregulatory capacity would have been exposed by the prolonged duration of the exercise, the relatively high exercise intensity that was fixed and did not allow for any behavioral response, the absence of drinking and of appropriate convective cooling (box 6.1, page 186), and the moderately severe environmental conditions. Yet these experimental conditions failed to find any such weaknesses. Instead, the athletes had no difficultly in maintaining rectal temperatures well below any that could be conceived as remotely dangerous. A not unreasonable conclusion might have been that trained athletes can exercise vigorously in hot, almost wind-still conditions for 2 hours without risk to their health even if they do not drink. But this would not be how the study was marketed. It would be 17 years before the U.S. Army Research Institute of Environmental Medicine (USARIEM) would report the research study (Ely, Ely, et al., 2009) that would begin to address the errors of this study.

The finding that humans can exercise vigorously in hot conditions without thermoregulatory failure is entirely compatible with our evolutionary history and the experience from the early, classic studies of marathon runners described in chapter 3. An important weakness of the 1992 study is that it failed to include a measure of the effects of these different drinking behaviors on cycling performance. To ensure that they did not lose any weight during exercise, the cyclists in this study would have had to carry a minimum of an added 2.3 kg for the duration of any 2-hour race (figure 6.4c). Rather obviously, the cost of this extra weight needs to be considered if the effects on athletic performance of drinking at such high rates are to be properly investigated.

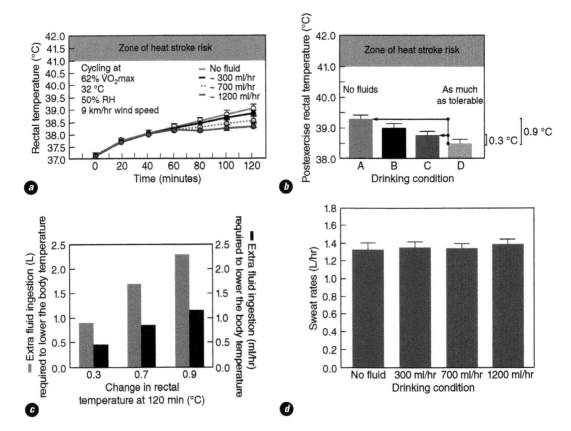

FIGURE 6.4 Response of the rectal temperature to prolonged exercise in the heat in athletes drinking fluid at 0, 291, 712, or 1190 ml/hr. *(a)* Fluid ingestion and rectal temperatures over the course of 2 hours of exercise in moderately severe heat with inappropriate convective cooling. *(b)* Drinking "to prevent any weight loss during exercise" produced a final rectal temperature that was only 0.9 °C lower than when no fluid was ingested during exercise. *(c)* The extra weight cost of lowering the body temperature by drinking at different rates. When athletes drank to prevent any weight loss during exercise, they needed to ingest 2.3 L (1.15 L/hr) more fluid than when they drank nothing during exercise. This lowered their body temperature by ~0.9 °C. *(d)* Sweat rates in the trials.

(a) Adapted, by permission, from S.J. Montain and E.F. Coyle, 1992, "Influence of graded dehydration on hyperthermia and cardiovascular drift during exercise," *Journal of Applied Physiology* 73(4): 1340-1350. *(b-d)* Data from Montain and Coyle 1992.

When I raised this uncomfortable point during my debate with Dr. Coyle at the 2001 ACSM Congress, I was informed that the performance of the heaviest drinkers had to be better according to the industry-directed logic that the lower the body temperature, the better. The counterargument that a higher core temperature improves heat loss and can be a water-conserving mechanism or that the weight loss might improve performance in weight-bearing activities like running and cycling was summarily dismissed without due consideration. As a result, it was hinted and actively advertised that drinking 1,200 ml/hr was the only way to achieve an optimal performance even though no such data were provided by that study. But drinking so much requires that extra weight be carried on the bicycle, in the form of water bottles carried on the bicycle frame and then as water stored in the body.

It is intrinsically obvious that those who do not drink during exercise will ultimately reach a point at which their performance is impaired. However, no one currently knows at what point the benefit of being lighter (as a result of not drinking during exercise) is outweighed by the biological effects on performance of becoming progressively more thirsty and dehydrated.

There was one other overlooked finding of the study: The rectal temperatures were increased in those who drank less despite the finding that all groups sweated equally (figure 6.4*d*). Since sweating is the principal method of heat loss during exercise and since each athlete's rate of heat production would have been the same in each trial (since each exercised at the same work rate), because they sweated equally, their body temperatures should also have been the same. This finding of higher body temperatures in the group when they drank nothing during exercise despite similar sweat rates was also reported in those studies of Costill and colleagues (1970) and Gisolfi and Copping (1974) that also make up this scientific trilogy.

The point is that the higher body temperatures in the no-drink trials cannot be explained by a reduced capacity to lose heat. Simply by sweating more, the body temperatures during the no-drinking trial could have been reduced to values measured in the "drinking to prevent any weight loss" trial. This must indicate that for whatever reason, the brain makes the decision to exercise at a higher body temperature when no fluid is ingested.

Drs. Montain and Coyle concluded, in keeping with Dr. Cade's model of human thermoregulation during exercise (figure 5.3, page 173), that the higher body temperatures in those who did not drink during exercise were (a) detrimental to their health and (b) due to a reduced blood flow to the skin. But this cannot be the answer because the sweat rate, the major determinant of body heat loss under these conditions, was not affected by dehydration. The real answer lies in the brain's choice to maintain the same sweat rate at the slightly higher body temperature. Thus, the brain had actively chosen *not* to increase the sweat rate in the no-drinking condition and to allow a higher rectal temperature during the second hour of the trial. But the extent of the temperature rise was still tightly controlled by the brain, and the exercise was terminated also by the brain before a dangerous rectal temperature was reached (figure 6.4).

The importance of this study was that it would provide the rationale for the 1996 ACSM drinking guidelines, which proposed that athletes should drink 1,200 ml/hr during exercise, the exact rate at which Cynthia Lucero drank during the 2002 Boston Marathon (table 1.1, page 7). Surprisingly, Dr. Coyle wrote subsequently (1994, p. 2), "To our knowledge, no studies have directly compared the effect on running or cycling performance of fluid replacement at rates that prevent dehydration versus rates voluntarily chosen by many endurance athletes (e.g. 500 ml/hr) who replace only 30-50% of fluid losses." But these authors would not ever study that question. Rather, any research that sought to evaluate the zero percent dehydration rule objectively and without prejudice would not be encouraged.

It would take 17 years before one of the authors of this study, Dr. Montain, would be associated with another study (Ely, Ely, et al., 2009), which would disprove the assumptions he and Dr. Coyle used to interpret the findings of their 1992 study. In their new study, the rectal temperatures of subjects were studied when they ran 8 km as fast as they could in either cool (16-17 °C) or hot (29-30 °C) environmental conditions on either an indoor (cool trial) or an outdoor (hot trial) track (which allowed proper convective cooling). In keeping with the prediction that it is the rate of heat production controlled by the exercise intensity that determines the body temperature during exercise, this new study showed that much higher body temperatures (40.3 °C) were achieved in the 8 km run in the heat that lasted less than 26 minutes than were reached (39.2 °C) in the 120-minute laboratory trial undertaken in even more unfavorable environmental conditions. The authors concluded, "Our observation that runners were able to sustain running velocity despite rectal temperatures >40.0 °C is evidence against 40.0 °C representing a 'critical' core temperature limit to performance" (p. 1519) (figure 6.5). It is more of a pity that Drs. Montain and Coyle had not reached the same conclusion in 1992 on the basis of the evidence that was already available then (see figures 3.6 and 3.8, pages 70 and 75).

Had this new (2009) interpretation been applied to their 1992 study, it would have led to only one conclusion: That the 1992 study did not prove that drinking "as much as tolerable" was any better than drinking nothing during 2 hours of vigorous exercise in the heat. Had that conclusion been drawn in 1992, the epidemic of EAH and EAHE that followed might have been averted.

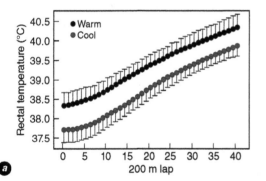 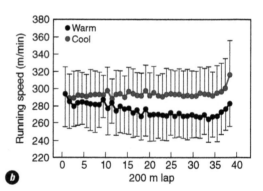

FIGURE 6.5 *(a)* Rectal temperatures every 200 m during hot and cool trials. In both conditions, the rectal temperature rose progressively, exceeding 40 °C after about 34 laps in the hot trial. *(b)* The average running speed sustained in cool and warm conditions. Note that in cool conditions, the final 4 laps were the fastest, whereas in hot conditions the athletes' paces varied much more and were inappropriately fast for the first 15 laps before slowing. Nevertheless, even in the hot condition, subjects were able to speed up in the final 2 laps when their average rectal temperatures were greater than 40 °C.

Reprinted, by permission, from B.R. Ely, M.R. Ely, S.N. Cheuvront, et al., 2009, "Evidence against a 40°C core temperature threshold for fatigue in humans," *Journal of Applied Physiology* 107(5): 1519-1525.

Water Versus Carbohydrate Ingestion

Two Gatorade-funded studies followed, which sought to determine which improved performance: the ingestion of more water or of carbohydrate.

Fourth Gatorade-Funded Study

"Fluid and carbohydrate ingestion independently improve performance during 1 hr of intense exercise."

Authors: P.R. Below, R. Mora-Rodríguez, J. González-Alonso, and E.F. Coyle. Published in *Medicine and Science in Sports and Exercise,* Volume 27, pp. 200-210, 1995.

The study of Below, Mora-Rodriguez, and colleagues (1995) showed whether the ingestion of more water or of more carbohydrate or the combination of both improved exercise performance of short duration. Subjects completed four trials in which they first cycled at a fixed work rate for 50 minutes during which they ingested the different solutions. This produced different levels of dehydration before the time trial in which subjects had to complete a certain amount of work in as short a time as possible (~10-15 min).

Exercise performance was worst when only a small volume (~200 ml) of fluid was ingested and was best when more fluid (~1,330 ml) with added carbohydrate (80 g) was ingested. But the ingestion of 80 g carbohydrate in a small volume of fluid produced essentially the same result as did the ingestion of a large volume of fluid without added carbohydrate. Performances in trials in which either no carbohydrate or a small volume of fluid was ingested were the same (10:56 vs. 10:55, respectively). Similarly, performance in trials in which either more carbohydrate or more fluid was ingested were also the same (10:13 vs. 10:14, respectively). Thus, adding carbohydrate to the solution or drinking more seemed to be equally effective in improving performance. Notably, *drinking less (~200 ml) of a carbohydrate-containing solution was as effective as drinking an extra 1.1 L of water.* This finding was not communicated to the athletic population.

Fifth Gatorade-Funded Study

"Water and carbohydrate ingestion during prolonged exercise increase maximal neuromuscular power."

Authors: R.G. Fritzsche, T.W. Switzer, B.J. Hodgkinson, S-H Lee, J.C. Martin, P.R. Below, and E.F. Coyle. Published in *Journal of Applied Physiology,* Volume 88, pp. 730-737, 2000.

This study was of a similar design to that of Below, Mora-Rodriguez, and colleagues (1995) except that the performance of subjects was evaluated during prolonged exercise (122 min at 62% $\dot{V}O_2$max) in the heat (35 °C, 50% RH, wind speed 2 m/s) when subjects drank either (a) 3.28 L of water, (b) 3.28 L of a solution containing 204 g of carbohydrate, (c) the same amount of carbohydrate in 0.49 L of water, or (d) 0.4 L of water with no carbohydrate (placebo group). Athletes exercised at a fixed work rate, but at 30, 60, 90, and 120 minutes of exercise they were asked to perform a bout of maximal exercise during which their peak power output was measured. When they ingested fluid at high rates during exercise, subjects lost 1.1% of their body weight, but when they drank little during exercise, they lost 4.2% of their body weight.

The study found that peak power output was the same in all groups after 30 minutes of exercise, but by 120 minutes power output in the group ingesting water and carbohydrate at high rates was significantly superior to performance in all the other trials. The ingestion of water alone was surprisingly effective and produced for the first 90 minutes of exercise a performance equivalent to that achieved when carbohydrate was also ingested at high rates. There was no difference in performance when either carbohydrate alone or placebo was ingested. Interestingly, the difference in performance when fluid was ingested at either fast or slow rates was only about 1%. This is substantially less than the numbers usually promoted by the industry.

Cardiovascular Model of Thermoregulation

An important question raised by the study of Montain and Coyle (1992) was how fluid ingestion causes a reduction in the rectal temperature during exercise. The results of the original study suggested that a reduced blood flow to the skin would explain this effect. This is in line with a set of original studies from the 1960s (Rowell, Marx, et al., 1964), which had concluded that the combined stresses of exercise and heat exposed the cardiovascular system to the dual stresses of attempting to maintain adequate blood flow to both the muscles (to maintain the exercise intensity) and to the skin (to maintain a safe body temperature). These studies concluded that cardiac output was reduced during exercise in the heat as the result of a redistribution of central blood volume to the periphery causing an impaired filling of the heart with the development of "cardiovascular strain." Since the oxygen consumption was not affected by exercise in the heat, the reduction in cardiac output must be due mainly to a reduced blood flow to the skin rather than to the exercising muscles (Rowell, 1983). As a result, "the failure to provide adequate increments in cardiac output constitutes an important contributory factor limiting man's capacity to work in the heat" (p. 1815). Subsequently it was shown that blood flow to the skin increased during exercise in more moderate conditions (24 °C) (Johnson and Rowell, 1975) in which there was no evidence for cardiovascular strain.

Modern researchers from the USARIEM also use this model to explain how heat exhaustion and dehydration cause collapse: "Maintaining high skin blood flow (during exercise in the heat) can impose a substantial burden on the cardiovascular system. High skin blood flow is associated with reduced cardiac filling, reduced right atrial pressure and reduced stroke volume. . . . This reduction in cardiac filling occurs because the cutaneous venous bed is large and compliant, and dilates during heat stress. In addition, sweat secretion can result in net body water loss (dehydration), thereby reducing blood volume. . . . During severe exercise-heat stress, cardiac output can decrease below levels observed during exercise in temperate conditions. This reduced cardiac output and vasodilated skin and muscle can make it difficult to sustain blood pressure and perhaps cerebral blood flow" (Kenefick and Sawka, 2007, p. 379).

All these studies evaluated cardiovascular and thermoregulatory function during exercise at a fixed work rate in which subjects were unable to make behavioral adaptations, in particular by reducing their work rates in order that the exercise might continue, albeit at a lower intensity but with an appropriate thermoregulatory response. In addition, conditions of extreme heat (43 °C) were required to produce this effect of cardiac strain (Rowell, Marx, et al., 1964).

Sixth Gatorade-Funded Study

"Fluid ingestion during exercise increases skin blood flow independent of increases in blood volume."

Authors: S.J. Montain and E.F. Coyle. Published in *Journal of Applied Physiology*, Volume 73, pp. 903-910, 1997.

For their study, Montain and Coyle (1997) used essentially the same design as for their previous study (Gonzalez-Alonso, Mora-Rodriguez, et al., 1997) in which subjects exercised for 2 hours in hot conditions when they ingested either nothing or 2.4 L of a fluid, presumably Gatorade. In this experiment, cardiac output and blood flow to the skin of the forearm were measured repeatedly every 20 minutes during exercise.

The study found that cardiac output fell when no fluid was ingested during prolonged exercise. Forearm blood flow was also lower for the last 30 minutes of exercise when no fluid was ingested, whereas the rectal temperature was higher for the final 60 minutes of the exercise when no fluid was ingested.

The authors also measured changes in blood sodium concentrations and in osmolality during exercise and again found that serum sodium concentrations rose significantly when no fluid was ingested during exercise but did not change when fluid was ingested at high rates. This response is reported frequently in the literature.

The authors concluded that fluid ingestion "attenuated" the hyperthermia of exercise by maintaining a higher blood flow to the skin. But they failed to consider the possibility that the higher rectal temperatures during exercise when no fluid was ingested are part of a regulated process in much the same way that the body temperatures of mammals in the desert are higher when they do not have access to fluid but are reduced (by sweating) when fluid is more freely available, the phenomenon known as adaptive heterothermy.

The reality is that (a) the rectal temperatures during exercise in these subjects were well below values at which heatstroke or hyperthermic paralysis occurs and (b) subjects could have reduced their body temperatures simply by sweating more. Studying the response of skin blood flow to fluid ingestion during exercise might be intellectually interesting, but it does not really answer the more pertinent question: How and why does the body regulate its core temperature at a higher value when no fluid is ingested during exercise?

Seventh to Twelfth Gatorade-Funded Studies (1995-1999)

Dr. Jose Gonzalez-Alonso was the first author of a series of articles that further evaluated the cardiovascular responses to exercise in subjects who either did or did not ingest fluids during exercise. These studies established Dr. Gonzalez-Alonso as a premier modern researcher of cardiovascular function during both prolonged exercise in the heat and also during maximal exercise of shorter duration. Dr. Gonzalez-Alonso believes that a limiting cardiac output determines maximal exercise performance (Gonzalez-Alonso and Calbet, 2003; Gonzalez-Alonso, Dalsgaard, et al., 2004), a conclusion that contrasts with our theory that maximal exercise always terminates before the heart reaches its maximal output since the performance of such exercise is regulated (Noakes and Marino, 2007) and must stop before there is a catastrophic failure of the functioning of any organ, including the heart (Noakes and St. Clair Gibson, 2004).

This series of studies established the following:

- Cardiac output and mean arterial pressure fell and systemic vascular resistance rose when prolonged exercise was performed without the ingestion of any fluid (Gonzalez-Alonso, Mora-Rodriguez, et al., 1995).
- The reduction in cardiac output and stroke volume and the increase in heart rate and vascular resistance are greater when fluid is not ingested during prolonged exercise (Gonzalez-Alonso, Mora-Rodriguez, et al., 1997).
- About 66% of the reduction in cardiac output during exercise in the heat without fluid ingestion is due to a reduced blood flow to the exercising muscles (Gonzalez-Alonso, Calbet, et al., 1998).
- This reduction in blood flow does not alter either the oxygen consumption (Gonzalez-Alonso, Calbet, et al., 1998) or the metabolism of the exercising muscles. As a result, "hyperthermia rather than altered metabolism is the main factor underlying the early fatigue with dehydration during prolonged exercise in the heat" (Gonzalez-Alonso, Calbet, et al., 1999, p. 577).
- Progressive increases in the levels of dehydration from 0% to 4% accentuate these cardiovascular changes (Gonzalez-Alonso, Mora-Rodriguez, et al., 2000).
- The graded effect of dehydration on these cardiovascular changes is increased during exercise in the heat but attenuated in the cold (Gonzalez-Alonso, Mora-Rodriguez, et al., 2000). Thus, during exercise in the heat, the fall in cardiac output and in stroke volume and the rise in heart rate increase as a function of increasing levels of dehydration. But during prolonged exercise in the cold, the cardiac output is not reduced even at a 4% level of dehydration.
- The effects of dehydration on some of these cardiovascular changes are present only during exercise in the upright position (Gonzalez-Alonso, Mora-Rodriguez, et al., 1999). During exercise when lying (supine position), there was no effect of even a 5% level of dehydration on mean arterial pressure, forearm blood flow, cutaneous blood flow, or systemic vascular resistance. In addition, the effects of dehydration on the fall in cardiac output and in

stroke volume and the rise in heart rate were substantially reduced during supine exercise.

▨ The rise in rectal temperature during exercise in the heat cannot be due to altered cardiovascular function (Gonzalez-Alonso, Mora-Rodriguez, et al., 1999), including a reduced blood flow to the skin, since the rise in body temperature was the same when subjects were dehydrated whether or not they exercised in the upright or lying positions (figure 6.6). But cardiovascular function, especially blood flow to the skin, was higher in dehydrated subjects when they exercised in the lying compared to the upright position. If forearm blood flow determines the core body temperature during prolonged exercise, in this study the core temperature should have been lower in supine than in upright exercise (independent of the state of hydration). It should have been the highest during upright exercise in the dehydrated condition, and it should have been very much higher in upright than in supine exercise in the dehydrated state (which it was not). This finding dissociates the effects of dehydration on cardiovascular and thermoregulatory function during prolonged exercise.

▨ Blood sodium concentrations remained relatively unchanged or decreased (Gonzalez-Alonso, Mora-Rodriguez, et al., 1995) when fluid was ingested during prolonged exercise but increased when little or no fluid was ingested (Gonzalez-Alonso, Mora-Rodriguez, et al., 1995; Gonzalez-Alonso, Mora-Rodriguez, et al., 1999; Gonzalez-Alonso, Mora-Rodriguez, et al., 2000).

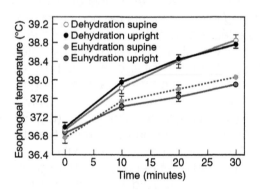
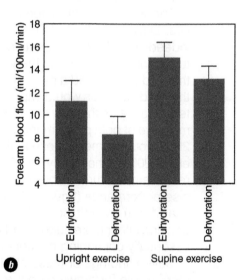

FIGURE 6.6 *(a)* The rise in esophageal (core body) temperature was the same in the (5%) dehydrated state when exercise was performed in either lying or upright positions. *(b)* But the state of hydration did not influence forearm (and cutaneous, not shown) blood flow during exercise in either the upright or the supine position. Rather, forearm blood flow was much lower in upright than in supine exercise.

(a) Reprinted, by permission, from J. González-Alonso, R. Mora-Rodríguez, and E.F. Coyle, 1999, "Supine exercise restores arterial blood pressure and skin blood flow despite dehydration and hyperthermia," American Journal of Physiology: Heart and Circulatory Physiology 277(2): H576-H583. (b) Data from González-Alonso, Mora-Rodríguez, and Coyle 1999.

Summary

In this chapter, we have looked at the evidence that fluid ingestion during exercise prevents dehydration, improves athletic performance, and prevents heatstroke. The studies of Wyndham and Strydom (1969), especially, promoted the belief that dehydration is a direct cause of heatstroke (figure 3.1, page 61). But this belief was not supported by their findings; rather, those authors simply interpreted their data according to what they believed must be true. Their bias had been acquired through decades of work in the South African gold mines during which their primary function was the prevention of heatstroke. Interestingly, they did not ever propose that an increased rate of fluid ingestion was the single most important factor necessary for preventing heatstroke in miners. Rather, they spent most of their academic careers, nearly 30 years, proving that multiple interventions were needed for reducing the incidence of heatstroke in the South African gold mines (Wyndham, 1973). Why, then, did they ever believe that one single intervention—drinking more fluid during exercise—would achieve the same result in millions of runners all over the world?

At the same time in the mid- to late 1960s, Dr. Cade drew the same conclusion, and this became his personal mantra explaining why the product that he developed would prevent heat illness and enhance sport performance. His three scientific studies conducted over 2 decades showed only that (a) it is perfectly safe to exercise without drinking during most forms of exercise and (b) carbohydrate ingestion improves exercise performance (in carbohydrate-adapted athletes).

The three original Gatorade-funded studies performed in the laboratories of Drs. David Costill, Carl Gisolfi, and Edward Coyle reviewed in this chapter did indeed show that the ingestion of fluid during exercise lowers the body temperature during exercise. But the value of this effect was not shown because none of the studies included a measure of performance. Rather, it was originally assumed that fluid ingestion would improve exercise performance if it also lowered the body temperature. In this way the body temperature during exercise became a surrogate measure of both performance and the risk that heat illness would develop. Only in 2009 would some of those authors undertake a study to test that theory (Ely, Ely, et al., 2009). That study disproved their original conclusion by showing that the rectal temperatures achieved in those studies would not have impaired their exercise performance (figure 6.5, page 200). The studies of Below, Mora-Rodriguez, et al (1995) and Fritzsche, Switzer, and colleagues (2000) did, however, show that drinking either more fluid or adding carbohydrate improved exercise performance, essentially confirming the conclusion from Dr. Cade's earlier studies.

Seven findings of these studies were, however, ignored, especially by those responsible for drawing up the 1996 ACSM drinking guidelines.

First, in all these trials, the control group that drank either nothing or little did not develop any evidence of illness even when they exercised in quite severe environmental conditions. None developed heatstroke; indeed, none had body temperatures elevated anywhere near the range present in patients with heatstroke. Rather, there was always a body temperature reserve of about 3 °C (39 vs. 42 °C) between the final body temperature at the end of exercise and that at which heatstroke develops. This is a common finding (box 5.3, page 171).

Since athletes began exercise with body temperatures of ~37 °C and finished exercise with temperatures of only ~39 °C, they had increased their body temperatures by about 40% of that needed to induce heatstroke. In contrast, athletes in real competitions frequently raise their body temperatures above 41 °C without showing any evidence of heat illness.

Second, one could argue that the most important finding of these studies is the remarkable ability of the human body to regulate temperature even when exercising in testing environmental conditions when no fluid is ingested, avenues for convective heat loss are suboptimal, and the exercise work rate is fixed so that the athlete is unable to modify her behavior specifically to prevent the development of heat illness.

The third finding that has been overlooked was the difficulty that subjects experienced when they tried to drink at the high rates necessary for preventing any weight loss when they exercised at high work rates as advocated by the 1996 ACSM drinking guidelines.

The fourth overlooked factor was that these findings were collected in studies of better-than-average athletes, some of whom might be sufficiently trained to sustain the high rates of heat production potentially necessary for generating heatstroke. Yet the results from these studies would be used as the "scientific" basis for drinking guidelines generalized to all classes of athletes, including joggers and walkers, whose slow running speeds ensure that they are unable to produce heat sufficiently rapidly to generate heatstroke in usual environmental conditions—except if they have some predisposing factors.

Fifth, in the Gatorade-funded studies in which blood sodium concentrations were measured (Fritzsche, Switzer, et al., 2000; Gonzalez-Alonso, Mora-Rodriguez, et al., 1995; Gonzalez-Alonso, Mora-Rodriguez, et al., 1999; Gonzalez-Alonso, Mora-Rodriguez, et al., 2000), all showed that when athletes did not drink during exercise, their blood sodium concentrations increased. This confirms the historical conclusion drawn from the original studies (table 4.2, page 129). It was not a finding that drew any comment from these authors.

Sixth, the studies of Gonzalez-Alonso and colleagues established that dehydration has a marked effect on cardiovascular function, especially blood flow to muscle and skin, during prolonged exercise. But these effects seem to be remarkably unimportant since they do not impair oxygen delivery to muscle, nor do they alter metabolism, nor do they influence thermoregulation (figure 6.6, page 205). Rather, they appear to be part of a beneficial adaptation that would be expected if humans evolved as hot-weather persistence hunters. This is not the manner in which these adaptations continue to be interpreted (Gonzalez-Alonso, Crandall, et al., 2008).

In the final distortion, the total absence of evidence that not drinking during exercise was dangerous would be used as the basis for drinking guidelines that, beginning in the 1990s, would encourage athletes to drink without restraint before, during, and after exercise.

CHAPTER 7

Early Drinking Guidelines

Thirst is a poor indicator of your child's need for fluids. By the time most active kids become thirsty, they have already lost important fluids and electrolytes and may be dehydrated. While a cool drink of water may feel satisfying, it doesn't supply the energy kids need to keep playing hard and having fun. A sports drink like Gatorade is the best way to keep kids both cooled and fueled.

Dr. Bob Murray (1999, p. 5), cofounder and director of the Gatorade Sports Science Institute (GSSI) 1985-2008

When Ron Hill won the 1970 Commonwealth Games Marathon in Edinburgh in 2:09:28, then perhaps the world's fastest time on an accurately measured course, he did not drink at all during the race and lost 3.9% of his body weight (Muir, Percy-Robb, et al., 1970).

He was not the first nor probably the last runner to win a major marathon foot race without drinking. In Emil Zátopek's first 42 km marathon and after winning gold medals in both the 5,000- and 10,000-meter races, he added a third Olympic gold medal when he won the marathon at the 1952 Helsinki Olympic Games in 2:23:03, also without drinking. Jim Peters set the (then) four fastest-ever marathon times in the world from 1953 to 1954, including his final world record of 2:17:39, without drinking in any of the races. Ethiopian Abebe Bikila also did not drink at all when he set the new Olympic and world marathon record of 2:15:16 in the

1960 Rome Olympic Games. The official history reports that none of these athletes appeared distressed when they finished these races, despite their high body temperatures and levels of dehydration. In fact, when Bikila repeated this feat 4 years later in the Tokyo Olympics, setting world and Olympic marathon records of 2:12:11, he spent the 4 minutes waiting for the second-place runner to finish by "doing postrace calisthenics to loosen up, his freshness making the race appear almost easy" (Martin and Gynn, 2000, p. 251).

Hill, with a PhD in chemistry, was known as one of the more intellectual world-class runners in the history of the sport. Hill was one of the first elite runners to adopt the carbohydrate-depletion, carbohydrate-loading diet, the potential benefits of which were first shown in the late 1960s (Hultman, 1967). Thus, if in 1970 Hill chose not to drink during the best race he ever ran in his life, it is quite possible that he had researched the topic and decided that this was the best approach. This must indicate that the advice to marathon runners that they should not drink during exercise, first advocated in the earliest book on marathon training published in English in 1910 (Sullivan, 1909), was still the prevailing opinion 60 years later.

If another 30 years later, in the first decade of the 21st century, marathon runners and other endurance athletes have received quite different advice, so that beginning in 1996 they were advised to drink upward of 1.2 L/hour or as much as can be tolerated, the question becomes this: What caused such a radical change in drinking behaviors during exercise—from avoidance to excess?

I have shown in chapters 3, 5, and 6 that this did not occur because of the publication of revolutionary scientific findings that proved that all these great runners were wrong. Rather, all those studies seem to show that, provided athletes drink according to the dictates of their thirst (ad libitum), which might include not drinking anything if they so choose, then there is no evidence either that they risk their health or that their performances would be impaired. The evidence that Jim Peters and Abebe Bikila, probably among others, established world-record marathon times even when they did not drink does not suggest that drinking would have allowed them to run much faster. Figure 3.19 (page 95) suggests that the fastest marathon runners are also those who lose the most weight during racing and so are the most dehydrated.

Yet scientists connected with Gatorade, the Gatorade Sports Science Institute (GSSI), and organizations sponsored by Gatorade would promote a different finding.

1975 ACSM Position Statement on the Prevention of Heat Injuries During Distance Running

Probably as a result of his original studies in 1975, Dr. David Costill was invited to produce the world's first drinking guidelines for distance running endorsed by a significant international sporting organization, the American College of Sports Medicine (ACSM). Costill, an honorable scientist absolutely resistant to commercial influence (box 6.2, page 193), could not have imagined where his well-intended act would finally lead.

The original ACSM position statement provided the simple advice that athletes should "be encouraged to frequently ingest fluids during competition" (American College of Sports Medicine, 1975, p. vii). *Frequently* was considered to be every 3 to 4 km in races of 16 km or longer, suggesting that fluid ingestion was deemed to be less important in races of less than 16 km. As I have argued, this is paradoxical, because the incidence of heatstroke is much greater in exercise of short duration and essentially negligible in marathon races.

But Costill's advice that runners in races longer than 16 km should be encouraged to ingest fluids was entirely appropriate in 1975 since, for the previous 100 years, athletes had received the opposite advice, specifically that they should avoid fluid ingestion during exercise. The rationale for fluid ingestion was to reduce rectal temperature and prevent dehydration. No specific reference was made to the possibility that fluid ingestion alone would influence the risk of, much less prevent, heat illness during exercise.

In retrospect, these guidelines contain little if anything that can be criticized. In particular, there was clear evidence from the studies of Cade, Costill, and Gisolfi that fluid ingestion during exercise does reduce the rectal temperature during exercise. But whether or not this reduction in rectal temperature was of any real value had not been established at that time. True to his belief that scientifically based guidelines should be just that—evidence based—Dr. Costill restricted his recommendation to those that he believed had been scientifically proven at that time.

The guidelines proposed that only solutions with low carbohydrate (<2.5% glucose) and electrolyte concentrations (sodium <10 mmol/L, potassium <5 mmol/L) should be ingested. This was based on the erroneous beliefs that (a) water rather than carbohydrate was the critical constituent of the ingested solution and (b) only hypotonic solutions containing low concentrations of glucose and electrolytes could be rapidly absorbed by the human intestine during exercise.

At the time, the only solution that had been tested during exercise was the ancestral Gatorade solution with a glucose concentration of 2.5% and a sodium concentration of 17 mmol/L (Cade, Spooner, et al., 1972). Dr. Costill would of course have known this since he had been the first to undertake research for the company that produced that product.

1976 New York Academy of Sciences Conference on the Marathon

The year 1976 was instrumental in marathon running because it was the year that launched marathon running into the stratosphere (figure 2, page xv). A crucial component was the running of the first New York City Marathon through the five New York boroughs, starting on Staten Island and ending in Central Park. To accompany the race, the New York Academy of Sciences held a conference devoted to the medical and scientific aspects of marathon running from October 25 to 28, 1976. Because this conference presented the state-of-the-art information on physiology of marathon running, it provides a historical record of the state

1 In hindsight, it is perhaps ironic that I also attended that meeting after running the marathon. I presented a paper on marathon running and heart disease, a forerunner of a more complete paper that disproved the theory of California pathologist Tom Bassler, also presented at the NYAS conference, that anyone who has completed a marathon race would henceforth enjoy total immunity from heart disease for the rest of their days.

of scientific knowledge on fluids and exercise in 1976.[1] In addition to other presentations on a variety of topics, there were four presentations relevant to thermal regulation and fluid balance before, during, and after exercise. These were given by Cyril Wyndham, David Costill, Carl Gisolfi, and Ethan Nadel's group from Yale University (Nadel, Wenger, et al., 1977).

Professor Wyndham (1977) presented a paper titled "Heat Stroke and Hyperthermia in Marathon Runners." He began by quoting Sir Adolphe Abrahams' 1936 statement about the risk of heatstroke in marathon runners: "I am of the opinion that in healthy subjects the only serious potential risk to life from violent exercise is heatstroke—a danger well exhibited by examples I have seen of alarming collapse and, on one occasion, death" (p. 128).

The striking point is that if in the 38 years since he began his long career with British athletics at the 1912 Stockholm Olympic Games, Sir Adolphe had encountered only one fatality from heatstroke, then clearly, while heatstroke might indeed be the only serious potential risk to the lives of marathon runners, the real risk had to be very small indeed. This becomes critical if guidelines are developed to prevent a condition that occurs with relative rarity, especially if the proposed intervention—drinking as much as tolerable—has no proven role in the prevention of the condition but may cause an even more dangerous condition in unimaginable numbers.

In fact, Ernest Jokl and L. Melzer (1940) reported, "In view of the statement made by Abrahams [1936] that athletes might become victims of heatstroke, it is noteworthy that to the writers' knowledge not a single fatal case of heatstroke in an athlete has yet been reported" (p. 4). As another speaker at the New York Academy of Sciences conference on the marathon, Dr. Nadel addressed the biological adaptations that protect humans from hyperthermia during exercise. He discussed the control of the primary mechanism for heat loss, sweating, and concluded that "the trained athlete has acquired a resistance to hyperthermia and an improved tolerance to a combined heat and exercise exposure" (Nadel, Wenger, et al., 1977, p. 108).

Nadel did not consider that this resistance to hyperthermia might have been acquired as a result of evolutionary selection rather than recent physical training. Nor did he discuss any role for fluid ingestion in protection against hyperthermia. Probably this was not an oversight; it simply reflected a general indifference to the value of fluid ingestion during exercise, an indifference that at that time was clearly shared by all the world's most eminent sport scientists with an interest in marathon running.

Little attention was paid to any special role of fluid ingestion during exercise. In particular, there was no specific lecture dedicated to the role of fluid ingestion during exercise. The value of carbohydrate ingestion during exercise was not yet realized, although mention was made of the potential ergogenic value of carbohydrate loading before marathon running; there was no suggestion that electrolytes must be ingested during exercise. In fact, Dr. Costill advised the opposite, and only Dr. Wyndham suggested a specific rate (900 ml/hr) of fluid ingestion during

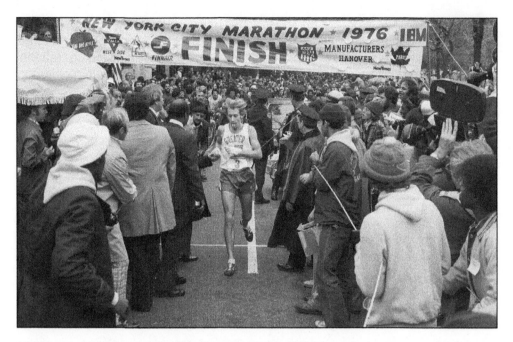

Bill Rodgers wins the New York City Marathon on 24 October, 1976. The race preceded the New York Academy of Sciences Conference on the Marathon, a landmark event in the science of marathon running.
AP Photo/LW

exercise. But his presentation focused on the medicinal value of fluid ingestion in the prevention of heatstroke. No one mentioned the possibility that fluid ingestion might improve performance in the marathon race.

It seems that by 1976, few scientists had yet to seriously consider that fluid ingestion during exercise might improve athletic performance. Clearly Dr. Cade's message had not yet reached the scientists interested in endurance exercise such as marathon running.

USARIEM: Water as a Tactical Weapon

Probably the two papers with the greatest influence on the drinking guidelines that would be produced by the ACSM and other organizations after the early 1980s were coauthored by three physiologists then working at the United States Army Research Institute of Environmental Medicine (USARIEM), Roger W. Hubbard, PhD, Milton Mager, PhD, and Morris Kerstein, PhD, and were published in 1982 and 1984.

1982 USARIEM Paper

Their hypothesis was stated succinctly in an internal military document (Hubbard, Mager, et al., 1982):

"Success in battle during hot weather operations requires maximal operational capability, flexibility, and effectiveness. In order to fulfill mission requirements, individuals must operate at optimal efficiency *yet remain free from the serious consequences of dehydration and heat illness* [my emphasis]. . . . New guidelines for the prevention of heat casualties were field-tested ('80 and '81) during large scale tactical maneuvers and found highly effective in meeting both operational and physiological requirements. This proposed doctrine requires field monitoring of environmental conditions by each unit with a simple small device (Botsball) and increasing individual water intake from 0.5 qt/hr during mild heat conditions (code 1) to 2.0 qt/hr during extreme heat conditions (code 4). During these changes in environmental conditions, simultaneous alterations in work-rest cycles from 50/10 (min) to 20/40 are necessary to maintain body temperature near normal. With these adjustments, commanders can operate in extremely hot conditions, albeit at a slower rate, and complete their missions without undue deterioration of their units' physical and mental capabilities" (p. iii).

These authors viewed water as a tactical weapon and recommended new guidelines for the prevention of heat casualties, which included increasing water intake and altering work-to-rest cycles to maintain body temperature near normal (table 7.1).

These guidelines were subsequently adopted by the U.S. Military in 1988 (Department of the Army, 1988).

These documents are significant for the following reasons:

- The doctrine is based on the implicit assumption that heat illness is due to inadequate fluid ingestion during activity and that it can be prevented by an increased fluid intake. Despite the authors' certainty that they had produced definitive evidence to substantiate their theory, the reality is that even today this theory remains unproven (chapter 5).

- The document suggests that modifying two variables—fluid ingestion and the amount of activity undertaken—reduced the incidence of heat illness during military maneuvers in the heat (Kerstein Mager, et al., 1984). But scientific truth can be detected only in those experiments in which only one

TABLE 7.1 **Water Intake, Work-to-Rest Cycles During Field Operations for Heat-Acclimated Unit**

Heat condition	Botsball WGT (° F)* (° C)	Water intake (qt/hr) (L/hr)	Work-to-rest cycles (min)
1. Green	80-83 (26.6-28.3)	0.5-1.0 (0.48-0.95)	50/10
2. Yellow	83-86 (28.3-30.0)	1.0-1.5 (0.95-1.43)	45/15
3. Red	86-88 (30.0-31.1)	1.5-2.0 (1.43-1.89)	30/30
4. Black	88 and above (>31.1)	2.0 (1.89)	20/40 **

*To convert WGT to wet bulb globe temperature (WBGT), add 2 °F (1.1 °C). Below 80 °F (26.6 °C) drink up to 0.5qt/hr, 50/10 work-to-rest cycles.

**Depending on condition of the troops.

variable is changed at a time. Instead in these experiments, two variables were changed simultaneously. Thus, it is not possible to determine whether both variables or just one contributed to the favorable outcome. For example, reducing the amount of activity soldiers are allowed to undertake each hour from 50 to 20 minutes would be expected to prevent all forms of heat illness for the simple reason that however much activity soldiers performed in any 20-minute exercise bout in the heat, their body temperatures would return to near-normal values in the 40-minute rest between exercise bouts. Regardless of how much fluid they ingested each hour, soldiers exposed to such a favorable work-to-rest ratio when active in the heat would be expected to be essentially immune from the development of heat illness.

- ■ It is not clear why the authors believed that the body temperature must be maintained "near normal" to produce a favorable outcome.

1984 USARIEM Paper

The study that evaluated the efficacy of this novel doctrine involved 6,010 U.S. Navy and Army reservists who participated in a 15-day exercise in the California desert in temperatures ranging from 49 °C to 54 °C (Kerstein, Mager, et al., 1984). Environmental conditions were sufficiently severe that military condition 4 (a state of voluntary or no activity) was achieved "frequently." The exercise was known as the Combined Arms Exercise (CAX 8-80). The goal of the study directed by Dr. Kerstein and his colleagues was to determine whether their guidelines for fluid intake and activity regulation would optimize performance and minimize the risk of heat illness under these severe environmental conditions. The experiment involved two groups of reservists: the control and the experimental groups.

The authors acknowledged that the experimental subjects "were selected for special treatment because they were considered highly motivated and could be expected to put forth maximal effort in the forthcoming exercise" (p. 651). In contrast, the control group came from the other units not involved in "high-risk" military activities.

The basis for any intervention trial is that subjects in both groups must be essentially identical and are then randomized to either the experimental or control groups. But this was certainly not the case in this study.

Before the trial, the experimental group was informed of "six physiological laws governing work in the heat." These six laws included the following (Kerstein, Mager, et al., 1984, p. 651):

- d. If the loss of body fluid by sweating is not replaced, dehydration follows which will hamper heat dissipation and lead to heat-stroke.
- e. The soldier . . . will not feel when he is *dangerously dehydrated* [my emphasis]. It is, therefore, forbidden to have the administration of fluids be dependent upon his thirst . . . Thus, the regular and timely administration . . . of fluids is the responsibility of the commander.
- f. The body temperature can rise because of excessively high . . . temperatures and continuous physical exercise, even when sweating and drinking. . . . To prevent this . . . rise in body temperature, it is mandatory to stop the heat production and provide adequate and recurrent rest periods.

In addition to this lecture, field leaders of this experimental group were then provided with an apparatus (the Botsball) to measure the environmental conditions so that they could implement the rest, activity, and drinking guidelines described in table 7.1. A Botsball thermometer measures the temperature of the thermal environment, as a combination of air temperature, humidity, wind, and thermal radiation.

It is not clear where these guidelines originated. It is fair to conclude that these guidelines were not evidence based and seem to be the individual constructs of the individuals conducting the study.

For the purposes of this experiment, the control group of soldiers did not receive the information provided to the experimental group. Instead, they were provided with the standard U.S. military information of how to conduct themselves when exercising in the heat. Nor was the fluid intake of the control subjects regulated as might be expected in a study purporting to determine whether fluid ingestion alters the risk of developing heat illness. Instead, fluid was provided "generously" to these soldiers at the "usual stopping sites." There is no record of exactly how many soldiers were included in the experimental and control groups.

During the experiment, 1387 soldiers (23% of the total) reported for medical care. Of these, 286 were considered to be heat related, and these included 110 cases of heat exhaustion, 53 cases of headache, 31 cases of cramps or nausea, 46 cases of nose bleeding, and 46 cases of eye irritations. Notice that the definition of what constitutes a heat illness was even vaguer than is usual. It is difficult to understand how these later categories, which comprised 176 cases (62% of the total of 286 cases), can seriously be considered heat illnesses.

The authors claimed that "the results clearly established the validity of the WBGT concept, Botsball use, in desert combat scenarios" (p. 652). There is no table in the text showing exactly how many subjects were in each group and the exact number who developed heat illness in the different categories. Thus, it is not possible to determine whether or not the apparent absence of cases of heat illness in the experimental group is a real finding.

Kerstein, Mager, and colleagues (1984, p. 655) concluded the following:

1. Water should be considered a tactical weapon.
2. Commanders, who modify the activity levels of their units as the heat stress level increases and, additionally, enforce drinking in the absence of thirst, can maintain a viable and efficient fighting force under any environmental condition encountered in the desert.

The purpose of publishing these data from a military exercise is to provide other investigators, *who treat full-time athletes, part-time athletes* [my emphasis], and individuals with heat-related problems, with the information that there are methods for preventing heat-related illnesses.

In discussing their results, the authors pay almost no attention to the role of fluid ingestion in the outcome of their studies. This is understandable because they had not measured the weights of any subjects during the exercises so they could not determine the levels of dehydration present in soldiers in the experimental and control groups. Nor had they recorded the soldiers' rates of fluid ingestion. Thus, they could have no idea how much or how little fluid subjects with or without heat illness had drunk during exercise and therefore if the apparent absence of cases of heat illness in the experimental group was because subjects in that group had drunk more and were therefore less dehydrated.

If there truly were no cases of heat illness in the experimental group, this could have been because (a) they were superior athletes with better motivation and therefore at low risk of seeking medical care for a heat illness, or (b) they exercised more carefully in the heat and rested more, or (c) they drank more and therefore became less dehydrated during the trial, or (d) a combination of a, b, and c. Just as had Wyndham and Strydom, the authors of this study concluded exactly what they were bound to conclude, even before the experiment began. Thus, they really had no need to undertake the study other than to convince others by publishing as a "scientific article" what they believed to be the truth independent of the facts.

The tragedy of this study was that it failed to establish that drinking at such high rates of up to 1.89 L/hr in more severe heat is beneficial. Instead, this novel doctrine was accepted without proper scrutiny, first by the USARIEM and then by the ACSM and GSSI.

1987 ACSM Position Stand on the Prevention of Thermal Injuries During Distance Running

Twelve years after the publication of the original ACSM drinking guidelines, the greatly expanded *ACSM Position Stand on the Prevention of Thermal Injuries During Distance Running* was published (American College of Sports Medicine, 1987). For the first time, apparent scientific "proof" was provided for the medicinal value of fluid ingestion during exercise in preventing heat illness: "Fluid consumption before and during the race will reduce the risk of heat injury, *particularly in longer runs such as the marathon* [my emphasis] (Costill, Cote, et al., 1975; Gisolfi and Copping, 1974; Wyndham and Strydom, 1969)" (p. 530).[2]

But there is no evidence base for this conclusion, since the three correctly cited foundational references, described in full in chapters 3, 5, and 6, do not include experiments that were designed to support that specific conclusion. Rather, all quoted studies evaluated the effects of different levels of weight loss and rates of fluid ingestion solely on the rectal temperature response either in a 32 km race or during laboratory exercise, and none studied the influence of different rates of fluid ingestion on the incidence of heat injury in distance runners competing in appropriate environmental conditions outdoors. So none could conclude that fluid ingestion reduces the risk of heat injury, however defined, in runners competing outdoors in appropriate environmental conditions.[3]

> **2** One of these studies was incorrectly referenced. Costill, Cote, et al., 1975, should have been referenced as Costill, Kammer, et al., 1970.

This stand, which introduced a fundamentally novel concept not present in the 1975 position statement, was not based on new evidence that had suddenly become available since 1975. To have produced novel, evidence-based information to support these guidelines, scientists would first have had to develop unambiguous criteria for diagnosing heat injury, specifically to ensure that only

3   While causation can be proven only by randomized, controlled, prospective (intervention) trials, an absence of causation can sometimes be inferred from cross-sectional studies. The value of cross-sectional studies is that they can identify apparent relationships that might be worth studying with definitive randomized, prospective, controlled (intervention) trials. Or, conversely, they might indicate which studies are not likely to prove a causal relationship.

The consistent finding in cross-sectional field studies has been that the level of dehydration that develops during exercise is unrelated to the postexercise temperature, even in American football players (Fowkes, Godek, et al., 2004) and, as described in chapter 3, that the fastest finishers in endurance events are frequently, if not inevitably, the most dehydrated. This could indicate that there is relatively little probability that a causal relationship between dehydration and either risk of heat illness or impaired running performance will ever be found in those who drink according to the dictates of thirst during exercise.

this condition was being studied. Certain that they were diagnosing exactly and exclusively the condition they had defined as heat injury, the scientists would need to study the incidence of this condition in the same group of runners on two or more occasions when they ran the same marathon at exactly the same pace, after exactly the same training and recovery periods, and under identical environmental conditions, but when they drank fluid at different rates.

Instead, this position stand quoted two studies in which runners ran for 2 hours on a laboratory treadmill drinking at different rates while their body temperatures were measured. This is an altogether different experiment that can only ever answer a much simpler question: What is the effect of different rates of fluid ingestion on the rise of body temperature in laboratory exercise performed under specific environmental conditions?

While the two laboratory studies were indeed randomized, controlled, prospective (intervention) trials and so were able to answer that specific question, the study of Wyndham and Strydom (1969) was uncontrolled and hence could not answer that question.

The second statement was as follows: "Such dehydration will subsequently reduce sweating and predispose the runner to hyperthermia, heat stroke, heat exhaustion, and muscle cramps" (Wyndham and Strydom, 1969, p. 530). This statement also is not evidence based because the quoted reference, the original South African study by Wyndham and Strydom (1969), studied neither the incidence of hyperthermia, heatstroke, heat exhaustion, or muscle cramps in marathon runners nor, in a randomized, controlled, prospective (intervention) trial, the effects of different rates of fluid ingestion on the incidence of those conditions.

Rather, as already described (figure 3.1, page 61), Wyndham and Strydom's study simply reported a relationship between the postexercise rectal temperature and the extent of weight loss in competitors in two 32 km running races, in which no experimental variable was controlled other than the distance the athletes ran. In addition, that study falls foul of the obvious criticism that association does not prove causation (box 3.1, page 62). Again, to provide evidence that the rate of fluid ingestion prevents hyperthermia, heat stroke, heat exhaustion, and muscle cramps, the experimental studies described previously would need to be undertaken in an appropriate group of runners at special risk of developing these conditions[4] when they exercised in appropriately hot environmental conditions.

Nor, as described in the previous chapter, is there any evidence from those and other studies that the dehydration that develops during exercise reduces the sweat rate (Armstrong and Maresh, 1998; Cheuvront and Haymes, 2001;

Costill, Kammer, et al., 1970; Saunders, Dugas, et al., 2005a). The functional studies of David Costill and colleagues (1970) showed that sweat rates were the same regardless of the rate of fluid ingestion. Furthermore, the authors of that paper concluded that fluid ingestion reduced the rectal temperature during exercise not as a result of superior thermoregulation but as a consequence of the cooling effect of the cold fluid that was ingested.

If the sweat rate is not reduced by dehydration, it becomes increasingly difficult to believe that dehydration can have a significant effect on thermoregulation during exercise because, under all but the most unusual conditions, sweating is the main avenue for heat loss during exercise in humans. Thus, another explanation must be provided to explain the higher body temperatures in dehydrated athletes exercising in the laboratory. One possibility is the inappropriately low circulating wind speeds provided in those studies (box 6.1, page 186).

But the most important question that invites an answer is the following: Why, from 1975 to 1987, did the desire suddenly arise to save all exercisers from the risks of hyperthermia, heatstroke, heat exhaustion, and muscle cramps given that (a) a decade earlier the NYAS conference on the marathon could advise only that marathoners should drink during exercise, in line with the 1975 ACSM guidelines, in order to prevent a fluid loss greater than 3% (in line with the theory of Wyndham and Strydom that only weight losses greater than 3% carry an increasing risk of heatstroke); and (b) there was a continuing absence of any evidence that these conditions are especially common in marathon runners and that they are preventable by an increased fluid ingestion during exercise? The answer to this question would solve the mystery of why Dr. Cynthia Lucero died.

The position stand also included guidelines on how much fluid should be ingested during exercise: "An adequate supply of water should be available before the race and every 2-3 km during the race. Runners should be encouraged to drink 100-200 ml at each station." (American College of Sports Medicine 1987, p. 529). For an athlete running a marathon in 2:04 who drinks 200 ml at each station situated every 2 km, this would equate to a rate of fluid intake of ~2 L/hr, whereas runners taking 6 hours to cover the same distance and drinking the same volume at each aid station would sustain a fluid intake rate of 666 ml/hr. Thus, this advice is that marathon runners need to drink at rates of 0.7 to 2.0 L/hr.

The reason this seemingly sound advice is so wrong when applied to runners whose running speeds during a marathon may differ by a factor of 4 has been

4 This is one of the more serious limitations of this type of research. If medical complications occur during exercise only in those who are biologically predisposed either genetically or because of the presence of a transient (intercurrent) condition, then experimental studies of interventions that may prevent those complications must include only those subjects who are biologically predisposed to developing those complications or who have that specific intercurrent condition at the time of the study.

We believe that clinically significant EAH and EAHE can occur only in those who not only overdrink during exercise but who also have at least two additional biological abnormalities (SIADH and abnormal regulation of exchangeable sodium stores, chapter 9). Thus if one wishes to determine whether or not the ingestion of an electrolyte-containing sports drink prevents EAH and EAHE in those who overdrink during exercise, then one must exclude from study those who do not have those biological predispositions. Studying those who do not have SIADH and abnormal regulation of their exchangeable sodium stores and who will therefore not develop the condition when they overdrink during exercise is an expensive waste of time that is likely to lead only to incorrect conclusions as, in my view, has happened frequently (Noakes, 2004; Noakes, 2006).

5 In retrospect, had Professor Wyndham's proposal been followed, lives would have been saved. In essence, he suggested that athletes should have access to fluids only every 20 minutes. Of course, since not all athletes run at the same pace (in a modern big-city marathon race, the last finisher will run three to four times slower than the winner), this solution would have been impractical because it would have required the placement of many more refreshment stations and then allowing the athletes to drink only at those they passed every 20 minutes. Instead, race organizers began to place seconding stations every 5 km (15 minutes running time for an elite marathon runner), then every 3 km (18 minutes running time for a 4:12 marathoner), and then every 1.5 km (15 minutes running time for a 7:00 marathoner). This calculation shows that the evolution of the placement of refreshment stations in big-city marathon races after 1976 was to ensure that even the slowest runner would have access to fluid every 15 to 20 minutes, as originally proposed by Wyndham. The problem was that, provided the athlete ran faster than 10 minutes per km, she would have access to fluid at least every 15 minutes. And if she ran the marathon in between 4:00 to 4:30—the group in which the risk of EAH begins to rise (chapter 10)—she would have access to fluid every 8 1/2 to 9 1/2 minutes, twice as frequently as Professor Wyndham's original proposal.

described.[5] It is logical to advise athletes to drink a certain number of times each hour, say two or three times, since it is extremely difficult to overdrink when drinking in this way because gastric distension will terminate the desire to drink as soon as ~300 to 400 ml is ingested. But when athletes were advised to drink after they had run quite short distances of 1.5 to 3 km, the opportunity for overdrinking was immeasurably increased. Even the very slowest athletes would reach a drinking station, at worst, every 15 minutes and the fastest runners every 4 to 5 minutes (if stations are placed 1.5 km apart).

Those who drew up these 1987 guidelines did not believe that overdrinking during exercise could be dangerous, which was perhaps reasonable since the data disproving that idea had been provided only 2 years earlier (chapter 8).

1996 ACSM Position Stand: Heat and Cold Illnesses During Distance Running

Nine years after the 1987 position stand had promoted high rates of fluid ingestion for the first time during prolonged exercise, the *1996 ACSM Position Stand: Heat and Cold Illnesses During Distance Running* (Armstrong, Epstein, et al., 1996) proposed that dehydration can "predispose the runner to heat exhaustion or the more dangerous hyperthermia and exertional heat stroke (Hubbard and Armstrong, 1989; Pearlmutter, 1986)" (p. iii). This statement is again not evidence based since the two referenced articles are literature reviews that do not provide any new findings, subsequent to the 1987 position stand, that would justify this new dogma that dehydrated runners are at increased risk of dangerous hyperthermia or heatstroke.

In particular, there were no fresh data from randomized, controlled, prospective (intervention) trials designed specifically to determine whether the incidence of dangerous hyperthermia or heatstroke is increased in runners who drink the least during a 42 km marathon race. Nor was there any new evidence showing that the incidence of medical complications is reduced when the same runners drink at higher rates while performing the identical runs under otherwise identical experimental conditions. Rather, these new guidelines projected an increasingly strident opinion even without new evidence from appropriately randomized, controlled, prospective (intervention) trials.

The 1996 position stand appears to be contradictory since it later states that "excessive hyperthermia may occur in the absence of significant dehydration, especially in races of less than 10 km, because the fast pace generates greater metabolic heat" (Armstrong, Epstein, et al., 1996, p. iv). That statement is indeed evidence based. There is clear evidence that heatstroke occurs more commonly in short-distance running events in which high rates of heat production occur in environmental conditions that limit the rate at which heat can be lost to the environment and are completed without the development of significant dehydration (Armstrong, Crago, et al., 1996; Noakes, 1982).

The 1996 position stand (Armstrong, Epstein, et al., 1996) also includes this statement: "Adequate fluid consumption before and during the race can reduce the risk of heat illness, including disorientation and irrational behavior, *particularly in longer events such as a marathon* [my emphasis] (Costill, Kammer, et al., 1970; Gisolfi and Copping, 1974; Wyndham and Strydom, 1969)" (p. ii). But the statement is not evidence based since the same three foundational references used in the 1987 position stand are again quoted in this position stand, and none is a randomized, controlled, prospective (intervention) trial that measured the effects of different rates of fluid ingestion on the incidence of heat illness, disorientation, or irrational behavior in any running races, including marathon races, conducted under appropriately controlled experimental conditions.

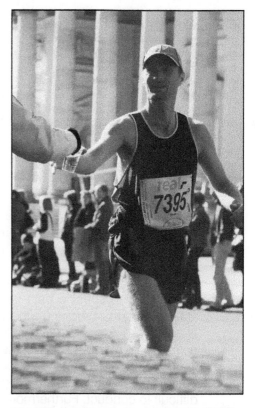

After 1996, marathon runners were advised to drink "as much as tolerable" in order to improve performance and prevent heat stroke. They were also advised not to lose any weight during exercise, also known as the zero % dehydration rule.

Karl-Heinz Spremberg/age fotostock

The 1996 position stand (Armstrong, Epstein, et al., 1996) also included this statement: "Intravenous (IV) fluid therapy facilitates rapid recovery (in runners with heat exhaustion) (Hubbard and Armstrong, 1989; Nash, 1985)" (p. iv). That statement is also not evidence based since it referenced two review articles, neither of which contain evidence from randomized, controlled, prospective (intervention) trials that compared the effects of the administration of IV fluids and another form of treatment on the rates of recovery in athletes with "heat exhaustion." Nor is it exactly clear what constitutes "heat exhaustion." Thus, no evidence-based information is provided to justify this widely promoted view.

The companion *1996 Position Stand on Exercise and Fluid Replacement* (Armstrong, Epstein, et al., 1996; Convertino, Armstrong, et al., 1996) extended these new claims by stating that the "most serious effect of dehydration resulting from the failure to replace fluids during exercise is impaired heat dissipation,[6] which

6 Since the sweat rate is *not* reduced in athletes who become dehydrated during exercise, dehydration does not impair the capacity of dehydrated athletes to lose heat during exercise. Instead, dehydrated athletes could simply sweat more if they wished to lose more heat. Rather, they choose to exercise at a higher, but regulated, temperature because this is a water-conserving mechanism. Other mammals with superior ability to live or exercise in the heat (African hunting dog, eland, oryx, ostrich, baboon, and camel) all show this same adaptation. Thus, the presence of this response indicates superior hot-weather running ability, not an impaired thermoregulatory response.

can elevate core temperature to dangerously high levels (i.e., >40°C)" (p. ii). Later the statement is made that dehydration during exercise "presents the potential for the development of heat-related disorders . . . including the potentially life-threatening heat stroke (Sutton, 1990; Wyndham, 1977). It is therefore reasonable to surmise that fluid replacement that offsets dehydration and excessive elevation in body heat during exercise may be instrumental in reducing the risk of thermal injury (Hubbard and Armstrong, 1989)" (p. ii).

But these conclusions are once again not evidence based because the information quoted in support of these new interpretations is from review articles and is not supported by properly conducted, randomized, controlled, prospective (intervention) trials. More important, none provided specific data from properly randomized, controlled, prospective (intervention) trials showing either that athletes who are dehydrated are at greater risk of heatstroke during exercise or that fluid ingestion during exercise can reduce the number of athletes who develop heatstroke under controlled experimental conditions.

Given that cases of heatstroke occur so infrequently in prolonged exercise in which dehydration is more likely to occur, such research would be extremely difficult to conduct. Furthermore, since it seems probable that individual factors are essential for the development of heatstroke during exercise, the only effective method of studying interventions that prevent heatstroke would be studying athletes who have already developed heatstroke and who are therefore likely to carry one or more genetic or other predispositions for the condition.

Both 1996 position stands advise that athletes should be encouraged to replace their sweat losses or consume 150 to 300 ml every 15 minutes (600-1200 ml per hour). But, again, no scientific rationale for this new guideline is provided.

These rates of fluid ingestion were different from those of the 1975 and 1987 position stands, even though the only new evidence came from the industry-funded studies of Montain and Coyle (1992) and Below, Mora-Rodriguez, and colleagues (1995) reviewed in chapter 6.

But neither of these studies evaluated the effects of a range of fluid ingestion rates on either the risk of developing heatstroke during exercise or on exercise performance. In particular, neither evaluated whether the usual manner in which athletes drink during exercise—that is, according to the dictates of thirst—was as good, better, or worse than these new much higher rates that were proposed.[7]

The greater error was that the consequences of these new drinking guidelines were not evaluated before they were made public. The safe therapeutic dose of the prescription—water or sports drink—was never tested because it was naturally assumed that all humans can safely drink at any rate during exercise. Thus, the possibility that this advice could produce a fatal outcome was not considered even though the evidence for such an effect was, by then, already well established in the scientific literature (chapter 8).

These essential studies were never undertaken because the prevailing belief was that the "perception of thirst, an imperfect guide of the magnitude of the fluid deficit, cannot be used to provide complete restoration of water lost by sweating" (Armstrong, Coyle, et al., 1996, p. ii).

As a result, the *1996 Position Stand on Exercise and Fluid Replacement* included the following: "During exercise, athletes should start drinking early and at regular intervals in an attempt to consume fluids at a rate sufficient to replace all the water lost through sweating (i.e., body weight loss) or *consume the maximal amount that can be tolerated*" [my emphasis] (Convertino, Armstrong, et al., 1996, p. i). It was proposed that this rate could be 600 to 1200 ml/hr, and the solution should contain 4% to 8% carbohydrate and, for exercise lasting more than 1 hour, approximately 0.5 to 0.7 g of sodium chloride (9 to 12 mmol) per L of water (Armstrong, Coyle, et al., 1996).

The *1996 Position Stand on Heat and Cold Illnesses During Distance Running* also included

7 The studies of Montain and Coyle (1992) and Below, Rodriguez, et al. (1995) violated a cardinal rule of comparative trials. If one wishes to determine whether a new treatment is superior to another, the comparison must be against the standard treatment that one wishes to replace. Since the majority of athletes in marathon and other races drink according to the dictates of thirst, it follows that the standard treatment against which to measure a new drinking guideline has to be the ad libitum condition. Instead the industry-funded studies reviewed in chapter 6 inevitably compared a new (higher) drinking protocol to either drinking nothing (figures 6.2, page 189; 6.3 and 6.4, pages 194 and 198) or drinking less than ad libitum (figure 6.5, page 200). The effect was that the ad libitum condition was ignored; instead, the advice athletes received changed from "nothing" to "maximal amount that can be tolerated" (Convertino, Armstrong, et al., 1996, p. i) without any evaluation of the value of intermediate rates of fluid ingestion.

this statement: "Excessive consumption of pure water or dilute fluid (i.e. up to 10 liters per 4 hours) during prolonged endurance events may lead to a harmful dilutional hyponatremia (Noakes, Goodwin, et al., 1985). . . . The possibility of hyponatremia may be the best rationale for inclusion of sodium chloride in fluid replacement beverages" (Armstrong, Epstein, et al., 1996, p. iii). But this advice was also not evidence based since there was then, as there is now (Noakes, 2011), no published evidence proving that sodium chloride ingestion can prevent the development of EAH or EAHE in those who overdrink during exercise. Rather, the only published evidence at that time showed that athletes with EAHE are no more sodium deficient than are controls.

In addition, the *1996 Position Stand on Exercise and Fluid Replacement* included the statement that "the perception of thirst (is) an imperfect index of the magnitude of the fluid deficit (and) cannot be used to provide complete restoration of water lost by sweating" (Convertino, Armstrong, et al., 1996, p. ii). But there is no conclusive evidence that the perception of thirst is inadequate during exercise because it is not known how much of the fluid lost during exercise needs to be replaced either during or immediately after exercise. The point is that since the prevention of any weight loss during exercise requires that athletes drink "ahead of thirst," once the zero % dehydration rule was decided on, then thirst had to be dismissed as an imperfect indicator of the real fluid requirements before and after exercise. No one bothered to ask this question: If thirst is an imperfect index of the body's fluid requirements, how is it possible that every (other) creature on Earth that relies solely on thirst to regulate fluid balance seems to achieve this balance rather well?

Summary

In three decades, advice about hydration during exercise had evolved from believing that no or ad libitum drinking was safe or even ideal to believing that the recommendation that drinking as much as 1.2 L/hour, if not more, was optimal. Had the 1996 guidelines been drawn up exclusively for elite athletes, they would have been safe, because elite runners would soon have discovered that such high rates of fluid ingestion are simply not sustainable especially during competitive running. Any athlete trying to drink at a rate of 1.2 L/hr when running at 20 km/hr would soon be unable to sustain that pace because of the development of uncomfortable gastrointestinal symptoms (Robinson, Hawley, et al., 1995), as occurred in the original study of Costill, Kammer, and colleagues (1970). Only cyclists might be able to sustain such high rates of drinking for more than an hour or two.

But slow runners with maximum sweat rates of only 500 ml/hr when running a 4:30 marathon (Twerenbold, Knechtle, et al., 2003) would be more likely to sustain such high rates of fluid ingestion relatively comfortably, especially if they had the capacity to absorb fluid rapidly through the intestine and if they also had syndrome of inappropriate antidiuretic hormone hypersecretion (SIADH). Without SIADH, they would be passing at least 700 ml of urine per hour and so would probably begin (eventually) to question whether it was really necessary to have to pass urine almost as frequently as they ingested fluid.

Thus, the error made by the authors of the 1996 ACSM position stands is strikingly obvious. The studies they cited were designed to measure the maximum rates of sweat loss and fluid ingestion that better-than-average athletes could sustain during prolonged exercise lasting about 2 hours in conditions that were hot enough to be categorized as either high or very high risk (for heatstroke) by the ACSM itself. Drinking guidelines based on those studies were then extrapolated to recreational runners and cyclists who run or cycle 2 to 4 times slower than these better athletes. Because they were exercising at much lower metabolic rates, the real fluid requirements of these recreational athletes were also 2 to 4 times lower than the fluid requirements of the subjects tested in those studies. And because they were exercising at much lower intensities, their much slower breathing rates allow only the slow-running athletes to ingest fluid at such high rates.[8]

[8] Elite athletes cannot ingest fluid at rates of 1.2L/hr for two reasons other than that they have no need. First, if they are runners, they are often smaller than the 72 kg (158 lb) giants studied by Montain and Coyle (1992). Their smaller size means that they will have smaller stomachs and intestines, with a lesser capacity to process fluid when ingested at such high rates. But more important, when running fast, the respiratory rates of these athletes are so high that they do not have time to ingest a large volume of fluid before they must take another breath. This behavior is easy to observe in world-class marathon runners. The better the athlete, the less he appears to ingest when running at 20 km/hr. In races of shorter distances, these world-class marathon runners do not usually ingest any fluid.

The opposite applies to recreational athletes. The only factor preventing a high rate of fluid intake in slow runners might be the inconvenience of having to stop communicating with their friends while they are drinking.

CHAPTER 8

Discovery of Exercise-Associated Hyponatremia (EAH)

It is difficult to visualise a survival incident in which the main hazard is an excess of water to drink.

W.S.S. Ladell (1965, p. 277)

Wyndham and Strydom's message began to influence my thinking in 1972 after I had run my first 42 km (26 mile) marathon and was preparing to run the 90 km (56 mile) Comrades Marathon. So I had developed an interest in the physiology of ultramarathon running, even presenting a paper on this topic at a student medical conference at the University of Cape Town. In this process I came across two other South African studies (Dancaster, Duckworth, et al., 1969; Dancaster and Wherat, 1971) of Comrades Marathon runners.[1] These studies concluded that the fluid intakes of these Comrades runners were "totally inadequate" since their water deficits were "very high." But "surprisingly none showed evidence of heat exhaustion or higher rectal temperatures." Nor, interestingly, was there any evidence that such "totally inadequate" fluid intakes and "alarming water deficits," which "in the majority . . . assumed dangerous proportions" had any significant effects on the runners' kidney function since no athlete developed kidney failure and their rates of urine production after the race were "surprisingly good." Furthermore, "in spite of the severe water deficits rectal temperatures of over 102 °F (38.9 °C) were not recorded" (Dancaster and Whereat, 1971, p. 150).

1 The first of these studies (Dancaster and Whereat, 1971) proved how safe it is to lose quite large volumes of fluid during the 90 km Comrades Marathon. Only 3 of the 24 runners who were studied lost less than 4% of their body weight (BW) during the race; 10 lost more than 6% BW, and 1 runner lost 8.2% BW. According to the Wyndham and Strydom theory, runners who lost more than 3% BW should have been at risk of developing heatstroke. But the postrace rectal temperatures of these Comrades runners did not support that theory. Nine runners whose body weights fell by more than 4%, finished with postrace rectal temperatures of 38.3 °C to 38.8 °C. These values are not much greater than those of the spectators watching the race (~37 °C) and much lower than values measured in athletes with heatstroke (>42 °C). Rectal temperatures in the two runners with the greatest weight losses of 7.1% and 8.2% BW were only 38.3 °C and 38.8 °C, respectively. All these temperatures were much lower than values predicted from Wyndham and Strydom's graph (figure 3.1, page 61). An independent observer might have concluded that these real data from Comrades Marathon runners disprove the theory that quite severe levels of dehydration (>7%) will cause the rectal temperature to rise to dangerous levels (>42 °C).

In retrospect, these two studies provide an interesting example of how preconceptions can blind scientists to the real meaning of their data. The authors had presumed that the model developed by the experts, Wyndham and Strydom (physiological model 1 in box 3.1, page 62), had to be correct. So perhaps to ensure that their work would be more readily accepted, they had interpreted their own findings according to the explanation that Wyndham and Strydom had introduced.

But as an impressionable medical student ignorant of the complexity of the scientific method and overenthused by all this talk of "alarming water deficits," "totally inadequate fluid intakes," and "heatstroke" caused by "dehydration," it was perhaps only natural that I should consider it my personal responsibility to ensure that all the world's runners must be encouraged to drink more during exercise if their lives were to be spared.

So it was that my first contributions to running books (Noakes, 1974; Noakes, 1978) and to the medical literature (Noakes, 1973) focused on what I had been taught to believe was the greatest danger to the health of runners: heat illness, specifically heatstroke. Thus, in 1974, my final year as a medical student, I wrote this: "The prime object of the marathon runner must be to avoid dehydration by drinking adequately during a run. My experience is that few runners know what is adequate. This problem arises because of the international ruling that stipulates when an athlete can drink or be sponged during a marathon, and is compounded by the practice of many world-class marathon runners *not* to drink during a race. Ron Hill ran the world's third fastest marathon without drinking any fluid. This practice is to be condemned as it sets an example for less-gifted runners, whose bodies are not capable of withstanding the heat stress as well as those of world-class runners.[2] It also makes runners careless in their attitude towards the longer races. In these races, very severe dehydration will occur, and the danger of heat injury is increased immeasurably. Five cases of heat-induced kidney failure occurred in the Comrades 57-miler in the years 1968 to 1972" (Noakes, 1974, p. 186).

Suffused by youthful arrogance, I then provided guidelines of how race organizers, international sporting bodies, the medical profession, and the athletes themselves could prevent heat illness during running. Athletes were informed

2 Such is the arrogance of ignorance. I suppose that since I had by then run the 90 km Comrades Marathon, I had enough experience to be certain of my correctness. In fact, less gifted runners have a lesser risk of heat illness because they run slower at a lower metabolic rate, and thus usually at lower body temperatures.

that they could lose 1 to 2 L of fluid as a result of sweating every hour that they exercised. To ensure that they did not become dehydrated by more than 3% body weight (BW) during marathon races, they were encouraged to drink at least 1 L (250 ml every 15 min) of cool fluid every hour that they ran. Doubt was expressed about the value of ingesting salt tablets during exercise. The article ended with a touching and patriotic tribute to "Professors Wyndham and Strydom of the Human Science Laboratory, Johannesburg, South Africa, whose inquisitive research has supplied most of our knowledge concerning exercise in the heat" (Noakes, 1974, p. 189).

My more detailed review of the physiology of running in the heat (Noakes, 1978), written for the lay public, again emphasized the "danger" of dehydration and referred to the study of Wyndham and Strydom (1969) who apparently "showed that the body temperatures of athletes, who become dehydrated by more than 3% of body weight, approached values previously only recorded in victims of heatstroke." The article noted that restrictions on fluid ingestion during marathon races had recently been relaxed, "allowing the 1976 Olympic Marathon to be the first run without restriction on the amount of fluid that athletes could drink during the race" (p. 250). The article again argued that there was little evidence that salt supplementation was necessary even during the Comrades Marathon since total salt losses in sweat were insufficient to cause adverse consequences. The article continued by introducing the concept of a "hyperthermic spiral" in which progressive dehydration would cause a reduction in blood flow to the skin and, as a result, a reduction in the sweat rate. This would then initiate a further rise in the body temperature and a continual reduction in sweat rate, progressing until the body temperature rose so high that heatstroke developed.[3]

I concluded with one flash of inspiration: "Fortunately, most athletes seldom reach this point because, due to fatigue caused by factors other than heat, they hit 'the wall' after about 30 miles (48 km) and start to slow down. By slowing down, the athlete immediately reduces his rate of energy production and is released from the hyperthermic spiral. Thus, 'relative' unfitness is paradoxically the safety factor that protects against heatstroke" (Noakes, 1978, p. 256). At the time, I could not have conceived that the brain might use fatigue specifically to prevent the development of heatstroke, a novel idea we first developed only years later.

The more that I ran in those years, the more convinced I became that my crusade was correct and that runners must be encouraged, indeed forced, to drink more during exercise. But my retrospective analysis undertaken more recently reveals that I did not follow my own advice. Thus I incurred a body weight loss of 4% during one 42 km marathon (Irving, Noakes, et al., 1986). Since my drinking pattern was the same during ultramarathon races, I more than likely finished some Comrades Marathon

3   I do not know how I arrived at this explanation. It is wrong because sweating is controlled by neural reflexes that are essentially independent of the amount of blood flowing to the skin. Thus sweating is impaired by factors that influence the nervous control of the sweat glands. Furthermore, dehydration at levels frequently measured in competitive athletes (1%-8% BW loss) is clearly not one of these factors because sweat rates remain high even in athletes who do not drink during exercise in the heat and who can develop high levels of dehydration (chapter 6). I now refer to this incorrect physiological model as the cardiovascular model of thermoregulation (CMT).

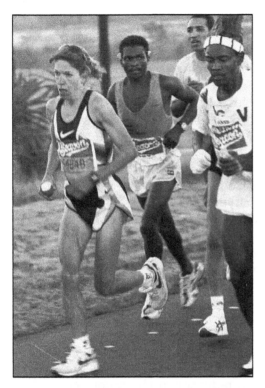

American ultramarathon runner and former world 100km world record holder, Ann Trason, competes in the Comrades Marathon, which she won in 1996 and 1997. The world's first case of EAHE was recognized in the 1981 Comrades Marathon.

AP Photo/Str

races with a weight loss closer to 8% to 10%. Despite this, my postrace rectal temperatures and kidney function, including my urinary calcium excretion, were all quite normal in those races in which I was studied.

But so convinced was I of my righteousness that in an article published in May 1981 I included drinking to prevent dehydration as one of the 5 keys to "improve the imperfect peak." To quote: "The fourth performance aid is to drink everything in sight during the race. And the fluid that doesn't go into the stomach must be doused over the head, abdomen, legs and arms" (p. 11). "Time was, of course, when to drink during a marathon race was to be something less than masculine. Thus the early marathoners were expected to be camels of the road. Fortunately, research by Professor Wyndham and Strydom of the former Chamber of Mines Human Sciences Laboratory in Johannesburg showed just how dangerous this practice is. For they found that the uncorrected dehydration of marathon runners caused their body temperatures to reach levels similar to those found in heat stroke victims. Furthermore we now know that adequate fluid ingestion during exercise will prevent an excessive rise in body temperature" (Noakes, 1981a, p. 11).

There is a touching innocence in such certainty. It was the last time I would ever be so certain of this or any other of my opinions.

For less than a month later in June 1981 I received letters from two female athletes who had run the 1981 90 km Comrades Marathon; one had almost died. They had written to me because at the time I wrote a regular medical column in the only running magazine then published in South Africa.

First Cases of EAH and EAHE

The medical condition both runners in the following letters described had not been reported previously by any athlete participating in any sport. At first I did not understand the full portent of what they had described. Nor could I have predicted the effect it would have on my academic career. I could not have known then that the work these letters initiated would, 25 years later, be rated as one of the 40 most important "persons or events" in running in the last 40 years (Gambaccini, 2006).

First Runner's Story

Having just completed the 1981 Comrades Marathon and, despite following all the advice with regard to dehydration, I "woke-up" to find myself in hospital five hours after the race had ended. I think that my story may be of value to other runners.

Comrades day started at 4am. I woke feeling really good and looking forward to the run. On the way to the start I drank 500ml of water. In addition, I carried 750ml of a mixture of Liquifruit [a 10% carbohydrate fruit drink] and water to cover the almost certain problems of getting something to drink at the first three [refreshment] tables. Thereafter, I drank a WEAK mixture of Coke and water at virtually every table. [Note: There were a total of 57 aid stations during the race, one every ~1.5km.] During the first 60km I probably made three or more pit-stops (to pass urine) so it seemed that I was drinking adequately.

My running time to the 40km was 55min slower than my normal marathon time (which is slow anyway) so I was really taking it easy. When I began to feel nauseous at the 40km mark I assumed that the reason was probably due to too much Coke. I switched over to straight water at that stage.

The nauseousness got progressively worse until by the 70 km mark I started to bring-up. Whenever this happened there was no dry retching—*I brought up a lot of water*. If I walked I seemed to be OK but the minute I began to run no matter how slowly, I was sick. The last 18km were heavy going for the above reasons, but otherwise my body felt fine.

I was glad to see the finish line! After receiving my finish-time card etc, I wandered through the cattle pen onto the grass and sat down. That was the last thing I was conscious of until 5 hours later when I "came-to" in a bed in Grey's Hospital.

When I passed out, I was carried to the first-aid tent where I was given 3 litres of saline drip. I did not appear to be recovering as rapidly as expected so I was given a blood test. This showed a low blood sugar level and I was put on a glucose drip for a while and then discharged.

I was carried to the car to be transported to a friend's flat. At the flat my pulse was taken and found to be very faint and rapid (in excess of 120 beats per minute). In addition, I still did not appear to be properly conscious.

I was carted off to Grey's Hospital where my blood pressure was found to be low (90/60mmHg). I was given another litre of saline drip and an injection of Stemetil to counteract the dry-retching. For the first time after sitting down at the finish, I knew what was going on.

From hospital, I was taken back to the flat and put to bed. During the night I made three or four trips to the toilet—understandable, I think, after all the saline drip I had been given.

When the alarm woke me at 4am the next morning I felt in good shape and, to the utter amazement of my friends, totally unaware of the drama that had taken place the day before. In fact, I didn't feel, from a physical point of view, that I had even had a run the day before—no trace of stiffness or pain in any muscle or joint. My body had obviously had a very comfortable and easy run but I had ended up in a coma.

Why? (Noakes, 1981b, pp. 8-9)*

*Reprinted from T.D. Noakes, 1981, "Comrades makes medical history—again," *S A Runner* 4(Sept): 8-10.

Second Runner's Story

I finished the 1980 (Comrades) race in good condition. For this year's race I had trained harder and felt fitter. However, at 30km I developed diarrhea. My husband was shocked at my condition when he saw me at 60km and begged me to stop but I was determined to finish. I have no recollection of even seeing him. At 70km my husband took me off the road and obtained assistance from a first aid station. I can vaguely recollect getting into an ambulance. I was then taken to Grey's Hospital where it was diagnosed that I was suffering from *dehydration*, and I was given a rapid electrolyte infusion. I was discharged from Grey's Hospital and my husband took me to Umhlanga Rocks by car. I was having convulsions during the ride. At the hotel I had another fit and the local doctor was called. I was rushed by ambulance to the nearest hospital.

4   By coincidence, I was involved in a study of blood glucose and hormonal changes in Comrades Marathon runners at that year's race and was present in the medical tent at the race finish from midmorning until late evening on the day that Eleanor Sadler (case 2) was treated there. At the time we failed to appreciate that since this was the first Comrades Marathon in which runners would be able to drink every 1.5 km, perhaps some might drink more than their thirst dictated. When Eleanor Sadler was admitted to the medical tent where we were working, the true nature of her condition was clearly not recognized by those treating her, presumably because her blood sodium concentration was not measured. And why would anyone have considered it necessary since we all "knew" that blood sodium concentrations "always" rise during prolonged exercise? It was the classic case of the unexpected appearance of the highly improbable, the black swan, described in the best-selling book of the same name by Nassim Nicholas Taleb (2007).

The doctors took blood tests and x-rays immediately and discovered I was suffering from water intoxication which was apparently due to lack of salt in my system caused by the diarrhea. They informed my husband that my condition was very serious and there was also a possibility of both brain and kidney damage. They also said that if I had taken four salt tablets during the race I would have been fine.

These doctors were wonderful and took care of me throughout Monday night and all day Tuesday until I came out of the coma on Wednesday. I was given oxygen and a slow sodium chloride and dextrose drip. The drip remained in until the Saturday. On the Wednesday the doctors were still uncertain whether I would have brain damage as I was having hallucinations and couldn't see or speak properly. On the Thursday everything cleared and the doctors said it was only because I was so fit and strong that I had recovered without brain or kidney damage. I was discharged on the Sunday after the doctors were satisfied that I was fine.

I am deeply grateful for the fantastic medical know-how and loving care of the staff of the hospital as they certainly saved my life.[4] (Noakes, 1981b, pp. 9-10)*

*Reprinted from T.D. Noakes, 1981, "Comrades makes medical history—again," *S A Runner* 4(Sept): 8-10.

My Investigation Begins

I have always been bored by the mundane and challenged by the unusual or unexplained. By 1981 I had regularly treated athletes at the finish of marathon and ultramarathon races and had served for some years as the medical doctor at the 56 km (35 mile) Two Oceans Ultramarathon in Cape Town. I had seen my share of unconscious patients after these races; most suffered from the typical range of medical emergencies, sometimes caused by abnormal heart function. I had also been among the first to measure blood changes in ultraendurance exercise

(Noakes and Carter, 1976); always we had found that blood sodium concentrations *rose* during exercise. With the exception of one study, discussed in chapter 4, the data of which must be erroneous, every other study at the time reported exactly the same finding—blood sodium concentrations always rose during exercise (table 4.2, page 129). But here were two cases in which the opposite had happened. The blood sodium concentration of the second runner had fallen so low that she had lost consciousness and almost died. In time we would establish that hers was the first case of exercise-associated hyponatremic encephalopathy (EAHE) to be described in the scientific literature.

I was immediately challenged to understand what had happened. There seemed to be only two possible explanations—either both ladies had lost excessive amounts of salt, as the second runner believed, or they had retained a large volume of fluid and diluted their blood sodium concentrations. At the time the first seemed much more probable—surely humans can lose large amounts of salt in their sweat during exercise. What is more, we all "knew" that it is dehydration, not overhydration, that causes ill health during long-distance running. Professors Cyril Wyndham and Nic Strydom among many others had taught us this, and their opinions were sacrosanct.

So within a month I wrote an article (Noakes, 1981b) describing these cases and explaining what I thought had happened. Even though I had formerly been convinced that it was impossible for a runner to develop this condition, I acknowledged, after having consulted with the doctors at Addington Hospital, that the second runner had, in fact, suffered from water intoxication. I explained how I thought two factors contributed to water intoxication: sodium depletion due to water loss from diarrhea or vomiting, and then intake of fluid without attention paid to the sodium loss. "The blood then becomes very diluted, its sodium content falls, and all the cells to the body, including the brain, become waterlogged causing the frightening symptoms you describe. And until the sodium deficit is corrected, the body is unable to rid itself of this extra fluid" (p. 10).

I explained that in order for water intoxication to occur in the Comrades Marathon, a runner would have to lose 60 g of sodium (a huge amount) and fail to replace it, by drinking only water and not eating anything, since most foods are laden with salt. Or a runner might develop water intoxication if he or she lost slightly less sodium but then was treated with non-sodium-containing intravenous fluids.

I calculated that since sweat contains 2 g of salt per L, a person would have to lose 30 L of sweat to lose 60 g of salt. But the highest sweat loss in a Comrades runner of which I was aware was 10 L. So sweating alone would not cause sufficiently severe salt depletion to result in water intoxication. I concluded that in the case of this runner, there must have been another source of salt loss, likely the diarrhea.

I then attempted to calculate whether it would be possible to lose another 40 g of salt in diarrheal fluid and concluded that in this case death would likely occur first as the result of a fatal loss of body water. Instead, I proposed the following:

> Alternatively, the runner may have been salt depleted before the race but that has also never been reported before.
>
> In summary, the sweat losses alone during the Comrades will never cause sufficient salt to be lost so that the majority of runners will never risk developing water intoxication

if they drink only water or non-salt containing drinks during the race. However, the message from this case must be that once one has diarrhea, salt losses may become substantial.

Only under such conditions would it seem advisable to take some salt. Incidentally, the amount of salt that would have been needed to prevent water intoxication in this case would probably have been about 60 grams (or 120 salt tablets as each contains 0.5 grams salt) (p. 10).

This explanation that water intoxication is caused by large sodium losses that are not replaced in those who drink only (sodium-free) water during exercise would, two decades later, become the staple of the GSSI, the ACSM, and the scientists who advise these organizations. My other possible explanation was that EAHE might occur when an athlete who was partially sodium depleted was treated inappropriately with large volumes of intravenous fluids during recovery. It did not occur to me that perhaps these athletes had simply drunk too much during the race. Clearly this was an intellectual jump for which my mind was not yet ready—and understandably so. It is not easy to discard a hallowed belief.

So my personal bias at the time was clear. In 1981 I did not yet believe that it was possible for an athlete to drink so much during exercise that she would develop water intoxication. How could I or anyone else believe this since we had become so conditioned to believe that dehydration was the real killer of athletes? But sometime between 1981 and 1984 when we submitted the paper describing the first cases of EAH and EAHE to a scientific publication, I had changed my mind; I had crossed a personal Rubicon. Perhaps my good fortune was that the athletes themselves continued to educate me after July 1981.

A few weeks later, an anesthetist wrote to me explaining his own experiences also at the 1981 Comrades Marathon. He admitted himself to the hospital when he became concerned that his level of consciousness was fluctuating. His blood sodium concentration on hospital admission was 118 mmol/L, indicating that he, too, was suffering from EAHE.

Then after the 1982 Comrades Marathon a 20-year-old university student developed an epileptic seizure an hour after finishing the race. His blood sodium concentration was 124 mmol/L, confirming the diagnosis of EAHE.

The next case occurred in an accomplished triathlete who, fortuitously, I knew well because she had previously consulted me. During what was then the longest (148 km, or 92 mile) triathlon in South Africa, she had developed shortness of breath and had been forced to walk the final 14 km of the running leg. On admission to the hospital, she was found to have fluid in the lungs (pulmonary edema) with a blood sodium concentration of 125 mmol/L. Thus, she had EAHE complicated by noncardiogenic pulmonary edema.

Fortunately, careful interrogation of these five cases provided all the evidence necessary to determine what had caused their condition.[5]

5 All five of these cases survived. Cases 1, 4, and 5 were in the hospital for 7, 4, and 4 days, respectively, while case 3 was released from the hospital after only 24 hours. Case 5, the most competitive of these athletes, completed the 1983 226 km Ironman Hawaii Triathlon 2 years later in 30th position in the women's race in 12 hours 19 minutes. During the race she drank 5.5 L (450 ml/hr) compared to a drinking rate of 800 ml/hr in the South African race in which she had developed EAHE. Her case illustrates that EAHE is not an inevitable consequence of prolonged exercise but must occur in some otherwise predisposed individuals when they drink to excess during prolonged exercise.

Determining What Causes EAH and EAHE

Scientists use different experimental techniques to determine truth. The gold-standard technique is the randomized, controlled intervention (clinical) trial (RCT). In this experimental model, a population of subjects is divided into two matching groups. During the experiment, only the subjects in the intervention group receive the intervention that is being evaluated (e.g., a drug designed to treat a particular disease). The subjects in the control group, identical in every conceivable way to the intervention group, do not receive the intervention. Instead, they receive a placebo intervention that is indistinguishable from that of the real intervention. In the case of a drug trial, the placebo will look, taste, and smell exactly the same as the real drug under investigation. Any differences that develop between the groups during the course of the trial are then considered to be caused solely by the intervention.

However, undertaking an RCT requires that there first be a testable hypothesis or theory. This usually requires that an observation has been made, which then stimulates the generation of a hypothesis. Most hypotheses have their origins in a single unusual observation that cannot be explained according to the scientist's current understanding. In other words, the observation cannot be predicted according to the scientist's model of how the world is meant to work. Instead, the observation is paradoxical.[6]

In medical science, this paradoxical observation is often based on a single case report or a collection of similar reports. These reports do not by themselves prove anything; they are essentially anecdotes (or stories)[7] that could have many different explanations. The explanation that is first offered will reflect the personal biases of the individual who develops the new model with which to interpret this paradoxical observation.

My personal biases would determine what I would ultimately conclude had caused EAHE to develop in these five athletes. At the time, these included the following (among many others of which I remain blissfully unaware):

> **6** A paradox is defined as a contradictory statement (or, in science, a research finding) that is nevertheless true. Paradoxes occur in science when the actual findings in an experimental study are the exact opposite of those that the scientist expected to find on the basis of the model that he or she uses to predict what should happen. Thus, our finding that athletes became very ill when they overdrank during exercise was paradoxical according to the model that predicts that underdrinking can cause athletes to die during prolonged exercise.

> **7** There is a famous scientific aphorism: "The plural of anecdote is not scientific data." Scientific proof requires that scientific data be collected in appropriately designed randomized controlled intervention trials.

- Although I believed that athletes should drink as much as possible during exercise, I never personally followed that guideline. In fact, I disliked drinking during exercise and had run my best 90 km ultramarathon race without drinking anything for the first 2 hours and then relatively little for the next 62 km. After 9 years of marathon and ultramarathon running, I had discovered that ingesting carbohydrate during exercise had a much more obvious effect on my running performance (Noakes T.D., 2003a) than ingesting fluid at rates greater than my thirst dictated. Carbohydrate ingestion (in the form of either the original FRN Squeezy or solid foods) always allowed me to maintain my ultramarathon pace with less mental discomfort. Not once did I experience the same benefit from fluid ingestion alone. The fact that it took me 8 years to learn this truth is a reflection of the power of the prevailing dogma at that time that dehydration caused by drinking too little fluid, rather than hypoglycemia (low blood glucose concentration) caused by ingesting too little carbohydrate, is the more important cause of fatigue during prolonged exercise (see note 1 in chapter 6, page 184).

■ I had only once ingested salt tablets during a running race. I had instantly felt better. The effect was so rapid that, in retrospect, it had to be due to a mental (placebo) effect and could not have been due to the negligible change in body sodium content produced by the tablets. More important in training, we did not ever ingest extra salt beyond that dictated by any increased craving for salt. I do not recall that I ever developed a craving for salt in all the years that I ran marathons and ultramarathons. But I did notice that my sweat became less salty the more I trained. When I trained little, my sweat tasted very salty; when I was highly trained, it tasted more like pure water. This would result from the sodium-conserving mechanisms described in chapter 4 as well perhaps as a shift to a less salty diet when training intensively.

■ During my medical training I had never seen a patient suffering from salt deficiency. Nor, with one exception, did I recall seeing patients with low blood sodium concentrations (hyponatremia). Such cases would most likely have occurred in surgical patients treated inappropriately with excessive fluids either orally or intravenously during their recovery from surgery. I recall that our professor of surgery had specifically warned us that patients retain fluid excessively after any stressful procedure, including surgery, because they have increased blood concentrations of the water-conserving hormone AVP/ADH. As a result, we were taught to monitor carefully the fluid status of our postsurgical patients. Subsequently, through my interests in EAHE I would learn that patients given large volumes of intravenous fluids after surgery recovered more slowly than those who received less fluid.

The singular patient with hyponatremia whom I recall treating during my medical training had developed an unusual form of lung cancer. Rarely such cancers can manufacture the hormone AVP/ADH and so retain water inappropriately causing hyponatremia. The condition is known as the syndrome of inappropriate ADH secretion (SIADH). It would have been helpful if years later I had better understood this condition (box 8.1). Clearly I had not paid enough attention to this condition of SIADH. I now find this surprising because, like many medical students, I had a natural affinity for remembering the most unusual information that is often of little real practical value. Indeed, the more bizarre the information, the more likely I was to remember it.

■ Even though I had managed to convince my examiners that I knew more than 50% of the required medical curriculum and was not a clear danger to an unsuspecting public, at the end of my medical training I clearly had only a cursory understanding of body sodium balance in health and disease. Probably this is because I must have developed the incorrect belief that

---

BOX 8.1   Mink and Schwartz Connect SIADH to EAH

Again, there was other evidence I missed because my mind was not yet properly prepared. Only now do I appreciate the full meaning of this evidence.

In 1989 I traveled to Aspen, Colorado, where I met Dr. Barry Mink. Subsequently, he sent me a copy of his paper describing a study of six runners in the 1988 Leadville Trail 100-mile (160 km) race (Mink and Schwartz, 1990), of whom only three completed the race. Although none of the six runners developed EAH or EAHE, blood AVP/ADH concentrations were decreased or unchanged in finishers but "greatly elevated in non-finishers" (p. 20); unfortunately, actual data were not reported. In contrast, blood aldosterone concentrations, the hormone regulating sodium in the kidneys, were significantly higher in finishers than in non-finishers. On average, runners lost 2 kg (~4 lb) during the race. The authors concluded that "... reports have suggested that long-distance runners may be drinking too much fluid and not taking in enough salt (Hiller, 1989). *Our study suggests another mechanism* [my emphasis]. Elevation of ADH levels in non-finishers, along with blunted elevations of aldosterone values, suggests that hormonal influences may play a role in successfully finishing an ultramarathon, as well as in the production of the hyponatremic syndrome. The inappropriate ADH syndrome is a medical phenomenon seen during acute and stressful illness (Goldberg, 1981). Running long distance is very stressful for some, and if the inappropriate ADH syndrome develops and persists after the race when the runner has the opportunity to drink copious amounts of hypotonic fluids, then significant hyponatremia and water intoxication can become a reality" (pp. 22-23). Thus, Mink and Schwartz concluded the following: "Inappropriate anti-diuretic hormone and blunted aldosterone responses may contribute to the phenomenon of hyponatremia and water intoxication observed rarely in long-distance runners" (p. 23).

In a letter to me dated September 13, 2006, Dr. Mink reminded me of this study and wrote this: "I hope you will find our humble study useful in the history of this condition and am grateful for your input and acknowledgement about our hypothesis at that time."

Clearly Dr. Mink and his colleague Arthur Schwartz were the first to propose that EAH and EAHE occur in those with inappropriate ADH secretion (the condition of SIADH) who also overdrink during exercise. Their ideas were correct and well ahead of the rest of ours. I have no idea why their correct conclusion made no impression on me at the time. We all have our blind spots! I trust Drs. Mink and Schwartz will accept my much-belated recognition of their prescience and their historical contribution.

---

sodium balance is seldom an issue in the management of medical disease (with the exception of patients with kidney failure and whose diseased kidneys are unable to excrete sodium normally).

■ Since I was essentially a teetotaler at the time (as I still am), I was unaware of the condition known as beer potomania, a form of water intoxication that occurs in those beer drinkers who ingest beer at faster rates than they can excrete the ingested water. But now I also suspect that beer potomania cannot occur in the absence of SIADH.

■ Generally in my training I had been taught a conservative medical approach in which we were cautioned to give the body every opportunity to cure itself before we began to intervene intensively. Only many years later would I begin to appreciate the wisdom of this approach. Then I was introduced to the fictional doctor, the Fat Man, a medical resident in *The House of God* (Shem, 2003), by Lewis Maharam, MD, whom I had helped develop the athlete management programs incorporated in the Rock 'n' Roll Marathon Series run under his direction, as well as the drinking guidelines of the International Marathon Medical Directors Association (Noakes, 2003b), that he established. Dr. Maharam considered my medical education to be incomplete until I had been introduced to the Fat Man, who taught the following: "The main source of illness in this world is the doctor's own illness: his compulsion to try to cure and his fraudulent belief that he can. . . . We hardly ever cure. We cure ourselves, and that's it" (Shem, 2003, p. 193). So perhaps early in my career I had either been taught or I instinctively understood that patients are best served by doctors who have first cured themselves of the doctor's disease—the pathological compulsion to try to cure.

■ On reflection I was probably so ignorant about the real causes of hyponatremia that it would have been difficult for me to have any major biases.

My approach to the solution of this problem was twofold: First, I exhaustively interviewed four of the five athletes and the medical staff who treated them to search for points of commonality in their stories (I was unable to identify and locate the first runner, the writer of the first letter). My medical training had taught me that patients usually have all the answers, although neither they nor their doctors initially know this. The doctor's responsibility is to ask the correct questions that will uncover the crucial information. Fortunately, two of the athletes provided the critical information that seemed to allow only one conclusion.

Second, I searched all the relevant scientific literature. This supported the general belief at the time that "sodium chloride replacement during marathon or ultramarathon racing is unnecessary," especially since five separate studies had shown that "the addition of sodium chloride to the optimum fluid replacement regimens fails to improve either work performance during exercise or the rate of heat acclimatisation" (Noakes, Goodwin, et al., 1985, p. 370). This information would have confirmed my personal bias that sodium supplementation is unnecessary since a state of sodium deficiency had never been reported in marathon or ultramarathon runners. In fact, when they drank little and did not ingest any sodium, the blood sodium concentrations of marathon and ultramarathon runners always rose (table 4.2, page 129), the opposite of the expected outcome if they were truly sodium deficient.

Third, I attempted to produce data to differentiate between the two opposing theories that EAHE must be caused either by large unreplaced sodium losses during exercise or by abnormal fluid retention[8] associated with smaller sodium losses. To do this, I needed to calculate the amount of sodium chloride that each athlete might have lost during the races in which they developed EAH or EAHE. This required an estimation of how much each might have sweated and the likely sodium chloride content of their sweat. Then I needed to estimate how much each had drunk and the likely sodium chloride content of their drinks. From this I would be able to estimate the extent of any deficit or excess of sodium chloride or water that each might have developed during the race. Since I knew their prerace weights, I could then predict what should have been their postrace blood sodium concentrations compared to the values that were actually measured (table 8.1, page 238).

Given the speculative nature of the estimations that I made, the predicted postrace blood sodium concentrations were sufficiently close to the values that were actually measured to suggest that they were not completely wrong. Thus, the predictions precisely matched the measured value (122 mmol/L) in one case, whereas in another it was too high by 7 mmol/L. In contrast, the predictions for the two other cases were too low by 6 and 8 mmol/L, respectively. But the crucial information was provided by cases 3 and 4.

Fortunately, case 3, the 20-year-old university student, was studied very carefully in the hospital so that his fluid intake and urine output were carefully measured; thus, we could calculate his fluid balance during his hospital stay with a reasonable degree of accuracy. The data showed that his urine output during recovery exceeded his intake by 5 L, indicating that his total body weight (TBW) must have increased by at least that amount when he was first admitted to the hospital. Thus, he was the first patient in whom the presence of fluid overload, produced by an excessive fluid intake during exercise, was clearly documented as the cause of his EAHE (box 8.2, page 239).

In addition, the urine he passed during recovery contained a high sodium content (115 mmol/L) and was of high osmolality (257 mOsmol/L), indicating that he was "wasting" sodium. If his EAHE was due to sodium deficiency, then his urine would have contained no sodium (chapter 4). My ignorance at the time prevented me from realizing that the presence of sodium in high concentration in his urine, like that of Cynthia Lucero, indicated the presence of fluid overload and SIADH. That I completely missed this very obvious clue did not invalidate our nascent theory that fluid overload caused EAH and EAHE. But it would have been a most valuable insight, the importance of which became apparent to me only two decades later (chapter 9).

Similarly, case 4, whom I knew had a special preoccupation with her body weight and how much she ate and drank, reported that she had gained 4.5 kg (9.9 lb) during the 148 km (92 mile) triathlon in which she developed EAH. As improbable as this information seemed at the time—recall that we then believed that athletes *always* lost weight during exercise so that it was impossible to gain weight during exercise—there was no reason to doubt the veracity of her observation. Even if different scales were used to measure her weight before and after the race, it seemed improbable that different scales would measure a spurious 4.5 kg difference in a woman of 57 kg (125.7 lb). It was more probable that she

8 In fact, both theories are the same since in both the volume of fluid in the extracellular space is abnormally large. I did not appreciate this at the time. The *total* body osmolality (both intra- and extracellular) is the protected variable, but the brain probably monitors only the osmolality of the extracellular fluid (ECF) present in the blood perfusing it. Total body osmolality is regulated by the total amount of (exchangeable) sodium and potassium present within and outside all the body's cells. The point is that if total body osmolality falls, it is because the body contains too much water relative to its total sodium and potassium contents, not just the content of the sodium in the ECF. Since the hormone AVP/ADH is the most important regulator of the body's water content, so it is that abnormalities in AVP/ADH secretion are likely to be the most common cause of disturbances in body osmolality of the type found in otherwise healthy athletes with EAH and EAHE.

TABLE 8.1   Estimated Water and Sodium Balance in Four Original Cases[*] of EAH and EAHE First Described in 1985

Case number	Body mass (kg)	Postrace [Na⁺] (mmol/L)	Predicted sodium chloride losses to explain postrace [Na⁺] (mmol)	Predicted fluid retention to explain postrace [Na⁺] (L)	Estimated fluid intake (L)	Predicted total sweat loss (L)	Estimated excess fluid intake (L)	Estimated total sweat sodium chloride losses (mmol)	Estimated sodium chloride intake required to return [Na⁺] to 140 mmol/L (mmol)	Estimated postrace serum [Na⁺]
1	49	115	676	5.4	6	4	2	240	722	122
2	75	118	900	7.6	12	9	3	540	960	118
3	73	124	1007	8.8	10	5	5	300	683	118
4	57	125	445	3.6	8	3.5	4.5	210	503	117

[*]Note that the first runner described on page 230 is not included in this table as her sodium and fluid balance could not be estimated.

Reprinted, by permission, from T.D. Noakes, N. Goodwin, B.L. Rayner, T. Branken, and R.K. Taylor, 1985, "Water intoxication: A possible complication during endurance exercise," *Medicine & Science in Sports & Exercise* 17(3): 370-375.

BOX 8.2 First Documented Cases of EAH

It is not clear which might have been the first case of EAH described in the medical literature. A study of 95 runners in the 1980 Comrades Marathon (Kelly and Godlonton, 1980) found that 89 lost weight during the race, whereas 6 gained weight, and one runner gained 2.5 kg. Perhaps that was really the first recorded case of overhydration in an ultramarathon runner. However, that athlete was without any symptoms (asymptomatic), even though his total body water content must have increased. We have since shown that up to 70% of athletes who gain weight during prolonged exercise do not develop EAH (Noakes, Sharwood, et al., 2005).

In 1982 Myhre, Hartung, and colleagues described blood electrolyte changes in six competitors in a marathon race run "in the southern part of the USA," presumably the Houston marathon. A 49-year-old woman weighing 52 kg (114.6 lb) stopped running at 35.5 km (22 miles, the same distance at which Cynthia Lucero and Hilary Bellamy stopped running), which she reached in 3:28 after she had drunk a total of 2.05 L (590 ml/hr). The authors noted the following: "Most notable among the non-finishers was runner 6, who *forced herself* [my emphasis] to drink regularly in an effort to resist hypohydration; she stopped with nausea and vomiting at 35 km after consuming a total of 2,050 ml of water" (p. 232).

Although this athlete's prerace blood sodium concentration had been measured and was abnormally low (130 mmol/L), her postrace value was not measured. Such a low prerace blood sodium concentration either is a measurement error or indicates that the athlete had either acute or chronic hyponatremia on the basis of recent or persistent overdrinking. Her fluid intake during the race was not excessive. But if she had a slow rate of intestinal fluid absorption and had begun the race with an intestine full of unabsorbed water (as a result of persistent overdrinking especially in the last few hours before the race), the added fluid she ingested during the race would have been sufficient to produce nausea and the vomiting of clear fluid. The authors failed to notice that this runner had hyponatremia even before she began the race.

Perhaps a stronger case can be made for two cases of heatstroke reported by Shibolet, Coll, and colleagues (1967). Their blood sodium concentrations on hospital admission were 125 and 120 mmol/L, both below the value of 130 mmol/L that was the bottom of the normal range for their laboratory at the time. The authors did not accord any special relevance to this finding, although they did classify these as "mild" cases of heatstroke. It is possible that either or both of these patients might have been suffering from EAHE rather than heatstroke but that this was not recognized at the time.

had indeed gained a substantial amount of weight during the race, whether or not it was precisely 4.5 kg.

Indirect support for this interpretation of water overload came from the realization that the alternative salt-deficiency theory was highly improbable. If sweat NaCl losses alone caused EAH and EAHE in these athletes, then their total NaCl losses would have been 445 to 1007 mmol, equivalent to 26 to 58 g of sodium chloride (NaCl, or salt). In contrast, their estimated sweat NaCl losses were much smaller, from 210 to 540 mmol (12-32 g). Thus, it seemed extremely unlikely, perhaps impossible, that sweat NaCl losses alone could have explained the development of EAH and EAHE in these subjects.

But if each athlete had retained 2 to 5 kg of water, then the extent to which their blood sodium concentrations had fallen could be reasonably explained by this combination of moderate sweat NaCl losses and water retention. But without the water retention, EAH could not have occurred (table 8.1).

Summary

Thus, we concluded the following: "The etiology (cause) of the condition appears to be voluntary hyperhydration with hypotonic solutions combined with moderate sweat sodium chloride losses" (Noakes, Goodwin, et al., 1985, p. 370) so that "*advice (on sodium replacement during exercise) should be tempered with the proviso that the intake of hypotonic fluids in excess of that required to balance sweat and urine losses may be hazardous in some individuals*" (p. 374) [my emphasis]. Finally, because I had forgotten the lesson of the single case of SIADH that I had observed in my clinical training, we also wrote this: "The reason why the fluid excess in these runners was not corrected by increased urinary losses is not known" (p. 370) "but may relate to the sodium and water conserving mechanisms that are activated by prolonged exercise (Costill, 1977)[9] and which probably last for at least 48 hours after exercise (Dickson, Wilkinson, et al., 1982). The high urine osmolality measured in case 3 for the first 24 hours after the race is compatible with this interpretation" (p. 374).[10]

When we submitted that paper in May 1984, we could not have foreseen the epidemic that was waiting in the wings. We had failed to ask the one critical question: What had caused these athletes to gain weight during exercise given that in the annals of recorded history, humans always lose weight and increase their blood sodium concentrations when they exercise?

9 Paradoxically, the quoted paper makes no reference to the role of AVP/ADH in the regulation of water balance during prolonged exercise. This is in part because the measurement of AVP/ADH is difficult; in this paper Dr. Costill and colleagues focused on the measurement of blood aldosterone concentrations as if aldosterone alone directs the body's water balance. Thus, I can transfer blame for my ignorance to my great friend and supporter, Dr. David Costill!

10 In fact, this is wrong. The high urine osmolality indicates a state of water conservation and urinary sodium loss diagnostic of SIADH. This point was hidden from me for 20 years until March 2005 when I met the world's authority on AVP/ADH, Dr. Joseph Verbalis (2003) from Georgetown Medical School in Washington, DC. He was one of the members of the First International Consensus Conference on EAH held in Cape Town, South Africa, from March 22 to 24, 2005. There he taught me that EAH and EAHE cannot occur without SIADH (or some similar abnormality that prevents the normal regulation of total body water content by the kidneys).

CHAPTER 9

The Biology of EAH

All things are hidden, obscure and debatable if the cause of the phenomenon be unknown, but everything is clear if this cause be known.

Louis Pasteur
(Pasteur and Lister, 1996, p. 112)

H ow much of what happens in our lives is preordained? And how much happens by chance?

Eleanor Sadler would not have written to me in June 1981 if at the time I was not writing a monthly column on medical matters for the South African running publication *SA Runner.* I would not have been writing that column if I was not myself medically trained and, more important, a runner who had by then run the same Comrades Marathon four times. In turn, I might not have been either a medical doctor or a runner if I had not finished my high school education, knowing only that I was not yet ready to make a decision on my life's work. Instead, I had taken South African citizenship; my birthplace in Zimbabwe and my parents' British citizenship meant that until then I was a British citizen. So directly after high school as a new national I spent 9 months discovering myself in the lowest ranks of the South African Defence Force.

From there I went to the United States to study for a year as an American Field Service (AFS) high school exchange student at Huntington Park High School in Los Angeles, California. There a number of crucial events occurred. First, I was exposed to a culture in which everything seemed possible; this contrasted with the more conservative outlook of my adopted country. Second, on Sunday afternoon, 3 December, 1967 while traveling back to Huntington Park from a trip to Capistrano, the news on the car radio announced that a South African doctor, Christiaan Barnard, had performed the world's first successful heart transplant at the Groote Schuur Hospital in my hometown of Cape Town. Three months later, while still in California, I awoke one morning informed by my brain that when I returned to South Africa I would apply to the University of Cape Town to study medicine at the facility in which Dr. Barnard worked.

Only decades later would I discover that it was never more than a racing certainty that Dr. Barnard would become the first to perform that iconic operation. More than a year earlier on 29 June, 1966, and again three days later on my birthday (July 2), an American surgeon, Dr. Adrian Kantrowitz, was on the verge of performing the first human heart transplant, only to discover that as he waited for the donor heart to stop beating so that he could comply with U.S. law and not be charged with killing the donor, the heart had become irreversibly damaged and so could not be transplanted (McRae, 2006).

I did not then appreciate that the South African legal definition of death was somewhat in advance of that in the United States since South African law recognized that a person's heart could still be beating but yet the body in which it beat could be (brain) dead. This meant that under South African law the surgeon could choose the optimal time to remove the still-beating donor heart once the donor was legally dead. As a result, the donor heart could be harvested before it suffered irreversible damage.

Had the law in the United States and South Africa been the same, Kantrowitz, or perhaps some other U.S. surgeon, but not Christiaan Barnard, would have been the first to transplant a human heart. Had that happened, I might never have studied medicine at the University of Cape Town. And this book would never have been written.

Another crucial event was the chance statement by a friend at Huntington Park High School who mentioned that he would start rowing when he went to college in the fall of 1968. This thought appealed to me. At the time I was aware of the heroic annual rowing race on the Thames contested by crews from Oxford and Cambridge. Mastering the physical challenge of rowing seemed a worthwhile endeavor. Rowing eventually led me to running, when I discovered that after 40 minutes of running, I developed an indescribably delicious mental buzz, subsequently described somewhat inadequately as the runner's high. I had finally discovered the activity for which my brain, if not my body, seemed perfectly suited. Later I would discover that runs of 3 or 4 hours would transport me to an even more incredible cerebral heaven.

So any number of choices would have caused Eleanor Sadler to write her letter to someone other than me. But her letter, crucial as it was, was only the first in a trilogy of events, all of which conspired further to channel my mind in a specific direction.

The second of the trilogy of epiphanous moments occurred three months after I had received Eleanor's letter. I was serving as the race doctor at the 1981 South African National Cross-Country Championships held in Cape Town at the end of winter on an unusually hot, cloudless, humid, and windless day. Three male athletes competing in the under-19, under-21, and men's open races collapsed unconscious shortly after each finished the race. Another male athlete, confused and convinced he was about to die, was also treated. A female runner staggered down the finish line after racing only 4 km. She collapsed but recovered without receiving any treatment. Fortunately all the affected athletes recovered consciousness within 10 to 20 minutes when cooled appropriately and given a small amount (500-1000 ml) of fluid intravenously.

I had not taken a thermometer with me to the race, so certain was I that I would never encounter a case of heatstroke in races of such short distances (4-12 km). So I could not measure the body temperatures of any of these athletes. Clearly I was still committed to the model of heatstroke promoted by Wyndham and Strydom. If dehydration is the sole direct cause of heatstroke, how could a runner possibly become sufficiently dehydrated to develop heatstroke when running for only 20 to 40 minutes?

Later, I published a report (Noakes, 1982) of these cases. It sought to warn that heatstroke can occur in highly trained athletes in short-distance races and not just in either "fun runners who are poorly trained, overweight, unacclimatized to heat and (who) ignore the warning symptoms of heatstroke as they fail 'to listen to their bodies'" (p. 145) or in those elite athletes who become "dehydrated" during exercise.

The letter drew a strong rebuke from Professor Wyndham's colleague and coauthor of their classic paper, Professor Nic Strydom. Strydom contended that my diagnosis of heatstroke "on-the-spot" constituted "nothing more than educated guesswork" (Strydom, Kielblock, et al., 1982, p. 537). He was also less than impressed with my choice of cooling method—the application of ice packs directly to the major arteries of the body. Rather, "the use of ice-packs, chilled water or ice baths is contraindicated for the simple reason that they are more likely to induce dermal vasoconstriction, an event tantamount to insulating the hot body core from its environment, than to achieve heat dissipation through conduction." So, according to Strydom, a person exercising in cold water would heat up, not cool down, because of an inability to transfer heat from the core to the skin because of a reduced skin blood flow caused by the low skin temperatures.[1]

Strydom forgot to mention that our treatment, ineffective as it should have been according to his theory, did in fact cure the patients. This exchange occurred 6 years before we published our first paper questioning the Wyndham and Strydom theory that dehydration is the direct cause of heatstroke.

My next epiphanous moment came in January 1983 on the final day of a 4-day 244 km (152 mile) surf-ski race contested on the east coast of South Africa between the cities of Port Elizabeth and East London. Our research team wished to study the effects of 4 consecutive days

1 Many others have shown that the most effective way to cool patients with heatstroke is to place them in ice-cold water for 20 to 30 minutes, and this is now the accepted practice. Ice-cold water cools the skin and the underlying muscles, conducting heat directly from the athlete's muscles to the water, causing the muscles to cool rapidly. To my knowledge, there has yet to be a case report of heatstroke occurring in a swimmer swimming in ice-cold water. On the other hand, some elite triathletes achieve their highest temperatures (~40 °C) after the swim leg of the Ironman Triathlon. Their temperatures then fell during the running and cycling legs. Why? Because they wore wetsuits in the swim and this limited their ability to lose heat. Fast swimmers able to sustain high metabolic rates are able to generate enough heat to raise their body temperatures substantially during the swim. Once they are on the bicycle, the increased rates of convection and evaporation will increase their rates of heat loss to the environment, producing a cooling effect.

of paddling at sea on the fluid and energy balance of a sample of competitors (Noakes, Nathan, et al., 1985).

As part of our study, we measured the competitors' body weights before and after each stage and drew a blood sample to measure various chemicals, including the blood sodium and glucose concentrations. Their kidney function was also studied by Dr. Tony Irving, who 5 years later would perform the definitive study of fluid and electrolyte balance in exercise-associated hyponatremic encephalopathy (EAHE).

The final stage of 50 km began with a tough paddle through large surf that would intimidate all but the most hardy. The race leader at that stage, 18-year-old Oscar Chalupsky,[2] had lost the two large water bottles containing the fluids he would drink during the 4 or more hours it would take him to paddle the 50 km.

But I knew nothing of this because as Oscar was at sea, I was traveling to the finish, ready to prepare the scale to measure his body weight, the syringe and needle to collect his blood sample, and the thermometer to be placed in his rectum to measure his core body temperature. These examinations revealed that Oscar had lost 4.2 kg (9.3 lb, 4.1% BW, sweat rate 0.96 L/hr). This was the greatest weight loss I had ever observed. Naturally, I assumed that since he was so dehydrated his rectal temperature would be sky-high, probably well over 40 °C, according to the Wyndham and Strydom model (figure 3.1, page 61).

Yet his measured temperature was only 38 °C, probably only 1 °C higher than when he started the day's paddle 4 hours earlier. I was astonished. I knew the measurement was not wrong. The only other explanation was that the Wyndham and Strydom theory had to be wrong. But was I prepared to challenge the authority of my two heroes—men whose word was gospel in the field of human thermoregulation during exercise?

So in less than 2 years I had written that athletes should "drink everything in sight" when they run (May 1981), a position that was merely an extension of essentially similar advice in the chapters I had contributed to two popular running books in the 1970s (Noakes, 1974; Noakes, 1978); a month later I received a letter from a lady who nearly died after the Comrades Marathon perhaps because she had drunk "everything in sight." I had then treated 4 athletes with heatstroke at the end of a 12 km cross-country race during which they could not have lost more than 1 L of fluid as sweat (sweat rate ~2 L/hr) and could therefore not have been sufficiently dehydrated to support the Wyndham and Strydom hypothesis that heatstroke is caused solely by dehydration. Thus, from these anecdotes I "knew" that heatstroke had to have more causes other than dehydration. Finally and conversely, I measured an unexpectedly low (38 °C) postrace rectal temperature in an ocean kayaker who had not drunk during 4.5 hours of vigorous exercise and who had lost 4.1% of his body weight. According to the Wyndham and Strydom theory, his rectal temperature should have been much higher, closer to 40 °C (figure 3.1).

In retrospect, it is clear that these three events triggered in my mind the following desires.

2 Full details of Oscar Chalupsky's remarkable kayaking achievements in the years since 1983 can be found at www.epickayaks.com/about/oscarchalupsky. He continues to compete at the highest level of the sport despite now being in his mid-40s.

1. To understand why Eleanor Sadler had developed EAHE. By 1984 I was pretty certain it was because she had simply drunk too much, becoming "waterlogged."
2. To understand what role, if any, dehydration plays in determining the rise in body temperature during exercise.
3. To understand how much and what athletes should drink during exercise, especially more prolonged exercise including marathons, ultramarathons, and the newest sport that was becoming increasingly popular in the early 1980s, the Ironman Triathlon. Multiday adventure races had yet to be invented in the 1990s.
4. To discover why athletes collapse during but especially after exercise and how best they should be treated.

Because almost all my medical and scientific colleagues already believed or would soon be encouraged to believe that the only danger during exercise is dehydration so that any medical condition that arises during exercise must be due to dehydration, I was unwittingly setting myself up for a long battle. Nor at the time did I anticipate that some would be less than pleased by these attempts to dislodge a hallowed dogma on which an entirely novel and extremely lucrative industry is based. The result of all this was that, when we submitted our paper titled "Water Intoxication: A Possible Complication During Endurance Exercise" to the journal *Medicine and Science in Sports and Exercise* (MSSE) in May 1984, I was sufficiently certain that exercise-associated hyponatremia (EAH) and exercise-associated hyponatremic encephalopathy (EAHE) were due to overdrinking that I began to make public statements to this effect.

Perhaps the first was shortly after the 1985 Comrades Marathon when the wife of an acquaintance, then a well-known public figure, collapsed during the race, slipped into a coma, and suffered an epileptic seizure. By then, I realized that her presentation was identical to that of our index case, Eleanor Sadler. In response to a newspaper reporter's inquiry, I suggested that she had drunk too much, not too little, during the race and so had developed EAHE. Of course this was an unpopular opinion since everyone believed then, as they still do today, that athletes collapse during exercise solely because they have become dehydrated.

A month or so later the lady consulted me for advice. Evaluation of the data from her hospital admission confirmed that she had indeed developed EAHE, not dehydration, during the Comrades Marathon. Thus, the correct advice was that in the future she should simply drink less. She was initially uncertain that the solution could be so simple. Surely if she had nearly died, there must be something seriously wrong with her? But slowly her confidence returned and she began to run again. In time, this advice allowed her to return safely to long-distance running. By then I already knew that the advice worked because all four athletes in our initial study had subsequently safely completed ultradistance events when they followed this advice to drink to thirst and not to drink more than 500 ml/hr (17 fl oz/hr). This included the most competitive athlete who had subsequently finished the 226 km Ironman Hawaii triathlon in 12:19 in 30th position without developing any symptoms, even though she drank only 450 ml/hr during the race.

In previous chapters I provided detailed findings on the role of dehydration in body temperature regulation and the causes of athletes' collapse. Although body temperature rises with increasing levels of dehydration during exercise, the effect is small, such that rectal temperature rarely reaches the levels found in patients with heatstroke, even with marked levels of dehydration. In fact, because of complex biological controls before their rectal temperatures reach near 42 °C, athletes most often slow down or stop exercising, thereby preventing heatstroke. Furthermore, athletes with heatstroke are rarely dehydrated; the two phenomena may be linked in time without being causally linked. The most common reason for collapse in athletes, especially postrace, is exercise-associated postural hypotension, which is easily cured by elevating the legs of the athlete above the level of the heart. In this chapter, I examine another question that had piqued my research interest: What are the causes of EAH and EAHE? Specifically, what roles do overhydration, dehydration, and sweat sodium losses play in the development of EAH and EAHE?

Three Studies Indicate the Real Causes of EAH and EAHE

Among many others, some of which were not intended to produce the same conclusions, the three landmark studies described here all clearly identify identical causes of EAH and EAHE. These three studies examine real athletes who developed EAH or EAHE and so are based on real data and not on hypothetical conjecture.

1988 Comrades Marathon

The 1988 Comrades Marathon provided the first group of athletes to determine the mechanisms causing this condition. My student, Tony Irving, whose doctoral work involved studying kidney function in marathon and ultramarathon runners, studied eight athletes who developed EAHE either during or after that year's race (Irving, Noakes, Buck, et al., 1991). Their mean blood sodium concentration was 122 mmol/L; three runners were unconscious with grand mal epileptic seizures; the remaining five presented with weakness, confusion, lack of coordination, and nausea.

All athletes subsequently reported that they had drunk heroically during the race; their estimated average hourly fluid intake was 1.3 L/hr (44 fl oz/hr; range 0.8-1.9 L/hr) sustained for 8 to 11 hours.

Balance studies revealed that, at the time of hospital admission, the hyponatremic athletes had a (minimum) positive fluid balance (i.e., a gain) of 2.9 L (range 1.2-5.9 L) compared to a negative fluid balance (i.e., a loss) of about 2.5 L in a group of control athletes who maintained normal blood sodium concentration during ultramarathon races. The estimated sodium deficit was the same in normonatremic and hyponatremic ultramarathon runners (153 mmol, 7 g) and was not higher than deficits measured in other exercisers (183 mmol, 8 g) who nevertheless maintained normal blood sodium concentrations during exercise (figure 9.1).

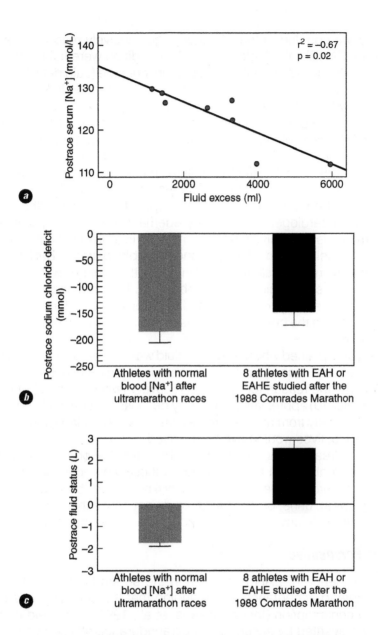

FIGURE 9.1 Data from 8 runners who developed either EAHE or EAH during the 1988 Comrades Marathon show that *(a)* their postrace blood sodium concentrations were linearly related to their calculated fluid excess at the time they finished. *(b)* This relationship is not spurious; the only other variable that could explain this phenomenon, the sodium chloride deficit at the end of the race, was not different in these 8 Comrades runners with EAH and EAHE compared to others who completed ultramarathon races with normal blood sodium concentrations. *(c)* Comrades runners with EAH or EAHE developed fluid excess at the end of the race, whereas other runners who completed ultramarathon races with normal blood sodium concentrations showed a postrace fluid deficit of ~2 L.

(a) Adapted, by permission, from T.D. Noakes, 1992, "The hyponatremia of exercise," *International Journal of Sport Nutrition* 2(3): 205-228. *(b, c)* Data from Irving, Noakes, Buck, et al., 1991.

Accordingly, we concluded that our study "conclusively resolves this issue [of what causes EAHE]." All subjects with the condition were fluid-overloaded but without evidence for abnormally large sodium chloride (salt) deficits. Hence, ". . . the hyponatremia of exercise results from fluid retention in subjects who ingest abnormally large fluid volumes during prolonged exercise" (p. 342).

These initial case reports established the typical features of this condition. Patients with EAHE have blood sodium concentrations that are reduced below the normal values of 135 to 145 mmol/L. Once the blood sodium concentration falls below about 128 mmol/L, affected athletes present with varying degrees of altered levels of consciousness, from mild confusion to frank coma (complete loss of consciousness), frequently associated with epileptic seizures. Other complications include noncardiogenic pulmonary edema with respiratory failure. The primary abnormality is excessive fluid accumulation in all the fluid compartments of the body—in the cells, around the cells, and in the bloodstream. But brain cells, encased as they are in a rigid skull, cannot increase their volume without causing a steep rise in the pressure inside the brain (box 9.1). The progressive increase in pressure inside the waterlogged brain cells interferes with their function, leading ultimately to death with the cessation of certain vital functions, in particular those of the heart and lungs.

No one had yet explained why this excess fluid was not rapidly excreted by the kidneys as is the usual case when a fluid excess is ingested (Noakes, Wilson, et al., 2001). Nor was the reason for the rapid recovery (within 8 hours) of Dr. Bob Lathan (see chapter 10) appreciated especially because the speed of his recovery differed so dramatically from all other treated cases of EAH. Had we understood this already in 1985, lives would have been saved.

But what had already been established absolutely beyond doubt was that (a) EAHE is due to abnormal fluid retention in those who voluntarily overdrink during prolonged exercise usually lasting at least 4 hours and (b) abnormal sodium losses either in sweat, urine, or diarrheal fluid do not cause this condition and in fact do not contribute in any way to the seriousness of the condition.

New Zealand Perspective

Whereas the incidence of EAH had fallen in the 90 km Comrades Marathon after the widespread acceptance of our finding that the condition was due to excessive fluid consumption (Irving, Noakes, et al., 1991) and could therefore be completely prevented by ensuring that ultraendurance athletes do not drink to excess during competition (Noakes, 2003a), an increasing incidence of the condition in New Zealand endurance athletes stimulated the next group of studies of EAHE conducted by New Zealand sports physician Dale Speedy between 1996 and 1998.

Dr. Speedy's interest in the condition was stimulated when he found an inverse relationship (linear relationship with a negative slope) between the body weight changes and postrace blood sodium concentrations in 48 athletes who completed the 233 km (145 mile) triathlon across the width of the South Island of New Zealand (Speedy, Faris, et al., 1997), the Coast to Coast One Day Triathlon Challenge, for which Dr. Speedy was the medical director.

BOX 9.1 Brain Swelling Causes EAHE Symptoms

Exercise-associated hyponatremic encephalopathy (EAHE) (brain dysfunction caused by the accumulation of fluid in the brain consequent to a reduced blood sodium concentration) is the condition that caused Dr. Cynthia Lucero to be admitted to a hospital on 15 April, 2002. This condition occurs when the blood osmolality falls as the result of a fall in the blood sodium concentration below 135 mmol/L (hyponatremia). This produces an osmolality difference between the lower osmolality in the ECF and higher osmolality in the ICF. This draws water into the ICF in order to equalize the osmolality inside and outside the cells. Water continues to move until the osmolality on both sides of all cell membranes in the body is again equal.

The brain is the organ at greatest risk when it swells because it is encased in a rigid skull (figure 9.2). Thus, any increase in brain size caused by swelling of the brain cells must cause the pressure inside the skull to increase. To limit the extent of this swelling as blood sodium concentration and osmolality fall, the brain cells begin to extrude sodium and other molecules into the surrounding fluid (Pasantes-Morales, Franco, et al., 2002), the ISF that together with the fluid component of the blood (plasma) makes up the extracellular fluid (ECF). The osmolality difference between the brain cells and the ECF is lessened so that the osmotic drive attracting fluid into the brain cells is somewhat reduced. But this effect is of value only when EAHE develops over days or weeks. In runners who develop EAHE within a few hours, this mechanism does not protect against brain swelling.

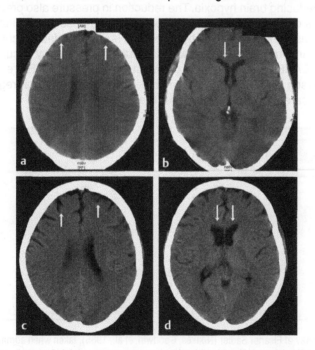

FIGURE 9.2   These scans show the extent of brain swelling in a triathlete who developed EAHE during the 2006 Frankfurt Ironman Triathlon but who survived because she received the appropriate treatment (Richter, Betz, et al., 2007) (case 1558 in appendix B). The top figures *(a* and *b)* show her brain at the time she was admitted to the hospital unconscious with EAHE. At that time, her blood sodium concentration was 111 mmol/L. The lower figures *(c* and *d)* show her brain 2 days later when she regained consciousness. The arrows point to natural spaces in the brain that are compressed in the top pictures but regained their normal volumes when her blood sodium concentration and level of consciousness returned to normal 2 days later.

Reprinted, by permission, from S. Richter, C. Betz, and H. Geiger, 2007, "Severe hyponatremia with pulmonary and cerebral edema in an Iron-man triathlete" (in German), *Deutsche Medizinische Wochenschrift* 132: 1829 -1832.

(continued)

BOX 9.1 **Brain Swelling Causes EAHE Symptoms** *(continued)*

Brain swelling also reduces the oxygen content of the brain cells, a condition known as cerebral hypoxia. This hypoxia is caused by a brain-directed reflex of unknown origin, which causes fluid to accumulate in the alveoli, the oxygen-transferring membranes in the lungs, whenever the pressure inside the brain increases. This condition is known as pulmonary edema (figure 9.3). Pulmonary edema is more often caused by heart failure, but there is no heart failure in EAHE. Thus, the pulmonary edema that develops in EAHE is called non-cardiogenic or neurogenic pulmonary edema (Ayus, Varon, et al., 2000). Laden with fluid, the alveoli are unable to transfer oxygen properly to the bloodstream, causing the oxygen content of the blood to fall. As a consequence, the blood perfusing the brain cells also has a reduced oxygen content. In this way, EAHE produces a secondary consequence, cerebral (brain) hypoxia, which compounds the original insult, increasing the probability for a fatal outcome unless the condition is correctly managed. Hypoxia lessens the capacity of the brain cells to extrude sodium and other molecules, thereby limiting the extent to which the brain can reduce its swelling when the osmolality of the ECF falls.

The key medical intervention in the management of EAHE is to urgently increase the osmolality of the ECF by infusing highly concentrated (hypertonic) saline solutions into the ECF. This reverses the movement of water from the ECF into the brain cells. The resulting reduction in pressure inside the brain reverses pulmonary edema, improving oxygenation of the blood and reducing brain hypoxia. The reduction in pressure also prevents extrusion of the lowest parts of the brain through the opening at the base of the skull, the foramen magnum. This extrusion, known as cerebellar coning, is uniformly fatal because it produces an instantaneous and irreversible cessation of breathing as probably occurred in some of the fatal cases of EAHE listed in appendix B. Most deaths from EAHE are caused by this mechanism. A person with EAHE who stops breathing rarely survives, regardless of the quality of medical care he or she may receive thereafter.

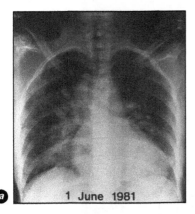
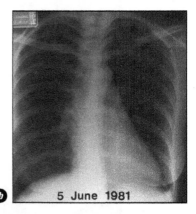

FIGURE 9.3 Chest X-ray of Eleanor Sadler (Noakes, Goodwin, et al., 1985), taken when admitted to the hospital in a coma on 1 June, 1981 (chapter 8), with a blood sodium concentration of 115 mmol/L, shows *(a)* shadowing in areas of both her lungs. This resolved on a second X-ray *(b)* taken on 5 June, 1981, when she regained consciousness and her blood sodium concentration was 140 mmol/L. The change in resolution of the X-ray confirms that the shadowing present on 1 June was due to fluid and not to some other cause such as infection, as occurs in pneumonia or tuberculosis.

Reprinted, by permission, from T.D. Noakes, N. Goodwin, B.L. Rayner, T. Branken, and R.K.N. Taylor, 1985, "Water intoxication: A possible complication during endurance exercise," *Medicine & Science in Sports & Exercise* 17(3): 370-375.

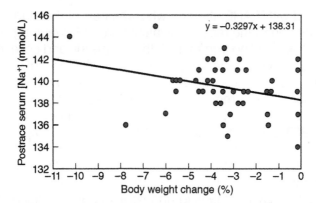

FIGURE 9.4 The original study from Dr. Dale Speedy's group showed a linear relationship with a negative slope between blood sodium concentrations and body weight changes in finishers in the 1996 Coast to Coast One Day Triathlon Challenge (233 km, or 144.8 miles).

Reprinted, by permission, from D.B. Speedy, R.M.B. Cambell, G. Mulligan, et al., 1997, "Weight changes and serum sodium concentrations after an ultradistance multisport triathlon," *Clinical Journal of Sport Medicine* 7(2): 100-103.

Blood sodium concentrations were again highest in those triathletes who lost the most weight during the race and might therefore have been the most dehydrated (figure 9.4). At the time, no one had yet noticed that the blood sodium concentration at any level of weight loss could vary quite substantially, about 10 mmol/L in this study for athletes who lost 3% of their body weight during the race. A possible explanation for this unexpected finding is provided later in this chapter.

Inspired by his finding that blood sodium concentrations were lowest in those who lost no weight during that race, Dr. Speedy and colleagues next performed a similar study in the 1996 New Zealand Ironman Triathlon. They studied triathletes before and after the race and again found an inverse relationship between the postrace blood sodium concentration and the change in percent body weight (BW) during the race (figure 9.5), confirming their original finding. Four athletes

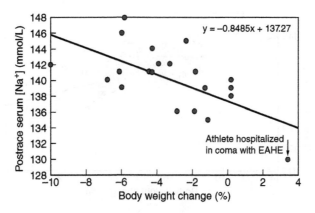

FIGURE 9.5 The study of the 1996 New Zealand Ironman Triathlon confirmed the usual linear relationship with a negative slope between postrace blood sodium concentration and body weight change during the race. The athlete who gained the most weight during the race (arrowed) was critically ill and was admitted to the hospital for treatment of EAHE. He survived without any long-term consequences.

Reprinted, by permission, from D.B. Speedy, J.G. Faris, M. Hamlin, P.G. Gallagher, and R.G.D. Campbell, 1997, "Hyponatremia and weight changes in an ultradistance triathlon," *Clinical Journal of Sport Medicine* 7(3): 180-184.

were hospitalized with EAHE; the one who was part of the study gained 2.5 kg (5.5 lb) of weight during the race, equivalent to a body weight gain of 3.5%.

At the 1997 New Zealand Ironman Triathlon, Speedy and colleagues reported the same finding in a very large sample (330) of triathletes (figure 9.6). Fifty-eight athletes (18% of the original sample of 330) finished the race with blood sodium concentrations below 135 mmol/L but were without symptoms (asymptomatic EAH). The details of two of these athletes were subsequently reported (Speedy, Noakes, et al., 2000). Both had gained weight (0.5 and 1.5 kg) during the race, even though their rates of fluid intake (733 and 764 ml/hr) were relatively modest. Of 115 athletes requiring medical care after the race, 26 (23%) were both hyponatremic and symptomatic (EAHE). Fourteen triathletes with EAHE were sufficiently ill to require hospitalization; the fluid and sodium balance during recovery was studied in seven of those athletes (Speedy, Rogers, et al., 2000a), along the lines of the original study by Dr. Tony Irving.

The New Zealand study produced essentially identical results to those of the South African study, although the extent of the fluid abnormality in the New Zealand triathletes was slightly less (Irving, Noakes, et al., 1991), presumably because the New Zealand triathletes were less ill. Thus, the median excess of fluid excreted during recovery was 1.3 L compared to 3.0 L in our study. The median postrace blood sodium concentration was also higher (128 mmol/L vs. 124 mmol/L) in the New Zealand study. The median postrace sodium deficits in the two groups of athletes were not statistically different, nor was the difference large enough to be of any biological significance: 100 versus 153 mmol, respectively. The authors concluded, as had we, that triathletes with EAHE "have abnormal fluid retention . . . without evidence for large sodium losses" (p. 272).

Even though all these athletes survived, Dr. Speedy and his team faced an usual problem. The Auckland municipality, under whose jurisdiction that triathlon was held, operates under a by-law that requires that a citywide state of emergency be declared if 15 patients are admitted to the hospital as the result of a single

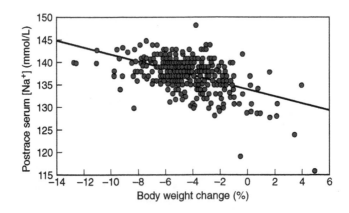

FIGURE 9.6 The study of 330 finishers in the 1997 New Zealand Ironman Triathlon showed the expected linear relationship with a negative slope between the postrace blood sodium concentration and weight change during the race. There was significant individual variability in this response. Athletes who showed a weight loss of ~4% showed a variation in postrace blood sodium concentrations of up to 28 mmol/L. The most seriously ill athlete gained the most weight (5%) and had the lowest blood sodium concentration (115 mmol/L).

Reprinted, by permission, from D.B. Speedy, T.D. Noakes, I.R. Rogers, et al., 1999, "Hyponatremia in ultradistance triathletes," *Medicine & Science in Sports & Exercise* 31(6): 809-815.

incident. Because 14 athletes were hospitalized after the 1997 New Zealand Ironman, a state of emergency had only just been averted. This possibility focused Dr. Speedy's mind because he would be accountable were such an emergency to occur in a future New Zealand Ironman Triathlon.

Dr. Speedy was forced to introduce changes that would reduce the availability of fluid during the 1998 race and would discourage athletes from overdrinking. As a result of these interventions, the incidence of EAHE in the following year's race was dramatically reduced (Speedy, Rogers, et al., 2000b).

Before the 1998 New Zealand Ironman Triathlon, Dr. Speedy warned the race entrants of the potential dangers of overdrinking. He encouraged them to drink only 500 to 1000 ml/hr during the race. In addition, the frequency of drink stations was decreased from every 12 to every 20 km on the cycle leg of the race and from every 1.8 to every 2.5 km on the run. As a result, whereas 25 athletes were treated for EAH or EAHE in the 1997 race (3.8% of starters), 14 in a hospital and two in an intensive care unit (ICU), only 4 triathletes in the 1998 race were treated for EAH or EAHE (0.6% of race starters) and none was admitted to ICU, compared to 2 in 1997. Continuation of these preventive practices has ensured that EAH is now a historical disease in the New Zealand Ironman Triathlon.

Other studies completed by Speedy's group showed that in response to forced overdrinking (3.4 L in 120 min, or 1.7 L/hr), Ironman triathletes with a history of EAH or EAHE increased their urine production to the same extent as did triathletes who finished those races without developing EAH (Speedy, Noakes, et al., 2001b). The authors concluded that "there does not appear to be any unique pathophysiological characteristics, at least when evaluated at rest, that explains why the study cases developed hyponatremia during ultradistance exercise" (p. 1441). But they suggested that this does not exclude the possibility that "during exercise there may be additional factors, such as an *inappropriate inhibition of diuresis* . . . that would increase the probability that hyponatremia will develop in those who ingest large fluid volumes during prolonged exercise" (p. 1441). In fact, this study shows that the inappropriate antidiuresis (SIADH) that develops in those who develop EAH or EAHE must be specific only for exercise; at rest they do not necessarily show evidence for SIADH.

2002 Boston Marathon

A study of 741 runners in the 2002 Boston Marathon first published in March 2005 (Almond, Shin, et al., 2005) calculated the percentage of participants with EAH and the risk factors for developing the condition. The study found that 13% of a sample of 488 race finishers had serum sodium concentrations below 135 mmol/L; 3 subjects were markedly hyponatremic with serum sodium concentrations below 120 mmol/L. This was also the race in which Cynthia Lucero developed EAHE (chapter 1). The two most important risk factors for hyponatremia were weight gain during the race (odds ratio, or OR, of 4.2) and race duration in excess of 4 hours (OR 7.4). The authors concluded the following: "Excessive consumption of fluids, as evidenced by substantial weight gain while running, is the single most important factor associated with hyponatremia" (figure 9.7, page 254) so that "efforts to monitor and regulate fluid intake may lead to a reduction in the frequency and severity of this condition, which, in rare cases, can be fatal" (p. 1556).

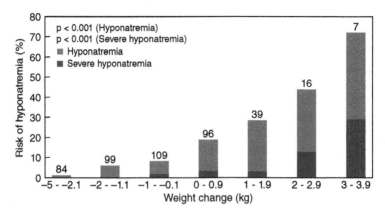

FIGURE 9.7 The risk of developing hyponatremia and severe hyponatremia in runners in the 2002 Boston Marathon rose with increasing weight gain. Runners who gained more than 3 kg (6.6 lb) had a 72% probability of developing hyponatremia.

Adapted, by permission, from C.S.D. Almond, A.Y. Shin, E.B. Fortescue, et al., 2005, "Hyponatremia among runners in the Boston Marathon," *New England Journal of Medicine* 352(15): 1550-1556. Copyright © 2005 Massachusetts Medical Society.

In fact, Dr. Speedy's interventions at the 1998 New Zealand Ironman Triathlon (Speedy, Rogers, et al., 2000b) had already proven that the regulation of fluid intake reduces the frequency and severity of EAH and EAHE. The same interventions at the 2000 and 2001 South African Ironman Triathlons resulted in only one case of EAHE, and it occurred in an athlete who chose to ignore that advice.

Compare the conclusion from the 2002 Boston Marathon with ours first drawn in 1985 (Noakes, Goodwin, et al., 1985): "The etiology of the condition appears to be voluntary hyperhydration with hypotonic solutions combined with moderate sodium chloride losses" (p. 370) and ". . . Thus, it would seem that a very strong case can be made that the etiology of the hyponatremia of exercise in these runners was due to overhydration" (p. 374) so that ". . . the intake of hypotonic solutions in excess of that required to balance sweat and urine losses may be hazardous in some individuals" (p. 374). The results of our study completed at the 1988 Comrades Marathon and published in 1991 verified these hypothetical proposals.

By 1991, we concluded the following: "The hyponatremia of exercise results from fluid retention in subjects who ingest abnormally large fluid volumes during prolonged exercise." All these points were restated in an editorial published two years earlier in the *British Medical Journal* in July 2003 (Noakes, 2003b): "The athlete most likely to develop hyponatremic encephalopathy is a female marathon runner, who runs those 42km races at speeds slower than 8-9km/hr (about 5mph). She gains weight during exercise because she drinks excessively both before and during exercise . . ." (p. 113).[3]

3 A study by Almond, Shin, and colleagues in the *New England Journal of Medicine* was accompanied by an editorial written by two cardiologists (Levine and Thompson, 2005). Some mistakes were included in the editorial, yet to their eternal credit, they correctly concluded the following: "Although there has been vigorous debate about the relative importance of fluid overload as compared with sodium loss due to sweating in the development of hyponatremia in runners, an extensive literature has accumulated over the past 20 years documenting that the *primary cause is water intake in excess of sodium loss*" [my emphasis] (p. 1517). They also warned, "It is important to recognise that currently available 'sports drinks' are not protective: most are hypotonic and provide far more water than salt. Similarly, the infusion of large volumes of hypotonic intravenous solutions into athletes who have an exercise-associated collapse, especially if it is performed without knowledge of the serum sodium concentration, may exacerbate the underlying pathophysiology and do more harm than good" (p. 1517).

Salty Sweating, Dehydration, and EAH

Because the principal abnormality in both EAH and EAHE is a reduced blood sodium concentration, it follows that the condition must be caused by abnormalities in either water or sodium balance or perhaps both, usually during but sometimes after prolonged exercise typically lasting more than 4 hours.

If one wishes to study a disease caused by these mechanisms, then logically the surest way must be to study water and sodium balances in athletes suffering from EAH and EAHE. This is not particularly challenging especially because athletes with EAHE must be hospitalized in order to have the complications of EAHE treated, including coma, convulsions, and respiratory failure. Thus, all that needs to be done is to measure the volumes and sodium (and potassium) contents of all fluids ingested or excreted by, or infused into, these athletes as they recover.

Provided these measurements are continued until the subject's blood sodium concentration returns to normal, it is possible to be certain that whatever disturbances in water or sodium balance caused the EAH and EAHE, the contribution of each will have been identified.

Furthermore, because patients with life-threatening EAHE are usually unconscious and so can receive fluids only intravenously, the problem of determining how much sodium and water are present in any food they might have ingested during their recovery does not arise. By the time the patient awakens from coma, it should be apparent what caused the EAHE (as I was able to establish in the triathlete whom I treated for EAHE after the 1998 Ironman Hawaii Triathlon). The athlete ingested too much fluid either before, during, or after the race. Or else the athlete lost too much sodium in sweat or perhaps in feces, if diarrhea developed. Or perhaps it is caused by a combination of both conditions.

Appendix B details the relevant information from more than 1,600 cases of EAH and EAHE that were either reported in the scientific literature as of September 2010, or had been documented in the Ironman Hawaii Triathlon from 1983 to 1998, or had come to my attention in other ways. What is astonishing is that only very few of these subjects were ever studied in order better to understand the causes of EAH and EAHE. Only two groups in the entire world, ours in Cape Town and Dr. Dale Speedy's group in Auckland, beginning in 1996, have systematically addressed this question.

In time we were to learn that our joint efforts were not particularly welcomed in certain parts of the world, especially by the sports drink industry and most particularly by Dr. Bob Murray, formerly director of the Gatorade Sports Science Institute (GSSI) and full-time employee of PepsiCo, who accused the only scientists ever to directly address this question of being "painfully uninformed" scientists who "stumble over basic thermoregulatory physiology," who ignore "over 50 years of scientific endeavor," who "enthusiastically manufacture" a "self-professed claim of 'case proven'" in a publication that suffers from "an absence of novel findings (and) does not qualify as science" since it is "rife with factual errors and unfounded inferences" and includes "blatant misrepresentations" and "unsubstantiated insinuations of impropriety" while presenting claims that are "ludicrous and without basis" (Murray, 2007, p. 106).

Perhaps we have earned the right to ask this question: How could we possibly have been so wrong? Was it because we had asked the correct and hence the inconvenient questions? Additionally, why do so many cases of EAHE occur in the Gatorade-sponsored Ironman Hawaii Triathlon, and why has a study of fluid and electrolyte balance in triathletes who developed EAHE in that race never been reported? Would those studies not produce the definitive data to end the debate?

Instead, it appears that the response of Gatorade and the GSSI was to develop another novel tale, the mythical salty sweater, a much easier option than discovering why, from 1983 to 1998, the Gatorade-sponsored Ironman Hawaii Triathlon produced more than 700 cases of EAH and EAHE.

Perhaps the fact that both Dale Speedy and I come from relatively less sophisticated countries in which a lack of resources places a greater emphasis on individual initiative and the simpler medical skills caused us to understand the potential value of these rather unsophisticated fluid balance studies in athletes with EAH and EAHE. And after those simple studies had been completed and we had come to the identical conclusion that EAH and EAHE are due to overdrinking, we were able to introduce preventive measures with the result that very few cases occurred thereafter in marathons and longer sporting events in either South Africa or New Zealand. This confirmed that we had indeed discovered the cause of both conditions. Instead, in other parts of the world where this advice was not followed, the number of cases of EAH and EAHE reported annually continued to escalate.

The cause we identified threatened a core concept on which an entire sports drink industry was based. So it was rather easier to continue arguing

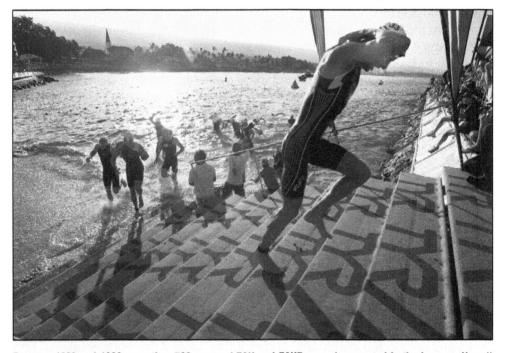

Between 1983 and 1998 more than 700 cases of EAH and EAHE were documented in the Ironman Hawaii Triathlon. Athletes in that race were encouraged to drink at high rates to maximize their performance and to prevent heat stroke.

AP Photo/Chris Stewart

that dehydration and salty sweating were much greater risks to the health of all endurance athletes competing in any event anywhere in the world. But what do the facts reveal?

The salty sweater concept—a theory developed by Dr. Randy Eichner (American Football Monthly Research Staff, 2004), a member of the Speakers Bureau of Gatorade and of the GSSI Sports Medicine Review Board—asserts that high rates of salt loss in sweat cause sodium deficiency, and this deficiency must be prevented by ingesting large amounts of dietary salt both before and after but especially during exercise. But recall from chapter 4 that sweat sodium losses are determined by the level of daily salt intake in the diet and that excessive amounts of salt in sweat indicate the presence of too much salt in the diet, not a need for more! In fact, it is very difficult to attain a true state of sodium deficiency, as shown in the experiment of Dr. McCance as well as the findings of other researchers described in chapter 4. In health, humans accurately regulate their total body sodium stores despite any short-term or long-term changes that may occur in the rates of either sodium intake or sodium losses.

Similarly, because the human body is designed for survival, recall from chapter 2 that studies of athletes competing in long-distance races before the introduction of novel drinking guidelines in 1996 established that the blood sodium concentrations of those athletes who became dehydrated always stayed the same or increased. In all these studies, subjects lost weight because they were advised to drink either nothing, or little, or ad libitum, or less than they lost as sweat. The data presented in table 4.2 (page 129) show unequivocally that the blood sodium concentrations of these athletes who had lost weight during exercise (thereby becoming dehydrated) either stayed the same or rose during exercise. This confirms that when athletes drink less than they sweat during exercise, their blood sodium concentrations either stay the same or they rise; they do not fall as would be predicted if dehydration were to cause EAH.

Because athletes did not usually ingest additional sodium during these races and because any solutions they ingested would have had a low or absent sodium content, all these athletes must also have developed sodium deficits during these races, as we measured in some of those studies (Irving, Noakes, et al., 1986; Irving, Noakes, et al., 1990a). Thus, the only logical conclusion that we could draw is the following: Provided they also develop a mild fluid deficit in the ECF especially, humans are quite able to tolerate a relatively large sodium deficit during exercise while maintaining or even *increasing* their blood sodium concentrations. This is exactly what we would predict if humans evolved as long-distance runners in the heat while surviving on low-sodium diets. Because I had contributed to these studies, including the first study of athletes competing in a 24-hour race (Noakes and Carter, 1976), in which athletes lost relatively little weight (~4% BW) but maintained their blood sodium concentrations in the normal range, I was pretty certain that the data were reproducible and logically consistent with our understanding of physiology; hence, they were probably true.

The reason blood sodium concentrations were so normal in all those studies was that this is the way the body is designed to function—to ensure that the blood sodium concentration and the blood osmolality are homeostatically regulated within a tight range. Logically, if a change, especially a reduction in the

4 Probably the cardinal error of the 1996 ACSM drinking guidelines was the suggestion that athletes should drink to "maintain their body weight during exercise," what I have termed the zero % dehydration rule. This was erroneous because the body does not regulate its weight during exercise; it regulates the osmolality of all the body fluid compartments. If the body loses any electrolytes during exercise, either through the skin or through the gastrointestinal tract, then to regulate its osmolality within the normal range, it must also lose some fluid and hence reduce its weight. Or else body osmolality must drop, causing fluid to enter the cells and risking the development of EAHE if the electrolyte loss is large and is not compensated by an equivalent loss of body weight.

5 The sole exception to this general rule appears to be some patients with cystic fibrosis (CF). These patients secrete sweat with a high sodium concentration, up to 110 mmol/L. But the concentration of sodium in their sweat is still less than in their blood. Even though they lose more sodium in their sweat than do those without this condition, people with CF are still secreting a sweat that has a *lower* sodium concentration than is present in their blood. As a result, the blood sodium concentrations of those with CF should still rise and not fall during exercise if salty sweating is the exclusive mechanism causing EAH. Therefore, some other mechanism must also be active to explain why some subjects with CF reduce their blood sodium concentrations during exercise. To my knowledge, this has not been investigated.

osmolality of the cells in the brain, can lead to death (box 9.1, page 249), then humans must have evolved strong controls to ensure that the body's and especially the brain's osmolality is always tightly regulated to ensure that this does not happen. This regulation is achieved by reducing the body's water content when electrolytes, especially sodium and potassium, are lost in sweat or by retaining water when body electrolyte content rises. The point is that to regulate their body osmolality, humans must allow body weight to change during exercise. *As a result, humans do not regulate body weight during exercise; rather, they regulate the osmolality of the body tissues and most especially that of their most important organ, the brain.*[4]

So the only conclusion one can draw from the original studies listed in table 4.2 (page 129) is that when subjects lose weight during exercise because they drink less than they sweat and so become dehydrated, reducing their body water content, their blood sodium concentrations will either stay the same or will rise. But there is no reason to believe that they will fall,[5] except according to an alternative explanation that has no basis in published scientific fact or logic.

If blood sodium concentrations rise or stay the same when athletes drink less than they sweat and if EAH and EAHE became increasingly prevalent after athletes began to be encouraged to drink more during exercise, then it would seem obvious that EAH and EAHE must logically have something to do with the act and consequences of drinking to excess during exercise.

Hiller and Laird Hypothesis

Shortly after we published our initial study of four cases of EAHE and proposed that all had suffered from water intoxication, Drs. Hiller and Laird, the race doctors at the Ironman Hawaii Triathlon, published a paper proposing an alternative hypothesis, specifically that EAH and EAHE are due to dehydration and large unreplaced losses in sweat sodium. This hypothesis of Hiller and Laird would then become the staple explanation offered by the GSSI and its scientists and would survive even into the 2007 ACSM position stand (Armstrong, Casa, et al., 2007). There is no published evidence to support this hypothesis. Instead, there is a great deal of evidence that disproves it.

Early in the evolution of this condition, before it had spread around the world, Dr. Hiller (1986) wrote the following: "Hyponatremia without overhydration obviously can occur in athletes replacing massive sweat losses with hypotonic fluids. Although the tendency to hyponatremia will be exacerbated by overhydration, we feel that the vast majority of athletes in ultraendurance races finish dehydrated. In treating athletes at the Ironman Hawaii Triathlon, it has been our experience that *almost all* [my emphasis] athletes requiring intravenous fluid therapy are clinically dehydrated. We feel that discouraging fluid intake during endurance or ultraendurance races is dangerous for some athletes. There can be no hyponatremia if salt intake during the race is adequate. We therefore recommend that ultraendurance athletes be encouraged to develop, train, and race with a palatable salt replacement plan" (p. 213). And: "At Ironman, up to 27% of athletes have been hyponatremic—75% of the athletes who require IVs were hyponatremic. The majority of these athletes were also dehydrated" (Hiller, 1988a, p. 213).

Subsequently, Hiller, O'Toole, and colleagues (1987) wrote the following: "Dehydration is the most common problem at the Ironman race. It is frequently compounded by hyponatremia. Dehydration, with or without hyponatremia, is the most common medical problem in ultraendurance races" (p. 166). Later, Dr. Hiller (1989) wrote, "It is clear, then, that exercise-induced hyponatremia is [caused by] a combination of massive unreplaced sodium losses associated with partially replaced massive water losses" (p. 220).

In a subsequently published discussion (Eichner, Laird, et al., 1993a) I provided the following counterarguments, among others:

- The development of hyponatremia requires that fluid be ingested at high rates for at least 4 hours; therefore, dehydration cannot be a cause of hyponatremia.

- I found no evidence to support the contention that large sodium losses are important in the etiology of hyponatremia. In fact, Dr. Irving's study found that total sodium chloride losses in runners who develop hyponatremia were no different from losses in other runners who completed the same ultramarathon races with normal serum sodium concentrations.

- A study by Armstrong, Curtis, and colleagues (1993) showed that a seriously ill soldier with EAHE they studied was profoundly overhydrated, not dehydrated

- "Usually, providing fluids to a collapsed hypernatremic athlete is innocuous. *However, giving intravenous fluid at fast rates to a subject with hyponatremia is definitely contraindicated and could be fatal* [emphasis added].[6] Perhaps the real danger of hyponatremia is that its seriousness is underestimated. In my opinion, hyponatremia is potentially the most dangerous current threat to the health of the

6 I take no pleasure in pointing out that these comments were published a few months before the first case of fatal EAHE occurred in a female runner in the 1993 Valley of the Giants Marathon (case 657, appendix B). She received isotonic saline intravenously, and the possible diagnosis of EAHE was first considered only 7 hours after she was first hospitalized when her blood sodium concentration was measured for the first time. By this stage, however, she could not be saved because she was already brain dead. Hilary Bellamy also died as a result of excessive intravenous fluid therapy after she collapsed in the 2002 Marine Corps Marathon (case 1416, appendix B), as did others listed in appendix B.

ultraendurance athlete because it is poorly recognized, it is difficult to treat, and it will be exacerbated by inappropriate treatment, as we have seen on more than one occasion in South Africa" (p. 4).

Drs. Hiller and Laird again disagreed with my points, and Dr. Hiller stated, "In prospective studies of more than 1000 athletes, we have had only one 'overhydrated' athlete, who gained 2 kg during the Hawaiian Ironman" (Eichner, Laird, et al., 1993a, p. 3).

I have been unable to find evidence that already by 1993 Dr. Hiller had measured weight changes during the race in more than 1,000 Ironman Hawaii triathletes. Instead, I could find evidence that 77 competitors were studied in the 1985 race (Laird, 1987; Laird, 1988; O'Toole, 1988), 37 in the 1989 race (figure 9.8a; figure 9.9, page 263) and another 30 in the 1991 race (O'Toole, Douglas, et al., 1995) (figure 9.8b). Blood sodium concentrations were measured simultaneously, showing a total of 144 measurements in these different studies. The results of these studies are the opposite of what Dr. Hiller remembers.

The 77 competitors (56 men and 21 women) were measured in the 1985 race, which was run in an air temperature of 29.5 °C (85 °F) with a relative humidity of 62%. The average weight loss was 2.8 kg; the greatest weight loss was 6.1 kg and the least was a weight gain of 1.6 kg in an athlete whose blood sodium concentration fell 5 mmol/L (O'Toole, 1988). This athlete apparently did not have EAH because he or she was not considered in the further discussion. After the race, 10 of the athletes developed EAH; 8 of these athletes were "hemodilated [sic] postrace according to hematocrit and hemoglobin measurements" (O'Toole, 1988, p. 95) and therefore suffering from overhydration, not dehydration. According to the authors, "None of the hyponatremic athletes were grossly overhydrated as judged by weight gain. Two of them were measured to have gained 0.5 lb each and the rest either stayed the same or lost weight" (p. 95). Although these changes in body weight may seem small, that is precisely the point: If the body weight does not fall by perhaps 2 to 3 kg during the course of an Ironman triathlon, then the athlete is already overhydrated by that amount. Thus, a weight gain of 0.5 lb means that the athlete is actually overhydrated by close to 3 kg. These findings should have convinced these authors of two clear observations:

1. Weight loss was lower in those with EAH than it was in those who maintained or increased their blood sodium concentrations
2. Athletes with EAH were more likely to be "hemodiluted" (overhydrated).

7 Data for figure 9.8a are courtesy of Dr. Robert Laird, which he personally entrusted to my care at the 1998 Ironman Hawaii Triathlon. These data have not previously been published. Because I know the data exist, it is my ethical duty to publish them, especially since they could affect the health of triathletes competing in future Ironman Hawaii Triathlons. I could reasonably be criticized for my failure to publish these data previously.

Data were collected in the 1989 Ironman Hawaii Triathlon, although they were not reported at the time. I analyzed those data only years later, and they are reported here for the first time (figure 9.8).[7]

The body weights were measured before and after the race in 37 triathletes. Their blood sodium concentrations were also measured but only after the race. The data (figure 9.8a) showed a linear relationship with a negative slope between the postrace blood sodium concentration and the change in body weight during the race so that those athletes who lost the most weight and were the most dehydrated (left side of the figure) had the highest blood sodium concentrations, whereas the athlete with the lowest blood sodium concentration of 128 mmol/L (arrowed) had gained about 1% body weight during the race. The change in body weight predicted 23% of the variance in the postrace blood sodium concentrations.

At the 1995 race Dr. Mary O'Toole and colleagues (1995) completed an identical study and reported their findings in the scientific literature for the first time. As was the case in the 1989 race, they showed the classic inverse relationship between body weight change and postrace blood sodium concentration (figure 9.8b). Thus, seven of the eight athletes whose postrace blood sodium concentrations were less than 130 mmol/L lost less than 2% of their body weight during the race. Furthermore, athletes with EAH lost significantly *less* (~0.6%) body weight during the race than did those who finished the race without EAH (~2.5% body

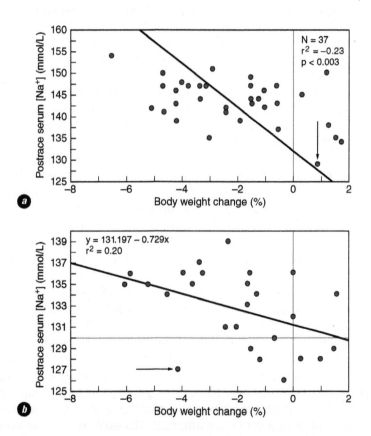

FIGURE 9.8 *(a)* A study of 37 triathletes in the 1989 Ironman Hawaii Triathlon showed a linear relationship with a negative slope between body weight change and postrace blood sodium concentrations. The only athlete with EAH (blood sodium concentration below 135 mmol/L—arrowed) had gained ~1% body weight during the race. *(b)* A study of 30 triathletes in the 1995 Ironman Hawaii Triathlon showed the classic linear relationship with a negative slope between body weight change and postrace blood sodium concentrations. One athlete (arrowed) developed EAH despite losing ~4% of his body weight during the race.

(a) Data from 1989 Ironman Hawaii Triathlon data set collected by Dr. Robert Laird and colleagues and made available to the author in October 1998. *(b)* Adapted, by permission, from M.L. O'Toole, P.S. Douglas, R.H. Laird, B. Hiller, and W. Douglas, 1995, "Fluid and electrolyte status in athletes receiving medical care at an ultradistance triathlon," *Clinical Journal of Sport Medicine* 5(2): 116-122.

weight), confirming that *dehydration protects against the development of EAH.* Again, the change in body weight during the race predicted 20% of the variance in the postrace blood sodium concentrations. Most of the variance in postrace blood sodium concentrations is unexplained and is perhaps influenced most by the release of sodium from the internal sodium stores into the extracellular fluid in order to offset any sodium lost in sweat and to increase the sodium content of the increased total body water content in those who overdrink during exercise. The athlete cannot control these internal sodium movements, but she can control how much she drinks.

In both figures 9.8*a* and 9.8*b*, the athletes who lost the most weight (left side of the graph) had the highest postrace blood sodium concentrations, whereas concentrations fell with increasing weight gain during the race (right side of graph). This finding disproves the hypothesis of Hiller and Laird that dehydration and large sodium chloride losses cause EAH to develop in Ironman Hawaii triathletes.

According to figure 9.8*b*, a tiny minority of Ironman Hawaii triathletes completed that race even mildly dehydrated. This confirms the interpretation that the abnormally high incidence of EAH and EAHE in the Ironman Hawaii Triathlon must be due to an overemphasis on the prevention of dehydration at that race with the result that overdrinking occurs in 10% to 20% of athletes in that race compared to a trivial incidence of overdrinking in Ironman Triathlons held in nontropical climates such as New Zealand and South Africa. Perhaps this explains why that race has produced a greater number of cases of EAH and EAHE than any other sporting event that has ever been studied.

The one measurement in figure 9.8*b* that conflicts with the general rule that dehydration protects against EAH has been identified with an arrow. That athlete developed EAH despite a body weight loss of ~4%. This anomalous finding could be explained if the athlete had a condition in which some of his circulating ionized sodium (Na^+) was osmotically inactivated by mechanisms that are currently poorly understood. The point, however, is that this athlete is the exception because his or her response is quite different from that of all the other subjects in this trial. Developing a general overreaching hypothesis that dehydration causes EAH on the basis of the single subject who responds differently to all others is an invitation to error. These authors would not be the sole perpetrators of this error.

Note that six triathletes (figure 9.8*a*, 16% of the sample) in the 1989 race gained weight during the race (right of the vertical line at 0% body weight loss) but that in this group there was a wide range of blood sodium concentrations. In the 1995 race, six athletes (figure 9.8*b*, 20% of the sample) gained weight during the race (right of vertical line at 0% body weight change), and in that group there was again a wide variation in postrace blood sodium concentrations. We also observed this finding many years later and have attempted to explain the reasons this can happen (see figure 9.15, page 288, and the subsequent discussion).

Acknowledging that EAH can be caused by overdrinking with fluid retention due to abnormal renal function and that athletes with EAH lost less weight than did those who did not develop EAH, the authors concluded "that a combination of both of these mechanisms [fluid retention and significant sodium losses] may be operative in causing EAH" (O'Toole, Douglas, et al. 1995, p. 121). They apparently saw no reason to warn Ironman Hawaii triathletes about the dangers of overdrinking during the race. Nor did they choose to prospectively study fluid and electrolyte balance during recovery in any of the 106 triathletes treated that year for EAH in the medical tent, including nine with postrace blood sodium concentrations below 128 mmol/L (figure 9.8). That would have been a valuable study for confirming or refuting the findings of Tony Irving's study. Their study was funded by the Quaker Oats company, then manufacturers of the sports drink Gatorade, the official sponsors of the (Gatorade) Ironman Hawaii Triathlon.

Further analysis of the data from the 1989 Ironman Hawaii Triathlon revealed that six (16%) of the athletes gained weight during the race and another 16 (43%) lost 3% or less of their body weight during the race and so were likely to be normally hydrated (Noakes, Sharwood, et al., 2005). The case can be made that 59% of all the athletes studied by these doctors were either normally hydrated or over-hydrated, whereas only one athlete lost more than 6% of body weight finishing the race in about 11 hours (figure 9.8*a*).

The incidence of overhydration (16%) in the runners they studied in this sample was similar to the proportion (15%) of patients they treated for EAH and EAHE (66 cases in 409 medical admissions; cases 291-356 in appendix B) after the race in the medical tent. The figure is also not too dissimilar to the incidence of EAH (13%) reported by Dr. Almond and colleagues in the 2002 Boston Marathon. Perhaps a minimum of 13% of people develop SIADH during exercise and are therefore at risk of developing EAH and EAHE if they overdrink during prolonged exercise.

We were also able to trace the finishing times of 29 of the triathletes from the 1989 Ironman Hawaii Triathlon. Figure 9.9 shows that there was no relationship between the percent body weight loss of the triathletes during the race and their finishing times. Thus, the fastest finisher in this sample lost 4% of his body weight during the race finishing in 9 hours, whereas the slowest finisher (16 hours) lost about 5% of his body weight. The 5 triathletes who gained weight during the race finished in 11.5 to 12.5 hours, well behind the race winner.

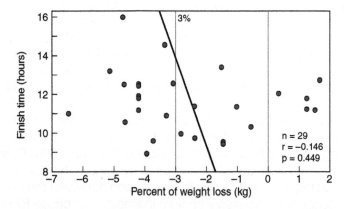

FIGURE 9.9 There was no relationship between BW changes and finishing times in 29 triathletes competing in the 1989 Ironman Hawaii Triathlon. Five athletes (17%) gained weight during the race, whereas another 9 (33%) lost less than ~3% BW during the race and hence were not substantially dehydrated (Noakes, Sharwood, et al., 2005). Exactly (50%) of triathletes who were studied finished the race either overhydrated or normally hydrated, and only one lost more than 6% body weight.

Data from 1989 Ironman Hawaii Triathlon data set collected by Dr. Robert Laird and colleagues and made available to the author in October 1998.

Of the 30 subjects reported in the 1995 paper, 6 (20%) gained weight, and two gained about 1.7% (figure 9.8). As also found in the 1985 survey, weight gain was associated with reduced, not elevated, blood sodium concentrations, the opposite of their conclusions. Thus, there is a discrepancy between what this group believed they observed on clinical grounds, specifically that "almost all" Ironman Hawaii triathletes finish the race clinically dehydrated, and what they actually showed when they measured body weight changes in the 67 athletes in the 1989 and 1995 races. Of their total sample of 144 race finishers in 3 different races studied over 8 years, 22 (15%) either did not lose weight during the race or developed evidence for dilution of their blood and so were overhydrated, not dehydrated, at the finish of the race. In addition, only 1 athlete in the 1989 race and 2 in the 1991 race lost more than 5% of body weight during the race. This contrasts with a much larger number of Ironman triathletes who developed much greater levels of weight loss in the New Zealand and South African Ironman races (figures 9.6, page 252, and 10.5, page 307), even though those races are held in cooler conditions.

We have since discovered why Drs. Hiller and Laird made this error. We have found that the level of dehydration of marathon runners cannot be determined by a clinical examination, that is, by looking at and feeling the patient, regardless of the thoroughness of that examination (McGarvey, Thompson, et al., 2010). Instead, the singular symptom of dehydration is thirst, and the sole way to detect the level of dehydration is to compare the athlete's weight before and after the race. Thus, Drs. Hiller and Laird were seeing exactly what they thought they should be seeing in these "massively" dehydrated Ironman triathletes, many of whom were actually overhydrated. So when these authors finally reported changes in blood sodium concentrations and body weight in Ironman Hawaii triathletes, they showed (figure 9.8), as has every other study, that blood sodium concentrations fall in those who lose the least weight during exercise, the opposite of their prediction. Indeed, they continue to follow their bias, even in 2005 (Pahnke, Trinity, et al., 2005) and beyond (Pahnke, Trinity, et al., 2010) as Dr. Hiller joined up with Ed Coyle, PhD, in a continuing search to prove that sodium deficiency is the sole cause of EAH and other medical conditions in Ironman Hawaii triathletes.

That series of Gatorade-funded studies subsequently undertaken by Dr. Coyle's group with the help of Dr. Hiller at a series of Ironman Hawaii Triathlons from 2003 to 2005 were singularly unsuccessful in advancing our understanding of sodium balance as a potential cause of EAH and EAHE. Certainly, they failed to support the Hiller and Laird hypothesis that sodium deficiency is the crucial factor causing EAH and EAHE. Rather, they confirmed the importance of fluid balance in determining the change in blood sodium concentrations even during exercise lasting up to 17 hours in hot conditions (Pahnke, 2004; Pahnke, Trinity, et al., 2010). Nevertheless, the Hiller and Laird hypothesis that EAH is caused by dehydration and massive salt losses in sweat soon achieved the status of fact.

But the evidence that excessive sodium losses do not cause EAH and EAHE had already been established by Tony Irving's 1988 Comrades Marathon study, published in 1991, and confirmed by Dale Speedy's group who studied New Zealand Ironman triathletes with EAH and EAHE (figure 9.10). We added to these data by showing (a) that a triathlete who developed EAHE during the 2000 South African Ironman because he gained 3.6 kg (case 1233 in appendix B) returned

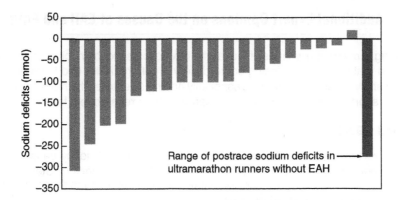

FIGURE 9.10 Range of postrace sodium deficits in published cases of EAH and EAHE. Note that the sodium deficits are not greater than values measured in other endurance athletes who finished similar races without developing EAH or EAHE. These deficits are also less than those measured in a number of laboratory studies in which subjects did not develop EAH or EAHE.

Data from Dugas and Noakes 2005; Irving, Noakes, Buck, et al., 1991; Noakes, Sharwood, Collins, et al., 2004; Speedy, Noakes, Rogers, et al., 2000; Speedy, Noakes, Kimber, et al., 2001b; Speedy, Rogers, Noakes, et al., 2000a.

his blood sodium concentration to normal without ingesting any salt just by passing 4.6 L of urine during the first 17 hours after the race (Noakes, Sharwood, et al., 2004) and (b) a cyclist who developed EAHE during the 2004 109 km Argus Cycle Tour (case 1504 in appendix B) when she gained 2.4 kg could have lost only ~100 mmol sodium in sweat during that race, far too little to cause the condition (Dugas, and Noakes, 2005).

In the course of normal science, these conclusions, based on a reasonable sample size of athletes studied on different continents and all of which showed the same response, should have been accepted as the initial truth until they were subsequently shown to be wrong. But this never happened. Instead, "expert" opinion in North America repeatedly stated and indeed continues to state that EAH and EAHE are caused by large sodium losses usually associated with dehydration (box 9.2, page 266). Since some of these experts also provide content for the GSSI and the ACSM, it is perhaps not surprising that this incorrect and disproven opinion continues to be widely promoted.

Models Predicting EAH

Instead of studying athletes in the field, the leading protagonists for the theory that EAH is caused by large sodium losses have produced modeling examples of what *might* happen to blood sodium concentrations in athletes who (a) exercise for prolonged periods (>6 hours), (b) lose sodium at a fixed rate in their sweat regardless of any developing sodium deficit, (c) do not have an internal store of sodium to replenish the ECF sodium content as it becomes progressively depleted by sweat losses, and (d) drink at prescribed rates and not according to the dictates of thirst during exercise.

Scott Montain, who together with Dr. Ed Coyle had produced the 1992 study (Montain and Coyle, 1992) that encouraged the ACSM to advocate that athletes should drink up to 1.2 L/hr during exercise and who then played an important

BOX 9.2   Additional Expert Opinions on the Causes of EAH and EAHE

It is interesting to review the writings of those who have expressed their opinions on this topic and to record that despite convincing contradictory proof, the Hiller and Laird hypothesis continues to enjoy widespread support, especially among scientists who have a relationship with the U.S. sports drink industry. Several examples from researchers follow.

Robert Lind (1988)

An early convert to the theory that dehydration and sodium deficiency cause EAH and EAHE was Robert H. Lind, MD, former medical director of the Western States 100-mile race, run annually in the Sierra Nevada Mountains since 1974. In 1988 Dr. Lind described his model of how EAH and EAHE develop:

> Hyponatremia may be frequently observed in athletes who have exercised for several hours in high temperatures. . . . Consider that a runner not trained for high temperatures secretes an arbitrary 60mEq [milliequilavent] of sodium per liter of sweat. Replacing that lost fluid with plain water could easily decrease the sodium concentration from 135mEq/L to 120mEq/L, putting the runner at risk for a seizure. A decrease in sodium concentration in the extracellular fluid of 15mEq/L X 42L = 630mEq total sodium loss. If our runner secretes 60mEq/L of sodium in sweat, only 10.5L of sweat is needed to lower the sodium in the blood to 120mEq/L. (p. 30)

Dr. Lind proposed that only by ingesting salt during exercise and by training in the heat to reduce the sweat sodium concentration could athletes prevent the development of EAH and EAHE. He also described the situation at the finish line of the 1985 American River 50-Mile Run, where

> two runners who experienced seizures were taken to the emergency room for hospitalization. Many runners who were vomiting and nauseated or extremely weak and unwilling to swallow anything were fed ice chips and potato chips in an attempt to get salt back into them. Lead runners have fewer problems than those in the middle or back of the pack . . . (who) may not concentrate as closely on fluid management, may not take in sufficient electrolytes in the form of fluids or food. (pp. 33-34)

This description appears rather more typical of athletes who have developed EAH and EAHE as a result of overdrinking and who develop nausea and vomiting as a consequence of the accumulation of unabsorbed fluid in their gastrointestinal tracts.

Dr. Lind's model of how EAH develops in those who replace their sweat losses during exercise by drinking only water would be adopted subsequently by scientists from the U.S. Army Research Institute for Environmental Medicine (USARIEM) and become the USARIEM model of sodium deficiency during exercise (see figures 9.11 and 9.12, pages 274 and 277).

Armstrong and Colleagues (1996)

Dr. Larry Armstrong is a prodigious writer of books on heat and exercise and has a long history of believing that any dehydration that develops during exercise is detrimental to both health and performance. He trained at the USARIEM, and his former student and current colleague, Dr. Douglas Casa, has received substantial funding from the GSSI.

As lead author of the *1996 American College of Sports Medicine Position Stand: Heat and Cold Illnesses During Distance Running,* Dr. Armstrong wrote the following:

> A primary rationale for electrolyte supplementation with fluid replacement drinks is, therefore, to replace electrolytes lost from sweating during exercise greater than 4-5 hours in duration (Armstrong, Curtis, 1993).[8]

... electrolytes (primarily NaCl) should be added to the fluid replacement solution to enhance palatability and reduce the probability for development of hyponatremia.

There is no published evidence showing that the ingestion of sports drinks containing sodium chloride at concentrations that are palatable can prevent the development of EAH or EAHE in those who overdrink and have SIADH.

Convertino and Colleagues (1996)

As lead author for the *1996 American College of Sports Medicine Position Stand: Exercise and Fluid Replacement*, Dr. Convertino wrote the following:

> Excessive consumption of pure water or dilute fluid (i.e. up to 10 liters per 4 hours) during prolonged endurance events may lead to a harmful dilutional hyponatremia (Noakes, Goodwin, et al., 1985) which may involve disorientation, confusion, and seizure or coma. The possibility of hyponatremia may be the best rationale for inclusion of sodium chloride in fluid replacement beverages (Armstrong, Epstein, et al., 1996). (p. 3)

Michael F. Bergeron (2000)

Dr. Michael Bergeron contributed an article for the GSSI titled "Sodium: The Forgotten Nutrient" (GSSI, 2000). Because sodium is one of the most avariciously consumed foodstuffs in the world, it is difficult to imagine that it has been forgotten.

After describing a case of EAH in a U.S. nationally ranked tennis player who had ingested "a considerable amount of water" on the advice of "tournament medical personnel," Bergeron began by stating the following:

> The precise mechanism underlying hyponatremia is somewhat unclear, but . . . it seems to be brought on by extensive sweating incident with and/or followed by repeatedly ingesting low-sodium-free fluids (e.g. water) for several hours or more. . . . (p. 2)
>
> Those with greater than average sweating rates and extensive sweat sodium losses may be at high risk. Such athletes are the ones most likely to develop a sodium deficit that is fostered by these characteristics in combination with an inappropriately low salt intake. However, excessive drinking of plain water (or other sodium-free fluids such as soft drinks) before, during and after exercise may be the most important cause of hyponatremia. (p. 2)
>
> . . . Thus, to prevent hyponatremia, one should consume an appropriate amount of fluid ... and adequate salt before, during, and after competition and training . . . particularly when competing or training for a long duration or multiple times on successive days in the heat. (p. 2)

Dr. Bergeron also suggested that drinking sports drinks, even with their low concentrations of sodium, and using GatorLytes, a prepackaged electrolyte mix, also helps to prevent heat cramps. He summarized his article as follows:

> Large sweat losses often mean extensive sodium losses. Such sodium losses can result in incomplete rehydration and may predispose the athlete to heat cramps during subsequent exercise. Moreover, rehydration with sodium-free fluids such as water can lead to hyponatremia in certain individuals. Thus, any time considerable sweating occurs or is anticipated, appropriate fluid intake with an accompanying increase in dietary salt can help prevent problems related to a sweat-induced sodium deficit and incomplete or inappropriate rehydration. (p. 3)

8 Here the authors used a reference to a case of EAHE caused by fluid overload alone (case 557 in appendix B) to argue that sodium must be ingested during exercise in order to prevent EAHE. Rather, the only lesson to be learned from case 557 is that overdrinking during exercise causes EAHE in the presence of SIADH. In actuality, there is no appropriate reference showing that electrolyte ingestion during exercise can prevent EAH and EAHE.

(continued)

Scott Montain, Michael Sawka, and Bruce Wegner (2001)

Drs. Scott Montain and Michael Sawka are employed as researchers at the USARIEM. Dr. Armstrong is a former employee of USARIEM; the past two editors (2004-2009) of MSSE have also been USARIEM employees. These close links may have caused all of the modern ACSM position stands to be unusually influenced by the opinions of this small group, all of whom are or have been employed by the same U.S. government agency.

In addition, Montain completed his PhD with Edward Coyle, PhD, at the University of Texas at Austin; together they produced the Gatorade-funded study that led to the theory that humans needed to drink 1.2 L/hr or "as much as tolerable," what I have called the zero % dehydration rule. In chapter 7 I review the evidence that it was the development of the theory of water as a tactical weapon by USARIEM in 1982 that was the single most important factor driving the adoption of the 1996 ACSM drinking guidelines, which fundamentally changed attitudes on drinking during exercise, especially in the United States.

Together these authors (Montain, Sawka, et al., 2001) wrote the following:

> Sweat electrolyte losses contribute to the development of the syndrome (of EAH), particularly if sweat sodium losses are high. The condition may also occur when individuals consume low-sodium or sodium-free water in excess of sweat losses during and/or shortly after completing exercise. (p. 113)
>
> In summary, both large salt losses via sweat and excessive water intake, singly or in combination, contribute to lowering serum sodium during prolonged exercise (p. 116).[9]
>
> Competitive and recreational athletes . . . should be taught that persistent excessive fluid intake can be harmful and that fluid intake should not exceed sweat losses. (p. 117)
>
> During prolonged exercise lasting in excess of 3-4h, snacks or fluids containing sodium chloride should be ingested to offset the loss of salt in sweat. The latter recommendation is especially prudent for individuals who know that they lose excessive amounts of salt in their sweat. (p. 117)

9   There is no scientific basis for these conclusions. Instead, the published record can be interpreted only to support a quite different conclusion.

Larry Armstrong (2000)

In his book *Performing in Extreme Environments,* Dr. Armstrong (2000b) wrote the following:

> Because the vast majority of exertional hyponatremia cases today result from overhydration, virtually all of these are preventable. Prevention and risk reduction can be accomplished by modifying sodium intake and moderating fluid intake.[10] (p. 133)
>
> People participating in prolonged endurance events (>4h), should ingest electrolytes (e.g. sodium, chloride, potassium, magnesium) via fluids and foods during and after exercise . . . This supports the rationale for including sodium in fluid replacement beverages, although the effect likely will be small. (p. 133)[11]
>
> The only certain method of preventing EH is to avoid overdrinking too much pure water or dilute fluid (Davis, Videen, et al., 2001; Irving, Noakes, et al., 1991; Noakes, 1992a; Speedy, Noakes et al., 2001c). (p. 135)
>
> Despite these dangers, few athletes realize that excessive fluid consumption may cause illness, hospitalization, cognitive impairment, or occupational disability. . . . Virtually all individuals who experience EH attempt to drink as much fluid as possible during and after exercise. . . . The simplest way to reduce the risk of EH is

10   The logic of this statement is not immediately clear. If overhydration causes the "vast majority" of cases of exertional hyponatremia, why is it necessary to modify sodium intake to prevent EAH?

11   This is an interesting admission that the effect of electrolyte ingestion is likely to be "small." In fact, it is so small that it is irrelevant. But preventing overdrinking will absolutely prevent EAH and EAHE, as Dr. Armstrong correctly includes in his next statement.

to ensure that fluid is consumed at a rate that equals or is less than the sweat rate. Post-exercise consumption of sodium-rich beverages and foods . . . also reduces EH risk. (p. 135)[12]

Tim Noakes (2002)

For historical context, I offer this summary in advance of providing Murray and Eichner's 2004 statements. In 2001 I was invited by Dr. Robert Sallis to contribute an article on EAH to *Current Sports Medicine Reports,* the journal of which he had recently been appointed the editor in chief. The journal appears to publish articles at the discretion of the editor, who may invite contributions from anyone he wishes. It does not appear to require rigorous peer review.

I had met Dr. Sallis at the 1998 Ironman Hawaii Triathlon, the only recent Ironman Hawaii Triathlon at which Gatorade was not a sponsor and to which I, perhaps therefore, was invited. Dr. Sallis has subsequently incorporated some but not all of our ideas into his teachings (Sallis, 2004). But he continues to believe that sodium deficiency contributes to EAH and EAHE (Sallis, 2008). I wrote the following:

> We have consistently proposed that symptomatic hyponatremia cannot occur in the absence of fluid overload, and the expected sodium deficit incurred during exercise probably plays an insignificant role. (p. 199)

I then traced three modifications through which the opposing theory for the etiology of EAH and EAHE had passed:

1. The first proposal was that EAH "occurs in athletes who develop dehydration and large sodium deficits . . . both as a result of high sweat rates sustained for very many hours during prolonged exercise" (p. 199). So athletes were advised "to drink larger volumes of electrolyte-containing sports drinks at higher rates during prolonged exercise" (p. 199).

2. The second iteration was that EAH "occurs in athletes who develop large sodium deficits during exercise but who fail to replace that deficit, even though they ingest large volumes of hypotonic fluids, especially water, at high rates" (p. 199) To prevent this condition athletes were advised to "continue to ingest fluid at high rates during prolonged exercise" and, in order to avoid the large sodium deficits, "to ingest only electrolyte-containing sports drinks during exercise and to supplement their sodium intakes from other sources both before and during exercise" (pp. 199-200).

3. The third modification was that "both large salt losses via sweat and excessive water intake, singly or in combination, contribute to lowering serum sodium during prolonged exercise (Montain, Sawka, et al., 2001," p. 200). I pointed out that this proposal was based on a set of theoretic calculations, but that those calculations "conflict with the actual findings in real patients treated for symptomatic hyponatremia" (p. 200).

> On the basis of recent publications, there is no longer any possibility to conceal the conclusion that fluid overload as a result of voluntary over-drinking, is the only important etiologic factor causing the hyponatremia of exercise. (p. 205)
>
> By limiting fluid intake during prolonged exercise, symptomatic hyponatremia is as preventable today as it was before 1981 when the condition simply did not exist. (p. 206)

12 There is no evidence for this statement. Athletes with EAH or EAHE immediately excrete any ingested sodium in their urine because they have SIADH and elevated, including levels of a variety of sodium-losing hormones like ANP that increase sodium losses. Ingesting any fluid that has an adequately low sodium concentration to make it palatable can only exacerbate the EAH or EAHE (since the fluid will be retained and the sodium excreted). Only salt solutions with a sodium chloride content of 3.0% (the concentration present in sea water) should be ingested by those with EAH or EAHE. But such solutions are utterly unpalatable. Athletes with low blood sodium concentrations must not drink anything until they begin to pass urine—indicating that their blood ADH concentrations have fallen and the state of SIADH has corrected itself.

(continued)

Bob Murray and Randy Eichner (2004)

Bob Murray, PhD, was, until July 2008, a full-time employee of PepsiCo with the responsibility of managing the GSSI. As a result, he was the main public face of the "science" behind the Gatorade brand and the GSSI "science of nutrition." Dr. Murray has no training in clinical medicine, so he has never treated a patient with EAH or EAHE. Nor has he ever personally undertaken any research that attempts to understand the factors causing the condition.

Randy Eichner, on the other hand, is medically trained. As a member of the Speakers Bureau of Gatorade and of the GSSI Sports Medicine Review Board, Dr. Eichner has traveled extensively across the United States, giving lectures on behalf of Gatorade and the GSSI. These lectures tout the dangers of dehydration and the importance of ingesting sports drinks at high rates during exercise. Interestingly, Dr. Eichner has not undertaken original studies of fluids and exercise (other than the use of sodium supplementation to prevent muscle cramping in American college football players) or of the cause, treatment, or prevention of EAH and EAHE. Yet he drew up drinking guidelines for competitors in the Ironman Hawaii Triathlon, including the advice that "heavy sweaters" in that race need to ingest 2 L/hr if they are to survive and optimize their performance.

This article was published in *Current Sports Medicine Reports*, perhaps to counter my article published 2 years earlier in the same journal. They began by describing three ways in which they deduced hyponatremia could occur (Murray and Eichner, 2004):

13 This is based on the theory that EAH and EAHE allegedly due to sodium deficiency occurs only in prolonged exercise like the Ironman Hawaii Triathlon, which is held in "tropical climes." There is no published evidence showing that sodium deficiency causes a unique form of EAH and EAHE that occurs solely in triathletes competing in the Ironman Hawaii Triathlon.

14 This is the dehydration myth for which there is no scientific evidence.

15 Athletes with EAH and EAHE have SIADH and elevated blood ANP concentrations, and the condition of cerebral salt wasting (CSW) will not retain the sodium ingested in a sports drink unless the salt content is so high (3%-5%) that the drink is utterly unpalatable. This advice will only cause the exacerbation of EAH and EAHE in those who overdrink because, like Dr. Cynthia Lucero, they believe they are protected from developing EAH and EAHE as long as they ingest a sports drink that contains at least some sodium.

1. From excessive water intake alone. . . . This form of hyponatremia . . . may be the main cause of the serious or lethal hyponatremia seen in some women marathon runners (p. 117).[13]

2. From excessive drinking and large sweat sodium loss . . . . This form of hyponatremia can occur even in the absence of overdrinking, . . . and seems more likely in very long events and in those who for genetic or other reasons have very salty sweat. (p. 118)

3. In dehydrated endurance athletes, from large sweat sodium losses and ingestion of low sodium beverages. This form of hyponatremia occurs despite under-drinking. . . . An athlete who loses 10 L of salty sweat and drinks 8 L of water will be both volume depleted (dehydrated) and hyponatremic. Hypovolemic hyponatremia is not the most common form of hyponatremia, but does occur in prolonged endurance events in tropical climes, such as some Ironman-distance triathlons. (p. 118)

Educating athletes about the dangers of excessive drinking and the need to ingest adequate sodium in their diets and during training and competition can help prevent hyponatremia. The goal of drinking during exercise is to minimize body weight loss and therefore reduce the risk that dehydration will impair performance and increase the risk of heat illness[14]. . . . During workouts and competition, athletes should favour sodium-containing drinks over water to assure an additional intake of sodium to help stabilize the sodium content of the ECF. (p. 118)[15]

In discussing the treatment of hyponatremia, the authors erroneously wrote the following:

If plasma sodium is low and the athlete is clinically hypovolemic (as in some triathletes in tropical climes), one can safely begin with intravenous normal saline. (p. 118)

This advice is entirely incorrect. Only hypertonic (3%-5%) saline solutions may be given to athletes with EAH or EAHE.

An article presenting identical arguments was also published in the lay magazine, *Marathon and Beyond* (Murray, Stofan, et al., 2004).

Scott Montain, Samuel Cheuvront, and Michael Sawka (2006)

These authors, all of whom are employed by the USARIEM, wrote the following in *Current Sports Medicine Reports* in 2006:

In summary, fluid intake in excess of sweating rate is the primary cause of hyponatremia associated with prolonged exercise. Thus preventive strategies to limit overhydration are warranted. The contribution of sweat sodium losses, however should not be ignored. People who secrete relatively salty sweat can tolerate less overdrinking before developing hyponatraemia. Furthermore, if they rely solely on water or weak electrolyte solutions for fluid replacement and consume only electrolyte solutions for fluid replacement and consume only electrolyte-poor foods, it is possible for them to become both dehydrated and hyponatremic. (p. 104)

This advice is essentially repeated in a subsequent paper also by Dr. Montain (2008).

Lawrence Armstrong, Douglas Casa, and Greig Watson (2006)

These authors (2006) wrote the following:

Two exercise-related forms of acute hypotonic hyponatremia have been observed among endurance athletes (Armstrong, 2003; Speedy, Noakes, et al., 1999). Hypervolemic hyponatremia involves fluid overload with a relatively small Na^+ loss; this expands the extracellular volume and results in edema. Hypovolemic hyponatremia involves a larger Na^+ loss with dehydration (no water excess and decreased body weight) and shrinkage of the extracellular volume, resulting from deficits of both total body Na^+ and water; edema is absent. Although both conditions involved reduced extracellular Na^+ concentrations and expanded intracellular volume, all previously published cases of symptomatic hyponatremic illness (HI) with encephalopathy (i.e. brain dysfunction involving an altered mental state) have involved hypervolemic hyponatremia. (p. 221)

The authors suggested that the answer to their rhetorical question, "How does exertional hyponatremia develop?" is "complex." (p. 222). To reduce the risk of HI, the authors proposed the following:

1. During exercise, attempt to lose no more than 1.5% of the pre-exercise weight.[16] (p. 222)

2. During exercise, fluids containing Na^+ maintain plasma Na^+ slightly better than pure water. However, consuming a large volume of a fluid-electrolyte beverage (5-10 L of a hypotonic Na^+ solution) may induce exertional hyponatremia (EH) or HI. Ultraendurance competitors may find it beneficial to take brief rest periods to consume Na^+-rich beverages and foods (e.g. low-fat soup or stew with crackers), in an attempt to maintain normal plasma Na^+. (p. 222)

3. Before and after exercise, consume food and fluids that contain Na^+ to offset Na^+ losses in sweat and urine. (p. 222)

16 There is no logic in this statement. EAH and EAHE are not caused by weight loss but by weight gain. Thus, the correct advice should be that athletes need to ensure that no weight *gain* occurs during exercise, not that the extent of weight loss needs to be less than 1.5% of the prerace body weight. An athlete who increases her body weight by 6% or more, as did Cynthia Lucero, would fulfill this criterion for safety described by these authors since, by gaining 6% of body weight, she also restricted her weight loss to less than 1.5%. But she still died. Thus, following this advice will not ensure that athletes do not develop fatal EAHE.

(continued)

Michael Sawka, Louise Burke, and Colleagues (2007)

The *American College of Sports Medicine Position Stand: Exercise and Fluid Replacement* (2007) was drawn up by 5 scientists who acknowledged they received funding or honoraria from the GSSI. Dr. Randy Eichner, the sole contributor with a medical training but who has yet to publish his first original study of EAH or of fluid balance during exercise, acknowledged that he is a member of the GSSI Speakers Bureau. Dr. Louise Burke, who was instrumental in assisting the entry of Gatorade into Australia, was included as a contributor for the first time but did not disclose her involvement with Gatorade and the GSSI. These authors wrote the following:

17 First, the paper Dr. Sawka and his colleagues quoted clearly shows a linear relationship with a negative slope between the amount of weight the athletes lost during the race and their postrace blood sodium concentrations. Thus, the fall in blood sodium concentrations in athletes competing in the Ironman Hawaii Triathlon is a function of how little weight they lose during the race, exactly as it is for triathletes competing in "nontropical" climes. There is nothing magical about the Ironman Hawaii Triathlon that it causes a unique form of EAH and EAHE, different from the type that occurs in athletes competing in nontropical climes. Second, it has been clearly shown that clinical observations cannot accurately detect whether or not marathon runners are dehydrated.

Contributing factors to exercise-associated hyponatremia include overdrinking of hypotonic fluids and excessive loss of total body sodium (Montain, Cheuvront, et al., 2006, p. 382).

There is no scientific basis for this statement. It is based purely on the predictions of the USARIEM model, which fails to predict what actually happens in real athletes. This model is discussed later in this chapter.

In tropical triathlons (e.g. Kona, HI), some participants may have been both dehydrated and hyponatremic based upon clinical observations. (p. 382)[17]

In longer ultra-endurance events, sodium losses can induce hyponatremia to levels associated with the onset of symptoms regardless if the individual is over- or underdrinking, so replacing some of the sodium losses is warranted. (p. 382)

Consumption of beverages containing electrolytes and carbohydrates can help sustain fluid-electrolyte balance and exercise performance. (p. 386)

Robert E. Sallis (2008)

Dr. Sallis is the editor in chief of *Current Sports Medicine Reports* as well as a former ACSM president. He wrote the following (2008):

Failure to match closely fluid and sodium loss with intake can result in dehydration and dysnatremias, along with a host of other problems. (p. 514)

… it is encumbent [sic] upon athletes to learn to approximate their sweat rate in various situations and environmental settings, in order to plan their drinking to try and match fluid loss. Athletes can learn their fluid requirements by weighing themselves before and after workouts with the difference being a good estimate of sweat losses and the amount of fluid needed to optimize performance. (p. 514)

(There is no evidence that humans need to ingest fluids to match closely their water and sodium losses during exercise; instead humans ideally drink according to thirst. We have survived precisely because we developed the appropriate biology.)

18 This is an interesting admission because it conflicts with the traditional Hiller and Laird theory and the position statement of the ACSM that Ironman triathletes competing in tropical climes develop EAH as a result of dehydration and large, unreplaced losses of sweat sodium chloride. Faster athletes are more likely to become dehydrated and so, according to all the evidence, would be protected from the development of EAH and EAHE.

These athletes with hyponatremia have often gained from their pre-race weight. Some athletes with hyponatremia, on the other hand, can also be dehydrated and volume depleted, having lost from their pre-race weight. This is probably due to partial replacement of sweat loss with hypotonic fluid. In my clinical experience, this hypovolemic type of hyponatremia is not as common as the hypervolemic type and is more often seen in faster runners who develop hyponatremia of exercise. (p. S16)[18]

Scott Montain (2008)

Dr. Scott Montain, who is the main instigator behind the USARIEM model of EAH, was also invited to publish an article in *Current Sports Medicine Reports* (2008). This particular issue of the journal, containing this paper, as well as that of Dr. Sallis and others, was widely distributed at no cost to all members of the ACSM in 2008. In his article, Dr. Montain again described his model and its predictions and concluded the following:

> Overdrinking, both in absolute (volume related) and relative forms (relative to sodium loss), predisposes individuals to EAH. The objective of fluid replacement should be to drink enough to prevent excessive dehydration (equivalent to >2% body mass loss) and never drink in excess of sweating rate. Individuals that secrete relatively salty sweat and participate in athletic events in excess of 6 h should consider inclusion of salt-containing food and drinks during the competition to attenuate the solute deficit that can accrue with multiple hours of continuous sweating. (p. S34)

This chapter explains why many of these statements are simply not true.

ACSM, ADA, and Dietitians of Canada (2009)

The joint position statement from the American College of Sports Medicine, American Dietetic Association, and Dietitians of Canada (2009) includes the following statement:

> Sodium is a critical electrolyte, particularly for athletes with high sweat sodium losses. . . . Many endurance athletes will require more than the UL for sodium (2.3 g/d). . . . Sports drinks containing sodium . . . are recommended for athletes especially in endurance events (>2 h). (p. 717)

Furthermore,

> hyponatremia (serum sodium concentration less than 130mmol/L) can result from prolonged, heavy sweating with failure to replace sodium, or excessive water intake. (p. 718)

There is of course no evidence that EAH can occur as a result of prolonged heavy sweating. Hence this statement, if evidence based, should have stated only that EAH is caused by excessive water intake.

Randy Eichner (2009)

In another article in *Current Sports Medicine Reports,* "Pearls and Pitfalls: Six Paths to Hyponatremia" (2009), Randy Eichner, MD, wrote that overdrinking during exercise, salty sweating, preventive drinking before exercise, forced or induced drinking, medicinal overhydration particularly during surgical interventions, or recreational overhydration as a result of beer drinking or in association with the use of the drug ecstasy are the six paths to hyponatremia (Eichner, 2009).

Thus, 18 years after we first proved that EAH is due to fluid overload and to which a sodium deficit plays no role, Dr. Eichner finally acknowledged that fluid overload is the common mechanism causing all forms of acute hyponatraemia. However, he still included salty sweating, which makes no contribution to the development of EAH and EAHE.

role in encouraging the U.S. military to *reduce* the high rates of fluid intake that USARIEM scientists had been advocating from 1982 to 1998 (Montain, Latzka, et al., 1999), developed one such model (Montain, Cheuvront, et al., 2006). Their model predicted that EAH caused by a developing sodium deficit could only ever develop under very specific circumstances (figure 9.11, page 274).

Figure 9.11*a* predicts that when drinking at 800 ml/hr (27 fl oz/hr), this athlete will always gain weight (panel A), causing his blood sodium concentration to fall progressively, reaching a value of 130 mmol/L (at which concentration significant

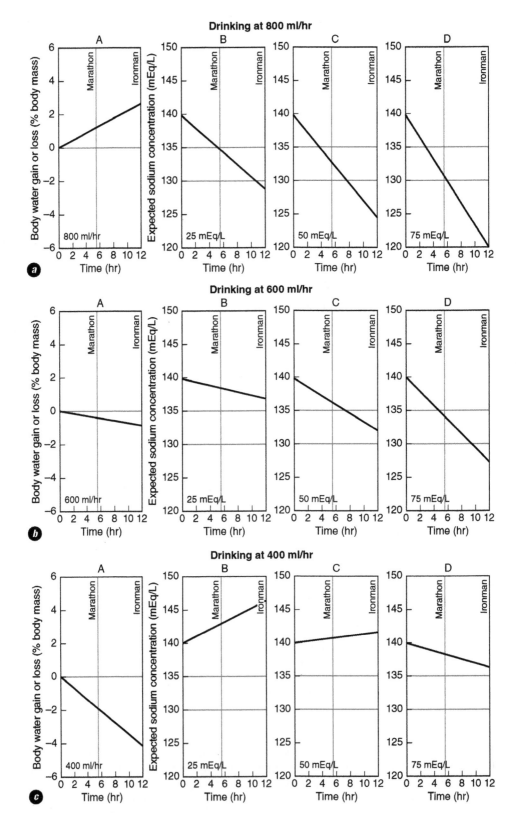

FIGURE 9.11 The model of factors causing EAH developed by the USARIEM exercise scientists predicts the duration of exercise required to produce EAH in a lean athlete of 70 kg running at 8.5 km/hr in cool conditions (18 °C) with sweat sodium concentrations of 25, 50, or 75 mmol/L. *(a)* Drinking at 800 ml/hr. *(b)* Drinking at 600 ml/hr. *(c)* Drinking at 400 ml/hr.

symptoms of EAHE are likely to occur) after about 10 hours if his sweat sodium concentration was 25 mmol/L (panel B); after about 8 hours if his sweat sodium concentration was 50 mmol/L (panel C); and after about 6 hours if his sweat sodium concentration was 75 mmol/L (panel D). This model requires that for any of these to happen, there can be no renal (kidney) compensation for overdrinking; that is, the athlete must also have SIADH and so is unable to excrete the excess fluid that in this example is the main cause of the EAH. In addition, this model ignores sodium losses in urine and assumes that the body has no mechanisms to curtail either sweat or urinary sodium losses during exercise. Instead, the model is catastrophic because it presumes that the body will simply continue to lose sodium without control until a catastrophic failure, even death, occurs.

Sweat sodium concentrations are dependent on dietary sodium intake (chapter 4) and can typically vary from 20 to 50 mmol/L. A value as high as 75 mmol/L in a trained athlete running ultramarathons would be uncommon because it would require that he habitually ingest an inordinate amount of salt to match what he was losing each day in his sweat. Another key weakness in this model is that the sodium lost in sweat during an ultramarathon is simply the excess that was ingested in the diet the day before and must be excreted to maintain daily sodium balance.

Figure 9.11b predicts that when drinking at 600 ml/hr (20.3 fl oz/hr), this athlete will lose very little weight so that even after 12 hours of running, he would have lost less than 1% of his body weight (panel A). If his sweat contained 25 mmol/L sodium, he could run for 12 hours without developing EAH (panel B). But if his sweat sodium concentration was 50 mmol/L, his blood sodium concentration would drop below 135 mmol/L after about 8 hours of running. If his sweat sodium concentration was 75 mmol/L, his blood sodium concentration would theoretically fall below 130 mmol/L after about 10 hours. This example predicts that dehydration and large sodium losses in sweat (and urine) can cause EAH. Other than this theoretical example, there is no evidence that these mechanisms cause EAH in humans. Nor is there evidence that many, if indeed any, healthy humans have such high sweat sodium concentrations.

Figure 9.11c predicts that when drinking at 400 ml/hr (13.5 fl oz/hr), this athlete will progressively lose weight (panel A) so that at the end of a marathon he would have lost about 2% of his body weight and about 4% at the end of an Ironman Triathlon. Such weight losses are quite mild in the Ironman Triathlon. This rate of drinking would cause his blood sodium concentration to rise progressively if his sweat sodium concentration was either 25 (panel B) or 50 mmol/L (panel C) but to fall somewhat if his sweat sodium concentration was 75 mmol/L (panel D). But according to this example, his blood sodium concentration would not drop below 135 mmol/L even after 12 hours of running (panel D), confirming that drinking at a rate less than the sweat rate so that a body weight loss of 2 to 4% is achieved prevents the development of EAH and EAHE.

Thus, a lean 70 kg (154 lb) athlete who drank at a rate of 400 ml/hr (13.5 fl oz/hr) would not develop EAH even if he ran for 12 hours (figure 9.11c). This, of course, fits with the experience in the South African and New Zealand Ironman Triathlons, in which athletes are encouraged to drink only to thirst and in which there is now a trivial incidence of EAH and EAHE. If the same athlete drank at 600 ml/hr, he would drop his blood sodium concentration to below 130 mmol/L, only if he ran for 9 hours and if his sweat sodium concentration was 75 mmol/L (figure 9.11b, panel D). Such a high sweat sodium concentration is highly improbable. In contrast, if the 70 kg athlete's sweat sodium concentration was either 25 or 50 mmol/L, values that are far more realistic and are in fact the values that the latest ACSM position stand considers to be correct, he would develop an equivalent degree of EAH only if he drank at a rate of 800 ml/hr or greater for 6 to 10 hours and gained weight progressively (figure 9.11*a*, panels B to D). But to gain this weight, the athlete would have to have SIADH. Without SIADH, the athlete drinking at 800 ml/hr would not have gained weight and so according to the USARIEM model would not have developed EAH.

Dr. Montain came to the following conclusions: ". . . drinking in excess of sweating rate rapidly can dilute plasma sodium, but drinking in excess of sweating is not the sole explanation for EAH.[19] Rather, it is overdrinking, both in its absolute (volume related) and relative forms (relative to sodium and potassium loss), that is the mechanism that leads to EAH" (Montain, 2008, p. S30).

19 But only according to their model. There is no published evidence showing that athletes with EAH have a sodium deficit that is greater than that achieved by control runners who do not develop EAH under the same exercise conditions (figure 9.10, page 265).

As result of this tortuous logic, the meaning of which is not entirely clear to me, Dr. Montain's practical conclusion was as follows: "As no single factor can be responsible for all EAH and, more importantly, symptomatic EAH cases, prevention strategies must consider the athletic event" (p. S30). In essence, athletes were encouraged not to overdrink in athletic events lasting less than 6 hours, whereas in longer-lasting exercise, "Individuals that secrete relatively salty sweat and participate in athletic events in excess of 6 h should consider inclusion of salt-containing foods and drinks during the competition to attenuate the solute deficit that can accrue with multiple hours of continuous sweating" (p. S34).

But the model and its predictions do not match what actually happens in the real world. Leaving aside for the moment our and Dr. Speedy's studies showing that a sodium deficit does not cause either EAH or EAHE, recall that Dr. Cynthia Lucero died from EAHE with a blood sodium concentration of 113 mmol/L even though she drank large amounts of Gatorade during the 2002 Boston Marathon. Indeed, the study of Almond, Shin, and colleagues (2005) found that the ingestion of Gatorade, although sodium containing, did not prevent the development of EAH in marathoners in the same race in which Dr. Lucero died. Thus, if they gained weight, it did not matter whether they drank Gatorade or water; the studied runners in the 2002 Boston Marathon were at risk of developing EAH if they overdrank enough to gain weight. All these studies show that weight gain is the single best predictor for the risk of developing EAH. Thus, it is clear that a single factor—specifically fluid retention—has been identified as the factor "responsible for all EAH and, more importantly, symptomatic EAH cases."

One can only wonder how a model that does not predict what actually happens in the real world could ever have been published in the scientific literature. A visual representation of the model is shown in figure 9.12*a*. The model as published in figure 9.11 was warmly embraced by the then-director of the GSSI, Dr. Bob Murray (2006), who complimented the authors for using a "unique and scientifically sound approach in developing a theoretical model to predict the development of hyponatremia under a variety of conditions" (p. 106). The report would also be widely quoted in articles originating from the GSSI and the ACSM because it

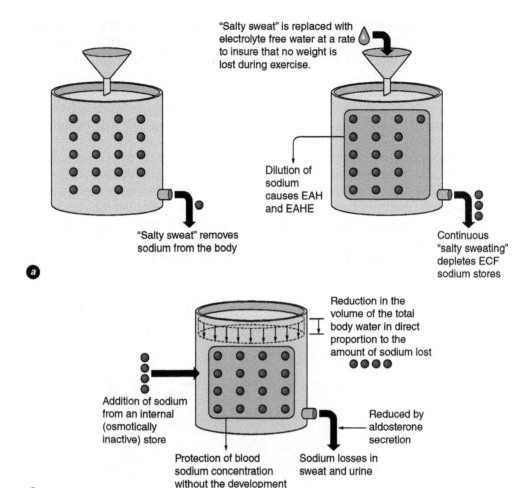

FIGURE 9.12 *(a)* The USARIEM model explaining how sodium deficiency leads to EAH and EAHE. This model uses the reservoir analogy to explain how the loss of sodium in sweat and its replacement with low-electrolyte-containing solutions like water will produce a progressive dilution of the ECF sodium concentrations. *(b)* The complex model that has evolved to ensure that humans can exercise for prolonged periods in dry heat while sweating profusely and regulating their blood sodium concentrations without developing EAH or EAHE.

"proved" that sodium deficiency contributes to EAH and that the ingestion of a sodium-containing sports drink like Gatorade can therefore prevent EAH.

The sodium deficiency predicted in figure 9.12a would develop in those who drink enough to prevent a reduction in body weight—in essence, who drink according to the 1996 ACSM guidelines, which advocates drinking to ensure that there is no loss of weight during exercise. In addition, Gatorade and other sports drinks contain less sodium (~18 mmol/L) than does the lowest sweat sodium concentration of 25 mmol/L used in this model. Thus, according to the predictions of this model, the ingestion of Gatorade must also lead to progressive hyponatremia during prolonged exercise.

Figure 9.12a is problematic for several additional reasons. First, the body does not regulate the volume of the reservoir; rather, it regulates the concentration of the electrolytes, especially sodium contained in the reservoir, the total body water. Second, the sweat sodium concentration is under hormonal control and is not constant during prolonged exercise. Should it so wish, the body can reduce its sodium losses in sweat during exercise by using the same hormones that regulate urinary sodium losses before, during, and after exercise. Third, it is probable that there are internal sodium stores that can be activated during exercise to balance sweat and urinary sodium losses should they threaten to cause the blood sodium concentrations to fall.

Figure 9.12*b* shows our model, which accurately predicts the blood sodium concentrations from experiments in which real data have already been collected from actual patients with EAH and EAHE. In this model, the size of the reservoir is not fixed, nor is it the primary variable that is regulated. Rather, the size of the reservoir is regulated to ensure that the concentration of the sodium it contains is held within a tight range of about 138 to 145mmol/L. When the concentration rises, thirst is generated, fluid is ingested, and the reservoir increases until its

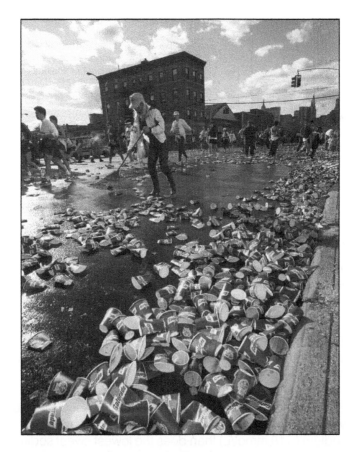

The false idea that high rates of fluid ingestion optimize performance and prevent heat stroke in marathon runners has led to a massive oversupply of sports drinks and water during these races. This in turn has contributed to the rise of cases of EAH and EAHE since 1981.
AP Photo/Kathy Willens

sodium concentration returns to the regulated range. This model also allows the amount of sodium lost in urine and sweat to be regulated by the action of specific hormones. In addition, if sweat and urine sodium losses are so excessive so that a reduction in the volume in the reservoir (to prevent the development of EAH) would threaten cardiovascular function, then additional sodium could be infused into the ECF from internal body stores found in bone or skin (Bergstrom and Wallace, 1954; Titze, Lang, et al., 2003). Conversely, addition of this sodium from internal body stores would explain why some athletes do not develop EAH even though they either maintain or increase the size of the reservoir by drinking to excess in the presence of SIADH. Abnormal fluid retention, not "massive" sodium losses, cause EAH and EAHE, which are therefore made worse, not prevented, by excessive fluid ingestion whether of water or a sports drink.

The body has evolved remarkable mechanisms for sodium conservation, and there is no reason to believe that these evolved either for a trivial reason or that they would not be activated if there was a real risk that a sodium deficit large enough to cause EAHE was in the process of developing (as required by the USARIEM model). By forcing humans to adopt a behavior for which our bodies were not designed—that is, full replacement of the fluid deficit as it develops, what I term immediate drinking—the scene was set for the development of EAH and EAHE in those athletes who followed this inappropriate behavior in response to the urgings of scientists who chose not to consider all the published evidence. Instead, they cherry-picked only the evidence that supported their preconceptions or biases.

Early Clues About Sodium Deficiency

Interestingly, 15 years earlier, Barr, Costill, and colleagues (1991) published a study that tested the prediction of Dr. Montain's model that an acute sodium deficiency can cause EAH and EAHE. This investigation was designed to differentiate between the two theories of what causes EAH: (a) excessive water intake and abnormal fluid shifts or (b) large losses of sodium through sweat and ingesting large volumes of low-sodium or sodium-free fluids.

In an attempt to differentiate between these two possibilities, Dr. Costill's group studied eight athletes who cycled for 6 hours at 55% of their maximum oxygen consumption while they drank, in random order, either nothing, plain water, or a 25 mmol/L sodium chloride solution, the latter two solutions at a rate that would prevent any weight loss during exercise. They found the following:

- When they did not ingest any fluid during exercise, subjects terminated exercise after about 4.5 hours, or 90 minutes before the trial was supposed to conclude.

- Their rectal temperatures at that point were ~39.0 °C. Thus, they did not stop because they were so hot that they were at risk of developing heatstroke. At that time, their rectal temperatures were about 1 °C above the values measured when they drank either water or the salt solution at rates sufficient to prevent any weight loss during exercise (figure 9.13, page 280).

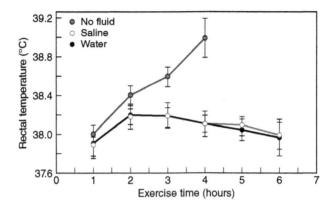

FIGURE 9.13 The rectal temperatures of athletes exercising for 6 hours when they ingested nothing, water, or a saline solution (Barr, Costill, et al., 1991). Note that the rectal temperatures of athletes who did not drink during exercise rose continuously during exercise and were about 1 °C higher than when the same athletes drank 1.15 L of fluid every hour during exercise. Athletes who did not drink terminated exercise about 90 minutes before the scheduled end of the exercise bout.

Reprinted, by permission, from S.I. Barr, D.L. Costill, and W.J. Fink, 1991, "Fluid replacement during prolonged exercise: Effects of water, saline, or no fluid," *Medicine & Science in Sports & Exercise* 23(7): 811-817.

- When they did not drink anything during exercise, subjects lost an average of 4.5 kg (9.9 lb), equivalent to an average body weight loss of 6.3%. According to the Wyndham and Strydom projections, at this level of dehydration their rectal temperatures should have been >41 °C (figure 3.1, page 61), not just 39 °C.

- Blood sodium concentrations *rose* in the group that did not ingest any fluids during exercise but *fell equally* (figure 9.14a) when either water or the salt solution was ingested during exercise. Thus, a sodium deficit cannot explain why athletes who do not ingest anything during exercise do *not* develop EAH.

  In figure 9.14a, note that the ingestion of the saline solution did not prevent a progressive fall in blood sodium concentrations essentially equal to what occurred when subjects ingested water at the same rate. This disproves the theory that the ingestion of a saline solution can prevent the development of EAH and EAHE.

  Figure 9.14c shows that sweat and urine sodium losses were lowest when no fluid was ingested during exercise. Overall sodium balance was lowest when saline was ingested during exercise but was greater when water was ingested during exercise than when no fluid was ingested. This is because fluid ingestion increased urinary sodium losses. The overall sodium deficit was unrelated to the blood sodium concentrations because the blood sodium concentrations rose when no fluid was ingested despite the large sodium deficit that developed. This again proves that a sodium deficit does not contribute materially to the development of EAH and EAHE during prolonged exercise.

- Rates of urine production were very different between trials (figure 9.14b). When drinking nothing, subjects essentially passed no urine. This would have been due to the increased blood osmolality activating AVP/ADH secretion causing complete water reabsorption by the kidneys.

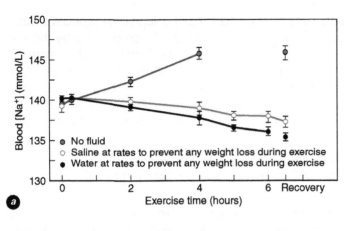

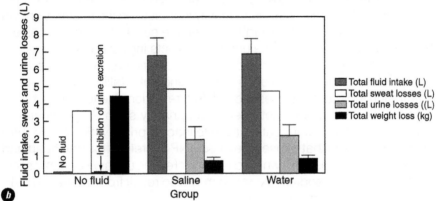

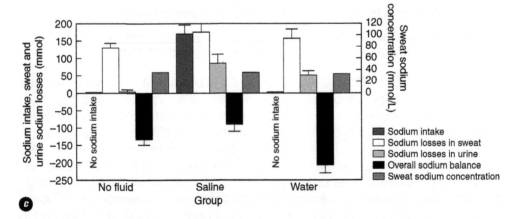

FIGURE 9.14 *(a)* Blood sodium concentrations rose when subjects did not drink anything during exercise but fell when they ingested water or a saline solution (25 mmol/L sodium chloride) at rates (1.1 5L/hr) to prevent any weight loss during exercise (Barr, Costill, et al., 1991). *(b)* Total fluid intake and sweat, urine, and total weight losses in the same three experimental conditions. Note that subjects who did not ingest any fluid during exercise did not pass any urine during 4.5 hr of exercise, whereas groups drinking enough to "prevent any weight loss during exercise" passed ~2 L of urine. *(c)* Total sodium intake, sweat and urinary sodium losses, overall sodium balance, and sweat sodium concentrations in the three experimental conditions.

(a) Reprinted, by permission, from S.I. Barr, D.L. Costill, and W.J. Fink, 1991, "Fluid replacement during prolonged exercise: Effects of water, saline, or no fluid," *Medicine & Science in Sports & Exercise* 23(7): 811-817. *(b, c)* Data from Barr, Costill, and Fink 1991.

In contrast, subjects passed 2.2 and 1.9 L of fluid in the respective water and saline trials (figure 9.14*b*). This would have been caused by the falling blood sodium concentrations and osmolalities inhibiting the secretion of AVP/ADH, allowing the passage of large volumes of urine necessary to "protect" the serum sodium concentration (figure 9.12*b*, page 277). But this response was not entirely effective because the blood sodium concentrations still fell in both these groups drinking to prevent any weight loss during exercise.

■ Subjects ingested about 6.9 L of water or the saline solution and passed about 2.0 L of urine so that 29% of the fluid they ingested was simply passed directly through the body as urine.

■ Because they passed large volumes of urine when ingesting enough fluid to maintain their body weight during exercise and because that urine contained sodium, urinary sodium losses were heavily increased in the heavily drinking groups (figure 9.14*c*) but were highest when the saline drink was ingested.

The presence of sodium in the urine of subjects ingesting either water or the saline solution indicates that none was salt deficient. Rather, the presence of sodium in the urine even in the presence of a falling blood sodium concentration indicates the presence of fluid retention due to levels of AVP/ADH in the blood that have not been appropriately suppressed since it is the increase in body water content (due to inappropriately high blood AVP/ADH concentrations) that causes elevated ANP secretion from the heart and brain (cerebral salt wasting), which directly increases urinary sodium losses. Inappropriate urinary sodium excretion may also result from increased AVP/ADH levels in the blood.

■ Sweat sodium losses were also highest in the group ingesting sodium and were lowest in the group that did not drink during exercise.

■ As a result, the net sodium deficit was only slightly lower in the group that ingested saline than in the other two groups (figure 9.14*c*).

The authors (Barr, Costill, et al., 1991) concluded that ". . . we would like to suggest that hyponatremia may be viewed as a syndrome and that both mechanisms proposed for its etiology *[i.e., sodium deficiency and abnormal fluid retention—my addition]* could be operative in different individuals" (p. 816). Even though their study showed that sweat sodium losses of 4.6 g "were not large enough to present a risk of hyponatremia during 6 h of exercise" yet "it is not inconceivable that cumulative sodium losses would be large enough to cause hyponatremia. . . . Accordingly, hyponatremia of exercise may occur in some individuals as a result of an abnormal response to fluid intake, and in others as a result of excessive sodium losses and low intakes, particularly over a period of several days" (pp. 816-817). They concluded that "sodium intake in amounts available in commercial beverages does not prevent a decrease in plasma sodium (*concentrations—in those who drink to maintain their body weight during prolonged exercise—my addition*). The results indicate that sodium replacement does not appear to be necessary during events of moderate intensity and 6h duration; nevertheless sodium losses were substantial" (p. 817).

I was so surprised by some of these authors' conclusions that I responded in a clinical commentary subsequently published in the same journal (Noakes, 1992b). I began by making the point that the only published study of sodium and water balance in patients with EAH and EAHE showed that the sodium chloride losses of runners who developed hyponatremia during a 90 km footrace were no greater than those of runners who maintained normal serum sodium concentrations during ultradistance foot races (Irving, Noakes, et al., 1991). Rather, the hyponatremia was associated with "retention of 3-5L of excess fluid ingested during exercise" (p. 403).

I next pointed out that their own data indicate "that fluid ingestion during exercise plays a critical role in the development of this condition, for the reason that serum sodium concentrations *rose* in their subjects who did *not* ingest fluid during exercise but *fell* equally in subjects who ingested fluid regardless of whether or not the fluid contained sodium" (p. 403). Thus, "far from preventing a fall in serum sodium concentrations during exercise, it was the fluid (and sodium) ingestion that actually caused serum sodium concentrations to fall during exercise. In addition, despite a less negative sodium balance, serum sodium concentrations in subjects who ingested saline were not higher than were those in subjects who ingested water" (p. 403).

"These findings are therefore not compatible with the interpretation that the hyponatremia of exercise is principally due to the development of a progressively increasing sodium chloride deficit during exercise" (p. 403). Now two decades later I finally understand what their data really did reveal.

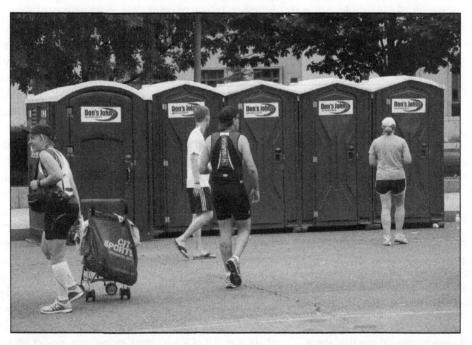

Athletes are often encouraged to drink before they are thirsty to ensure that their urine is clear. But drinking to the dictates of thirst both before and during exercise prevents excessive urine production as occurred in the study of Barr, Costill, et al., 1991.

The first finding, the importance of which I did not understand two decades ago, was the large volume of urine excreted when subjects tried to drink to replace all the weight they lost during exercise (figure 9.14*b*). There has to be a reason for this because the kidneys excreted essentially no urine in the no-drinking trial.

The logical explanation is that subjects excreted this fluid excess in order to regulate their blood sodium concentrations and osmolalities to ensure that their brains were not exposed to an excessive change in the osmolality of the blood. In the no-drinking condition, their high AVP/ADH concentrations resulting from the high blood sodium concentrations would have prevented any urine production. But when they drank more than they required even if the fluid contained sodium so that their blood sodium concentrations fell, they were (fortunately) able to reduce their AVP/ADH secretion just enough (since none of the tested subjects had full-blown SIADH) and so excrete most of the excess, preventing the development of EAHE. But because their blood sodium concentrations fell during exercise, they were not able to turn off AVP/ADH secretion appropriately so that they could excrete all the urine they needed to in order to prevent a fall in their blood sodium concentrations. As a result, their ECF volume increased out of proportion to its sodium content, causing blood sodium concentrations to fall progressively over 6 hours, reaching concentrations of ~136 mmol/L at the termination of exercise (figure 9.14*a*). This increase in body water content would have increased the secretion of ANP, increasing the loss of sodium in the urine (Leaf, 1962a; Leaf, 1962b).

But if any subjects had SIADH, their kidneys would have been unable to excrete that 2 L by which their fluid intake exceeded their requirement during exercise. As a result, EAH would have developed. In retrospect, it is perhaps profoundly unfortunate that none of these subjects had SIADH. If some had developed EAH or even EAHE when they drank enough "to prevent any weight loss during exercise" even with a drink containing some sodium, then the debate would have been resolved and there could never again have been any further argument of what causes EAH and EAHE during exercise. This randomized, controlled, prospective (intervention) trial would have established that EAH and EAHE are due to overdrinking in the presence of SIADH and to which sodium losses in sweat (and urine) play no part.

The second message hidden in the data was that during 6 hours of exercise humans must lose about 2 kg (4.4 lb) of weight if they wish to retain a state of normal fluid balance. This is shown by the "excess" urine excreted in the full- versus the no-fluid replacement trials. This seems to bolster the theory first proposed in the 1940s that the body has a fluid reserve of about 2 L (2 kg) that does not need to be replaced to prevent dehydration (Ladell, 1943; Ladell, 1947).[20]

20 A contentious topic in fluid replacement during exercise is whether or not a certain volume of water, about 2 L (Ladell, 1943; Ladell, 1947), can be lost from the body without requiring immediate (acute) replacement because it is a "reserve." This fluid may exist in the bowel as free water; a 700 kg camel may store 84 L of fluid in the gut (Macfarlane, Morris, et al., 1963). If the same applies to humans, the intestine of a 50 to 80 kg human could contain 2 to 4 L of free fluid. Free water may also accumulate with glycogen stored in muscle and the liver. This could be as much as 2.2 L in athletes who carbohydrate-load before competitive exercise (Olsson and Saltin, 1970). Ladell's (1955) inability to find any deleterious physiological effects of water losses of up to 2.5 L during exercise convinced him that about 2 L of water (equal to 2 kg of weight loss) does not need replacement during exercise.

The third message was that drinking fluid at high rates produces a substantial urinary sodium loss. Drinking water or the saline solution at high rates during exercise caused a loss of sodium in urine greater by 69 and 46 mmol, respectively, than when nothing was drunk. Similarly, sweat sodium losses were greatest when salt was ingested and lowest in the no-fluid trial.

This question then arises: Why does the body not extract all the sodium it can from sweat and urine to ensure that it minimizes sodium losses and maintains the blood sodium concentrations when subjects try to drink enough to prevent any weight loss during exercise? That the kidney is able to secrete a sodium-free urine when the dietary sodium intake is low is well established.

The answer is that this is the wrong question! Because in the short term, it is not the whole-body sodium balance that the kidney (or brain) is trying to protect; rather, it is the blood osmolality that must be regulated if life is to be preserved. So when the fluid intake exceeds requirement, the brain attempts to ensure that the kidney immediately excretes that fluid excess to ensure that the osmolality of the brain cells does not fall. But in this case, the human design seems not to be absolutely perfect because it is not able to respond perfectly to a fluid excess ingested during exercise. This would be entirely understandable if our evolutionary history designed us to exercise for prolonged periods in dry heat without ingesting much fluid (chapter 1). This exposure could not have prepared our physiology adequately for exercising in cool conditions when drinking to excess. The manner in which this *should* be achieved is by the complete suppression of AVP/ADH secretion. But AVP/ADH secretion is not regulated purely by changes in blood osmolality. As a result of the action of certain nonosmotic regulators of AVP/ADH secretion (see figure 4.2, page 110), the secretion of this hormone is not always completely suppressed as it should be when the serum osmolality and the blood sodium concentration fall.

In such a case, excess water will be retained and the amount of exchangeable sodium (and potassium) within the body will be insufficient to maintain the whole-body osmolality and the blood sodium concentration within the normal range, leading to EAH and EAHE. In summary, the true relevance of this study has never been appreciated. It showed already in 1991 that subjects who tried to drink to replace all the weight they lost during exercise were forced to excrete ~30% (2 L) of that fluid in order to prevent their blood sodium concentrations from falling too low. Since they could have completed that exercise without passing any urine, their rate of fluid intake was clearly too high by ~2 L. Presumably, the extra 2 L that they ingested was stored in some exchangeable fluid reserve that does not need to be filled in order to maintain sodium and fluid homeostasis during exercise. This is in keeping with the theory that the body has a 2 L fluid reservoir that does not need to be replaced acutely during exercise.

Unfortunately, the authors (Barr, Costill, et al., 1991) concluded that athletes should be advised "to replace fluid in no more than amounts lost" (p. 816). This advice, incorporated into the 1996 ACSM guidelines, might have encourage some athletes to overdrink during exercise, potentially with dire consequences.

Then they also showed that the ingestion of a salt-containing drink does not influence the extent to which the blood sodium concentration falls during prolonged exercise in those who drink to excess so that sodium intake in amounts available in commercial beverages does not prevent a decrease in plasma sodium. Since blood sodium concentrations rose substantially (figure 9.14*a*, page 281) when nothing was drunk during exercise, the authors were correct to conclude that sodium losses of the magnitude they measured did not present "a risk of hyponatremia" (p. 816).

The reason these authors and many others have missed this truth is that they have tried to reduce the complex biological regulation of the blood sodium concentration to the effects of a single variable, in this case the amount of sodium lost in sweat or ingested during exercise. But the problem is not one of sodium balance but one of fluid balance in those whose kidneys are unable to excrete a fluid excess when their blood sodium concentrations and osmolalities are falling. The primary error that causes EAH and EAHE lies in the behavior that produces overdrinking in association with abnormal regulation of AVP/ADH secretion by the brain. Ultimately, it is the brain that causes EAH and EAHE.

International EAH Consensus Development Conference

In our minds, we had already proven in 1991 that EAH and EAHE are both caused by abnormal fluid retention in athletes who drink to excess during and sometimes after exercise lasting at least 4 hours. We were also certain that sweat sodium losses played no significant role.

Perhaps because we were so frustrated that what seemed very obvious to us was still not being conveyed to the athletic population even though fatal cases of EAHE continued to occur, in March 2005 we convened the 1st International Exercise-Associated Hyponatremia Consensus Development Conference at the Sports Science Institute of South Africa in Cape Town. After 2 days of deliberations, the conference arrived at the following consensus (Hew-Butler, Almond, et al., 2005):

> Current evidence strongly indicates that EAH is a dilutional hyponatremia, caused by an increase in total body water relative to the amount of total body exchangeable sodium. . . . The primary etiologic factor appears to be the consumption of hypotonic fluids (water or sports drinks) in excess of . . . fluid losses. (p. 209)
>
> Therefore, it follows, that any individual participating in endurance exercise, . . . should avoid overconsumption of fluids. (p. 210)
>
> . . . to insure that weight gain does not occur during exercise: [athletes should] (1) drink only according to thirst (i.e., ad libitum) or (2) use the USATF guidelines, or analogous methods, to estimate hourly sweat losses during exercise and to avoid consuming amounts greater than this during endurance exercise events. (p. 210)
>
> There is no currently available evidence to support the suggestion that sodium supplementation prevents the development of EAH nor is there any evidence that consumption of electrolyte-containing hypotonic fluids (i.e., sports drinks) can prevent the development of EAH in athletes who drink to excess (p. 211).
>
> Strategies aimed at preventing the over consumption of hypotonic fluids (water or sports drinks) . . . need to be communicated to coaches and athletes. . . . Aid stations should be placed at appropriate distanced intervals. . . . Medical directors should ensure the availability of onsite sodium analysis to screen for EAH before medical treatment is initiated. (p. 211)

I learned two critical lessons from the interaction with these world authorities. First from Professor Joe Verbalis, I finally learned why athletes are unable to excrete the water excess that they must accumulate to develop EAH and EAHE. He used some of our own data to make the point.

In papers published in 2001 (Noakes, 2001b; Noakes, Wilson, et al., 2001) we showed that at rest, humans are able to excrete urine at rates of ~800 ml/hr. This was confirmed by Dr. Speedy's group, who showed that triathletes who had developed EAH or EAHE in previous New Zealand Ironman Triathlons were able to excrete, at rest, urine at similarly high rates that were not different from rates measured in control triathletes who had finished the same Ironman Triathlon without developing EAH (Speedy, Noakes, et al., 2001a). From other studies undertaken by Dr. Tony Irving, we also knew that rates of urine production during marathon and ultramarathon running are not different and are certainly not lower than rates measured at rest (Irving, Noakes, et al., 1986; Irving, Noakes, et al., 1990a). Together these data suggested that *(a)* a reduced rate of urine production is not an expected consequence of prolonged exercise and *(b)* renal function of athletes who develop EAH and EAHE is normal during the first 24 to 48 hours of recovery (Irving, Noakes, et al., 1991) or when studied some weeks later (Speedy, Noakes, et al., 2001a).

Dr. Verbalis posed this question: Why do athletes with EAH and EAHE not excrete the fluid excess before it accumulates since their normal renal function (which should not be affected by exercise) should be able comfortably to excrete any excess even in athletes drinking 1,800 ml per hour (since they could easily lose up to 1,000 ml/hr as sweat and another 800 ml/hr as urine)? The answer, he said, is that they have SIADH (Baylis, 2003; Hew-Butler, 2010), a condition about which he is an acknowledged world authority—with which the scales that had hidden the obvious from my eyes for 24 years suddenly disappeared (see box 8.2, page 239).

Dr. Louise Weschler provided the second critical piece of information. She had just published an extensive mathematical review (2005) of the probable causes of EAH and EAHE, concluding that "fluid overload predominates over electrolyte loss in the etiology of exercise-associated hyponatremia (EAH) and why the excretion of electrolyte-dilute urine is highly effective in correcting EAH. . . . Sports drinks will, if overconsumed, result in hyponatremia. Administration of a sports drink to an athlete with fluid overload hyponatremia further lowers the plasma sodium concentration and increases fluid overload. Administration of either a sports drink or normal (0.9%) saline increases fluid overload" (p. 899).

Weschler (2006) introduced me to the (still not universally accepted) concept of the osmotically inactive sodium stores of which I had previously been ignorant. It appears that in humans, as in other mammals, only about 68% of the sodium in the body exists in an exchangeable pool that is detectable by radio-labeled tracers in living humans (Forbes and Lewis, 1956). Whereas the exchangeable sodium concentration so measured in live humans is about 55 mmol/kg, the concentration of sodium directly extracted from human cadavers is higher, 60 to 70 mmol/kg. Total exchangeable sodium in a 57 kg (126 lb) female would then be 3,135 mmol, whereas the total amount of sodium in her body would be closer to 3,990 mmol or perhaps even higher, even up to 5,000 mmol (Garnett, Ford, et al., 1968). If her ECF volume was 12 L, then the total amount of osmotically active sodium it would contain would be only 1,680 mmol, or 54% of her exchangeable sodium but only 42% of her total body sodium stores. This indicates that there is more than enough sodium in the body to prevent the development of EAH. But the sodium must be activated for it to be of any value. Conversely, the inappropriate inactivation of circulating ionized sodium and storage in the osmotically inactive stores would worsen EAH, as perhaps happened in the case of Cynthia Lucero.

When I first concluded that sweat sodium losses were not sufficient to produce EAH or EAHE (table 8.1, page 238) unless there were also additional unrecognized losses (Noakes, Goodwin, et al., 1985), I wondered whether perhaps sodium could be temporarily displaced within the body into what is known as a "third space." Dr. Weschler's suggestion of the possible existence of an osmotically inactive sodium store within the body raised this question: Could this be the repository of the extra sodium "loss" necessary to explain the development of EAH and EAHE in those who had not lost sufficient sodium in their sweat or urine to lower their blood sodium concentrations below 135 mmol/L during prolonged exercise?

Another important outcome of the 1st International EAH Consensus Development Conference was our decision to pool all our data in which we had measured body weight changes during, and blood sodium concentrations after, various long-distance sporting events, including marathons, ultramarathons, long-distance cycling races, and Ironman triathlons. We were able to collect data on 2,135 individual sporting performances (Noakes, Sharwood, et al., 2005).

When we plotted the postrace blood sodium concentrations against the weight change during the race for all those data (figure 9.15), we again found, not unexpectedly, that the postrace blood sodium concentration was a linear function of the body weight change during exercise. But our closer examination of those data led

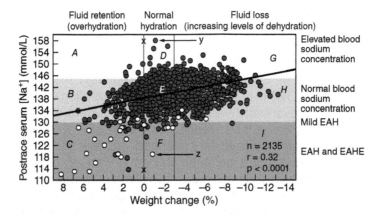

FIGURE 9.15 Data of 2,153 individual athletic performances in marathon and ultramarathon running races, Ironman triathlons, and long-distance cycling events showed the usual linear relationship with a negative slope between body weight change during the race and the postrace blood sodium concentration. Notice the wide range in individual responses. Clear dots represent athletes with severe EAHE, most of whom would have required hospital treatment.

Adapted from T.D. Noakes, K. Sharwood, D. Speedy, et al., 2006, "Three independent biological mechanisms cause exercise-associated hyponatremia: Evidence from 2,135 weighed competitive athletic performances," *PNAS* 102(51): 18550-18555. Copyright © National Academy of Sciences, U.S.A.

to the conclusion that three independent biological mechanisms must be present to cause EAH or EAHE to develop in any person during prolonged exercise.

The data in figure 9.15 predict that to maintain a normal blood sodium concentration of 140 mmol/L, an athlete would need to lose about 2% body weight during exercise. The most serious cases of EAHE occurred in block C of figure 9.15 in those athletes who had gained the most weight. In contrast, athletes with elevated blood sodium concentrations (hypernatremia) were found in block G (athletes who lost the most weight during exercise). Therefore, the data confirmed what we had speculated in 1985 and had already proven in 1991 (figure 9.1, page 247) that EAH and EAHE becomes increasingly more probable in athletes who lose the least weight or who gain weight during prolonged exercise. As a result, we were able to show that no cases of EAH occurred in any athlete who lost more than 6% of body weight during these races, whereas athletes who gained more than 4% body weight during exercise had 45% and 85% probabilities of developing EAHE and EAH, respectively (figure 9.16). These data look remarkably similar to those that Chris Almond and colleagues collected at the 2002 Boston Marathon (figure 9.7, page 254).

These data again disprove the theory first proposed by Dr. Doug Hiller and colleagues that dehydration causes EAH and EAHE since no one who lost 6% or more of their body weight during any of these races developed EAH.

We concluded that deliberate and sustained overdrinking is the first biological mechanism necessary to cause EAH and EAHE. But without SIADH, this overdrinking would not cause an increase in body weight; rather, the fluid would simply be excreted during exercise, causing the athlete to spend valuable time searching for appropriate places to pass urine. Presumably overdrinking is a self-limiting process in athletes without SIADH because those athletes must soon realize that their drinking behavior hardly aids their performance, and it simply causes them

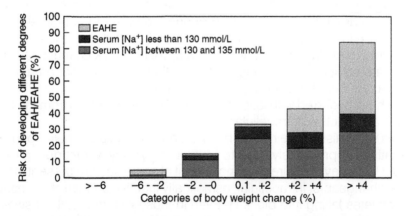

FIGURE 9.16 The probability of developing different levels of EAH according to body weight change during exercise. The data for this figure come from figure 9.15. There was a 0% prevalence of EAH in athletes who lost more than 6% of their body weight during prolonged exercise. Increasing levels of weight gain were associated with increasing probability that EAH or EAHE of increasing severity would develop: 80% of those athletes who reduced their blood sodium concentrations below 135 mmol/L increased their body weights by more than 4%. Similarly, 45% of those athletes with symptomatic EAHE increased their body weights by more than 4%.

Data from Noakes, Sharwood, Speedy, et al., 2005.

to waste time passing urine at the side of the road. SIADH is the second biological mechanism necessary to cause EAH and EAHE in athletes who voluntarily overdrink during prolonged exercise.

Closer examination of individual responses in figure 9.15 disclosed a third possible biological mechanism necessary to cause EAH and EAHE. We noticed that there was a remarkable range in the individual responses of blood sodium concentrations to similar changes in body weight. Subjects arrowed as Y and Z in figure 9.15 both lost ~0.5% of their body weight during these races. But their postrace blood sodium concentrations differed by ~34 mmol/L. If both had the same total body water after the race, athlete Z with the lower postrace blood sodium concentration must have lost approximately 1,360 mmoles more sodium (31 g of sodium or 80 g of salt) than athlete Y. It seems improbable that this difference could be explained purely by higher sweat sodium losses in athlete Y or a greater sodium intake during the race by athlete Z, or some combination of both. Something else appears to be involved

In addition, we found that only 69 (30%) of the 231 athletes who gained weight during the race (subjects to the left of line x-x in figure 9.15) developed EAH or EAHE. Thus, another factor protected 70% of those who overdrank and gained weight during exercise (because they also had SIADH) from developing EAH or EAHE.

On the basis of this and other evidence, we therefore speculated that the third factor that will determine whether EAH or EAHE develops in those who overdrink during exercise and who gain weight because they have SIADH is either the loss into or gain of ECF sodium from a "third space," in this case, the intracellular, osmotically inactive exchangeable sodium stores. Thus, "The only possibility is that some athletes can mobilize . . . sodium from internal sodium stores, the so-called exchangeable sodium stores (Nguyen and Kurtz, 2004). Alternatively, some athletes may prevent the inappropriate osmotic inactivation of sodium during exercise" (Noakes, Sharwood, Speedy, et al., 2005, p. 18554).

Referring back to figure 9.15, athletes who finished in blocks A and B because they both overdrank and retained fluid during the race did not develop EAH or EAHE because they were able to mobilize sodium from the intracellular, exchangeable sodium stores. In contrast, athletes with EAHE (block C) must have had an inappropriate sodium response to SIADH so that there was not an appropriate entry of sodium from the exchangeable stores into the ECF. In fact, the reverse may even have occurred with loss of osmotically active sodium from the ECF into an osmotically inactive, intracellular store.

Athletes who finished the race in blocks E and H regulated their blood sodium concentrations appropriately despite some loss of body weight during exercise. This would likely have required the movement of some sodium present in the ECF into the exchangeable, intracellular, osmotically inactive sodium store, especially in those athletes falling into block H. Even in those with the "saltiest sweat," the magnitude of the sweat sodium losses during exercise would not have been sufficient to prevent a rise in blood sodium concentrations during exercise in those athletes in block H. Thus, athletes who finished those races in blocks D and G must have been unable to translocate sufficient osmotically active sodium from the ECF into the osmotically inactive intracellular sodium stores in order to maintain normal blood sodium concentrations.

In contrast, athletes who finished with reduced blood sodium concentrations even though they lost some weight during exercise (blocks F and I) may also have abnormal regulation of the exchangeable body sodium stores with the translocation of some sodium from the ECF into the intracellular osmotically inactive stores, causing EAH. The USARIEM model (figures 9.11 and 9.12, pages 274 and 277), which does not consider most of these influences, argues that athletes who finish prolonged exercise in blocks F and I do so because of dehydration and large unreplaced sweat sodium losses.

In summary, we concluded that EAH and EAHE will occur only in those who overdrink persistently during prolonged exercise (figure 9.16); who also have SIADH or some related condition that prevents the development of a normal diuresis in response to persistent overdrinking; and who osmotically inactivate circulating sodium, storing it in an osmotically inactive, intracellular store. More recently we have suggested that genetic factors may also influence drinking behaviors during exercise. The Second International Exercise-Associated Hyponatremia Consensus Development Conference held in Queensland, New Zealand, in November 2007 confirmed these conclusions and emphasized the importance of appropriate acute management of those with EAHE (Hew-Butler, Ayus, et al., 2008).

Finally this question may be asked: If dehydration and sodium deficiency did indeed cause EAH and EAHE, what would be the nature of the relationship between body weight changes during exercise and the postrace blood sodium concentrations? The answer is shown in figure 9.17. Instead of a straight-line relationship, the line describing this relationship would be in the form of an inverted U, with low blood sodium concentrations in those who are either dehydrated or overhydrated.

The fact that this relationship cannot be found in data from 2,153 individual athletic performances in marathon and ultramarathon races, in Ironman triathlons, and in endurance cycling races confirms that the existence of a separate condition of EAH and EAHE caused by dehydration and salt losses is simply a myth sustained by the sports drink industry and its scientists.

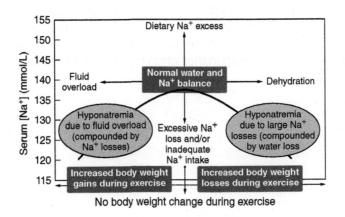

FIGURE 9.17 If EAH and EAHE can be caused by either overhydration or by dehydration with large sodium chloride losses in sweat and urine, then the relationship between body weight change and the postexercise blood sodium concentration would be in the form of an inverted U. But this does not happen.

Summary

The evidence presented here is absolutely conclusive: EAH and EAHE occur only in predisposed individuals when they ingest fluid to excess during prolonged exercise, usually lasting more than 4 hours. There is no original evidence that a sodium deficiency contributes to the development of either condition. The only such "evidence" is based on a biological model that is implausible and does not explain the observed phenomena.

It is more likely that internal movement of sodium to an exchangeable store makes it appear *as if* sodium losses in sweat could contribute to the development of EAH and EAHE.

Since neither EAH nor EAHE can occur unless there is SIADH (or similar but perhaps yet unrecognized conditions that produce the same outcome by preventing water excretion when the blood osmolality falls), then it follows that the only way to prevent the condition is to prevent SIADH during exercise. There is currently no practical mechanism for achieving this, although the first class of drugs that partially block the action of AVP/ADH on the kidney tubules is being developed (Verbalis, 2002).

But the use of this or any other drug is unnecessary because the most effective way to prevent EAH and EAHE is to ensure that predisposed individuals do not overdrink during prolonged exercise. This is not merely a theoretical concept. It has been proven. The incidence of EAH and EAHE was reduced in the New Zealand Ironman Triathlon when triathletes were encouraged to drink less and when fewer aid stations were provided on both the cycling and the running legs of the triathlon.

Similarly, the incidence of EAH and EAHE in the 90 km South African Comrades Marathon, the race in which the condition was first described, is now negligible despite the fact that the race lasts for 12 hours and includes ~10,000 runners. Had this race been held in the United States in 2002, when the incidence of EAH in the Boston Marathon was 13%, perhaps as many as 25% of the field, close to 2,500 Comrades Marathon runners might have developed EAH and EAHE, a catastrophe of unimaginable proportions. The sole conclusion must be that the epidemic of EAH and EAHE that struck especially North America in the 1990s was created by factors that caused those at risk to drink to excess during exercise, whether they were participating in marathon running, triathlons, or hiking or were serving in the U.S. military.

CHAPTER 10

EAH and EAHE on a Global Scale

Funny how we solve one problem—dehydration, and people go overboard and create another problem. The pendulum swings from one direction to the other—dehydration to overhydration.

John Sutton, MD, PhD, president of the American College of Sports Medicine, 1986-1987

Six months after the 2002 Boston Marathon, Hilary Anne Bellamy, a 35-year-old mother of two and first-time marathon runner, collapsed into the arms of her husband at the 33 km (20.5 mile) mark of the 2002 Marine Corps Marathon held in Washington, DC (Thompson and Wolff, 2003). Bellamy had prepared for some months with an organized training group and was running to raise funds for the National AIDS Marathon Training Program sponsored by the Whitman Walker Clinic. She did not miss a single training session. She always kept a water bottle on her desk at work "because she was quite aware of the dangerous effects of dehydration over the course of 26-plus miles. . . . Bellamy followed her training regimen, apparently drinking as much as she could hold" (Nearman, 2003, p. 1). Apparently she had never been warned that overdrinking during exercise can be fatal. Rather, she had been advised to drink ahead of thirst—"as much as she could hold."

Bellamy was a political activist who wrote policy research reports for Health Systems Resources, Inc., in Washington, DC. Her reports focused on the lack of access to medical care for children and the elderly in her district.

She had planned to finish the marathon in 5:45:50 (a pace of 13 minutes a mile or ~8 minutes per km). On the course, aid stations were placed every 2 miles, allowing athletes ample opportunity to drink as much as they could hold. In the race she reached halfway in 2:32:55, slowing slightly to reach the 18-mile (29 km) mark in 4:02:19. At mile 19 (30 km) she complained that she had a bad headache and blurred vision. She ran another mile before she left the course, where she collapsed in the company of her husband, her brother, her 3-year-old daughter, and her 9-month-old son.

The trip to the hospital took 2 hours, during which she was treated with oxygen and 0.9% normal saline by the medical personnel who "originally believed that she was suffering from a heat casualty" (Nearman, 2003, p. 2) even though her blood pressure was elevated (178/102 mmHg) and her pulse was 62 bpm, indicating that her cardiovascular system was functioning effectively. Since she was not in a state of shock, her condition did not need to be "improved" by intravenous fluids.

On hospital admission 2 hours after her collapse, she was conscious enough "only to state her name and follow simple instructions" (Nearman, 2003, p. 2); her blood sodium concentration was 123 mmol/L. Her mental status rapidly deteriorated; she had pulmonary edema, abnormal heart rhythms, and respiratory failure requiring mechanical ventilation. Within another 30 minutes she developed fixed, dilated pupils.

A brain scan indicated diffuse brain swelling causing compression of vital brain structures. Because there was no evidence for higher brain function, she was declared brain dead approximately 30 hours after she had begun a race for which she had trained diligently, had been in apparently perfect health, and had every prospect of a long and fulfilling life. She died even though she drank exactly as she had been advised during the race. A blood sample analyzed subsequent to her death revealed a blood AVP concentration of 6.7 picograms per milliliter (pg/ml), confirming the presence of SIADH.

As a result of the deaths of Cynthia Lucero and Hilary Bellamy, prior to the 2003 Boston Marathon, the Boston Athletic Association issued 20,000 pamphlets advising runners to "Drink to stay hydrated, don't overdrink" (Nearman, 2003, p. 2). This was exactly the advice we had first proposed 18 years earlier. Indeed, Dr. Joe Verbalis commented, "If she had followed the guidelines adopted by the USA Track and Field in April [2003] she wouldn't have had this problem. All these cases could have been prevented. The guidelines weren't available at the time" (p. 1).

The full-length paper describing our first four cases of EAH was submitted in May 1984 and published in *Medicine and Science in Sports and Exercise* (MSSE) in March 1985 (Noakes, Goodwin, et al., 1985).[1] At the time, I thought it would only ever be an interesting medical curiosity: Why ever would other athletes wish to overdrink in the future?

1 This paper would ultimately become a "citation classic," having been quoted more than 100 times in the scientific literature by 2007. It was reprinted in full in 2005 in *Wilderness Medicine* (Noakes, Goodwin, et al., 2005) with an accompanying editorial (Rogers I.R., 2005). In that editorial, Australian emergency medicine physician Ian Rogers wrote, "The detailed description, accompanied by an erudite discussion, predicted the outcomes of much of the research that followed over the next two decades—research that has now elucidated the epidemiology, etiology and preventive strategies for exercise-associated hyponatremia" (p. 219). He concluded by adding, "Tim Noakes was right in 1985, and the passage of two decades has done nothing to diminish the accuracy of his conclusions."

But, as described in chapter 9, debate ensued in the scientific literature and athletes were sent mixed messages, the loudest of which was to drink as much as could be tolerated. The deaths of Hilary Bellamy and others, along with the thousands of incidents of EAH and EAHE, illustrate that the scientific community failed to serve the needs of athletes.

Figure 10.1a shows the cumulative annual incidence of EAH and EAHE as best as I could trace it. These cases are listed in appendix B and were either reported in the scientific literature at the time of this writing (September 2010), had been documented in the Ironman Hawaii Triathlon from 1983 to 1998, or had come to my attention in other ways. It is likely that many other cases occurred but were not identified or reported. Figure 10.1b shows the growth in sales of Gatorade during a similar period.

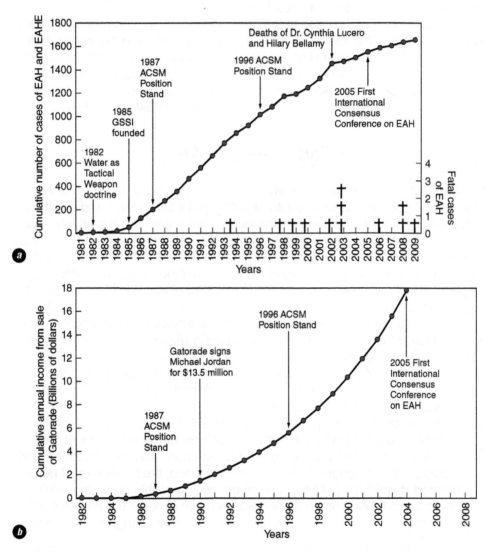

FIGURE 10.1 (a) The cumulative annual incidence of EAH and EAHE based on the data reported in appendix B. (b) The cumulative annual income ($18 billion) from the sale of Gatorade from 1982 to 2006.

(b) Data from D. Rovell 2005.

As can be seen in figure 10.1, the number of cases of EAH and EAHE reported annually accelerated after 1984 and began to decrease after 1998, perhaps because I was unable to access data on the number of cases of EAH and EAHE in the Ironman Hawaii Triathlon after 1998. Notwithstanding that consideration, there is a clear decline in the rate at which new cases of EAH and EAHE were reported after 2002. Sadly, 8 of 12 fatalities occurred after 2000 just as the epidemic had reached its peak. Cynthia Lucero died in 2002; the First International Consensus Conference on EAH was held in 2005 shortly after the publication of the paper of Almond, Shin, and colleagues (2005), showing that the incidence of EAH in the 2002 Boston Marathon was 13%. The graph suggests that it was the deaths of Cynthia Lucero and Hilary Bellamy that finally turned the tide and that the First International Consensus Conference on EAH in 2005 happened after the annual incidence of the condition had already peaked.

Note that the rate of increase in the cumulative number of cases of EAH and EAHE accelerated after the founding of the GSSI in 1987 and the publication of the 1987 ACSM position stand but was little affected by the publication of the 1996 ACSM position stand. It is important to remember that the finding that two events occur simultaneously does not prove causation. In fact, the sales of Gatorade grew faster in this time than did the number of cases of EAH and EAHE.

Early Cases of EAH

The May 1985 issue of MSSE, in which our first full-length paper on EAH was published in March, included an abstract written by Dr. Doug Hiller and colleagues (1985). They reported blood sodium concentrations measured in triathletes competing in a standard (52 km) triathlon, in an 8-hour laboratory simulation of an Ironman triathlon (5 hours cycling, 3 hours running), and in the actual Ironman Hawaii Triathlon. Whereas all the pre- and postevent blood sodium concentrations were normal in the first two events, 20% (27 of 136) of Ironman Hawaii triathletes had postrace blood sodium concentrations below 135 mmol/L, diagnostic of EAH. The authors did not report whether or not these athletes had symptoms. They also suggested that Ironman triathletes requiring medical care should receive intravenous solution containing glucose and 0.9% sodium chloride. Dr. Hiller and his coauthors, Drs. Mary O'Toole and Bob Laird, would become firm advocates of the theory that athletes with EAH are dehydrated and must be treated with intravenous sodium chloride solutions.

Because, as shown in the previous chapters, EAH is due to fluid retention, not to dehydration, treatment in the form of administering intravenous sodium chloride solutions is incorrect and potentially very dangerous. Although treatment with intravenous sodium chloride solution is recommended, the solution must be very concentrated (hypertonic): At the time of the writing of this book, the advice is that subjects with EAHE should immediately receive either a 100 ml bolus of 3% hypertonic saline intravenously or an amount of 1 ml per kilogram body weight per hour.

The next reported cases of EAHE occurred in the Fifth Annual American Medical Joggers Association (AMJA) 80/100 km Ultramarathon in Chicago on 2 October 1983 (Frizzell, Lang, et al., 1986). Dr. Tyler Frizzell, then a 24-year-old medical student, finished second in the 100 km (62 mile) ultramarathon in a time of 8:36. He had drunk approximately 300 ml (10 fl oz) at each of the aid stations, which, as in the case of the 1981 Comrades Marathon, were placed 1.6 km (1 mile) apart. His estimated total fluid intake during the race was 20 L. Immediately on completing the race, he became disorientated and was admitted to the hospital, where his blood sodium concentration was found to be 123 mmol/L. He was treated with an intravenous infusion of 0.9% NaCl; shortly thereafter he had a grand mal epileptic seizure and stopped breathing transiently. He remained in a semicoma for 36 hours before regaining consciousness. He was discharged from the hospital only 5 days after admission. His recovery rate was similar to those of our index cases who were treated with the same isotonic NaCl solution.

In the same race, Atlanta physician Bob Lathan also drank 240 to 360 ml at each aid station and walked the last 24 km of the 80 km race. His total fluid intake during the race was estimated at about 24 L in the 10:36 that he required to complete the distance. Thirty minutes after completing the race, he became disoriented and confused with slurred speech and was admitted to the hospital; his blood sodium concentration was found to be 118 mmol/L. He was treated with a hypertonic (3%) saline solution intravenously. This treatment resulted in a net excess fluid loss from the body of 2,000 ml (67.6 fl oz.) within 8 hours, by which time his blood sodium concentration had normalized and he was fully conscious. He was discharged from the hospital after 8 hours in the emergency room, a very rapid recovery compared to those experienced by Dr. Frizzell and the three most seriously affected athletes in our original study (Noakes, Goodwin, et al., 1985). Dr. Lathan was back at work in his Atlanta medical practice within 24 hours of finishing the AMJA ultramarathon.

Athletes in that race were encouraged to "push fluids" and "to drink more than their thirst dictates, since thirst may be an unreliable index of fluid needs during exercise" (Frizzell, Lang, et al., 1986, p. 774). Guidelines for that specific race recommended that runners drink 300 to 360 ml of fluid at each aid station. For an athlete running at world-record pace (~16 km/hr), this advice would have produced rates of fluid intake of 3.0 to 3.6 L/hr. The authors, who were initially unaware of our 1985 paper, nevertheless drew essentially the same conclusions as we had: "The two runners consumed such large quantities of free water during the race that apparent water intoxication developed. . . . The hyponatremia was caused primarily by increased intake and retention of dilute fluids and contributed to by excessive sweat sodium loss" (p. 772). The authors referred to three other cases of EAH in North American ultramarathon runners competing in the 1984 Western States 100-mile (160 km) endurance run in the Sierra Nevadas and an 80 km ultramarathon near Sacramento, California.

Nine of the 12 runners admitted to the hospital after the 1985 Comrades Marathon were reportedly suffering from overhydration (Godlonton, 1985). One of these patients, a 28-year-old female, was admitted in a coma, with both pupils dilated and her eyes deviated to the left, indicating that she was within minutes of dying. Her blood sodium concentration was 112 mmol/L, one of the lowest values yet reported in an endurance athlete who survived. The clinical diagnosis was severe EAHE with imminent "coning" of that part of the brain, the cerebellum, that lies directly above the large opening at the base of the skull, the foramen magnum. Protrusion of the cerebellum through the foramen magnum is uniformly fatal.

Treated intravenously with diuretics, hyperosmolar mannitol (20%), and hypertonic (5%) saline solutions to reduce brain swelling, she regained consciousness within 24 hours after hospital admission, and her blood sodium concentration returned to normal within 48 hours. For a patient at death's door and in whom any minor diagnostic or therapeutic error would have proved fatal, this was an exceptional outcome. The runner estimated that she drank 13 L (439.6 fl oz) during the Comrades marathon. During the first 48 hours in the hospital, she passed 9.5 L of urine (200 ml/hr). Her intake was not measured but was likely much less than 9.5 L, probably more like 2 to 4 L, the more usual rate at which fluid is provided to unconscious patients in the hospital. If correct, this would suggest that she was overhydrated by at least 6 kg (13.2 lb, or ~10% BW) when she collapsed after the race.

Studies at the medical tent at the finish of the 1986 and 1987 Comrades Marathons revealed that 10 and 34 runners finished those respective races with blood sodium concentrations less than 135 mmol/L; 14 were below 127 mmol/L after the 1987 race. On the basis of these data, we (Noakes, Norman, et al., 1990) concluded that EAH developed in approximately 0.3% of all the starters in that race.

In chapter 9 I described the research of Tony Irving on 8 athletes who developed EAH in the 1988 Comrades Marathon. It was that study that proved that the subjects had developed hyponatremia because of fluid overload, not sodium deficits.

An Epidemic of EAH and EAHE

At the same time that the first cases of EAHE were being reported in ultramarathon runners in South Africa and North America and in competitors in the 226 km (140.4 mile) Ironman Hawaii Triathlon, a dramatic revolution in the running world was taking place. Previously the chosen activity of a very few, most of whom were highly trained and obsessively committed to physical fitness and athletic performance, in the late 1970s and early 1980s a marathon running craze began in many major cities, including New York, Chicago, Boston, Los Angeles, London, and Berlin. Influenced by the growth of the sports drink industry (especially in the United States) and the invention of a novel, potentially fatal (non)disease called dehydration, race organizers began to ensure that ample fluid was available at multiple aid stations along the routes of these races. In addition, prerace publicity, increasingly supplemented by a media frenzy, emphasized the athletes' need to drink fluid at high rates to ensure that they did not suffer a fatal attack of "dehydration." This indeed was the advice given at the 1983 AMJA Ultramarathon at which Bob Lathan and Tyler Frizzell both developed EAHE. It is perhaps ironic that the first reported cases of EAHE in North America occurred to two members of the U.S. medical profession running in a race catering exclusively to medical and allied professionals.

Simultaneously there was also a large increase in the number of marathon runners seeking medical attention (Adner, Scarlett, et al., 1988) at the finish of those, by then, big-city marathon races. According to the Wyndham and Strydom foundation myth (box 3.1, page 62) that by then had been assimilated into the fluid replacement guidelines promoted by several influential organizations, it became the uncontested dogma that collapsed runners were still not drinking enough to prevent this dehydration-induced collapse. As a result, efforts to encourage athletes to drink even more during marathon races were intensified. And those who collapsed because of "dehydration" required resuscitation with the rapid intravenous infusion of often large volumes of fluid. Such fluids should, according to this advice, continue to be given until the patient has recovered.[2] Of course, if the athletes were suffering from overhydration rather than dehydration, then this treatment would be ineffective and potentially very harmful.

It was at this very time in the mid- to late 1980s that EAH and EAHE, previously reported infrequently and only in ultraendurance events like the 226 km Ironman Hawaii Triathlon and the 90 km Comrades Marathon, suddenly appeared in two novel populations—recreational runners who walked and jogged 42 km (a standard 26-mile marathon) in 5 or more hours, often to raise money for charity, and members of the U.S. military. The common feature was that both populations had been indoctrinated into the belief that their health could be ensured only if they drank copiously during exercise.

The first such report was of a 21-year-old man who ran the 1986 Pittsburgh marathon, his first. He completed the race in 5.5 hours, drinking at each of the 16 refreshment stations on the course. He drank 1.5 to 2 L more after the race. Four hours after finishing the race, he was found "wandering in his room in a confused state" (Nelson, Robinson, et al., 1987, p. 80; Young, Sciurba, et al., 1987, p. 73). On hospital admission, he was in pulmonary edema with a blood sodium concentration of 123 mmol/L. A brain scan showed increased pressure indicating brain swelling (edema). He was intubated and ventilated with gases containing a high oxygen concentration. During the first 3 hours of hospital admission he received ~3 L of intravenous fluids, 2 L of a low (0.45%) and 1 L of a 0.9% isotonic saline solution, for treatment supposedly of dehydration despite clear evidence that the athlete was edematous likely due to fluid overload. Since he received the same inappropriate treatment also given to Dr. Tyler Frizzell, predictably his blood sodium concentration returned to normal only on his third day in the hospital. Fortunately, 24 hours after hospital admission, he began to pass large volumes of urine; in the face of incorrect treatment, this diuresis (due to a suppression of inappropriate AVP/ADH secretion) likely saved his life. He was discharged from the hospital on the seventh day, fortunate to have survived.

A 57-year-old ultramarathon runner dropped out after he had run 88 km (55 miles) of a 100-mile (160 km) race in Vermont. He stopped because of painful blisters (Surgenor and Uphold, 1994). After stopping, he ingested 2 to 3 pints (~950-1370 ml) of a cool drink and began to complain of dizziness; his speech was slurred. Shortly thereafter, he lost consciousness and may have had a seizure. On hospital admission his

2 Intravenous fluids given without control to an athlete whose collapse is not due to dehydration but to overhydration will lead ultimately to brain death as has occurred in cases reported in this chapter.

blood sodium concentration was 111 mmol/L. Treated with 3% sodium chloride (and mannitol), he was released from the hospital after 3 days, fully recovered. During the first 12 hours of his treatment he passed a fluid excess of 900 ml.

Interestingly, after he had run 48 km (30 miles), this athlete complained to his son that he had a decreased urine output despite having already drunk 2 gallons (7.6 L) (estimated rate of fluid ingestion >1,500 ml/hr). He had also ingested 6 to 8 nonsteroidal anti-inflammatory drugs (NSAIDs). Only later would it become clear that the inappropriate use of NSAIDs during prolonged exercise increases the sensitivity of the kidney to the action of AVP/ADH, thereby promoting water retention and favoring the development of EAH (Baker, Cotter, et al., 2005; Wharam, Speedy, et al., 2006).

Even though we had established the cause of EAH 3 years earlier (Irving, Noakes, et al., 1991), Surgenor and Uphold (1994) concluded that the reasons why EAH occurred were "uncertain." But they had treated the patient correctly with a 3% sodium chloride infusion. They also drew an important conclusion: "A massive uptake of fluids after the completion of the race is also not the total explanation because the renal system should be able to handle such loads without difficulty. Therefore, inappropriate renal function and increased antidiuretic hormone (ADH) release were likely mechanisms, but this has not been clearly shown" (p. 443). They also concluded, "Hyponatremia may be one of the greatest risks to the health of participants in very prolonged athletic events" (p. 444). This was certainly insightful and conflicted with the popular view at the time that heatstroke is the greatest threat to the health of marathon runners, despite the absence of any evidence that heatstroke occurs commonly in marathon runners (table 5.1, page 159).

The first recorded fatality from EAHE occurred in a 32-year-old woman in the 1993 Avenue of the Giants Marathon in California. Her full case report was never recorded in the medical literature, perhaps because it might have identified inappropriate medical care as a factor in her death. A California physician who knew the runner but had not been involved in her medical care after the Avenue

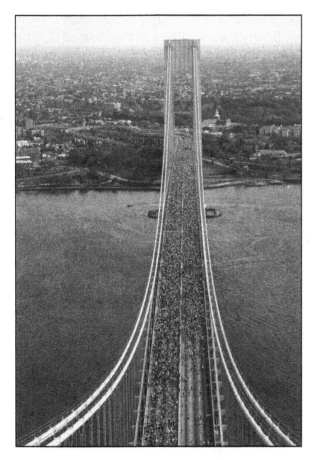

Runners crossing the Verrazano-Narrows Bridge at the start of the 1982 New York City Marathon. The explosive growth in the popularity of marathon running after 1976 is associated with the development and rise of EAH and EAHE, especially in North America.

AP Photo/Richard Drew

of the Giants Marathon told me that immediately after finishing the marathon, she had complained that she was very thirsty. She had drunk 1 to 2 L of a cola drink. Some time thereafter, she had developed an epileptic seizure and was admitted to the hospital, where she was treated for dehydration with an intravenous 0.9% saline solution. A chest X-ray showed pulmonary edema. In view of her abnormal neurological symptoms, a brain scan was performed. This showed brain swelling (edema) and other nonspecific findings. Since the clinicians were unaware of the diagnostic features of EAHE, they concluded that she had ruptured a blood vessel in her brain (cerebrovascular accident). Only 7 hours after she had collapsed was her blood sodium concentration measured for the first time. It was 117 mmol/L (Ayus, Varon, et al., 2000). But by then it was too late; she was in a deep coma without evidence for any higher brain functions. She was declared brain dead some time thereafter.

The U.S. military enacted novel drinking guidelines sometime in the late 1980s (chapter 7) that forced soldiers to replace their fluid losses as they developed. These replaced existing guidelines that focused on daily, not hourly, rates of fluid intake. These guidelines forced soldiers to drink up to 1.8 L/hr when they were exposed to hot environmental conditions (dry bulb temperature >32 °C). It was not long before the tragic consequence of this inappropriate advice would become apparent. The following case report (appendix B, case 1040) highlights how unquestioning devotion to an untested dogma can lead to death:

In early July, a male trainee was admitted to hospital with acute onset of rapidly progressing weakness that led to unresponsiveness. On the morning of admission, he moved with his unit to the rifle range. . . . At mid morning he complained of light-headedness and nausea, and he vomited. His supervisors suspected that he was suffering a heat injury. They moved him to the shade . . . and instructed him to drink 1Qt (909ml) of water every 30 minutes, as specified in the regulations. He began to vomit repeatedly. Unit members continued to encourage oral rehydration . . . during the next 2 hours he attempted to drink 10Qt (9090ml) of water while vomiting repeatedly. By mid afternoon, he was obtunded and was transported to the hospital. Medics administered normal saline intravenously during transport. The soldier arrived at the emergency department in respiratory distress. He was not hyperpyrexial. Initial laboratory tests revealed a blood sodium concentration of 121 mmol/L. A chest radiograph revealed diffuse pulmonary edema. Computed tomography revealed dilated lateral and third ventricles and edematous changes in the pons, with obliteration of the pons cistern. Despite intensive medical care, the soldier did not regain consciousness. A post-mortem examination documented severe cerebral and brainstem edema and hydrocephalus. (O'Brien, Montain, et al., 2001, p. 406)

This death occurred for the following reasons:

1. The soldier was at no risk of developing heatstroke since he was on the shooting range and not exercising vigorously.
2. He did not have a heat illness.
3. Drinking does not protect against heat illness.
4. The treatment of heat illness is cooling and not the provision of inordinate volumes of fluid orally and intravenously.

3 Vomiting is common in those who overdrink during marathon running. The vomiting of clear fluid indicates the presence of a large volume of unabsorbed fluid in the intestine. This occurs in those who drink at rates exceeding those at which their intestines can absorb the ingested fluids. It seems that few people can absorb fluid more rapidly than about 1,000 ml per hour. Some runners I have treated for nausea and vomiting during exercise have improved only when they drink less than about 250 ml per hour, suggesting that during exercise the intestines of these specific athletes may be unable to absorb fluid at rates faster than about 250 ml per hour.

But vomiting does not occur in dehydrated athletes, although of course persistent vomiting for some hours from whatever cause may cause dehydration, in which case the arrow of causation is reversed.

5. The vomiting of clear fluids indicates the presence of unabsorbed fluid in the intestine, a key sign that the patient is likely suffering from overhydration, not the fictitious condition of dehydration-induced heat illness.[3]

Sadly, at least three more fatal cases would be reported in the scientific literature in the following decade (appendix B).

During the course of an experimental study of heat acclimatization involving daily 8-hour exposures to intermittent exercise in the heat, a 21-year-old subject developed fatigue and nausea after 4 hours (Armstrong, Curtis, et al., 1993). During this time he had drunk 7.5 L of fluid (1.88 L/hr) and had passed 1 L of urine and 3 L of sweat, accumulating a fluid excess of 3 L. One hour later he had reportedly drunk another 3 L of fluid, increasing his fluid excess to 4.5 L. He stopped drinking and completed the remaining 2 hours of exercise finishing with a fluid excess of 3 L.

Three hours later, he complained of fatigue and malaise and was hospitalized. His blood sodium concentration was 122 mmol/L. He was treated with a 5% intravenous sodium chloride infusion and was released from the hospital the next morning. This rapid recovery was identical to that of Bob Lathan after the 1983 AMJA Ultramarathon (80 km). Unusually, the authors measured blood AVP/ADH concentrations during the experiment; these were markedly elevated (>250 pg/ml), indicating that the subject was suffering from SIADH. The authors correctly concluded that the intake and retention of a large volume of fluid explained the development of EAH, whereas sodium losses in sweat were normal and served only to "exacerbate" the hyponatremia (p. 543). In fact, we had already established in 1991 that sodium losses from the body during exercise play no part in the causation of EAH. The authors failed to identify the critical importance of SIADH for the development of EAH and EAHE, as had I.

Kelly Barrett, a 43-year-old pediatric dentist and mother of three young children, was discovered in a confused state at the 38 km mark of the 1998 Chicago Marathon (Zorn, 1999a). She had been running for about 5 hours and complained of headache, nausea, and vomiting. In training for the race, she had been advised to drink enough fluids and water to ensure that her urine was a clear color at all times, the same advice that Hilary Bellamy would receive. Her family stated that she had drunk "gallons and gallons of water every day for about 2 weeks" according to the dictum "Drink until your eyeballs float" (p. 1). Sadly, that is exactly what happened. When seen at the race medical tent, she was initially conscious and "did not seem extraordinarily distressed when paramedics brought her to the medical tent at the finish line in Grant Park." According to the race medic, "She looked dehydrated. She was dizzy, lightheaded and nauseated and it's not uncommon to see that." But when treated for "dehydration" with intravenous fluids, "she unexpectedly stopped breathing" (p. 1). She was resuscitated and admitted to the hospital, where her blood sodium concentration was 121 mmol/L. During the first 8 hours of hospitalization, she passed 6.7 L of fluid, 2.3 L more than she received intravenously. She was declared brain dead on the third hospital day and she died the same day.[4]

At about this time, between 1996 and 1998, Dr. Dale Speedy in New Zealand was studying the incidence and causes of EAH in New Zealand endurance athletes (see chapter 9). Eight athletes developed EAH in the 1996 New Zealand Ironman Triathlon and four were hospitalized with EAHE; 25 triathletes were diagnosed with EAH in the 1997 race, 14 of whom were hospitalized with EAHE.

As described in chapter 9, changes to reduce the availability of fluid in the 1998 New Zealand Ironman Triathlon in order to discourage overdrinking led to a significant decrease in the incidence of EAH: Only four triathletes in the 1998 race required treatment for EAH or EAHE (0.6% of race starters).

The next reports of significant numbers of athletes with EAH and EAHE came from the 1998 and 1999 Suzuki Rock 'n' Roll Marathons in San Diego (Davis, Videen, et al., 2001). These races were promoted to capture the new market of charity marathoners who wished to complete the marathon in between 4:30 and 6:00 and who were more interested in enjoying the event than establishing a personal-best time. Recall that before 1976, the goal of most marathon runners was to finish the race as quickly as possible, not to enjoy the social occasion.

A total of 26 runners in the 1998 and 1999 Rock 'n' Roll Marathons were admitted to hospital emergency departments in San Diego for the treatment of EAHE. Fifteen patients had severe EAHE; three had seizures requiring admission to the intensive care unit. Interviews with affected athletes revealed that "virtually all had attempted to drink 'as much as possible' during and after the race exceeding the race packet recommendations" (Davis, Videen, et al., 2001, p. 51). That is, they had drunk according to the drinking guidelines promulgated by the American College of Sports Medicine (ACSM) in 1996 and extensively promoted by the GSSI (Murray, 1996; Murray, 1999). Other risk factors for the development of hyponatremia were slow finishing times, female sex, and the use of NSAIDs.

The study also showed that the symptoms of EAHE could be readily reversed within hours and the blood sodium concentrations corrected within 5 to 8 hours with the use of a concentrated (3-5%) saline solution infused slowly (~100 ml/hr). Using this treatment, even the most severe cases of EAHE were "cured" within 5 to 8 hours

4   In the run-up to the 1999 Chicago Marathon, Eric Zorn, who wrote a regular column for the *Chicago Tribune*, phoned me to ask why Kelly Barrett had died in the 1998 Chicago Marathon. He subsequently wrote two columns for the *Chicago Tribune* titled "Runner's Demise Sheds Light on Deadly Myth" and "Water Intoxication Rare but Runners Should Pay Heed" on October 11 and 12, 1999. Rereading those columns now after so many more avoidable deaths from EAHE fills one with a mixture of great sadness and some anger.

A year earlier, after Kelly Barrett's death, the medical director of the 1998 Chicago Marathon had sent an e-mail "circulated to interested parties" (Zorn 1999b, p. 1) stating, "Do not tell the public to worry about fluid overconsumption. The public will be very difficult to counsel on how not to overconsume, then at the same time how not to underconsume fluids" (Zorn 1999b, p. 1).

Zorn concluded, "The simple, now-pervasive message 'hydrate, hydrate, hydrate' is easier to remember than a formula for moderation and a better slogan that 'water killed Kelly Barrett'" (Zorn 1999b, p. 1).

of hospital admission. This compares rather favorably to the 5 to 7 days required to treat the first cases (Frizzell, Lang, et al., 1986; Noakes, Goodwin, et al., 1985) but confirmed what had already been shown with the treatment of Rob Lathan after the 1983 Chicago AMJA Ultramarathon and the female athlete in the 1987 Comrades Marathon. This information was first published in the form of an abstract (Davis, Marino, et al., 1999) 3 years before the deaths of Cynthia Lucero and Hilary Bellamy in the 2002 Boston and Marine Corps Marathons, respectively.

The 2000 Houston Marathon was the next race to report a significant incidence of EAH and EAHE (Hew, Chorley, et al., 2003) with subsequent reports from the 2001-2003 races (Hew, 2005). Twenty-one athletes reporting to the medical facility at the end of the 2000 race were found to have EAH, although none had EAHE. Risk factors for hyponatremia included an increased number of cups of fluid drunk during the race, whether water or a carbohydrate-containing drink (figure 10.2), and longer finishing times. Fifty-three percent of hyponatremic athletes trained with a beginner's marathon training program that promoted aggressive drinking during exercise. Participants were encouraged to "drink until your urine is clear" and "do not wait until you are thirsty to drink" (p. 46).

Subsequent analysis of 60 runners with EAH in the 2000 to 2003 Houston Marathons revealed that female runners drank more than males of the same weight (Hew, 2005). Runners with EAH drank significantly more fluid than those who maintained normal blood sodium concentrations; they lost less weight during the race and had a significantly greater fall in their blood sodium concentrations. Compared to males, female runners with EAH were significantly lighter, ran slower, lost less weight, dropped blood sodium concentrations more so that they finished with lower postrace blood sodium concentrations, but consumed the same number of cups of fluid as did the males. There was also a linear relationship with a negative slope between the change in blood sodium concentrations and change in

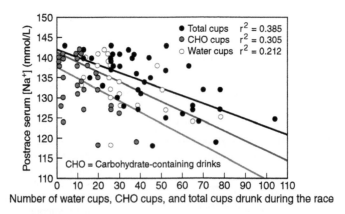

FIGURE 10.2 A study of athletes completing the 2000 Houston Marathon found a linear relationship with a negative slope between the postrace blood sodium concentrations and either the total number of cups or the number of cups of water or carbohydrate-containing drinks that the athletes reported they drank during the race. The total number of cups of fluid drunk during the race explained 39% of the variance in the postrace blood sodium concentrations.

Adapted, by permission, from T.D. Hew, N. Chorley, J.C. Cianca, and J.G. Divine, 2003, "The incidence, risk factors, and clinical manifestations of hyponatremia in marathon runners," *Clinical Journal of Sport Medicine* 13(1): 41-47.

body weight during the race (figure 10.3). There was no difference between men and women in the response of their blood sodium concentrations to changes in body weight during marathon running. Change in body weight could explain 36% to 44% of the variation in blood sodium concentrations during the race.

Hew (2005) also found that the ingestion of a sports drink with some added sodium chloride did not influence the extent to which the blood sodium concentrations fell in those who drank to excess during the race (figure 10.4). The change in body weight could explain 47% to 56% of the variation in the postrace blood sodium concentrations.

Not included in those subjects from the Houston Marathon were another four runners treated for pulmonary and cerebral edema after the 1999 marathon and a further four after the 2000 race (Ayus, Varon, et al., 2000). All survived and the majority were treated with hypertonic saline solutions that raised their serum sodium concentrations by ~10 mmol/L within 12 hours, reversing their symptoms equally quickly.

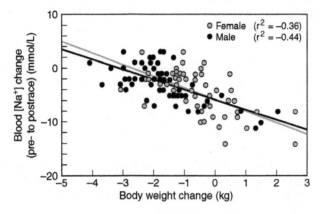

FIGURE 10.3 The relationship in the change in body weight and the change in blood sodium concentrations in male and female runners in the 2000 to 2003 Houston Marathons.

Reprinted, by permission, from T.D. Hew, 2005, "Women hydrate more than men during a marathon race: Hyponatremia in the Houston Marathon: A report on 60 cases," *Clinical Journal of Sport Medicine* 15(3): 148-153.

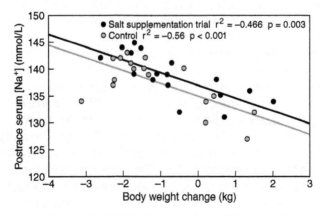

FIGURE 10.4 The ingestion of a drink with an increased sodium chloride content did not influence the relationship between the postrace blood sodium concentrations and changes in body weight during the race in those who either ingested (dark line) or did not ingest (light line) additional sodium chloride during the 2002 Houston Marathon.

Reprinted, by permission, from T.D. Hew, 2005, "Women hydrate more than men during a marathon race: Hyponatremia in the Houston Marathon: A report on 60 cases," *Clinical Journal of Sport Medicine* 15(3): 148-153.

A subsequent analysis of these data (Chorley, Cianca, et al., 2007) found that the risk of developing EAH was sevenfold higher in runners whose weight decreased by less than 0.75 kg during the Houston Marathon, that is, in runners who either gained weight or who lost relatively little weight during the race. Other risk factors included increased fluid intake during the race (measured as both the total number of cups of fluid ingested and the rate of fluid ingestion) slower finishing times, and lighter body weights. As a result of those studied, the organizers of the Houston Marathon reduced the number of refreshment stations to 16 placed every 1.5 miles (2.4 km) for the 2003 race.

Three (5.6%) of the runners requiring on-site medical care at the 2000 Pittsburgh Marathon had EAH (Hsieh, Roth, et al., 2002). In contrast, no cases of EAH were identified in a subset of faster runners (Nelson, Ellis, et al., 1989) in the 1987 Pittsburgh Marathon 13 years earlier.

Interestingly, the medical directors of the Houston Marathon tended to focus on sodium replacement rather than fluid restriction in the prevention of EAH. Houston Marathoners were advised to "train with a sports drink containing sodium. If you only drink water, you can make the situation worse." They were also encouraged to "eat salty foods before, during, and after training and competition. Increase salt intake several days before endurance training and competition." Finally, prospective marathoners were advised, "Understand your individual fluid needs. 'Listen to your body—don't drown your body with water'" (Honig, 2003, p. 9).

At the 2000 (figure 10.5a) and 2001 (figure 10.5b) South African Ironman Triathlons, only one athlete developed EAHE. He was also the only triathlete to gain significant weight during either race (Noakes, Sharwood, et al., 2004) (arrowed in figure 10.5b) because he ignored the prerace advice that athletes should drink according to the dictates of thirst and so avoid overdrinking. Change in body weight during the race could explain 20% of the variation in postrace blood sodium concentrations in these triathletes.

Thus the incidence of EAHE in the 2000 and 2001 South African Ironman Triathlons was 0.16% (1 in 610 finishers) (Sharwood, Collins, et al., 2002; Sharwood, Collins, et al., 2004) compared to a minimum probable rate of about 5% in the Ironman Hawaii Triathlon between 1983 and 1998 and 13.8% (62 cases in 447 studied athletes) in the 1997 and 1998 New Zealand Ironman Triathlons.

Nine of 39 finishers in the 246 km 2001 Spartathlon run between Athens and Sparta developed severe hyponatremia with blood sodium concentrations below 130 mmol/L (Kavouras, Anastasiou, et al., 2003). There was a linear relationship with a negative slope between body weight change during the race and the postrace blood sodium concentration. Furthermore, subjects with EAH lost less weight (0.6 kg) during the race than did those who finished the race with postrace blood sodium concentrations greater than 130 mmol/L (2.4 kg). The authors concluded that "hyponatremia is a common biochemical disturbance in ultramarathon runners . . . possibly due to a fluid overload" (p. S246). Interestingly, the first author would become a key spokesperson for Gatorade, fronting the product's advance into the UK market, by which time he had become convinced that excessive sodium loss, reduced by the ingestion of a sports drink during exercise, was the most important cause of EAH (Anastasiou, Kavouras, et al., 2009).

During the 2002 Boston Marathon, Dr. Cynthia Lucero developed EAHE and later died from the condition. Her story is told at the beginning of chapter 1. Recall

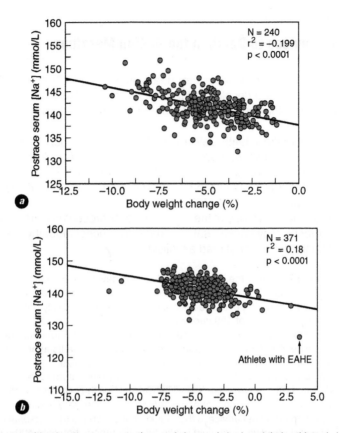

FIGURE 10.5 Postrace blood sodium concentrations and changes in body weight in athletes in both the *(a)* 2000 and the *(b)* 2001 South African Ironman Triathlons. The sole athlete to develop EAHE was also the only athlete to gain significant weight (>2.5%, arrowed) during the race.

(a) Adapted, by permission, from K. Sharwood, M. Collins, J. Goedecke, G. Wilson, and T. Noakes, 2002, "Weight changes, sodium levels, and performance in the South African Ironman Triathlon," *Clinical Journal of Sport Medicine* 12(6): 391-399. *(b)* Adapted by permission from BMJ Publishing Group Limited. *British Journal of Sports Medicine*, T.D. Noakes, K. Sharwood, M. Collins, and D.R. Perkins, 38(4), E16, 2004.

from chapter 9 that Dr. Almond found that 13% of a sample of 488 race finishers had serum sodium concentrations below 135 mmol/L; 3 subjects were markedly hyponatremic with serum sodium concentrations below 120 mmol/L (Almond, Shin, et al., 2005). The two most important risk factors for hyponatremia were weight gain during the race and race duration over 4 hours. Dr. Lucero's death spurred much-needed changes and brought reactions from all sides (box 10.1, page 308).

Unfortunately, incidents of EAH and EAHE continued to mount. From 2000 to 2010, 483 occurrences of EAH or EAHE were recorded in the literature. Several of the most illustrative or unique cases are described here.

A study of 16 competitors in the 2000 Iditasport 100-mile (160 km) ultraendurance race in Alaska found that 7 developed EAH during the race (Stuempfle, Lehmann, et al., 2002). Whereas weight fell significantly in athletes who maintained their blood sodium concentrations during the race, the weights of subjects who developed EAH did not fall. The authors concluded that "hyponatremia is common in an ultraendurance race held in extreme cold, and may be caused by excessive fluid consumption and/or inadequate sodium intake" (p. 51). Interestingly, EAH occurred even though the rates of fluid intake were low (500 ml/hr). No athletes

BOX 10.1 **Responses to Death in the Boston Marathon**

Stunned by Cynthia Lucero's unnecessary death, in 2003 USA Track and Field adopted the drinking guidelines I had developed for the International Marathon Medical Directors Association (IMMDA) (Noakes, 2003; Noakes and Martin, 2002) for all U.S. races under their jurisdiction.

I decided that Dr. Lucero's death justified one final attempt to publish an editorial on the dangers of overdrinking, which had been rejected by the *Annals of Internal Medicine,* the *Journal of the American Medical Association,* and the *New England Journal of Medicine.* At long last, the editorial was published by the *British Medical Journal* and can be found in full at www.bmj.com/content//327/7407/113.full.

The editorial summarized many of the same concepts presented in this book, especially that advice to overdrink may cause fatal hyponatremic encephalopathy (EAHE) in endurance athletes. In part, the editorial read as follows:

> Aside from military personnel, the athlete most likely to develop hyponatremic encephalopathy is a female marathon runner, who runs those 42km races at speeds slower than 8-9km/h (about 5mph). She gains weight during exercise because she drinks excessively both before and during exercise, sometimes in excess of 100 cups of fluid during the race (about 15 litres of fluid during 5-6 hours of exercise). She does not develop a marked sodium deficit, nor does she have evidence of inappropriate secretion of antidiuretic hormone, although antidiuretic agents are clearly active. Since the cause of the condition is now known, prevention is possible.
>
> To protect all exercisers from this preventable condition, rational and evidence based advice must be provided. In particular, exercisers must be warned that the overconsumption of fluid (either water or sports drinks) before, during, or after exercise is unnecessary and can have a potentially fatal outcome. Perhaps the best advice is that drinking according to the personal dictates of thirst seems to be safe and effective. Such fluid intake typically ranges between 400ml and 800ml per hour in most forms of recreational and competitive exercise; less for slower, smaller athletes exercising in mild environmental conditions, more for superior athletes competing at higher intensities in warmer environments.

This editorial did not go unnoticed in the Chicago headquarters of Gatorade. Robert Murray, PhD, then director of the GSSI, posted a response on the GSSI website on the same day that the editorial appeared in the print media.

The GSSI article was titled "Gatorade Sports Science Institute Refutes Hydration Advice in British Journal of Medicine [sic] report." In it, Dr. Murray stated that my editorial did not "factor in the very real dangers associated with the more common condition of dehydration" (p. 1). Portions of the article read as follows:

> Noakes' contention that the ACSM guidelines encourage excessive fluid consumption is simply untrue. The American College of Sports Medicine (ACSM) position statement on Exercise and Fluid Replacement recommends that athletes drink enough fluid during exercise in an attempt to replace what is lost in sweat, with those who sweat heavily being encouraged to drink as much as they can comfortably tolerate so they can get close to normal hydration.
>
> In summary, there is no doubt that hyponatremia is a rare but dangerous condition that affects a very, very small subset of the population. However, dehydration and heat illness occur far more frequently and represent the greater threat to anyone who is physically active in a warm environment.
>
> The scientific guidelines now in place provide clear and valuable advice: drink to stay well hydrated, but don't overdrink.[5]

When athletes drink according to the dictates of thirst, as I advised in my editorial, they will avoid dehydration. Furthermore, chapters 3 and 8 established that there is no published evidence showing that fluid ingestion during exercise has any role at all in the prevention of heatstroke. Instead, there is a great deal of evidence suggesting that fluid ingestion cannot play any such role since the causation of heatstroke is far more complex than simply the development of dangerous dehydration.

As proven in chapters 2, 3, and 8, it is also factually incorrect to argue that "dehydration and heat illness occur far more frequently and represent the greater threat to anyone who is physically active in a warm environment."

On 11 April 2006 at 1:12 p.m. ET, the Gatorade Sports Science Institute released "Hydration Recommendations for Boston Marathon Runners" (GSSI, 2006). The article again emphasized the dangers of dehydration, listing both dehydration and hyponatremia as serious concerns. Chris Troyanos, ATC, medical coordinator for the Boston Marathon, was quoted, "It's essential that runners keep hydration top of mind,

5 In fact, our subsequent analysis (Beltrami, Hew-Butler, et al., 2008) has established that the GSSI itself has continued to promote overdrinking even 5 years later in 2008. An analysis of drinking advice provided by GSSI websites in various countries revealed that most continue to promote overdrinking. For example, many include a fluid loss calculator reportedly formulated around "scientifically based evidence." However, this calculator predicts that a 70 kg athlete performing intense exercise in 35 °C would need to drink 1,400 ml/hr or 1,150 ml/hr if exercising in 20 °C. Both these guidelines far exceed the upper limit of the current ACSM guidelines.

I take pride in the fact that the world's athletes now follow the drinking guidelines that I developed in 2003, and they have subsequently been adopted by the ACSM when the proof we had presented could no longer be ignored.

and make sure to drink enough to prevent dehydration but avoid overdrinking" (p.1). The article continued: "The recommendations developed by GSSI focus on the importance for runners to gauge their own fluid needs, rather than drinking according to thirst or following a specific rule of thumb for fluid intake."

The GSSI again recommended "ingesting sodium during a marathon, especially for heavy sweaters and salty sweaters" (p. 1). In addition, "'The two most important things runners can do to protect themselves from hydration-related problems is [sic] to drink according to their individual fluid needs and make sure to consume adequate sodium,' said Dr. Bob Murray, director of the Gatorade Sports Science Institute."

The article promoted Gatorade Endurance Formula because it "contains approximately twice the amount of sodium (200 mg/8 oz) of Gatorade Thirst Quencher to meet the needs of athletes during prolonged exercise" (p.1) and stated that the Boston Marathon would be providing Gatorade Endurance Formula on the course at the 2006 race.

Because EAH is caused by fluid overload, not by sodium deficiency, drinking copious amounts of such a product cannot prevent hyponatremia in those predisposed athletes with SIADH who will develop the condition if they drink to excess.

From 1996 to 2007, the GSSI and the ACSM promoted the concept that athletes should drink beyond thirst by ingesting "the maximal amount that can be tolerated" (Convertino, Armstrong, et al., 1996, p. i). Indeed the GSSI sponsored the advertisement in the January 2002 issue of *New York Runner* magazine that encouraged *all* athletes to drink at least 1.2 L/hr during exercise "or else your performance will suffer" (n.p.). Only in 2007 did the ACSM alter its guidelines, whereas the U.S. military, presented with exactly the same evidence, modified its drinking guidelines specifically to prevent fatal EAHE already in April 1998, almost a decade before the ACSM acted similarly.

developed EAH in the 2001 race (Stuempfle, Lehmann, et al., 2003). The average rate of fluid intake during that race was lower: 300 ml/hr.

A study of competitors in a 109 km cycling race in Cape Town in 2003 detected one 57-year-old female athlete who developed EAHE (Dugas and Noakes, 2005) and whose postrace blood sodium concentration was 129 mmol/L. She complained of headache, dizziness, and difficulty in concentrating. During the race her weight increased 2.4 kg (3.6% of BW) even though she drank only 735 ml/hr. Her calculated sweat rate during the race was 270 ml/hr. Laboratory studies showed that she had a normal sweat sodium concentration (~68 mmol/L) so that her total sweat sodium chloride loss during the cycling race was only 70 to 105 mmol, far too little by itself to cause EAHE.

The study of 196 cyclists in the race showed the classic inverse relationship with a negative slope between the postrace blood sodium concentrations and body weight change during the race (figure 10.6). As was the case in the South African Ironman Triathlon, the only subject to gain significant weight during the race developed EAHE.

In the first report from Asia, three Indian physicians reported the case of non-cardiogenic pulmonary edema and EAHE in a 33-year-old female runner after she had run cross-country for 35 km (Kashyap, Anand, et al., 2006). Her blood sodium concentration was 119 mmol/L. She was treated with a 5% intravenous sodium chloride solution and recovered completely within 18 hours.

Several years after the event, studies from the Boston Marathons of 2001, 2002 (Kratz, Lewandrowski, et al., 2002), and 2003 (Kratz, Siegel, et al., 2005) concluded that blood sodium concentrations should be measured before intravenous fluid therapy is initiated. Thus, the authors cautioned "against institution of (intravenous) treatment until laboratory tests determine the patient's sodium status" (Kratz, Siegel, et al., 2005, p. 227). This reiterated what I had been arguing since at least 1988 and is a substantial change from the usual advice of that race (Adner, Gembarowicz, et al., 2002) that "severe hypohydration in the absence of hyperthermia is a more common occurrence [than heatstroke—my addition] at the Boston Marathon" (Adner, 1988, p. 6). Thus, signs of progress were finally apparent in the medical care of athletes, at least at the Boston Marathon.

A 41-year-old man completed the 2006 South African Ironman Triathlon in 10:49 (Hew-Butler, Anley, et al., 2007). During the race he drank more than 10 L on the cycle leg (~1.7L/hr) in order to "stay ahead of thirst." He experienced 3 bouts of diarrhea during the running leg, which he completed in 3:51. He became lethargic, sleepy, and disinterested in his surroundings after the race. One hundred minutes later his mental state was unchanged. Because his blood

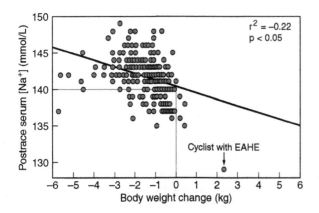

FIGURE 10.6 The expected linear relationship with a negative slope between the postrace blood sodium concentration and the weight change during a 2003 109 km cycling race in Cape Town.

Reproduced from *British Journal of Sports Medicine*, J.P. Dugas and T.D. Noakes, 39(10), E38, 2005, with permission from BMJ Publishing Group Limited.

sodium concentration had fallen to 132 mmol/L, medics decided to treat him with a 50 ml bolus of a 5% hypertonic saline solution. Five minutes after the infusion began, his mental state improved dramatically. He became awake and alert and began to converse with the medical staff. When the infusion was completed after 20 minutes, he wished to stand up to urinate. Ten minutes later, he was discharged from the medical tent fully recovered. To our knowledge, this is the first report of the successful use of a hypertonic solution to reverse mild EAHE rapidly in the field setting. Subsequently we reported a larger series in which hypertonic saline infusion reversed symptoms in athletes with more severe EAHE (Hew-Butler, Noakes, et al., 2008).

A 45-year-old female developed an epileptic seizure after completing the 2006 Frankfurt Ironman Triathlon (Richter, Betz, et al., 2007). Her face and ankles were swollen and her blood sodium concentration was 111 mmol/L, a very low measurement. She had pulmonary and cerebral edema and an elevated urine osmolality, indicating the presence of SIADH. She was treated with hypertonic saline but developed respiratory arrest for which

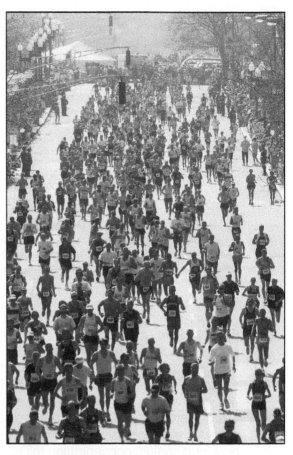

Runners in Boylson Street near the finish of the 2002 Boston Marathon, the race in which Dr. Cynthia Lucero developed fatal EAHE and in which 13% of a sample of runners developed EAH (Almond, Shin, Fortescue, et al., 2005).
AP Photo/Michael Dwyer

she required mechanical ventilation. Seven days later, she was released from the hospital fully recovered. One year later she completed another Ironman triathlon. She was advised to avoid excessive drinking and to ingest additional salt. Her blood sodium concentration at the end of the race was 141 mmol/L. The authors concluded that "a moderate fluid intake during and after endurance exercise is very important" (p. 1832).

Eleven of 88 runners studied in the 2006 London Marathon developed EAH during the race (Kipps, Sharma, et al., 2011). Factors predicting EAH were a larger fluid intake during the race (3683 vs. 1924 ml) and a faster rate of fluid ingestion (843 vs. 451 ml/hr). Runners with EAH also reported drinking more fluid after the race and before blood sampling. Runners with EAH also gained weight during the race (1.65 kg), whereas those without hyponatremia lost 1.46 kg. There was predictably a significant linear relationship with a negative slope between the postrace serum sodium concentration and weight change during the race, whereas there was the same relationship with a positive slope between the postrace blood sodium concentration and the total volume of fluid ingested during the race (figure 10.7, page 312).

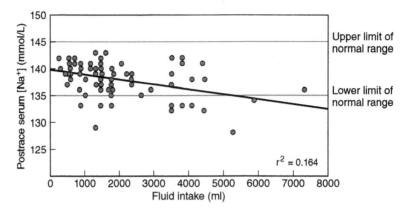

FIGURE 10.7 In the 2006 London Marathon, there was a linear relationship with a negative slope between the postrace blood sodium concentration and the total volume of fluid ingested during the race so that those who drank the most had the lowest postrace blood sodium concentrations.

Reproduced from *British Journal of Sports Medicine*, C. Kipps, S. Sharma, and D.T. Pedoe, 45(1), 15-19, 2011, with permission from BMJ Publishing Group Limited.

A runner in his 30s completed the London Marathon (date unspecified) in 4:30 (Petzold, Keir, et al., 2007). For 6 hours after the race he had a persistent headache and admitted himself to a London teaching hospital. He was fully alert with a normal blood pressure (130/70 mmHg) and his heart rate was appropriately elevated (80 bpm) for his postrace recovery. His initial blood sodium concentration was 133 mmol/L, indicating EAH due to fluid overload. Despite this, he received 1 L of isotonic (0.9%) saline and 1 L of a concentrated glucose solution (5% dextrose) intravenously, presumably for the treatment of dehydration. Predictably, his blood sodium concentration fell to 130 mmol/L. Four hours later he became confused, his level of consciousness fell, and he stopped breathing. A brain scan indicated that his brain stem had herniated through the foramen magnum at the base of the skull as a result of brain swelling, secondary to intravenous fluid therapy, and an unexpected abnormality preventing normal drainage of the fluid spaces (ventricles) within the brain, leading to hydrocephalus.[6] He was declared brain dead the following morning.

6 Hydrocephalus, literally water on the brain, occurs when the fluid secreted within the cavities inside the brain is unable to drain properly and accumulates. This causes the pressure inside the brain, the intracranial pressure, to rise. An athlete with hydrocephalus would have a higher-than-normal intracranial pressure. If the athlete were to develop EAH, that pressure would be raised even further. As a result, the athlete would develop the cerebral symptoms of EAHE at much higher blood sodium concentrations than a person without the condition and might develop cerebellar coning even though the blood sodium concentration was not as low as might be expected. The rapidity with which the male runner and Kelly Barrett went into a coma and stopped breathing raises the possibility that they may have had a condition causing an abnormal elevation in intracranial pressure.

Brain herniation does not usually occur at a blood sodium concentration of 130 mmol/L. This patient therefore had a predisposing factor (hydrocephalus due to impaired drainage of his cerebral ventricles) that reduced his brain's ability to accommodate the increase in its volume caused by voluntary overdrinking and inappropriate intravenous fluid therapy. Unnecessary treatment for a nondisease (dehydration) had caused the death of this runner because he had an unexpected and essentially undetectable abnormality in his brain's anatomy.

Five runners in the 2007 London Marathon were admitted to the hospital with EAHE (Doberenz, Nalla, et al., 2009). Despite treatment with hypertonic saline, mannitol, and a diuretic (furosemide), one athlete with an initial blood sodium concentration of 123 mmol/L died within 48 hours (case 1591 in appendix B).

A 31-year-old woman had completed 23 miles of the 2007 Chicago Marathon when the race was terminated after 3.5 hours on account of the severe environmental conditions (31.1 °C, 88 °F, 88-100% RH) and the unavailability of sufficient water at the aid stations (Rawlani and Noakes, 2008). She was participating in a research study in which her body weight and changes in blood and urine sodium concentrations were measured. Surprisingly, despite a reported "absence" of sufficient fluids on the course, she had nevertheless drunk sufficiently to increase her body weight by 0.8 kg during the race, causing her blood sodium concentration to fall by 8 mmol/L to 135 mmol/L. Her estimated rate of fluid intake during the race was 800 to 1,200 ml/hr. She did not urinate until after the race; at that time her urine osmolality was high (605 mOsmol/L), indicating the presence of SIADH.

On the advice of the medical staff at the race finish, in the next 24 hours she drank 8,000 ml in order to treat her symptoms of muscle soreness, which were reportedly due to "dehydration." Despite increasing abdominal pain, malaise, and mental confusion, she continued to drink at a high rate (13,000 ml in the next 24 hours). Seventy-two hours after completing the race, she became lethargic, her speech was slow and slurred, and she was unable to concentrate. Her husband took her to the hospital, where her blood sodium concentration was 125 mmol/L and her urine osmolality remained elevated (125 mmol/L). She was treated with a 3% hypertonic saline solution intravenously; her confusion resolved within 3 hours and her blood sodium concentration returned to 136 mmol/L 48 hours later.

A 34-year-old female runner sought nutritional guidance in 2007 at a New York sports medicine facility (Glace and Murphy, 2008). She reported that 1 month earlier she had been hospitalized for the treatment of "dehydration" after competing in a 21 km half marathon. She had drunk "copious" amounts of fluid before the race and another 4 L of water during the race. After the race, she felt nauseated and confused. Assuming that these symptoms were due to dehydration, she continued drinking copiously. She was brought to the hospital at 11:00 a.m. by a neighbor who found her disorientated.

The physician who examined her noticed that her wrists were swollen. Her blood sodium concentration was 119 mmol/L and there was evidence that her blood volume had expanded. Despite this, she was treated for dehydration and hyponatremia with 800 ml of normal saline intravenously. At 4 p.m. she suffered a grand mal epileptic seizure, for which she received another 2 L of normal saline in the next 90 minutes; she became unresponsive and was admitted to intensive care, where she immediately received 25 ml per hour of hypertonic saline. She suffered a second grand mal seizure. Thereafter she developed a profound diuresis, passing 5.4 L in the next 24 hours. She subsequently developed muscle cell breakdown (rhabdomyolysis) and was discharged from the hospital 8 days after her admission. She was advised to drink less in the future, in particular to drink according to thirst. Treatment with normal saline almost killed this young lady.

A 29-year-old man participating in his first Ironman Triathlon collapsed ~32 km into the run (Hew-Butler, Noakes, et al., 2008). During the 180 km cycle, he drank ~8 L of fluid (~1.5 L/hr). He also ingested approximately 7.3 g sodium chloride (~317 mmol or 8 mmol/L of fluid consumed) in the form of tablets, fluid, and foodstuffs. He did not remember urinating during the race. On admission to a hospital emergency room, his blood sodium concentration was 115 mmol/L, falling to 112 mmol/L 4 hours later. He was treated with 150 ml of a 15% mannitol solution and normal saline but remained in a coma for 4 days with persistent pulmonary and cerebral edema even though his blood sodium concentration had returned to 136 mmol/L within 24 hours of hospital admission. He recovered fully but later wondered "why my sodium levels were so low if I was taking sodium supplements specifically designed to have replaced any lost salt?" (p. 351). Clearly, like many, he was unaware that EAHE is a disease of fluid retention and fluid overload, not of sodium deficiency.

A study of the 2008 Rio Del Lago 100-mile (161 km) Endurance Run in Granite Bay, California, found that 16 of the 45 runners in the race developed asymptomatic EAH during the race, whereas another 5 developed symptoms compatible with a diagnosis of EAHE (Lebus, Casazza, et al., 2010). This is the highest incidence of EAH and EAHE yet reported in any ultramarathon race anywhere in the world.

Surprisingly, changes in body mass did not predict the postrace serum sodium concentrations as is the usual finding described in this chapter. Instead, blood sodium concentrations were reduced even in runners who lost weight during the race. This finding is unique and currently unexplained. Many runners in California ultraendurance events, including the Western States 100-mile (160 km) race, believe that large sodium losses in sweat are detrimental to both health and performance even though there is no scientific support for this belief. As a result, a culture has developed that promotes high sodium intakes both before and during these races. Perhaps unnaturally high sodium intake impairs the regulation of blood sodium concentrations during ultraendurance events lasting 12 or more hours. Nevertheless, the change in body mass during that race predicted race finishing time so that those runners who lost the most weight ran the fastest.

Races With a Low Incidence of EAH

It follows that if EAH is the natural and unavoidable consequence of prolonged exercise, aided perhaps by salty sweating, then the incidence of the condition should be the same in all similar events regardless of where they are held. Yet the minimum incidence of EAH and EAHE in the Ironman Hawaii Triathlon is at least 30 times higher than the incidence in the 2000 and 2001 South African Ironman Triathlons because the incidences in those races are respectively 5% and 0.16%. One difference is that I was the medical director of those two South African races, whereas the medical directors of the Ironman Hawaii Triathlon believe that drinking as much as tolerable optimizes performance and prevents EAH.

More recently two European ultraendurance races have shown an absence of any cases of EAH. Thus, there were no cases of EAH in 15 male ultramarathon runners competing in a 24-hour run in Basel, Switzerland (Knechtle, 2010), or in 11 female competitors in another Swiss running race of 100 km (Knechtle, Senn, et al., 2010). The authors of the latter paper conclude that "ad libitum drinking protects against exercise-associated hyponatremia" and that the reported higher incidence of EAH in women "is not really a gender effect but due to women being more prone to overdrink" (p. 83). The study also showed that prerace weight predicted running speed during the race and that the postrace blood sodium concentration was inversely related to the postrace total body water (TBW) content so that blood sodium concentrations were lowest in those runners with the greatest TBW after the race.

Similarly, there was only one case of asymptomatic EAH in 272 finishers in the 2008 Hong Kong Marathon (Au-Yeung, Wu, et al., 2010). Surprisingly, a number of runners gained weight during the race, but this was not associated with a reduction in the blood sodium concentrations—a not unexpected finding because we have also shown this phenomenon in our large cohort of endurance athletes (figure 9.15, page 288). Our explanation is that the mobilization of sufficient sodium from the internal (nonosmotic) sodium stores would prevent the development of EAH in those whose total body water content is increased as a result of overdrinking and fluid retention (due to SIADH).

The Special Case of the Ironman Hawaii Triathlon

The Ironman Hawaii Triathlon, involving a 3.8 km swim, 180 km cycle, and 42.2 km marathon, was first held on the island of Oahu on 18 February 1978. The steady growth of the race caused the organizers to move the race to Kailua-Kona on the island of Hawaii in February 1981, where it has been held ever since. It is one of the iconic sporting events in the world; for the athletes who race to win, it is perhaps the hardest one-day sporting event in the world. Over the years it has also produced more cases of EAH and EAHE than any other sporting event in the world, even far exceeding the number of cases in the military discussed subsequently (page 321).

Data on blood sodium concentrations in Ironman Hawaii triathletes were first collected in the 1983 race, and all those data up to the 1998 race were made available to me in 1998. This is a remarkable data set. Recall that in 1983, I and most others believed that it was pointless measuring blood sodium concentration in endurance athletes because blood sodium concentrations always rose during prolonged exercise. Thus, it is not immediately clear why the Ironman Hawaii medical team had the foresight to measure blood sodium concentrations already at the 1983 race.

Those data indicate that the first identified cases of EAH occurred in the 1983 race, although it would only be after the 1984 race that cases of EAH in that race were described for the first time (Hiller, O'Toole, et al., 1985).

At 6:51 p.m. on the afternoon of the 1983 race, a 28-year-old male finisher presented to the medical facility at the race finish complaining of dizziness. He was treated with 3 L of a 5% dextrose and Ringer's lactate solution containing 130 mmol/L of sodium on the grounds that he was probably dehydrated, with a low blood glucose concentration (hypoglycemia). But his blood sodium concentration was 127 mmol/L and his blood osmolality was 265 mOsmol/L, indicating the presence of EAH with the expected reduction in blood osmolality due to a dilution effect.

At 7:30 p.m. on the same day, a 35-year-old male presented to the medical tent complaining of nausea and "tingling." He, too, was diagnosed as suffering from dehydration and was treated with 3 L of a 0.9% sodium chloride and Ringer's lactate solution. His blood sodium concentration was 134 mmol/L and his blood osmolality was also reduced (282 mOsmol/L). An hour later a 24-year-old man presented with essentially the same symptoms and a blood sodium concentration of 134 mmol/L. He was treated with 2 L of a 0.9% sodium chloride and 5% dextrose solution for dehydration and hypoglycemia. Of 18 athletes treated in the medical tent at the 1983 Ironman Hawaii Triathlon and in whom blood sodium concentrations were measured, 3 had EAH, 2 more than the number of cases reported in the 1981 Comrades Marathon.

Over the next 14 years up to 1998, excluding 1984 and 1997 for which no records remain, blood sodium concentrations were recorded in all athletes seeking medical care at the race finish. During this period, 5,081 triathletes were seen in the medical tent and blood sodium concentrations were measured in 2,405 (42%) of these triathletes. Because during those years there were 19,207 finishers in that race, blood sodium concentrations were measured in 12.5% of all finishers in those years, about 172 triathletes per race. Of these blood samples, 761 were below 135 mmol/L, of which 231 were below 128 mmol/L, indicating more severe EAH.

Whereas some of the triathletes with blood sodium concentrations below 135 mmol/L may have had symptoms due to postural hypotension rather than EAH, it is almost certain that the symptoms experienced by athletes with blood sodium concentrations below 128 mmol/L—in particular, their altered levels of consciousness—were due to EAHE and not to postural hypotension. Twenty-three athletes had blood sodium concentrations below 120 mmol/L, indicating the presence of significant fluid overload with the real risk of a fatal outcome if the condition was treated inappropriately. That no EAHE deaths have been reported in the Ironman Hawaii Triathlon race is clearly a tribute to the physicians treating this large number of cases.

Figure 10.8 shows the *cumulative* number of athletes with different levels of EAH treated each year from 1983 to 1998 at the Ironman Hawaii Triathlon. Also included are the cumulative data for those with blood sodium concentrations

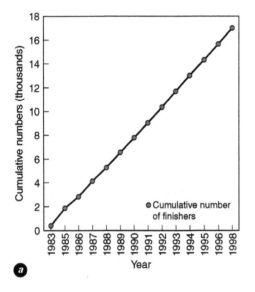

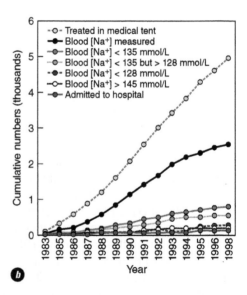

FIGURE 10.8 *(a)* The cumulative number of finishers in the Ironman Hawaii Triathlon, 1983-1998. *(b)* The cumulative number of athletes treated in the medical facility at the finish of the Ironman Hawaii Triathlon from 1983 to 1998 with different blood sodium concentrations.

above 145 mmol/L. Athletes with these elevated blood sodium concentrations have usually lost weight during exercise and are therefore dehydrated. Thus, the number of athletes finishing the race with blood sodium concentrations greater than 145 mmol/L provides an estimate of the number of runners who had lost more weight during the race and whose symptoms might therefore have been due to increased blood sodium concentrations.

Whereas 761 (31.6%) of these triathletes developed EAH during the race, only 231 (9.6%) finished with blood sodium concentrations above 145 mmol/L, which would occur with body weight losses of more than 3%. Thus, EAH was 3.3 times more likely to occur in Ironman Hawaii triathletes treated in the medical tent than was dehydration. Yet the message from the race sponsor, Gatorade, through its science affiliate, the GSSI, and their spokespersons has always been that dehydration poses the greatest risk for Ironman triathletes.

These data establish that at least between 1983 and 1998, the Ironman Hawaii Triathlon provided the world's richest source of clinical material for the study of EAH and EAHE, but little attempt was made to understand the true cause of the condition in that competition. In fact, athletes continued to be advised to drink at high rates during exercise in order to prevent heatstroke and to optimize performance.[7] Yet overdrinking was the precise cause of the extraordinarily large number of cases of EAH and EAHE in that race.

Even as I presented Dr. Tony Irving's data at the 1990 ACSM annual conference and continued through the years to present evidence and publish articles proving that EAH and EAHE are caused by fluid retention in those who overdrink during exercise and to which a sodium deficiency plays no role, Drs. Laird, Hiller, and others continued to assert that most participants in the Ironman Hawaii Triathlon who are hyponatremic are also dehydrated and that hyponatremia is caused by large losses in sweat and urine sodium, coupled with ingestion of large volumes of sodium-free fluids. But the data in figures 9.8 (page 261) and 10.8 show otherwise.

One of my early responses to these arguments, published in *The Physician and Sportsmedicine* (Pacelli, 1990), still applies: "Too often, people make the mistake of assuming that anyone who comes into a medical tent after a race looking pale and weak is simply dehydrated" (p. 30). Instead, I said that postural hypotension due to pooling of blood in the legs immediately after one stops running is often "mistaken for dehydration" so that "It is dangerous, maybe even life-threatening,[8] to give such people fluids. You ought first to try having them elevate their legs and pelvis and see if that helps. Most often, it does."

7 The idea that crippling dehydration causes heatstroke and impairs performance is at the center of what I have called the dehydration myth. Unpublished data measured in finishers in the 1994 Ironman Hawaii Triathlon provided to me in 1998 showed that their postrace rectal temperatures ranged from 37.0 to 40.2 °C, indicating that none was at any great risk of developing heatstroke. This is because the exercise intensity is relatively low in most Ironman Hawaii triathletes, because many take more than 4 hours to complete the marathon leg of the race. Since the metabolic rate determines the rectal temperature during exercise (chapter 3, figure 3.3, page 62), it is predictable that the majority of Ironman Hawaii triathletes are at extremely low risk for developing heatstroke regardless of how much they drink during the race.

8 Twelve years later, Hilary Bellamy would be treated inappropriately with intravenous fluids when she was in a coma with EAHE (Thompson and Wolff, 2003). She subsequently died. I have a feeling that most deaths from EAHE likely occur because these collapsed athletes are treated inappropriately with intravenous fluids on the assumption that they are dehydrated.

In 1993, the Gatorade Sports Science Institute published a roundtable discussion titled "Hyponatremia in Sport: Symptoms and Prevention" (Eichner, Laird, et al., 1993), in which I, Dr. Laird, Dr. Hiller, and Dr. Randy Eichner, who would subsequently become the medical spokesperson for Gatorade and the GSSI, presented our opinions of what causes EAH and how it should be treated and prevented. I, of course, restated my conviction based on the findings in Dr. Tony Irving's study that the primary cause of EAH was overdrinking, whereas Drs. Hiller and Laird reiterated their premise that athletes with hyponatremia at the Ironman Hawaii Triathlon were also dehydrated, so that their cases of EAH were due to "high sodium losses in association with inadequate sodium and fluid intake" (p. 3).

Interestingly, at that time, Dr. Eichner was more inclined to our interpretation: "The strongest hypothesis, in my opinion, is voluntary overhydration with water (and/or other very hypotonic fluids) in the face of moderate sodium losses in sweat. This seems to explain the most severe cases on record, such as those reported by Dr. Noakes in 1985 and 1990" (Eichner, Laird, et al., 1993, p. 2). He would later modify this opinion (box 9.2, page 266) such that his stated comments mirrored those of the GSSI.

So it seems that the illusion of knowledge—that EAH is caused by dehydration and large losses of sodium chloride—may have explained why no one involved with the Ironman Hawaii Triathlon ever asked this question: Why is the incidence of EAH and EAHE higher in the Ironman Hawaii Triathlon than in any other race in the world (box 10.2)?

Eventually in 2003, the GSSI finally funded a study to determine the factors that predict changes in blood sodium concentrations during the Ironman Hawaii Triathlon. The study was conducted by Dr. Edward Coyle. It found that "changes in serum sodium concentrations during endurance exercise can be largely attributed to changes in mass in male and female subjects and the rate of relative sweat sodium loss in males" (Pahnke, 2004, p. 84). Thus, 32% of the change in blood sodium concentrations in men and 40% in women could be explained by the change in mass during the race (figure 10.9, page 320), the expected finding. Furthermore, the authors found that subjects who decreased their mass by 2.88 kg or 4.1% of body mass maintained their blood sodium concentrations at the prerace value. They concluded that this was because these athletes were actually normally hydrated (not dehydrated) as a result of mass losses due to the irreversible oxidation of stored fuels and by depletion of the 2 L of fluid reserve discussed in chapter 9.

The data in figure 10.9 confirm that the same factor—excessive fluid consumption with weight gain—causes EAH in the Ironman Hawaii Triathlon, just as it does in all other events. These data disprove the Hiller, Laird, and GSSI hypothesis that EAH in the Ironman Hawaii Triathlon is caused by additional factors unique to that race, in particular high rates of sodium loss in salty sweaters.

Surprisingly, sweat sodium losses as calculated in this indirect manner explained about 13% of the change in blood sodium concentrations in men during the race but 0% in the women. According to my interpretation, the finding in the women is the expected finding on the basis of the entire body of published literature so that the finding in the men is likely to be an artifact of the indirect methods used and the established finding that if enough variables are studied, by chance alone some will inevitably appear to be related.

BOX 10.2 Experiences at the 1998 Ironman Hawaii Triathlon

The Ironman Hawaii Triathlon has enjoyed a number of title sponsors over the years. Bud Light was the first sponsor, from February 1982 until October 1990. Gatorade took over for an initial 5-year period in October 1991. For reasons best known to them, Gatorade relinquished that sponsorship for the 20th-anniversary race in 1998 before resuming in 1999. That choice would have an unpredictable consequence.

As long as the race was funded by Gatorade, I would not be a welcome guest. But when the Gatorade sponsorship was withdrawn, members of the 1998 Ironman Hawaii Triathlon medical staff invited me to talk at their prerace medical conference held during the week before the race. Interestingly, they did not originally invite me to speak on EAH and EAHE. I was also asked to act as a medical consultant on race day. During the prerace medical conference, a European doctor working at the German Ironman Triathlon showed a slide of an unconscious Ironman triathlete with EAHE being transported to the hospital. The unfortunate athlete was receiving intravenous fluids from drips placed in both forearms. The doctor stated that the cause of EAH is "unknown" but that affected athletes are "dehydrated" and require rapid intravenous fluid therapy.

I became so infuriated that I demanded to speak on the topic of EAH and EAHE. Naturally, I presented our data from the study of Irving, Noakes, and colleagues (1991) completed a decade earlier, which showed that EAH and EAHE are diseases of fluid overload in those who are encouraged to overdrink during exercise and is not caused by dehydration and sodium deficiency.

But what made the trip especially worthwhile at the time was my interaction with an elite triathlete who finished the race in a confused state in a little over 10 hours and with a blood sodium concentration of 125 mmol/L. When asked by the physician attending him what was required, I suggested that provided the athlete began to pass urine within 30 minutes, little needed to be done. Fortunately, that was precisely what happened. Over the next 6 hours, the patient spontaneously passed 5 L of urine and recovered fully, leaving the medical tent just before midnight.

When he asked me what had happened, I told him that he had drunk at least 5 L more during the race than he required. He confirmed that he had drunk heroically during the cycling and running legs. After 4 hours on the bicycle, he had started to vomit clear fluid. This, he "knew," indicated that he was "dehydrated" and needed to drink more. His run had been the worst of his career, which was not surprising if he was carrying 5 kg more weight than usual.

It was interesting to watch him shrink as he lost 5 kg in a few hours. He also informed me that he had loosened his watch strap during the race and that his Ironman identification tag had begun to feel progressively tighter during the race. I realized that these might be useful signs of a developing water intoxication in other athletes.

Two triathletes with EAH failed to develop a spontaneous diuresis and were treated with 1 L of 0.9% sodium chloride by other doctors, against my advice. Since they ultimately recovered sometime after receiving fluids intravenously, the treating doctor's bias that they were suffering from "dehydration" was confirmed. More probably, both recovered when they developed a spontaneous diuresis as their blood AVP/ADH concentrations fell appropriately.

These two patients had a common feature: They were completely withdrawn, responding poorly to questioning and wishing only to lie with eyes closed in the fetal position, while avoiding any contact with other humans. I have since realized that these are the typical behaviors of patients with EAHE. Once seen, these signs are not easily forgotten. Patients with these symptoms usually respond dramatically within minutes to the intravenous infusion of hypertonic saline solutions (Hew-Butler, Anley, et al., 2007) even before their blood sodium concentrations have normalized.

Probably these patients have a disproportionate rise in the pressure inside the brain (caused by brain swelling) relative to their blood sodium concentrations. Their rapid response must indicate that the hypertonic saline solution rapidly withdraws water from their soggy brain cells, lowering the pressure inside the brain and almost miraculously reversing their symptoms.

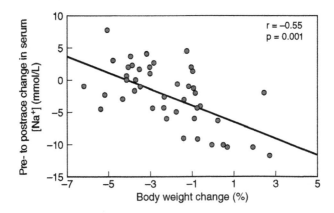

FIGURE 10.9   There was a significant linear relationship with a negative slope between the prerace to postrace change in blood sodium concentrations and change in body weight in competitors in the 2005 Ironman Hawaii Triathlon.

Adapted, by permission, from M.D. Pahnke, J.D. Trinity, J.J. Zachwieja, et al., 2010, "Serum sodium concentration changes are related to fluid balance and sweat sodium loss," *Medicine & Science in Sports & Exercise* 42(9): 1669-1674.

As I expected when these findings were published in *Medicine and Science in Sports and Exercise* (Pahnke, Trinity, et al., 2010), the authors focused on the role of sodium losses in men as the main determinant of the change in blood sodium concentrations during the Ironman Hawaii Triathlon while ignoring the fact that the change in body mass was the principal determinant of this change in male and female triathletes as found by all previous studies. The final publication of this work in *Medicine and Science in Sports and Exercise* still managed to fudge the issue by stating, "Changes in serum sodium concentrations during an ultraendurance triathlon are significantly related to interaction of fluid balance, sweat sodium loss, and sodium ingestion" (p. 1669). This, despite my insistence as a reviewer of the paper that the study again proved that fluid balance, not sodium ingestion, determines the postexercise blood sodium concentration. This statement is false because it did not apply to the female athletes in the study, the group at highest risk for the development of EAH and EAHE. In women, fluid balance alone explained measured changes in blood sodium concentrations during the race.

Fortunately, the incidence of EAH and EAHE has now dropped substantially in the Ironman Hawaii Triathlon. At the 2010 race, just 3 athletes finished with blood sodium concentrations below 130 mmol/L, and another 5 were between 131 and 134 mmol/L. But the race medical director, Dr. Bob Laird, was still uncertain of the etiology of EAH and EAHE. In his prerace lecture (Laird, 2010, p. 1) he said, "Experience at Ironman has shown that the sicker triathletes are probably dehydrated and/or hyponatremic." But he does now acknowledge that "While dehydration is common, some athletes may experience dilutional hyponatremia, with fluid retention and neurologic symptoms. This potentially serious condition is more likely to occur in athletes who have consumed excessive amounts of water and/or other fluids, especially the slower athletes who are able to take in more fluid relative to sweat loss" (p. 1). One must presume that the lower incidence of EAH in Ironman Hawaii triathletes in recent years is because these athletes have finally learned that drinking to excess during the race is not only detrimental to performance but also potentially very dangerous.

EAH and Fatal EAHE in the United States Military

The U.S. military provided another group of exercisers who suffered from an explosive incidence of EAH and EAHE in the 1980s (Montain, Latzka, et al., 1999). From 1989 to 1996 there were a total of 125 hospital admissions (~19 cases annually) for the treatment of EAHE, including at least 4 deaths. This epidemic followed closely the adoption of novel drinking guidelines for fluid replacement by the U.S. army sometime after 1991 (Burr, 1991; Montain, Latzka, et al., 1999).

These new guidelines described in chapter 7 required soldiers to drink more than 1.89 L/hr when exposed to environmental temperatures in excess of 30 °C (86 °F). In this heat soldiers were allowed to exercise for only 20 minutes of each hour and would presumably spend the next 40 minutes "rehydrating" by drinking more than 1.89 L of fluid. These guidelines were based on the hypothesis that only by drinking at high rates can heat illness be prevented. When followed as a military order, the predictable outcome could only be fatal as demonstrated by the tragic case report described earlier in this chapter (page 301).

Presuming that their new guidelines were at fault and were the probable cause of these tragedies, the U.S. military expeditiously introduced steps to ensure that more conservative drinking guidelines were introduced (Gardner, 2002; Montain, Latzka, et al., 1999). These ensured that soldiers were allowed to drink no more than 1.5 quarts (1,400 ml) per hour and no more than 12 quarts (11.4 L) per day (Craig, 1999). These guidelines were approved by the U.S. army medical leadership in April 1998. As a result, the incidence of new cases of EAH in the U.S. army began to fall after 1997, and most of the reduction occurred at Fort Benning, the U.S. army's infantry training center (Craig, 1999).

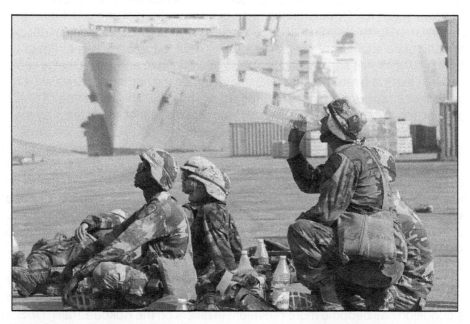

The introduction of novel drinking guidelines to the U.S. military after 1988 was followed by the sudden appearance of EAH, including fatal cases of EAHE. A reversal in 1998 to the drinking guidelines of the 1960s reversed this trend. U.S. military personnel are now advised about the dangers of drinking too much.

AP Photo/John Gaps

By 2002, Gardner was able to acknowledge that "further deaths from hypo-natremic encephalopathy in the United States Army will reflect the failure of the system to protect adequately its personnel through policy, procedures, and imple-mentation. Every military hospitalization for hyponatremia should be reviewed as a potential sentinel event that generates thorough review of policy develop-ment, with resultant intensive enforcement of life-saving preventive measures" (p. 434). This decisive action by the U.S. military in April 1998 (Craig, 1999) was not matched until very recently by the civilians charged with the care of runners and triathletes, especially in the United States—and then only after substantive lobbying in the scientific and lay press.

EAH in Hiking and Other Activities

A rising incidence of EAH has been reported in hikers including, paradoxically, those walking in the desert. The overriding conclusion from these studies is that EAH and EAHE occurred in those who reported very high rates of fluid intake when exercis-ing in the heat. The goal of such high rates of fluid intake was clearly to prevent heat illness and heatstroke. Yet Backer, Shopes, and colleagues (1993; 1999) did not encounter a single case of heatstroke in a period in the early 1990s when they treated 11 cases of EAH and EAHE in hikers in the Grand Canyon in Arizona. They concluded that "hyponatremia is much more common than heatstroke and in our experience is the most common cause of serious illness related to exercise in the heat" (Backer, Shopes et al. 1999b, p. 538), even though exercise was undertaken at high environmental temperatures (35-40 °C, or 95-104 °F). They noted that "this paucity of heat stroke cases is intriguing" (p. 536) (see note 3 in chapter 6, page 189).

The other significant observation by Zelingher and colleagues (1996) and Galun and colleagues (1991) was that the urine of hikers with EAH and EAHE contained substantial amounts of sodium. If patients with EAH and EAHE are sodium deficient, then their urine should not contain any sodium since the body has a remarkable capacity to conserve sodium and is able to secrete urine and sweat that is sodium free when there is a real sodium deficiency. Rather, the finding of urine with a high osmolality because of a high sodium content indicates the presence of SIADH. However, the importance of this finding was again overlooked, at least by me.

The incidence of EAH has also increased on the Kokoda Trail, a 96 km single-file thoroughfare that travels through the Owen Stanley Range in Papua New Guinea. In the 1950s, Australian world 1-mile record holder and the second man to run the mile in less than 4 minutes, John Landy, reinvigorated interest in the trail by covering it in 4 days with the help of carriers and guides. The number of people hiking the trail increased from 76 in 2001 to more than 5,600 in 2008. In 2008, a case of EAHE was described in a 44-year-old female hiker, Debra Paver (case 1612, appendix B). In 2009 four Australian hikers died while on the trail, but the autopsy findings were inconclusive.

Dr. Sean Rothwell, the physician who described the first case of EAHE on the trail (Rothwell and Rosengren, 2008) (case 1575 in appendix B), explained why the condition has become more prevalent in hikers on the Kokoda Trail ("Dr. Sean Rothwell," 2010): "The condition (EAHE) has been in endurance events for the last 25 years. One theory about this phenomenon is that athletes have been encour-aged to drink more fluids over this period. . . . There is no evidence that electrolyte containing sports drinks prevent this condition. The best treatment is prevention: the best prevention is to only drink while you are thirsty. . . . The jury is out with regards to (the preventive role of) salt supplementation. Avoiding overdrinking remains the best way to prevent EAH" (pp. 2-3).

EAH and EAHE have also been reported in Israeli military personnel who drank large quantities of water before a 2.4 km swim in open water (Weiler-Ravell, Shupak, et al., 1995); the Nijmegen Four Day Marches in the Netherlands, the largest walking event in the world with more than 45,000 participants annually (Eijsvogels, Thijssen, et al., 2008); and marathon cycling spinning in Sweden (Lorraine-Lichtenstein, Albert, et al., 2008). In the Nijmegen event, predictors of EAH were the usual candidates: weight gain during the walks, high rates of fluid ingestion, and prolonged finishing times.

Figure 10.10 shows the main activities associated with the development of EAH and EAHE. The most striking feature is that 55% of cases have occurred in the Ironman Hawaii Triathlon and another 14% in the U.S. military.

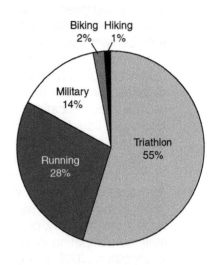

FIGURE 10.10 The proportion of cases of EAH and EAHE occurring in triathletes especially in the Ironman Hawaii Triathlon, in runners, in hikers, in the U.S. military, and athletes in other activities. The data are based on the individual cases collected in appendix B.

EAH in American Football

Even though American football players are encouraged to drink at high rates during training and competition in order to prevent heatstroke (Berning, 2008; Gatorade, 2007; GSSI, 2002), there are surprisingly few reports of EAH or EAHE in this group of athletes. Perhaps this is because practices usually last less than 2 hours, providing insufficient time to develop a profound fluid overload. Alternatively, it may be difficult to play or practice a vigorous contact sport with an intestine that is full of unabsorbed fluid. Yet some cases have been described.

A 22-year-old college football player was admitted to the hospital after he had received 8 L of hypotonic fluid, 5 intravenously, for the treatment of muscle cramps secondary to dehydration (Herfel, Stone, et al., 1998, p. 257). On this treatment, he developed pulmonary edema and EAHE; his blood sodium concentration was 121 mmol/L. He was discharged fully recovered 3 days later.

A 27-year-old National Football League player was admitted to the hospital after he suffered an epileptic seizure on the first day of training for the new season (Dimeff, 2006). His blood sodium concentration was 116 mmol/L. After training, he complained of feeling ill with nausea, excessive fatigue, and a diffuse headache. He drank 60 oz (1.7 L) of a sports drink; this induced vomiting. He was sent home and encouraged to consume sports drinks "as tolerated." His wife reported that during the evening he complained of increasing headache and nausea, becoming increasingly more disorientated before suffering the seizure. He regained consciousness 28 hours later and recovered fully. On questioning, he admitted to drinking 2 to 3 gallons (8-11 L) of water every day because "this is what he had been advised to do growing up in Texas and throughout his college and professional football career." He had also been taught that "water is the best replacement fluid" (p. 174).

In August 2008, Patrick Allen, a football player on the Bakersfield (California) Christian High School team, died as a result of EAHE caused by drinking too much water, according to the autopsy report: "The cause of death was determined to be due to complications of electrolyte imbalance including hyponatremia due to excessive liquid ingestion during marked physical exertion" ("Coroner: BCHS Student Died from Chemical Imbalance. . ." 2008, p. 1).

The coroner's report on the cause of death was absolutely specific since it made no reference to any contribution of salt deficiency to the cause of death: "Hyponatremia occurs when the sodium in your blood is diluted by excess water. Hyponatremia may result from medical conditions that impair excretion of water from the body, or by a significant increase in water consumption, such as athletes competing in marathons and other high-endurance events" (Ratliff and Youngblood, 2008, p. 1).

Unhelpfully, the media reported it differently. One report claimed incorrectly that "While Allen was consuming water, officials said he was sweating all of his sodium or salt out of his body and not replenishing that sodium—which they said is needed by the body's organs in order to run. [One must wonder which officials these were.] ABC23 spoke to an area pediatrician who said a good way to replenish sodium lost [sic] in the body is to consume sports drinks or to take

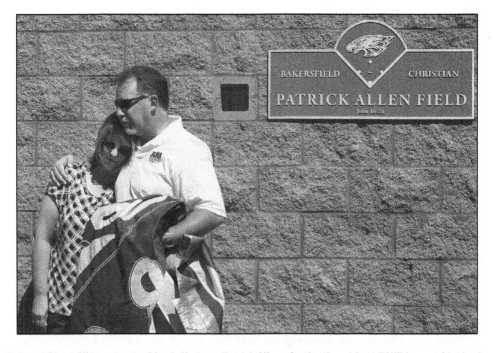

Bob and Diane Allen, parents of football player Patrick Allen who developed fatal EAHE by overdrinking in an attempt to treat his muscle cramping. The field where their son played football is now named the Patrick Allen Field at Bakersfield Christian High School, Bakersfield, CA.
Zuma Press/Icon SMI

salt tablets—especially for those working out for more than two or three hours and those sweating in high temperatures" ("Electrolyte Imbalance Blamed in Death of Football Player," 2008, p. 1).

The medical director of an emergency room in South Carolina also suggested that the condition could have been prevented if the player had ingested a sports drink: "If you drink water it can kind of leak out of the vessels and pull salt and other electrolytes with it. . . . You need to drink a lot of Gatorade, or 10k Powerade, something that has some substance to it because that type of fluid stays in the vessels. Drinking water doesn't" (Davis, 2008, p. 1). The doctor had clearly not studied the case of Cynthia Lucero.

This case indicates the extent to which, 27 years after Eleanor Sadler first developed EAHE and 6 years after Cynthia Lucero died from the identical condition that killed Patrick Allen, the dominant myth remains that it is unsafe to exercise without drinking to excess (box 10.3).

BOX 10.3 "You Think You Are Doing Everything Right"

When Robert Allen learned that his son Patrick had died from drinking too much, he was reportedly incredulous (Creamer and Hagedorn, 2009): "What do you do when you have cramps? You drink lots of water and rehydrate. You think you are doing everything right and then this still happens" (p. 1).

When their son came home from football practice and complained of muscle cramps, he drank water and Gatorade. When he started to vomit, his parents called an ambulance to take him to the hospital. He died two days later after experiencing "fluid in the lungs and surgery to relieve pressure on his brain" (Creamer and Hagedorn, 2009, p. 3). A local sport physician was reported as saying that as a result of this case it "would be madness" to avoid hydrating out of fear of developing fatal EAHE. Instead, he suggested that athletes under severe physical stress should drink fluids that contain electrolytes, "like Gatorade" (p. 4).

Robert Allen's wish was that "Hopefully we will learn something from this, so no other family has to go through this" (Creamer and Hagedorn, 2009, p. 2). Yet the advice that the "local experts" came up with would do little to prevent further tragedies—they advised that players should "drink fluids with electrolytes, like Gatorade, or take salt pills with water during heavy exercise" (p. 2). In addition, they advised athletes to be fit before they start football practice and to acclimatize to heat for at least 2 weeks, according to the advice of the Gatorade-funded National Athletic Trainers' Association.

No one had the courage to say that fluids play no part in the prevention of muscle cramps (chapter 4) or heatstroke (chapters 2 and 3) or that EAH is prevented simply by always drinking to thirst. Instead, "Research conducted by the Gatorade Sports Science Institute (GSSI) found that as many as 70 percent of high school football players could show up for practice inadequately hydrated. The recommendation of drinking fluids prior to practice increased the number of players appearing to be adequately hydrated upon arrival to practice. Scientific research has shown that dehydration or poor hydration increases the risk of heat illness" (Gatorade, 2007, p. 1).

Like Cynthia Lucero, who overdrank to prevent a condition that her slow running speed and the prevailing environmental conditions ensured she could never suffer, Patrick Allen died because he drank to excess in the mistaken belief that this was the correct treatment for a benign condition that resolves with time. But there is no evidence that fluid balance plays any role in either the causation or cure of exercise-related muscle cramps (chapter 4).

Non-Exercise-Related Hyponatremia

The content of this book has focused on the unexpected consequence of advising athletes to drink as much as tolerable during exercise. But was there a measureable consequence of the related advice to the general public that they should drink at least 8 glasses of water each day? Australian exercise scientist Frank Marino thinks he may have found such evidence in Australia.

Marino and King (2010) collected data from Australian hospitals for hospital admissions with a diagnosis of either hyponatremia or heat illness (figure 10.11). The data showed that from 1994 to 2007 the annual number of hospital admissions with a diagnosis of heat illness was essentially unchanged (lower line in figure 10.11: 1293 cases from 1994 to 2000 and 1523 cases from 2001 to 2007). In contrast, the annual number of admissions for a diagnosis of hyponatremia has increased progressively since 1994. This includes all types of hyponatremia, not just exercise-associated hyponatremia. As a result, in the years 1994 to 2000 there were 7,476 cases of hyponatremia, whereas in the following 7 years to 2007 this had increased by 63% to 20,348 cases. Marino wondered whether the same dramatic increase in the number of hospital admissions for hyponatremia has occurred in other countries in which the "healing" benefits of overdrinking have been marketed.

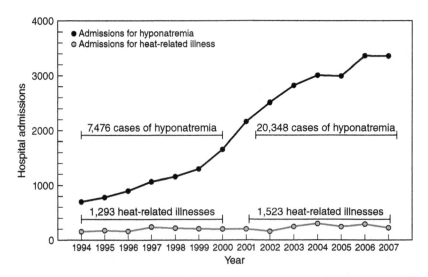

FIGURE 10.11 The annual number of admissions to Australian hospitals for a diagnosis of hyponatremia or heat illness.

Reprinted, by permission, from F.E. Marino and M. King, 2010, Limitations of hydration in offsetting the decline in exercise performance in experimental settings: Fact or fancy? In *Chocolate, fast foods and sweeteners: Consumption and health*, edited by M.R. Bishop (Hauppauge, NY: Nova), 63-73.

Summary

This chapter describes the rising incidence of EAH and EAHE as reflected in publications in the scientific literature and reports in the lay press. By July 2010, 12 fatalities and more than 1,600 cases of EAH and EAHE have been reported (appendix B). It is probable that many, many more cases have not been reported. Thus, the cases collected here represent the proverbial tip of the iceberg.

During this time, EAH became the single greatest risk to the health of endurance athletes (Verbalis, 2007), disproving the often-stated myth that "dehydration and heat illness . . . represent the greater threat [than EAHE] to anyone who is physically active in a warm environment" (GSSI, 2003, p. 1). During the same period, I was unable to find a single case report of death or ill health in an athlete in whom dehydration was established as the sole causative mechanism. Nor was any evidence published to show that dehydration is an important factor causing heatstroke.

The large number of cases of EAH and EAHE in the Ironman Hawaii Triathlon is of particular interest. That other Ironman triathlons around the world, especially those in New Zealand and South Africa, have by comparison contributed a trivial number of cases shows that these conditions are not the inevitable consequence of completing an Ironman triathlon. There is nothing specifically wrong with "fragile" humans, for example the condition of so-called salty sweating, that makes it inevitable that they will develop EAH and EAHE whenever they compete in an Ironman triathlon. Instead, we are the most enduring mammals specifically designed to exercise for prolonged periods in the heat with inadequate water and sodium replacement.

The Fat Man (chapter 8) was correct: We are not all about to self-destruct simply because we might wish to run the Comrades Marathon or to complete the Ironman Hawaii Triathlon. We are rather more robust. And imperfect health has always been perfect health (Shem, 2003).

CHAPTER 11

Guidelines
for Fluid Intake
and Diagnosis of EAH

But most of all I listen to my body and try
to unlearn being an educated specialist.
It's a lifetime work, this becoming a simple
and seamless whole.

George Sheehan (1975, p. 94)

S cientists failed the endurance athlete because they did not consider all of the
    evidence. Incorrect dogmas regarding fluid requirements during exercise,
all disproven by the totality of the published literature available already in the early
1990s, were actively sustained for more than two decades. In this book, I have
presented a thorough review of the research on the thirst mechanism, dehydration, thermoregulation, sodium balance, and the biology of exercise-associated
hyponatremia (EAH) and exercise-associated hyponatremic encephalopathy
(EAHE). My experiences as a runner and our discovery of EAH in the 1980s led
me to unexpected places in my research and professional life. It has not always
been an easy road. In the process I learned that very few of my colleagues are
prepared to support anyone who challenges an established mind-set, especially
one that is supported by powerful commercial interests because it underpins
an entire industry. But my instinct is to search for the truth. And that is what has
sustained me for the past two decades since I received that life-changing letter
from Eleanor Sadler in 1981. This brings us to this final chapter, wherein I present
the best and safest guidelines on hydration for health and performance during
endurance exercise, along with steps that medical professionals should take in
diagnosing and treating EAH and EAHE.

How Much Should You Drink?

In chapter 7, I described the drinking guidelines formulated mainly in the 1980s and 1990s, culminating in the *1996 American College of Sports Medicine Position Stand: Heat and Cold Illnesses During Distance Running.* The errors of these guidelines have been explained in previous chapters. In this chapter we look at the guidelines established in 2002 by the International Marathon Medical Directors Association (IMMDA). We also examine the 2007 American College of Sports Medicine (ACSM) position stands, on which many organizations' hydration guidelines are based. Although the ACSM corrected several errors in their 2007 position stands, crucial revisions have yet to be made. I advise marathon and other long-distance athletes to follow the IMMDA guidelines.

IMMDA Guidelines for Fluid Replacement During Marathon Running

In about March 2001, I was invited by the president of IMMDA, Lewis Maharam, MD, to present a paper at the annual IMMDA conference to be held in association with the 2001 New York City Marathon. He wanted me to discuss appropriate drinking during marathon racing, including the prevention of EAH and EAHE.

Dr. Maharam reminded me that about 5 years earlier at an ACSM annual conference he had asked my advice on handling the fluid requirements of marathon

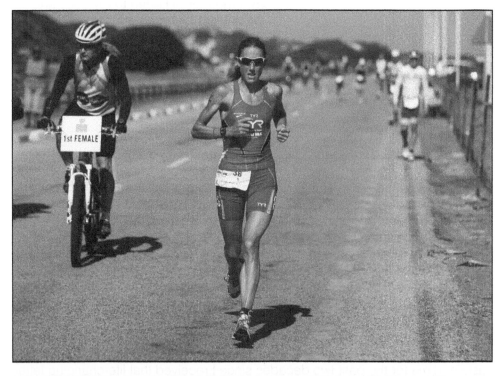

In the 2011 South African Ironman, Chrissie Wellington set a new world Ironman Triathlon record for women, finishing in 8:33:56. The race was managed according to the IMMDA guilines. Fluid availability was restricted on the course, and triathletes were encouraged to drink only according to the dictates of thirst.

Richard Stabler/Getty Images

runners and treating collapsed athletes. I gave him the advice that we had developed in South Africa over the years. At the time I did not have the evidence from the 2000 and 2001 South African Ironman Triathlons, which established that these guidelines are associated with the lowest rate, yet recorded, of triathletes seeking medical care after the race or that their care is simplified when these guidelines are followed (Sharwood, Collins, et al., 2002; Sharwood, Collins, et al., 2004).

Following are the key points of the advice I gave him (Mayers and Noakes, 2000; Speedy, Noakes, et al., 2003):

- Athletes should drink to thirst during the race and not more than 800 ml/hr.
- Athletes who collapse *during exercise* have one or more serious medical conditions and must be treated by the appropriate medical experts, knowledgeable in the management of these conditions in nonathletic populations.
- In contrast, the majority of athletes who collapse *after exercise* have EAPH and require no treatment other than to recover while lying supine with the head below the level of the heart and pelvis.
- The two most likely exercise-related causes of collapse during exercise are heatstroke and EAHE. They are differentiated by measuring the rectal temperature and the blood sodium concentration. Heatstroke is treated by immersion in a bath of ice-cold water, whereas EAHE is treated with concentrated (hypertonic) saline solutions and diuretics.
- Intravenous fluid therapy must be "earned" and may not be given unless measurement of the athlete's blood sodium concentration indicates that he or she has an elevated level (hypernatremia). However, there are very few indications for the use of intravenous fluids in collapsed marathon runners.

Dr. Maharam told me that when he had applied these guidelines in the marathon races at which he was the medical director, including the New York City Marathon, the incidence of EAH and EAHE was low and the management of collapsed runners was significantly simplified. After I presented the paper, he asked whether I would produce drinking guidelines that IMMDA could implement at all the marathon races at which their members were responsible for the medical care of the competitors.

The original guidelines (Noakes and Martin, 2002) were subsequently republished (Noakes, 2003a). They made the following points:

- That the nature of marathon running had changed since the 1970s as a result of the creation of the "big-city" marathons. The increased number of participants in these events had resulted in an enormous expansion of medical and allied support services. Much of this expanded support was provided in the form of "aid stations" along the course at which massive volumes of fluid were freely available. This had resulted from the fundamental change in the advice of how much athletes should drink during marathon races—from very little prior to the 1970s to "the maximal amount that can be tolerated" (Convertino, Armstrong, et al., 1996, p. i) after the publication of the 1996 ACSM guidelines, supported by those produced by the NATA and the American Dietetic Association and the Dietitians of Canada.

The second change was in the distribution of finishing times in U.S. marathon races from 1975 to 2001. Whereas 100% of 1,818 finishers in the 1975 Boston Marathon completed the race in less than 3:30, in the 2001 New York City Marathon only 10.8% of the 23,651 finishers completed the race within that time. Furthermore, 69.8% of athletes took more than 4 hours to finish the race and 23% more than 5 hours.

The athletic abilities of the athletes entering the race, the amount of training each was likely to undertake, and the running speed that the "average" athlete could sustain during the race had changed dramatically. Since a runner's speed determines his metabolic rate, which determines his sweat rates and body temperatures during these races (box 3.1, page 62), his fluid requirements would differ greatly depending on whether he is finishing the race in 2:07:43 (first finisher in the 2001 New York City Marathon) or in a time slower than 8:30, the time of the final finisher. Thus, these guidelines had to cover the requirements of athletes whose running speeds differed by a factor of ~4 and whose body weights differed probably by as much as threefold (40-120 kg).

■ That the usual drinking guidelines that advised athletes to drink as much as tolerable (e.g., the 1996 ACSM guidelines) were based on the findings in laboratory studies, not in studies of outdoor exercise, including competitive marathon races. Many of those studies were performed in environmental conditions that approximate those found in the more tropical countries, such as those of the Pacific Rim, whereas many marathons are run in the morning in cool to temperate spring or fall conditions in North America and Europe. In addition, many of these laboratory studies were completed without adequate convective cooling and therefore magnified many of the supposedly detrimental physiological effects of not drinking during exercise.

■ That the risk of heat illness is greatest in the elite runners running in short-distance races, not in those taking 5 or more hours to run or walk the same distance. Thus, it makes little sense to encourage those at little or no risk of heat illness to undertake the potentially dangerous practice of drinking as much as tolerable, a practice that in any case has no proven role in the prevention of heatstroke (chapter 3).

1 Although technically correct, we now believe that the rate of heat production in athletes who develop heatstroke may result not just from how vigorously they exercise but also by the onset of abnormal thermogenesis (heat production) in their skeletal muscles, probably as the result of some genetic predisposition. When associated with one or more internal triggers, prolonged exercise then initiates an explosive thermogenesis that produces a cataclysmic rise in body temperature leading to heatstroke (Rae, Knobel, et al., 2008). Thus, we now argue that just as EAHE cannot occur without the presence of at least two genetic variants, so heatstroke cannot occur unless there is also a genetic predisposition to this explosive thermogenesis.

I noted that "the risk of developing heat stroke is increased when exercise intensity is highest" (more likely in shorter-distance races) "in athletes with greater body mass" (because they generate more heat than lighter athletes), when environmental temperature and air humidity are high, and especially when there is little air movement so that there is limited convective cooling (Noakes 2003a, p. 312). I failed to add the proviso that heatstroke is likely due to excessive endogenous heat production.[1]

I added that four compelling pieces of practical clinical experience suggest that athletes should never be advised to drink as much as tolerable.

First is the evidence showing a marked rise in the incidence of EAH and EAHE in "back of the pack" athletes who finish marathon races in a state of fluid overload when advised to drink as much as tolerable.

Second is the evidence that encouraging athletes to drink more during exercise does not seem to have reduced the number of athletes seeking medical care at the end of marathon races. On the other hand, more conservative drinking policies may lead to fewer admissions if for no other reason than the incidence of EAH and EAHE will be reduced.

The third body of evidence is that athletes typically lose 2 to 3 kg of body weight during marathon races and that most of this weight loss could be due to fluid and other losses that do not contribute to dehydration and thus do not need to be replaced. If correct, this suggests that athletes drinking according to the dictates of thirst during exercise accurately anticipate how much they need to drink. Furthermore, these data confirm that athletes do not regulate their body weights during exercise; rather, they regulate the osmolality of their body tissues (figure 9.12*b*, page 277).

The fourth piece of evidence is that elite athletes drink sparingly during marathon races and that this does not appear to interfere with their performances or increase the risk that they will develop heatstroke.

The article then provided a set of five guidelines:

Guideline 1. Be careful to make accurate diagnoses so that the treatment plan can be optimally effective rather than inappropriate. (p. 314)

The point was that slow runners are essentially at no risk of developing heat illness (however defined) during marathon running. Since slow runners constitute the majority of those seeking medical care during or after marathon races, it makes no sense either to treat them for a condition they do not have or to advise them to adopt a behavior (drinking beyond the dictates of thirst) that has no proven value in preventing a condition for which they are essentially at no risk.

Guideline 2. Considerable individual difference in responsiveness exists for tolerable fluid ingestion during exercise. . . . It is neither correct nor safe to provide a blanket recommendation for all athletes during exercise. (p. 314)

I made the point that each human carries the necessary controls to ensure that he or she drinks appropriately during exercise; it is called the thirst mechanism. Provided athletes are told to drink according to thirst, they will perform optimally and will not be at risk of ill health induced by either over- or underdrinking during exercise.

Guideline 3. A diagnosis of heat illness should be reserved only for patients who have clear evidence of heat stroke, the diagnostic symptoms of which are a clear alteration of mental function, either confusion or loss of consciousness, associated with a body temperature >41 °C, and the successful treatment of which requires active whole body cooling. If the rectal temperature is not elevated to >41 °C so that the patient recovers fully without the need for whole body cooling, a diagnosis of heat illness cannot be sustained, and an alternative diagnosis must be entertained. (pp. 314-315)

The bases for this argument were presented in chapters 2 and 3. In brief, my belief is that EAPH is by far the most common condition causing athletes to collapse after marathon races. EAPH is also simply a normal physiological response to the sudden cessation of prolonged exercise, especially if it is performed in the heat. This condition requires no treatment because spontaneous recovery always occurs (Noakes, 2007a).

It is incorrect to presume that all athletes who collapse after exercise are suffering from a disease (heat illness) that is caused purely by dehydration. Rather, I suggested a more critical assessment of the clinical evidence and the use of only those forms of evidence-based treatments that are appropriate for each specific diagnosis. The best form of treatment is usually masterful inactivity (Noakes, 1988a; Noakes, 1988b).

> **Guideline 4.** Athletes who collapse and require medical attention *after* completing long distance running events probably are suffering more from the sudden onset of postural hypotension than from dehydration. (p. 315)

Again, the point was that there is no evidence that this condition of postexercise collapse is due to dehydration, nor that it should be treated with intravenous fluid therapy. There are no published randomized controlled clinical trials to show that intravenous fluid therapy is more effective than masterful inactivity.

Instead, I presented our South African evidence showing that we had been able to provide a high level of medical care to 33,000 runners in four consecutive 56 km ultramarathons and approximately 1,000 finishers in the South African Ironman Triathlon without once requiring the use of aggressive intravenous rehydration.

> **Guideline 5.** Runners should aim to drink *ad libitum* 400 to 800 ml/hr [13.5 to 27 fl oz/hr] with the higher rates for the faster, heavier runners competing in warm environmental conditions and the lower rates for the slower runners/walkers completing marathon races in cooler environmental conditions. (p. 316)

Athletes usually drink ~500 ml/hr during exercise, but EAH becomes increasingly more likely in those slower athletes who ingest more than 1 L/hr.

Thus, the final advice was that athletes "should drink *ad libitum* [at one's own discretion] and aim for ingestion rates that never exceed about 800 ml/hr" (p. 317).

USATF Endorses IMMDA Guidelines

In a press conference held in the week before the 2003 Boston Marathon, one year after the death of Cynthia Lucero, the USA Track and Field (USATF) announced that they would be adopting the IMMDA guidelines that I had developed, with immediate effect (USATF, 2003). They stated the following:

> For athletes in general and especially for those completing a marathon in more than four hours, USATF recommends consuming 100 percent of fluids lost due to sweat while racing. This marks a significant change from the understanding most runners have that they should be drinking as much as possible and following the guideline to stay ahead of your thirst, which has been held as the standard recommendation for many years.
>
> Simply put, runners should be sensitive to the onset of thirst as the signal to drink, rather than staying ahead of thirst. Being guided by their thirst, runners prevent dehydration while also lowering the risk of hyponatremia (low sodium), *a potentially dangerous condition increasingly seen as runners have erroneously been instructed to over-hydrate* [my emphasis].

The 2007 ACSM Position Stands

In 2007 the ACSM released their updated position stands on exercise and fluid replacement (Sawka, Burke, et al., 2007) and exertional heat illness during training and competition (Armstrong, Casa, et al., 2007). Since by then I had begun to focus on the issue of conflict of interest, I noted that the six authors of the first document all enjoyed close working relationships with Gatorade and the GSSI.

The 2007 position stands included one crucial change from the 1996 guidelines. Instead of encouraging athletes to "consume the maximal amount that can be tolerated" (Convertino, Armstrong, et al., 1996, p. i) during exercise in order to replace all the weight lost during exercise, these new guidelines proposed that "The goal of drinking is to prevent excessive (>2% body weight loss from water deficit) dehydration and excessive changes in electrolyte balance to avert compromised performance" (Sawka, Burke, et al., 2007, p. 377). Furthermore, the guidelines now recognized that "because there is considerable variability in sweating rates and sweat electrolyte content between individuals," it is not possible to provide blanket guidelines that cover all individuals under all circumstances. Thus individualized "customized fluid replacement programs are recommended." The guidelines also noted that "consuming beverages containing electrolytes and carbohydrates can provide benefits over water under certain circumstances."

Dehydration and Performance　The revised guidelines provided a more balanced review of the effects of different levels of weight loss on exercise performance, concluding that levels >2% are increasingly more likely to produce an impaired performance. However, the guidelines still fail to acknowledge that this conclusion is still at variance with the clear evidence that the best athletes often win major sporting events while drinking little and developing the highest levels of dehydration.

My conclusion is that there is no magical single level of dehydration above which the exercise performance of all humans will begin to be affected. Rather, the best athletes will be those who are least affected by fluid loss during exercise and who may therefore produce an optimal performance, perhaps even at weight losses in excess of 8%. This leads to the conclusion that it is the presence of thirst, not the level of dehydration, that is the important determinant of whether performance will be affected by the extent of drinking, including its absence during prolonged exercise (Sawka and Noakes, 2007). Hopefully, when the ACSM produces its next position stand, this will be the accepted position since it is the only one that best explains all the current evidence.

Hydration and Health　The revised guidelines note that while "dehydration is more common," "overdrinking— with symptomatic hyponatremia—is more dangerous" (Sawka, Burke, et al., 2007, p. 381). The guidelines include the principle, incorrectly stated in the 1996 ACSM position stand, that dehydration increases the risk for heat illness and heatstroke. As argued in chapter 3, there is no scientific evidence to support this conclusion. Furthermore, none of the studies that were referenced as evidence to support these guidelines was a randomized controlled clinical trial, and some actively disproved the relationship. Two quoted studies (Carter, Cheuvront, et al., 2005; Epstein, Moran, et al., 1999) reported cases of

2 The 2007 position stand also claims that the very serious condition of rhabdomyolysis (muscle cell breakdown with release of toxic chemicals into the bloodstream) may also be associated with dehydration. Similarly, kidney failure may also be associated with dehydration whether or not there is also rhabdomyolysis. As for all these associations, there is no scientific evidence that the relationship is causal. Rather, the finding that all these conditions—heatstroke, rhabdomyolysis, and kidney failure—occur so infrequently suggests that they must be due principally to an individual susceptibility that is exposed by the exercise, plus other environmental triggering factors, which are currently unknown.

heatstroke in which dehydration could not have been an important cause in the majority; yet they interpreted the data to support an exactly opposite conclusion.

The authors also contend that skeletal muscle cramps "are believed associated with dehydration, electrolyte deficits and muscle fatigue" (Sawka, Burke, et al., 2007, p. 381), so that "three factors are usually present in exercise-associated muscle cramping (EAMC): exercise-induced muscle fatigue, body water loss and large sweat Na⁺ losses" (Armstrong, Casa et al. 2007, p. 564). Neither of these statements is particularly meaningful since association does not prove causation. Instead there is a great deal of evidence showing that muscle cramping is a neuromuscular condition, completely unrelated to dehydration and electrolyte deficits[2] (chapter 4).

The new position stand provides no new information to prove that dehydration increases the risk of ill health. Rather, the position stand sustains the dehydration myth without addressing the concerns I have raised.

Overhydration The section dealing with exercise-associated hyponatremia begins with an incorrect statement that EAH was first described in the 1971 Comrades Marathon. In fact, as discussed in chapter 4, the data from that study are likely incorrect, in that the authors did not note symptoms of EAH in any of the competitors before, during, or after the race. Nor did the term *hyponatremia* appear anywhere in their article.

This section continues by acknowledging that overdrinking causes EAH and EAHE but continues to sustain the unproven hypothesis that "excessive loss of total body sodium" (Montain, Cheuvront, et al., 2006) can also cause these conditions.[3] As a result they conclude that: "In longer ultra-endurance events, sodium losses can induce hyponatremia to levels associated with the onset of symptoms regardless if the individual is over- or underdrinking, so replacing some of the sodium loses is warranted" (Sawka, Burke, et al., 2007, p. 382).

3 The position stand quotes a publication (Montain, Cheuvront, et al., 2006) describing a model that predicts that EAH might develop under certain specific conditions (figure 9.12a, page 277) and ignores published evidence from real-life studies (not theoretical models). This model requires that the sweat glands continue to "pour" out salt even as the body develops a sodium deficit and without any attempt by the body to prevent the development of a significant sodium deficit that will ultimately kill the person. But this seems unlikely because there are highly developed systems to ensure that the kidneys and sweat glands are able to conserve sodium very effectively when salt intake is low (box 4.5, page 133).

There is no evidence that these statements are true, whereas there is a great deal of evidence ignored by the authors, which disproves them (chapter 4). The position stand does not include reference to the landmark studies of Irving, Noakes, and colleagues (1991) and Speedy and colleagues (2000), both of which showed that EAHE is due to fluid overload in which a sodium deficit plays no part.

Rates of Fluid Intake During Exercise The authors concluded that the IMMDA/ USATF guidelines that athletes should drink ad libitum at rates of 400 to 800 ml/hr "are probably satisfactory for individuals participating in marathon length events" (Sawka, Burke, et al., 2007, p. 385). This is a relief since we have known since 1988 (Noakes, Adams, et al., 1988) that this is exactly what athletes do when they run marathons.

The science of hydration, it seems, has after nearly 20 years and a dangerous detour finally come to its senses. The guidelines for carbohydrate and sodium intake were the same as those included in the 1996 guidelines.

Interestingly, the senior author of the position stand had said in 1991, "I am less optimistic than Ethan Nadel about our ability to develop a model for fluid replenishment. . . . We have used a number of different models for sweating, and an important part of that is just simple metabolic rate . . . what really impressed me was the big difference in the metabolic rates required for different subjects to run at a given grade and speed. They are so diverse that . . . I think we can give advice on glucose and sodium concentrations, but the proper volume for fluid replacement is really an individual factor" (Lamb and Williams, 1991, p. 78).

Clearly something happened between 1991 and 2007 to make Dr. Sawka change his opinion on this matter.

Erroneous Assumptions

To understand truth, one must first appreciate that all truths are model dependent. This was best described by Stephen Hawking (1993): "A theory is a good theory if it is an elegant model, if it describes a wide class of observations, and if it predicts the results of new observations. Beyond that it makes no sense to ask if it corresponds to reality, because we do not know what is reality independent of a theory. . . . It is no good appealing to reality because we don't have a model independent concept of reality" (p. 38). Thus, to understand another's truth, one must first understand the model that the other uses to underpin his or her particular concept of reality. The model of reality on which the 1987 and 1996 position stands and, to a much lesser extent the 2007 ACSM position stands, are based makes at least six erroneous assumptions.

■ *Erroneous assumption 1:* All of the weight lost during exercise must be replaced if health is to be protected (by the prevention of heat illness) and performance is to be optimized.

■ *Erroneous assumption 2:* Fluid ingestion alone can prevent serious heat illness during exercise regardless of the circumstances in which the exercise is undertaken.

■ *Erroneous assumption 3:* Uniquely in humans, although apparently not in any other of God's creatures, the sensation of thirst underestimates the body's real fluid requirements before, during, or after exercise. As a result, humans will always drink too little before, during, and after exercise.

Were this true for all other creatures, all would be perpetually dehydrated and hence dogged by the ill health caused by chronic dehydration.

■ *Erroneous assumption 4:* The fluid requirements of all athletes, big and small, fast and slow, are sufficiently similar during all forms of exercise that a universal guideline (drink 600-1,200 ml/hr—the 1996 ACSM guidelines—or 400-800 ml/hr—the 2007 ACSM guidelines) is possible.

Measured sweat rates in humans during exercise vary enormously from as little as 100 ml/hr in ultramarathon runners in freezing Alaska (Stuempfle, Lehmann, et al., 2003) and who adjust their running speeds (and hence metabolic rates) in an attempt to remain dry when exercising (since sweat freezes in subzero conditions and increases the probability that hypothermia will develop) to about 3,000 ml/hr in huge (150 kg, or 330 lb) American football players training in hot conditions (Fowkes, Godek, et al., 2004) or in the much smaller Haile Gebrselassie when he set the current world marathon record (Beis, Fudge, et al., 2012). Thus, it is ludicrous to attempt to provide specific drinking rates that will cover all athletes under all conditions. Instead, such guidelines will cause some to drink too much and others too little.[4]

4 Indeed, EAH has occurred in some, especially female athletes, who drank less than our guidelines advise (i.e., at relatively low rates of fluid intake). For example, Dugas and Noakes (2005) reported the development of EAHE in a cyclist who drank only at a rate of 735 ml/hr during the 5 hours that she required to complete a 109 km cycling race. Since her sweat rate was only 270 ml/hr, she managed to increase her total body weight by 2.5 L in 5 hours, dropping her blood sodium concentration to 129 mmol/L (case 1504 in appendix B). Two cases of EAH also occurred in female competitors in the New Zealand Ironman Triathlon (Speedy, Noakes, et al., 2001), even though they drank at rates of less than 750ml/hr, well within all these apparently safe guidelines. Thus, the development of EAHE does not always require the heroic drinking rates of >1.2 L/hr.

■ *Erroneous assumption 5:* Athletes can safely ingest any volume of fluid both at rest and during exercise without harmful consequences.

The maximum capacity of the intestines to absorb fluid and the kidneys to excrete urine is about 1,200 ml/hr, whereas maximal sweat rate is ~3,000 ml/hr. Thus, we are designed to sweat at a much faster rate than we could absorb fluid or excrete urine.

■ *Erroneous assumption 6:* Human physiology is designed for failure. According to the catastrophe model of human exercise physiology, humans function as if they are brainless. Thus, we exercise without the protection of a brain whose function is to ensure that we survive. Instead, we must expect our bodies to betray us and to fail whenever we expose them to any stress that we find somewhat uncomfortable, such as running a marathon or completing an Ironman Triathlon or hiking through the Grand Canyon. Under these conditions the brain, rather than acting as our protector, becomes the agent of our destruction.

When I started running in 1969, there were few runners and hence no industries to exploit *our* passions for *their* commercial gain. Later, as I was running marathons and ultramarathons, we followed the dictums of gurus like Dr. George Sheehan, who advised that we should follow the "wisdom of the body," a concept I suspect he discovered from the great U.S. physiologist Dr. Walter B. Cannon, who wrote a book with the same title (Cannon, 1939). Sheehan also seems to have applied the phrase "listen to your body" to athletics (box 11.1).

If only we had been encouraged to listen to our internal voices, thirst included, EAH and EAHE could never have occurred.

BOX 11.1 George Sheehan

Dr. George Sheehan was the runners' iconic philosopher from 1968 until his untimely death from cancer in 1993 at the age of 74, four days before his 75th birthday. He trained as a cardiologist and served in World War II in the South Pacific as a doctor on the destroyer *U.S.S. Daly*. In his 40s, Dr. Sheehan became disillusioned with success and bored with his profession. He turned to the philosophers, and through his voracious reading he was inspired to run in order to become "fully functioning," after the writings of Ireneus, an early church father. Five years later, he was the first person 50 years or older to run a mile in under 5 minutes. He completed it in 4:47.

Dr. Sheehan wrote the classic books about the philosophy of running *Dr. Sheehan on Running, Running & Being, Medical Advice for Runners, This Running Life, Personal Best*, and *Running to Win*. He completed his final book, *Going the Distance*, during his illness, and it was published after his death.

Many runners knew Dr. Sheehan from his columns written as the medical editor for *Runner's World* magazine. Sheehan seems to have coined the term "listen to your body" or at least to have applied it to athletics. It is a concept that seems to have become increasingly foreign to those born in recent times. I recall Sheehan once telling me that one day people will want to be told how they must walk. He had little patience with such dependency.

What Should You Drink?

Although much of this book and our early research involved investigating how much to drink, every long-distance athlete wants to know *what* to drink, and rightly so. Our mental state and performance may well depend on it. Most sports drinks include some combination of electrolytes and carbohydrate. While the inclusion of electrolytes seems to have stemmed from misplaced conventional wisdom, the use of carbohydrate, at least by carbohydrate-adapted athletes,[5] is beneficial and has a foundation in sound research studies.

Sodium Chloride

What contribution, if any, does the addition of electrolytes, especially sodium chloride, have on performance? Sodium chloride (salt) was added to the ancestral Gatorade solution because of a study (Malawer, Ewton, et al., 1965) showing that the addition of this electrolyte slightly increases the rate at which the intestine absorbs water and glucose from the ingested solution; however, adding glucose had a much greater effect (chapter 5).

5 The common belief that *all* human athletes perform best when they eat high-carbohydrate diets and ingest additional carbohydrate during exercise has been challenged on the grounds that humans evolved as carnivores whose principal source of food energy was fatty meat, not carbohydrate (Cordain, Brand Miller, et al. 2000; Cordain, 2011; Cordain and Friel, 2005; Volek and Phinney, 2011). According to this interpretation, human athletes who eat a diet that excludes almost all carbohydrate—the so-called paleo diet—become fat adapted and can perform all forms of exercise without the need to ingest any more than trace amounts of carbohydrate either before or during exercise. Although this theory has yet to be properly evaluated by randomized controlled clinical trials, its advocates quote an impressive body of anecdotal evidence to support this interpretation (Cordain and Friel, 2005).

In that study, the test solution was added directly to the small intestine without first passing down the throat and through the stomach. The rate of fluid absorption was also measured over a small section of the small bowel that had been isolated from the rest of the bowel. A subsequent Gatorade-funded study (Gisolfi, Summers, et al., 1998) performed in humans who ingested either water or 6% glucose solutions with varying concentrations of sodium chloride showed that the addition of sodium chloride to any solution that is ingested via the normal route (and not infused artificially) does *not* alter the rate of water and glucose absorption by the intestine from that solution. This finding has been confirmed repeatedly (Jeukendrup, Currell, et al., 2009). Those studies therefore established that sodium chloride does not need to be present in the ingested solution in order to maximize the rate of water absorption from that solution. Rather, it is the carbohydrate content of the solution that determines the rate of water absorption (Shi, Summers, et al., 1995), but this effect is probably maximized from a 6% carbohydrate solution (Jeukendrup, Currell, et al., 2009). In concentrations at which it is still palatable in a fluid, the ingestion of sodium chloride during exercise appears to be without any biological advantage.

The 2005 International Consensus Conference on Exercise-Associated Hyponatremia (Hew-Butler, Almond, et al., 2005) "found that only during very prolonged exercise (such as the 226 km Ironman triathlon) undertaken in more extreme environmental conditions, *might* an acute sodium deficit contribute to exertional hyponatremia. Thus the consensus opinion is that only under those unique conditions of very, very prolonged exercise in more severe environmental conditions, might an increased sodium intake *during* exercise be beneficial. However, there currently are no studies to support this hypothesis and two that actively contradict it (Hew-Butler, Sharwood, et al., 2006; Speedy, Thompson, et al., 2002)" (Noakes, 2007b, p. 790).

In chapter 4, I presented the evidence showing that humans adapt very quickly to a low sodium intake by reducing the amount of sodium they lose first in urine and then in sweat. On the basis of this normal human biological response, I conclude that the sodium present in the urine and sweat during exercise represents the dietary excess ingested in the days before exercise and that must be excreted in order to maintain a safe sodium balance. As a result, any sodium ingested during exercise will be excreted in urine because it simply adds to that excess (figure 4.10, page 141).

So in the absence of any substantive evidence that sodium ingestion during exercise plays any role other than perhaps a possible placebo effect on performance, my advice is to limit sodium intake during exercise to only that which optimizes the palatability of the ingested fluids. There is also no need to increase daily sodium intake above that dictated by appetite. For those who are habituated to a high sodium intake or to ingesting sodium during exercise, it requires only a few days for the body to adapt to the lower sodium intake that I advise.

Carbohydrate

By 1981, I was certain that the ingestion of water alone would not optimize performance especially in ultramarathon races. The basis for this certainty was a number of races I had run in which I developed an unexpected symptom usually after 30 to 36 km in races of 42 to 56 km, and after about 60 km in the 90 km Comrades Marathon. The symptom was that in the space of a few hundred meters I would suddenly lose the desire to finish the race. This would be replaced with the perception that the finish of the race was desperately far away and I could not conceive, feeling as bad as I did at that moment, how I would be able to drive myself for the next 1, 2, or 3 hours that I would need to finish those races.

In time, I began to suspect that this symptom probably meant that my blood glucose (sugar) concentration had fallen too low and that this could perhaps be both prevented and cured by ingesting the most appropriate carbohydrate source in the optimal concentration during long-distance races.

Interestingly, there are indeed individual differences in sensitivity to hypoglycemia during exercise so that those who are accustomed to eating a high-carbohydrate diet or ingesting carbohydrate during exercise, as most athletes are, may be much more sensitive to the negative effects on their performance of falling blood glucose during exercise (Claassen, Lambert, et al., 2005).

We began to study the effects of hypoglycemia on exercise performance in distance runners at the same time that I had just begun my teaching career as a lecturer in sport science at the University of Cape Town. Our first experimental approach was to measure blood glucose concentrations at the finish of various South African marathon and ultramarathon races, continuing the approach we had begun in 1976. We found that 2% of the athletes we studied had measurably low blood glucose concentrations at the end of a 42 km marathon; this incidence rose to 6% after the 56 km Two Oceans Marathon and to 11% after the 1981 90 km Comrades Marathon.[6] This seemed to confirm my personal experience that the longer the race, the more probable it was that hypoglycemia would develop, causing the disabling symptoms I had experienced. It also suggested that carbohydrate ingestion during exercise might be a crucial factor in improving performance, especially during ultramarathon races.

The winner of the 1981 90 km (56 mile) Comrades Marathon, Bruce Fordyce, participated in that study. That was the first time I had met him. He would go on to win an unprecedented nine Comrades Marathons, a feat not likely to be repeated. In time he would tell me of his experience in the 1979 Comrades Marathon in which he had finished third and his potential for greatness had been exposed for the first time.

Bruce recalled that in that race he had begun to feel weak about 20 km from the finish and was passed by other runners. Fortunately his father, a medical doctor who was assisting him, knew that his son's fatigue was due to hypoglycemia, which could be corrected with a stiff dose of sugar. So he forced his compliant son to drink a very high-carbohydrate drink (Coca-Cola with added sugar at a concentration of probably about 10 g added sugar per 100 ml of Coca-Cola). The results were quite dramatic. Within a few minutes Bruce recovered and he surged forward, finishing strongly in third place. And so, thanks to his

6   This was also the race in which Eleanor Sadler developed EAHE. The remarkable realization is that our team did extensive analysis of blood samples from about 100 athletes who were in the medical tent at the end of race because they either sought medical care or they wished to be part of our study. But we did not think it necessary to measure blood sodium concentrations. Why should we? EAH had never been described before. And when we had measured blood sodium concentrations in the 1979 Comrades Marathon, the values had been boringly normal.

Perhaps the point is that in 1981 we were more interested in the carbohydrate intake of marathon and ultramarathon runners in order to prevent hypoglycemia and that probably we believed that they were already drinking sufficient fluid. But we had absolutely no idea that soon many would be drinking too much. I always regret that we had not measured blood sodium concentrations in that race, because we likely would have discovered some instances of EAH.

7 When I spoke to Bruce Fordyce in 2008, he told me of his experience during his final victory in the 1990 Comrades Marathon. During that race, he had organized more helpers than ever before. And each had been so effective in providing him with fluid during the race that toward the end of the race he began to feel and hear water sloshing around in his intestine. He felt, he told me, as if he had "water right up to his throat." Yet he continued to drink frequently lest he appear ungrateful to those who had given up their time to help him. It was his most difficult race, perhaps because he had overdrunk during the race.

father's intervention and a few grams of sugar, Bruce began to develop the belief that he would win the race sometime in the future.

Having discovered the value of sugar, Bruce asked me the next year if sugar was the most effective carbohydrate he could add to the Coca-Cola he would continue drinking during the Comrades Marathon. By this time he had already concluded that he was unable to run his best in the Comrades Marathon unless he ingested a high-carbohydrate solution, especially in the second half of the race.[7]

In fact, there was good reason to believe that sugar was not the ideal form of carbohydrate to add to the drink ingested during exercise. This is because a drink made from sucrose has a higher osmolality than one in which the carbohydrate in the drink is more complex, made up of long chains of glucose molecules, so-called glucose polymers. Since at that time we believed correctly that solutions with higher osmolality are emptied from the stomach more slowly than are solutions with a lower osmolality, we suggested to Bruce that he should instead prepare his Comrades Marathon drink using glucose polymers rather than sugar.

Perhaps as a result of this collaboration, in 1983 we were contacted by the manufacturers of the Leppin line of nutritional supplements to assist in the development of carbohydrate drinks and supplements for use by endurance athletes, including Bruce Fordyce. This became known as the FRN range, with the letters standing for the three—(Bruce) **F**ordyce, (Bernard) **R**ose, and (Tim) **N**oakes—who were involved in the intellectual development, testing, and promotion of the product.

We then began a series of experiments to determine the optimal solution for ingestion during exercise. Our approach differed from that adopted by Gatorade and its scientists who seem to have accepted that the solution developed by Dr. Cade in 1966 was ideal and did not require modification. As a result, the ingredients in Gatorade have changed very little in the past 40 years. We decided to begin from the beginning by building the solution one ingredient at a time.

Our starting assumption was that athletes would generally drink 400 to 800 ml/ hr. Thus, our solution would need to provide sufficient carbohydrate to optimize performance when ingested at that rate. Our first step then was to determine the optimal carbohydrate source for the drink. We assumed that this would be the carbohydrate most rapidly used by the exercising muscles.

To reach the muscle where it can be used (oxidized) as an energy source, the carbohydrate must first empty from the stomach, a process known as gastric emptying, before it is initially digested (intestinal digestion) and then absorbed by the intestine (intestinal absorption), transported to the liver where it may be either stored as glycogen or converted to glucose (if the ingested carbohydrate is fructose), after which it travels in the arterial blood to the muscles.

We discovered that simply ingesting large amounts of carbohydrate during exercise will not increase the rate at which the muscle will use that carbohydrate. There will be a limit determined by the factors that maintain the blood glucose concentration within the prescribed homeostatic range.

Thus, we established that the factor limiting the rate at which ingested carbohydrate can be used by the muscle is the level at which the blood glucose concentration is naturally regulated. Only by artificially increasing the blood glucose concentration could the rate of glucose oxidation by the exercising muscles be substantially increased.

As a result, we and others have shown that the nature of the carbohydrate ingested during exercise really does not matter; when ingested individually, many types of carbohydrate (glucose, maltose, glucose polymer, starch) are used by the muscle at essentially the same peak rate. Thus, we originally concluded that all carbohydrate will produce equivalent results when ingested during exercise.

Only more recently has it been shown that a specific mixture of carbohydrates (glucose and fructose) (Jentjens, Shaw, et al., 2005; Jentjens, Underwood, et al., 2006) ingested at high rates can produce very high rates of carbohydrate oxidation of up to 1.75 g/min (Jentjens and Jeukendrup, 2005). Such high rates of carbohydrate ingestion have also been shown to improve cycling performance during a 1-hour time trial (Currell and Jeukendrup, 2008), although as yet we have been unable to show the same effect.

During this period we also evaluated the rates of gastric emptying from different carbohydrate solutions (Sole and Noakes, 1989) but concluded that it was not the type of carbohydrate or its concentration that was the most important determinant of the rate of gastric emptying. Rather, the volume of fluid ingested is the more important determinant (Noakes, Rehrer, et al., 1991). We concluded that provided the athlete is prepared to start the race with a stomach loaded with 400 ml of even a highly concentrated (18%) carbohydrate solution and if he were to drink 100 ml of that same solution every 10 minutes each hour, his intestine would receive 600 ml and 108 g of carbohydrate. Both of these values exceed the athlete's needs in almost all conceivable circumstances.

We concluded that it is not the carbohydrate type or its concentration that determines how much carbohydrate is delivered to the athlete's muscles during exercise but rather the athlete's drinking behavior. In particular, the extent to which the athlete is prepared to run with a partially filled stomach during exercise will determine how much ingested carbohydrate his muscles receive during exercise (Noakes, 2003b).

So my advice is the following: If you are habitually adapted to eating a high-carbohydrate diet, then the research evidence is clear: Your performance will be improved by ingesting carbohydrate during exercise. The best evidence is that ingesting about 60 grams of carbohydrate per hour optimizes this effect in events lasting more than 2 hours; lesser intakes can achieve the same effect in races of shorter distance. Conversely, I am aware that some world-class triathletes are able to ingest more than 100 grams per hour during the last few hours of the Ironman Triathlon, but these athletes are unique, as are their requirements. I would not advise marathon or ultramarathon runners to attempt such high rates of ingestion.

To achieve an intake of 60 grams of carbohydrate per hour requires that one drink 600 ml (20.3 fl oz) of a 10% carbohydrate solution. This can easily be achieved if one's ad libitum fluid intake during exercise is 600 ml or more per hour. If it is less, then the athlete must drink either a more concentrated carbohydrate solution during exercise or else the athlete can supplement carbohydrate intake by ingesting one or more carbohydrate gels each hour during exercise. Most gels are usually packaged in sachets containing 20 to 25 g of carbohydrate.

At present, we do not know whether athletes habitually adapted to a low-carbo-hydrate ketogenic diet will also benefit by ingesting carbohydrate during exercise. My bias is to believe that such ingestion might be detrimental in exercise lasting less than 2 hours but may have some role in the latter stages of more prolonged exercise like ultramarathons or the Ironman Triathlon.

Symptoms of Exercise-Associated Hyponatremia

Having established how much and what endurance athletes should drink to optimize health and performance, we now turn to the defining characteristics of EAH and EAHE.

A review of the symptoms reported by real patients with clinically documented EAH or EAHE shows that the symptoms they develop are specific, common, and unmistakable. The order in which these diagnostic symptoms typically appear is usually the following:

1. Impaired exercise performance

This probably occurs at quite low levels of weight gain (>1% BW gain) and is due either to swelling of the brain cells or to an increased pressure within the brain (intracerebral pressure), either or both of which impair brain function.

While an acute weight loss of greater than 2% may impair exercise performance if it is associated with an uncorrected thirst (Sawka and Noakes, 2007), we and others have measured levels of dehydration of 6% or greater in winning athletes in ultramarathon races (Sharwood, Collins, et al., 2002; Sharwood, Collins, et al., 2004), as was typically the case in the 1950s and '60s when athletes were actively discouraged from drinking during exercise. In contrast, athletes who gain 6% or more of their body weight during exercise are likely to be close to death.

2. Nausea and vomiting

These symptoms result either from an increased intracerebral pressure caused by brain swelling or the presence of a large volume of unabsorbed fluid in the stomach and intestine, or perhaps a combination of both.

Especially the vomiting of large volumes of clear fluid (water) can occur only if the rate of fluid intake has been excessive. Similarly, the presence of excess unabsorbed fluid in the gut will cause a sensation of fluid sloshing around in the intestines. Neither of these symptoms can occur in dehydration, since in dehydration the content of water lying free in the intestine is reduced.

Indeed, one theory, discussed in chapter 9 (see note 20, page 284), is that humans can sustain a substantial (~2 kg) water loss without any noticeable effects. Spare fluid could lie freely in the intestine where it serves little real function except to act as a biological reserve in humans who practice delayed drinking. Delayed drinking, you will recall, is the likely adaptation our ancestors were forced to make once the size of the human gastrointestinal tract was reduced as we became increasingly more successful long-distance hunters. The body may first mobilize this water reserve stored in the gut before it begins to activate its defenses against dehydration.

Thus, by definition, dehydration cannot be the direct cause of the vomiting of large volumes of clear fluid from the gastrointestinal tract since the first consequence of water loss in humans is to reabsorb the fluid that lies freely within the intestine.

3. Headache

This results from the increased intracranial pressure caused by brain swelling in EAHE. Since dehydration reduces the fluid content of the brain, it cannot cause headache by this mechanism. Whereas headache might be an expected feature of EAHE, there is no reason for it to develop in dehydration. Headache is not listed as a common symptom in cholera, the disease causing the most rapid onset of profound and life-threatening dehydration in humans.

4. Altered level of consciousness

Athletes with mild EAHE become sullen, sleepy, and withdrawn; they avoid social interaction, close their eyes, and turn away from the light seemingly because they have photophobia (dislike of light). When addressed, they appear confused and somewhat dull; they are unable to hold a conversation of substance. They have difficulty concentrating and speak only when addressed directly. They have no interest in conversation. They appear to be either intoxicated or to have suffered a head injury causing concussion.

In those with mild EAHE, all these symptoms can be reversed almost miraculously within minutes by the administration of a hypertonic (3-5%) saline solution (Hew-Butler, Anley, et al., 2007; Hew-Butler, Noakes, et al., 2008). Observing the miraculous effects of this form of treatment taught me that EAHE makes clever people appear (temporarily) rather stupid. After questioning one confused patient with EAHE, I concluded that he was definitely not a rocket scientist. Minutes later, after he received 100 ml of 3% saline intravenously, he suddenly became fully alert, recognized me, and introduced himself as a highly qualified businessman. He wanted to know what had possibly caused his problem.

Mild dehydration of the type found in modern athletes causes none of these symptoms. This is readily confirmed by interviewing the hordes of "dehydrated" runners treated in the medical facilities at any endurance event anywhere in the world. While mentally fatigued, none show these classic features of being dull, sleepy, confused, withdrawn, and disinterested in their surroundings. These characteristic mental features always indicate that the athlete has either EAHE or another real medical condition, such as heatstroke or diabetic precoma.

The fact that dehydration does not cause any of these mental symptoms and especially the altered state of consciousness diagnostic of EAHE was noted already in 1947 in the famous U.S. military studies in the Nevada Desert (Adolph, 1947). Brown wrote, "In general, men cannot continue to walk in the desert heat unless they replace the water lost in the form of sweat. In some way dehydration augments the signs of physical fatigue until merely standing erect is an intolerable strain. Men dehydrated to this extent retain their mental faculties; they are not crazed by thirst. . . . Contrary to the popular legend . . .

when the unfortunate victim of water shortage is first incapacitated he is neither delirious nor in agony from 'mouth thirst'; he simply is incapable of even mild physical effort" (p. 143).

Those who had not read Brown's work promoted the fatally erroneous idea that dehydration also causes the altered level of consciousness found in those with EAHE. As a result, many athletes with EAHE received intravenous fluids for the treatment of altered states of consciousness supposedly caused by dehydration. And some died.

5. Seizure (convulsion)

This is caused by a marked increase in intracerebral pressure. Since dehydration reduces the intracerebral pressure, it cannot cause a convulsion by this mechanism. People who are lost in the desert without water do not develop seizures. Instead, they become confused and lapse into coma, most likely because of a progressive reduction in blood flow to the brain associated with the accumulation of toxic substances in the blood secondary to kidney and liver failure. Since the mild levels of dehydration (3-8%) encountered in ultramarathon runners and Ironman triathletes do not cause kidney and liver failure, so coma and convulsions in endurance athletes are not caused by dehydration.

6. Bloating and swollen hands, legs, and feet

These are usually first noted by the athlete's spouse or other relative or friend. Athletes may notice that their watch straps or race number bracelets become tighter as they become progressively overhydrated. In contrast, dehydration will cause the opposite—athletes will look as if they have become thinner, and their watches and race number bracelets will become less tight.

7. Muscle cell breakdown (rhabdomyolysis) with the development of acute kidney failure

Although there have been isolated reports of rhabdomyolysis and EAH occurring at the same time, the study of Bruso, Hoffman, and colleagues (2010) is the first to define this relationship in five competitors in the 2009 Western States 24-Hour/100-Mile Endurance Run. Blood sodium concentrations ranged from 127 to 134 mmol/L and all had blood creatine kinase activities in excess of 40,000 U/L (normal postrace values are up to ~2,000 U/L), indicating the presence of severe muscle cell breakdown; the highest value was >95,000 U/L. Three developed acute kidney failure; the most severely affected athlete required 12 days of hospital care.

Thus, far from protecting against acute kidney failure, aggressive drinking sufficient to produce EAH can, by mechanisms that are currently unknown, induce muscle cell damage that is sufficient to cause kidney failure. It is reasonable to assume that any level of overhydration will impair muscle cell function and hence athletic performance, and in some this effect will be sufficient to produce significant muscle cell damage.

Following are symptoms that are not a feature of either EAHE or dehydration:

1. Dizziness and fainting

Dizziness and fainting are caused by inadequate blood flow to the brain as the result of reduced blood pressure. An altered blood flow to the brain does not occur in EAHE or in dehydration at the mild levels measured in endurance athletes. Postexercise dizziness is due to EAPH, which is unrelated to the level of dehydration in athletes but is caused by an impaired regulation of the circulation when exercise terminates suddenly.

2. Muscle cramping

This is a separate condition that is caused by an altered nervous control of the muscles and is not due to overhydration, dehydration, or sodium deficiency in salty sweaters (chapter 4).

3. Wheezy breathing

This is a feature of asthma or similar respiratory conditions and is unrelated to EAHE or dehydration. Athletes with pulmonary edema due to EAHE may complain of shortness of breath and cough up a blood-stained sputum. Dehydration does not cause pulmonary edema.

Distinguishing Fluid- and Heat-Related Illnesses

Table 11.1 (page 348) lists the symptoms that are specific to the two conditions, EAHE and EAPH, that occur in endurance athletes. The only symptom of the nondisease of dehydration is thirst. Also included is a fourth set of symptoms that may be present during the first 5 days of heat acclimatization or when exercising for up to 60 minutes in "impossible" environmental conditions that cause exercise termination with "heat exhaustion."

In my view, the term *heat exhaustion* is a misnomer for a number of reasons. It is used purely to describe the circumstances (heat) in which a person chooses to stop exercising. This is then labeled as exhaustion even though the athlete may have no symptoms or other evidence of illness. But there is one feature that is constant in athletes with heat exhaustion: All have body temperatures that are too low for a diagnosis of heatstroke. Instead, their body temperatures are exactly appropriate for the intensity of exercise that they have sustained. Thus, an elevated internal body temperature has nothing to do with heat exhaustion and, unlike the situation in heatstroke, it cannot in any way be a factor causing the condition. Even if one believes (incorrectly) that fluid ingestion during exercise reduces the risk that heatstroke will develop, such fluid ingestion cannot influence the risk of a different "disease"—heat exhaustion—in which there is no abnormal heat retention.

Remember that experienced sport physicians cannot predict the extent of dehydration (or volume depletion) by simply examining the turgor of the skin,

TABLE 11.1 Symptoms of Conditions Associated With Collapse in Endurance Athletes

Condition	Symptoms
EAHE	1. Impaired exercise performance 2. Bloating and swollen face, hands, legs, and feet 3. Nausea and vomiting 4. Headache 5. Altered level of consciousness 6. Seizure (convulsion)
Dehydration	1. Thirst (box 2.2, page 49) 2. Impaired exercise performance, but only when thirst is present
EAPH*	1. Dizziness and faintness 2. Nausea caused by reduced blood flow to brain (cerebral ischemia) secondary to reduced blood pressure (hypotension) 3. Vomiting (occasionally), which is also due to cerebral ischemia
Heatstroke	1. Impaired exercise performance 2. Altered level of consciousness: confusion, loss of control, aggression 3. Collapse 4. Coma
Heat exhaustion during the first 5 days of heat acclimatization or when exercising for up to 60 minutes in "impossible" environmental conditions that cause exercise termination with heat exhaustion	1. Fatigue 2. Headache 3. Dizziness, especially when erect 4. Shortness of breath 5. Loss of appetite 6. Nausea 7. Vomiting 8. Abdominal cramps

*These symptoms are reversed the instant the athlete lies flat. In contrast, lying flat does not alter any of the symptoms of EAHE; nor does it cure thirst in those who are truly dehydrated. Nor does it reverse the symptoms present in the first 5 days of heat acclimatization.

the state of hydration of the mucous membranes in the mouth, the presence of sunken eyes, the ability to spit, and the sensations of thirst (McGarvey, Thompson, et al., 2010).

The only way to accurately determine the level of an athlete's state of hydration after prolonged exercise is to measure the body weight before and after exercise or, better, to measure the change in body water content. Urine color cannot be used in diagnosing dehydration (Cheuvront, Ely, et al., 2010) because it is a measure of the brain and kidneys' response to changes in blood osmolality. It does not tell us the exact blood osmolality (the true measure of the body's fluid status) and whether it is raised, lowered, or normal. For example, because they have SIADH, athletes with EAH typically excrete concentrated urine even though they are severely overhydrated with blood osmolalities that are greatly reduced (and should be excreting very dilute urine).

Postural hypotension is a common feature of collapse in unacclimatized subjects exposed to unusually demanding exercise in warm to hot conditions. In fact, the development of EAPH is the most important factor causing postexercise collapse (Noakes, 2010).

Dr. Lucy Holtzhausen directed our research on EAPH and developed management protocols that would become the world standard (Holtzhausen and Noakes, 1997; Noakes, 2000). We concluded the following (Holtzhausen, Noakes, et al., 1994): "On the basis of these findings, we hypothesize that the most likely mechanism for exercise-associated collapse (EAC) is a syncopal episode resulting from postural hypotension (Bethell, Jewell, et al., 1991) caused by a sudden cessation of exercise and loss of the skeletal muscle pump in the lower extremities. It is possible that a number of other factors, including mild dehydration, excessive racing effort and a training-induced reduction in the vasoconstrictor response to any hypotensive stress, may contribute to EAC. Hyperthermia would likely be a more important factor in shorter races run at higher exercise intensities (Noakes, Myburgh, et al., 1991) under more severe environmental conditions. . . .The modern management of EAC should take account of these several possibilities, rather than assuming that one single factor, in particular dehydration, is the sole etiological factor for EAC" (p. 1100). This was published in a North American journal in 1994, eight years before Hilary Bellamy was inappropriately treated for dehydration in the ambulance that transported her to Georgetown University where she died from EAHE.

Athletes who collapse at the finish of running races are no hotter or more dehydrated than are other runners who finish those races without collapsing. Thus, neither dehydration nor hyperthermia can explain why those runners collapse. Other evidence supports this conclusion: If athletes collapsed only because their cardiovascular function had been strained as a result of dehydration, which affects their hearts' ability to function, they would logically collapse when their hearts were working the hardest, that is, *during* the exercise bout and not immediately afterward when their hearts and circulation were recovering and returning to the resting state. Similarly, if an excessive accumulation of heat was the problem, why would it wait to strike only after an athlete had already finished the race, when her rate of heat production was already falling (box 11.2, page 350)?

Thus, athletes who collapse after exercise and who constitute the majority of cases treated in the medical facilities at endurance sporting events cannot be suffering from dehydration-induced heat illness, preventable and treatable simply by ingesting more fluids before, during, and after exercise. In short, encouraging athletes to drink more fluids during exercise in order to prevent the nondisease dehydration-induced heat illness makes no sense.

Instead, we have shown that the majority of athletes who collapse after exercise do so because they have developed exercise-associated postural hypotension (EAPH) resulting from an impaired regulation of blood pressure the moment exercise terminates. The optimal treatment of EAPH is to have athletes lie flat with the feet and

BOX 11.2 The Case of the Australian Open

The ACSM guidelines propose that exercise should not be performed when the air temperature exceeds about 30 °C (86 °F). Were this rule to be applied in Australia, some events like the Australian Open (tennis tournament) held annually in Melbourne at the height of summer would not exist. The on-court temperature usually exceeds those values on many days, sometimes with readings above 40 °C (104 °F).

But no game has ever been cancelled because of excessive heat, and no player in that competition has ever died of heatstroke. Thus, heat is a lesser threat to the conduct of the Australian Open than is rain to the Wimbledon Tennis Championships in London. In an attempt to explain this apparent paradox, John Brotherhood, PhD, and his PhD student, Susan Morante, chose to study the body temperatures and behaviors of tennis players when playing at various environmental temperatures. They showed that the temperatures of players were homeostatically regulated and remained below 40 °C regardless of the temperature in which the matches were played. Players achieved this by altering their behaviors so that they slowed down and rested more as the air temperature rose.

Although the presence of this anticipatory behavior was already shown in the study of Wyndham and colleagues, published in 1974,[8] it was perhaps the work of my PhD student Ross Tucker (Tucker, Marle, et al., 2006; Tucker, Rauch, et al., 2004) and that of Tatterson and colleagues (Tatterson, Hahn, et al., 2000) at the Australian Institute of Sport that reinvigorated interest in this concept in humans after 2004. Unlike human exercise physiologists, animal and insect biologists accept the cardinal role of anticipatory behavior in the regulation of body temperature in creatures other than humans (Heinrich, 1993).

8 Despite misinterpretations about dehydration and rectal temperature, Professor Cyril Wyndham was a good and innovative scientist. In experiments conducted in the 1950s (Strydom, Wyndham, et al., 1963; Wyndham, 1974), Wyndham documented anticipatory behavior among miners in South Africa. During these experiments, miners shoveled as much rock as they could into one-ton mine cars for a period of 5 hours in environmental conditions that varied from 27 to 36 °C (80.6 to 96.8 °F) with a relative humidity of 100% and wind speed that varied from 0.5 to 4.0 m/sec. Work output fell as an exponential function of environmental temperature, and at 36 °C with low wind speed (0.5 m/sec) only 20% of what could be produced at temperatures of 28 °C or below was produced. Productivity at the lower air temperatures was improved by the presence of an effective supervisor. But at the higher temperatures, the supervisor made no difference to the amount of work the miners performed. These studies show that humans regulate the amount of work they perform in an anticipatory manner. They do not simply work as hard as they can until they develop heatstroke.

What these new studies have shown is that when humans are exposed to an increased external heat load, they almost immediately reduce their exercise intensity (figure 11.1), just as they do when exposed to a sudden reduction in the oxygen content of the air that they breathe.

When subjects exercise at their own chosen paces during 20 km time trials performed in either hot or cool conditions, they begin to reduce their power output after about 5 minutes (after about 10% of the distance has been covered) in the heat compared to their performance in the cool conditions (figure 11.1a). We conclude that this is because the brain calculates that to continue exercising at the original pace in the heat would be suicidal. So it reduces the mass of muscle that it chooses to recruit in the exercising limbs, reducing the power output and thus the rate at which the athletes produce heat.

Interestingly, the brain might have chosen to sweat more to allow the athletes to exercise at the same pace in both environmental conditions, but it did not. Instead, the sweat rate remained the same so that the body temperatures of the athletes rose almost identically when they exercised in either the heat or the cold (figure 11.1b). In both conditions, there was a marked end spurt (even though rectal

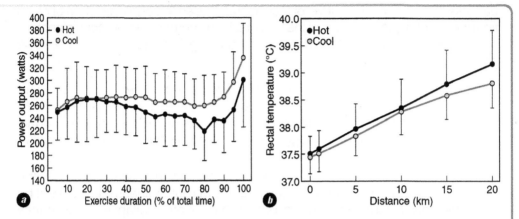

FIGURE 11.1 *(a)* Power output and *(b)* rectal temperatures during self-paced cycling time trials in cool and hot conditions.

With kind permission from Springer Science+Business Media: *Pflügers Archiv—European Journal of Physiology,* "Impaired exercise performance in the heat is associated with an anticipatory reduction in skeletal muscle recruitment," 448(4), 2004, 422-430, R. Tucker, L. Rauch, X.Y. Harley, and T.D. Noakes, figures 1 and 2, © Springer-Verlag 2004.

temperatures were high at that point) and subjects terminated the exercise with final rectal temperatures below 40 °C.

So all these experiments show that humans, like insects and other mammals, do not continue to exercise regardless of the outcome; they do not exercise mindlessly until the catastrophe develops and they die of heatstroke. Rather, the subconscious brain anticipates the danger the instant it appears and takes remedial action essentially immediately, specifically to ensure that the catastrophe is diverted. It achieves this by increasing the level of discomfort associated with continued exercise at that intensity. As a result, the easiest option is to slow down. If an athlete overrides the symptoms of discomfort, as Paula Radcliffe did in the 2004 Olympic Games in Athens,[9] eventually hyperthermic paralysis will develop to ensure that no further activity can be undertaken. As a result, heat production by the exercising muscles ceases and body cooling begins the moment the exercise terminates.

Perhaps it is clear that exercise is a behavior regulated in the brain to ensure whole-body safety. The brain almost always ensures this outcome. The only exceptions are medical conditions such as heatstroke and heart attack, which occur because of sudden bodily changes that the brain is unable to predict or expect.

So it may be extremely unpleasant to play tennis in the heat of Melbourne in January, but as decades of competition have shown, it is safe.

9 Later Radcliffe would report that she ran with difficulty throughout the race even though the average pace was 11 minutes slower than her world record. Her discomfort would be expected if she was progressively accumulating body heat and her subconscious brain was attempting to slow her down—in effect trying to warn her that if she wanted to finish the race she would need to run more slowly. But Radcliffe ignored the wisdom of her body and instead attempted to stay with the lighter Noguchi, whose rate of heat accumulation would have been considerably slower because she was 30% lighter.

Eventually at 36 km, Radcliffe's brain decided that she had had enough, forcing her to stop running. Later Radcliffe said, "I knew I was in big trouble. I could hardly pick my legs up at all; they were like lead weights. I felt so empty. It got to the point where I couldn't put one foot in front of the other. And I stopped" (Bryant, 2005, p. 12). In contrast, the diminutive Noguchi ran on apparently undisturbed by the conditions, indeed increasing her pace in the toughest section of the course.

buttocks elevated above the level of their hearts. This encourages the return of blood from the periphery to the center of the body, restoring normal cardiovascular function.

Two obvious conclusions can be drawn regarding fluid intake and postexercise collapse:

1. The amount of fluid an athlete ingests during exercise will not influence his risk of collapsing during or after the race. Rather, that risk is determined by factors that we do not fully understand but impair the ability of certain predisposed athletes to regulate their blood pressures immediately after they stop exercising.

2. Since dehydration is not the most common reason athletes collapse after exercise, then treating collapsed athletes with intravenous fluids cannot be the optimal form of treatment. But if some athletes collapse because they drank too much developing EAH and EAHE, then treating those specific individuals with intravenous fluids could produce a fatal outcome.

Following are the best ways to prevent fluid-related problems during exercise:

1. Encourage athletes to drink *only* according to their sensations of thirst during exercise.

2. Limit the amount of fluid that is available during competitive races. This can be done by providing aid stations only every 5 km during all road races, most especially during marathons or longer races when the problem of overdrinking becomes increasingly probable. A number of European marathon races, influenced by the IMMDA guidelines, now follow this practice.

3. Ensure that medical (including ambulance) personnel treating collapsed athletes first make a proper diagnosis before blindly instituting intravenous fluid therapy for the treatment of dehydration. Especially important is the measurement of the blood sodium concentration because, if low, it indicates the presence of overhydration and excludes a diagnosis of dehydration.

4. Athletes who collapse after exercise with EAPH should be placed on a bed, the foot of which has been elevated so that the legs and pelvis are above the level of the heart. This aids the return of blood to the heart and rapidly reverses the state of low blood pressure, instantly reversing the athlete's symptoms.

Treatment of EAH

Already in 1986 it had been shown that an athlete, Dr. Bob Lathan, who was treated with a 3% sodium solution for EAHE, recovered within hours, whereas the younger Dr. Tyler Frizzell recovered only after 4 days when treated with an isotonic 0.9% sodium solution (chapter 10). But it would take nearly 20 years and the hard work of Dr. Carlos Ayus[10] before this form of treatment would become the accepted global standard (Hew-Butler, Ayus, et al., 2008; Hew-Butler, Noakes, et al., 2008; Hew-Butler, Almond, et al., 2005; Siegel, 2007).

Thus, the present advice is that subjects with EAHE should immediately receive either a 100 ml bolus of 3% hypertonic saline intravenously or an amount of 1 milliliter per kilogram of body weight per hour. The sodium elevates the sodium

10   Dr. Juan Carlos Ayus' interest in EAHE arose when he was moonlighting in the medical services of the Argentine army. He tells the story of the wife of an army general who died after routine surgery. Autopsy revealed that she had died of gross brain swelling. Intrigued by something he could not explain, Ayus has spent much of his life understanding hyponatremic encephalopathy and how best to treat and prevent it.

In a series of scientific studies, Ayus and his colleagues have produced the fundamental finding that EAHE is best treated with 3% saline solutions and that the rapid correction of the low blood sodium concentration with concentrated (3%) sodium infusions in EAHE does not cause brain damage, as is usually presumed (Ayus, Arieff, et al., 2005; Ayus and Arieff, 1997; Ayus and Arieff, 1999; Cluitmans and Meinders, 1990). Rather, it is the delayed or inappropriate treatment with sodium solutions of lower concentrations (such as 0.9% sodium chloride) that is dangerous.

concentration of the arterial blood perfusing the brain. This develops an osmotic gradient between the brain cells and the blood perfusing those cells. As a result, fluid moves from the cells to the blood, increasing the volume of blood in the ECF. This then stimulates water excretion by the kidneys. The effect is rapid. Within minutes of beginning an infusion of hypertonic saline, urine flow increases in patients with EAH and EAHE and recovery has begun.

Summary

In this book I have described my odyssey of three decades that began when I received Eleanor Sadler's letter in June 1981. During this journey I have learned how science is meant to work and conversely how it often does work—a quite different reality. This has been a bitter lesson.

Over this period of 30 years I did, however, learn the real science of hydration:

- Your body will tell you what it needs, if you just listen.
- So drink only ad libitum—that is, according to the dictates of thirst.
- Dehydration is not a disease. Nor does dehydration contribute in any way to any illnesses associated with prolonged exercise like road, marathon, and ultramarathon running races and triathlons.
- If you are carbohydrate adapted, to optimize your performance during more prolonged competitive exercise, you will need to ingest some carbohydrate or perhaps preferably a favorite food (see also note 5, page 339).
- There is no need to increase your habitual daily sodium intake above that dictated by your appetite.
- There is no need to ingest additional sodium during exercise.
- Understand that much of what you believe about your personal well-being is the result of targeted manipulations by industries whose principal focus is their commercial fitness and not necessarily your health or safety.

I trust that the wisdom in this book will help you understand the exact how and why of drinking during exercise, free of any biases other than my own and those of the other scientists whose work it describes.

APPENDIX A

Deaths From EAHE

32-year-old female	1993 Valley of the Giants 42 km Marathon
18-year-old male	1997 U.S. Military
Kelley Barrett (43-year-old female)	1998 Chicago Marathon
19-year-old male	1999 U.S. Air Force
19-year-old male	2001 U.S. Military 42 km March
Dr. Cynthia Lucero (28-year-old female)	2002 Boston Marathon
Hilary Bellamy (35-year-old female)	2002 Marine Corps Marathon
Unknown male	2002 Half-Standard (26 km) Triathlon, Arkansas
25-year-old male	2005 U.S. Police
30-something male	2007 London Marathon
22-year-old male	2007 London Marathon
Patrick Allen (17-year-old male)	2008 U.S. Football

APPENDIX B

Cases of EAH and EAHE

The following are cases of EAH and EAHE reported in the scientific literature or to the author or occurring in the Ironman Hawaii Triathlon from 1983 to 1998.

Number	Age	Sex	Event or service	Blood [Na+] (mmol/L)	TREATMENT IV [Na+] (%)	Diuretic	Recovery time	Outcome	Presentation	Documented weight gain (kg) or fluid retention (L)	Reference
1	46	F	1981 90 km Comrades Marathon	115	0.9		7 days	Survived	Grand mal seizure.		Noakes, Goodwin, et al., 1985
2	37	M	1981 90 km Comrades Marathon	118	0.9		1 day	Survived	Altered LOC.		Noakes, Goodwin, et al., 1985
3	20	M	1982 90 km Comrades Marathon	124	0.9		4 days	Survived	Grand mal seizure.		Noakes, Goodwin, et al., 1985
4	29	F	1983 148 km Durban Ultratriathlon	125	0.9	Yes	4 days	Survived	Pulmonary edema.	+4.5 kg.	Noakes, Goodwin, et al., 1985
5	24	M	1983 100 km AMJA Ultramarathon	123	0.9		5 days	Survived	Grand mal seizure.	Drank 20 L.	Frizzell, Lang, et al., 1986
6	45	M	1983 80 km AMJA Ultramarathon	118	3.0		8 hr	Survived	Altered LOC.	Drank 24 L.	Frizzell, Lang, et al., 1986
7-9			1983 Ironman Hawaii Triathlon	127-134				Survived	Treated in medical facility at race finish.		Unpublished data
10	57	F	1984 Western States 100-mile run	124				Survived	Altered LOC.		Frizzell, Lang, et al., 1986
11-16			1984 Ironman Hawaii Triathlon	112-125				Survived			Laird, 1987; Laird, 1988
17			1984 Ironman Hawaii Triathlon	115			>4 days	Survived	Coma		Laird, 1987; Laird, 1988
18			1985 Sacramento 80 km race	124				Survived			Frizzell, Lang, et al., 1986
19			1985 Sacramento 80 km race	122				Survived			Frizzell, Lang, et al., 1986
20-28			1985 90 km Comrades Marathon					Survived	Altered LOC.		Godlonton, 1985
29-36			1985 Ironman Hawaii Triathlon	119-133				Survived	Treated in medical facility at race finish.		Unpublished data

(continued)

Number	Age	Sex	Event or service	Blood [Na⁺] (mmol/L)	IV [Na⁺] (%)	Diuretic	Recovery time	Outcome	Presentation	Documented weight gain (kg) or fluid retention (L)	Reference
					TREATMENT						
37-46			1985 Ironman Hawaii Triathlon					Survived	Participating in a study of changes in BW and blood sodium concentrations.	Two athletes gained weight during race (0.2 kg) and the rest stayed the same or lost weight.	O'Toole, 1988
47			1985 London Marathon					Survived	Grand mal seizures.		Goudie, Tunstall-Pedoe, et al., 2006
48-58			1986 90 km Comrades Marathon	125-134				Survived	Treated in medical facility at race finish.		Noakes, Norman, et al., 1990
59	21	M	1986 Pittsburgh 42 km Marathon	123	0.9; 5 dextrose	Yes	7 days	Survived	Altered LOC. Coma. Pulmonary edema.		Young, Sciurba, et al., 1987
60			1986 South African 186 km Triathlon	131				Survived	Asymptomatic (part of surveillance study).		Noakes, Norman, et al., 1990
61-116			1986 Ironman Hawaii Triathlon	115-134				Survived	Treated in medical facility at race finish.		Unpublished data
117-130			1986 Ironman Canada Triathlon Championship	125-134				Survived	Treated in medical facility at race finish.		Novak, 1988
131-166			1987 90 km Comrades Marathon	121-134				Survived	Treated in medical facility at race finish.		Noakes, Norman, et al., 1990
167	28	F	1987 90 km Comrades Marathon	112	20 Mannitol; 5 sodium chloride	Yes	2 days	Survived	Unconscious. Eyes deviated to right. Imminent cerebellar coning.	Passed 7.5 L in first 17 hr in hospital.	Noakes, Norman, et al., 1990
168-202			1987 Ironman Hawaii Triathlon	121-134				Survived	Treated in medical facility at race finish.		Unpublished data

	Age	Sex	Race		IV saline infusion of unknown concentration (probably 0.9)				Altered LOC. Fatigue. Dizziness.	+5 kg. Drank 2 bottles at every aid station on bicycle and run section of race. Drank 1.5 L per hr for 4 hr plus heavily before race and 1 L sports drink postrace.	Personal communication
203 SM		M	1987 Hotter 'n' Hell Hundred Cycling Race	118			24 hr	Survived	Altered LOC. Fatigue. Dizziness.		Personal communication
204	56	M	1988 90 km Comrades Marathon	113	0.9	Yes	3 days	Survived	Grand mal seizure. Pulmonary edema. Respiratory arrest.	+4.1 L.	Irving, Noakes, et al., 1991
205	35	M	1988 90 km Comrades Marathon	122	0.9		1 day	Survived	Altered LOC.	+3.3 L.	Irving, Noakes, et al., 1991
206	37	M	1988 90 km Comrades Marathon	113	0.9	Yes	3 days	Survived	Grand mal seizure.	+5.9 L.	Irving, Noakes, et al., 1991
207	42	M	1988 90 km Comrades Marathon	124	0.9		1 day	Survived	Altered LOC.	+1.5 L.	Irving, Noakes, et al., 1991
208	38	F	1988 90 km Comrades Marathon	127	0.9		9 hr	Survived	Altered LOC.	+1.5 L.	Irving, Noakes, et al., 1991
209	35	F	1988 90 km Comrades Marathon	124	0.9		1 day	Survived	Altered LOC.	+2.8 L.	Irving, Noakes, et al., 1991
210	41	F	1988 90 km Comrades Marathon	128	0.9		9 hr	Survived	Altered LOC.	+3.3 L.	Irving, Noakes, et al., 1991
211	46	F	1988 90 km Comrades Marathon	128	0.9		9 hr	Survived	Altered LOC.	+1.2 L.	Irving, Noakes, et al., 1991
212 Jan Ripple	32	F	1988 Ironman Hawaii Triathlon					Survived		+5 kg. Drank 2 bottles at every aid station on bike and run sections of race. Drank 22 bottles of a sports drink during bike leg of race.	Public domain
213-274			1988 Ironman Hawaii Triathlon	117-134				Survived	Treated in medical facility at race finish.		Unpublished data

(continued)

Number	Age	Sex	Event or service	Blood [Na+] (mmol/L)	TREATMENT			Outcome	Presentation	Documented weight gain (kg) or fluid retention (L)	Reference
					IV [Na+] (%)	Diuretic	Recovery time				
275-290			1989 U.S. military					Survived	Treated in U.S. military hospitals.		Montain, Latzka, et al., 1999
291-356			1989 Ironman Hawaii Triathlon	117-134				Survived	Treated in medical facility at race finish.		Unpublished data
357		F	1990 London Marathon					Survived	Grand mal seizures.		Goudie, Tunstall-Pedoe, et al., 2006
358 PM	32	M	1990 Ironman Hawaii Triathlon					Survived	Altered LOC. No memory of last 3 hr of the run in which he covered 22.5 km.	+5 kg. Drank 16.5 L during bike leg of race.	Personal communication
359	42	F	1990-1992 Hiking Grand Canyon	123	0.9 Ringer's lactate		4 hr	Survived	Weakness. Nausea. Vomiting.		Backer, Shopes, et al., 1993
360	29		1990-1992 Hiking Grand Canyon	126	0.9 Ringer's lactate		2.5 hr	Survived	Weakness. Diarrhea. Vomiting. Muscle cramps.		Backer, Shopes, et al., 1993
361-376			1990 U.S. military						Treated in U.S. military hospitals.		Montain, Latzka, et al., 1999
377-465			1990 Ironman Hawaii Triathlon	119-134				Survived			Unpublished data
466	49	F	1990-1992 Hiking Grand Canyon	107	3.0	Yes	5 days	Survived	Weakness. Dizziness. Coma.		Backer, Shopes, et al., 1993
467-476			1991 Ironman Hawaii Triathlon	126-129				Survived		3 athletes with hyponatremia gained weight (0-2%) during race.	O'Toole, Douglas, et al., 1995
477-540			1991 Ironman Hawaii Triathlon	118-134				Survived	Treated in medical facility at race finish.		Unpublished data

Case	Age	Sex	Event				Duration	Outcome	Symptoms	Notes	Reference
541-556		M	1991 U.S. military					Survived	Treated in U.S. military hospitals.		Montain, Latzka, et al., 1999
557	21	M	1992 8 hr laboratory study	122	5.0		12 hr	Survived	Nausea. Malaise.	+2.8 L.	Armstrong, Curtis, et al., 1993
558	51	F	1992 Hiking Grand Canyon	108	0.9		5 days	Survived	Grand mal seizures x 2.	+0.1 L. Evidence of SIADH.	Backer, Shopes, et al., 1993
559-573			1992 U.S. military					Survived	Treated in U.S. military hospitals.		Montain, Latzka, et al., 1999
574-656			1992 Ironman Hawaii Triathlon	118-134				Survived	Treated in medical facility at race finish.		Unpublished data
657	32	F	1993 Valley of the Giants 42 km Marathon	117	0.9		Died within 24 hr	Died (1)	Altered LOC. Coma. Brain stem herniation. Cardiopulmonary arrest.		Ayus, Varon, et al., 2000
658	57	M	1993 Vermont 160 km Ultramarathon	111	3.0	Yes	3 days	Survived	Altered LOC. Seizure.	+0.9 L (first 12 hr).	Surgenor and Uphold, 1994
659	50	F	1993 Hiking Grand Canyon	117	0.9; 3.0		3 days	Survived	Weakness. Vomiting. Seizure.	Evidence of SIADH.	Backer, Shopes, et al., 1999
660	64	F	1993 Hiking Grand Canyon	109	3.0; 0.9		4 days	Survived	Vomiting. Diarrhea. Seizure.	Drank large amounts of water. Evidence of SIADH.	Backer, Shopes, et al., 1999
661	19	F	1993 Hiking Grand Canyon	117	0.9		4 days	Survived	Dizziness. Vomiting. Altered LOC. Nausea.	Drank 10.5 L water. Evidence of SIADH.	Backer, Shopes, et al., 1999
662	21	F	1993 Hiking Grand Canyon	127	0.9		1 day	Survived	Headache. Dizziness. Nausea. Vomiting. Seizure.	Drank 4-6 L water.	Backer, Shopes, et al., 1999
663	52	F	1993 Hiking Grand Canyon	124	0.9		2 days	Survived	Lethargy. Dizzy. Nausea.		Backer, Shopes, et al., 1999
664	45	F	1993 Hiking Grand Canyon	127		Fluid restriction	6 hr	Survived	Dizziness. Nausea. Altered LOC.	Drank 8-9 L sports drink.	Backer, Shopes, et al., 1999

(continued)

Number	Age	Sex	Event or service	Blood [Na⁺] (mmol/L)	IV [Na⁺] (%)	Diuretic	Recovery time	Outcome	Presentation	Documented weight gain (kg) or fluid retention (L)	Reference
					TREATMENT						
665	23	M	1993 Hiking Grand Canyon	122	0.9		2 days	Survived	Altered LOC. Diarrhea. Vomiting. Combative. Muscle rigidity.	Drank 4 L water, 2 L sports drink. Evidence of SIADH.	Backer, Shopes, et al., 1999
666–681			1993 U.S. military					Survived	Treated in U.S. military hospitals.		Montain, Latzka et al., 1999
682–769			1993 Ironman Hawaii Triathlon	120–134				Survived	Treated in medical facility at race finish.		Unpublished data
770 Julie Hamilton	31	F	1993 Detroit Marathon	Hyponatremia diagnosed			2 days	Survived	Sluggish after 16 km. Face and hands swollen. Coma.	Week before marathon, always had water nearby. Drank at every station during race.	Public domain
771 CC		F	1994 Ironman Canada Triathlon	112			3 days	Survived	Altered LOC. Vomiting. Tiredness. Lethargy. Grand mal seizures.	Was told to drink plenty of fluids during exercise to avoid heat illness.	Personal communication
772–787			1994 U.S. military					Survived	Treated in U.S. military hospitals.		Montain, Latzka et al., 1999
788–857			1994 Ironman Hawaii Triathlon	119–134				Survived	Treated in medical facility at race finish.		Unpublished data
858			1995 London Marathon					Survived	Grand mal seizures.		Goudie, Tunstall-Pedoe, et al., 2006
859	15	F	1995 Hiking Israel	117	3.0		2 days	Survived	Malaise. Headache. Seizure.	Drank large quantities of water. Evidence of SIADH.	Zelingher, Putterman, et al., 1996
860	19	M	1995 Hiking Israel	115	0.9	Fluid restriction		Survived	Nausea. Vomiting. Seizure.	Evidence of SIADH.	Putterman, Levy, et al., 1993

861	19	F	1995 Hiking Israel	123	3.0		Survived	Nausea. Vomiting. Dizziness. Fatigue. Altered LOC.	Evidence of SIADH.	Putterman, Levy, et al., 1993
862	14	F	1995 Hiking Israel	121	3.0		Survived	Nausea. Vomiting. Dizziness. Fatigue. Altered LOC.	Drank >6 L water.	Zelingher, Putterman, et al., 1996
863	18	F	1995 Hiking Israel	120	0.9 Ringer's lactate		Survived	Vomiting. Generalized seizures.		Zelingher, Putterman, et al., 1996
864	18	M	1995 Hiking Israel	116	0.9 Ringer's lactate		Survived	Altered LOC.	Evidence of SIADH.	Zelingher, Putterman, et al., 1996
865	12	M	1995 Hiking Israel	117		2 days	Survived	Vomiting. Nausea. Altered LOC. Grand mal seizures \x 2.	Evidence of SIADH.	Zelingher, Putterman, et al., 1996
866-874			1995 U.S. military	114-133			Survived	Nausea. Vomiting. Confusion.	Each had drunk 9-21 L water in short time.	Gardner, 2002
875-890			1995 U.S. military				Survived	Treated in U.S. military hospitals.		Montain, Latzka, et al., 1999
891-920			1995 Ironman Hawaii Triathlon	122-134			Survived	Treated in medical facility at race finish.		Unpublished data
921	30	M	1996 New Zealand Ironman Triathlon	130	Fluid restriction		Survived	Nausea. Malaise. Fatigue. Headache. Dizziness.	+2.5 kg.	Speedy, Faris, et al., 1997
922	24	M	1996 New Zealand Ironman Triathlon	129	Fluid restriction		Survived	Nausea. Malaise. Fatigue. Headache. Dizziness.		Speedy, Faris, et al., 1997
923	27	F	1996 New Zealand Ironman Triathlon	132	Fluid restriction		Survived	Nausea. Malaise. Fatigue. Headache. Dizziness.		Speedy, Faris, et al., 1997
924	25	M	1996 New Zealand Ironman Triathlon	134	Fluid restriction		Survived	Nausea. Malaise. Fatigue. Headache. Dizziness.		Speedy, Faris, et al., 1997

(continued)

Number	Age	Sex	Event or service	Blood [Na⁺] (mmol/L)	TREATMENT		Recovery time	Outcome	Presentation	Documented weight gain (kg) or fluid retention (L)	Reference
					IV [Na⁺] (%)	Diuretic					
925	36	F	1996 New Zealand Ironman Triathlon	131	Fluid restriction			Survived	Nausea. Malaise. Fatigue. Headache. Dizziness.		Speedy, Faris, et al., 1997
926	22	M	1996 New Zealand Ironman Triathlon	122	Fluid restriction			Survived	Nausea. Malaise. Fatigue. Headache. Dizziness.		Speedy, Faris, et al., 1997
927	44	F	1996 New Zealand Ironman Triathlon	126	Fluid restriction			Survived	Nausea. Malaise. Fatigue. Headache. Dizziness.		Speedy, Faris, et al., 1997
928	57	M	1996 New Zealand Ironman Triathlon	131	Fluid restriction			Survived	Nausea. Malaise. Fatigue. Headache. Dizziness.		Speedy, Faris, et al., 1997
929			1996 London Marathon					Survived	Grand mal seizures.		Goudie, Tunstall-Pedoe, et al., 2006
930-945			1996 U.S. military					Survived	Treated in U.S. military hospitals.		Montain, Latzka, et al., 1999
946-1013			1996 Ironman Hawaii Triathlon	115-134				Survived	Treated in medical facility at race finish.		Unpublished data
1014-1029			1997 New Zealand Ironman Triathlon	117-134				Survived	Treated in medical facility at race finish.		Speedy, Noakes, et al., 1999
1030	35	M	1997 New Zealand Ironman Triathlon	116	0.9; 3.0		8 days	Survived	Generalized seizures.	+3.2 kg.	Speedy, Rogers, et al., 2000
1031	30*	F	1997 New Zealand Ironman Triathlon	131				Survived	Asymptomatic.	+0.5 kg.	Speedy, Noakes, et al., 2000
1032	39*	F	1997 New Zealand Ironman Triathlon	130				Survived	Asymptomatic.	+1.5 kg.	Speedy, Noakes, et al., 2000
1033		F	1997 New Zealand Ironman Triathlon	130			1 day	Survived	Altered LOC.	+3.7 L.	Speedy, Rogers, et al., 2000a
1034		F	1997 New Zealand Ironman Triathlon	119			1 day	Survived	Altered LOC.	+3.8 L.	Speedy, Rogers, et al., 2000a

ID	Age	Sex	Event	[Na]	Treatment	Duration	Outcome	Symptoms	Fluid Balance	Reference
1035		F	1997 New Zealand Ironman Triathlon	124	0.9	1 day	Survived	Altered LOC	-0.7 L.	Speedy, Rogers, et al., 2000a
1036		M	1997 New Zealand Ironman Triathlon	128	0.9	1 day	Survived	Altered LOC.	+0.4 L.	Speedy, Rogers, et al., 2000a
1037		F	1997 New Zealand Ironman Triathlon	128		1 day	Survived	Altered LOC.	+2.2 L.	Speedy, Rogers, et al., 2000a
1038		M	1997 New Zealand Ironman Triathlon	134		1 day	Survived	Altered LOC.	+0.8 L.	Speedy, Rogers, et al., 2000a
1039		F	1997 New Zealand Ironman Triathlon	129		1 day	Survived	Altered LOC.	+1.3 L.	Speedy, Rogers, et al., 2000a
1040	18	M	1997 U.S. military	121	0.9; Mannitol		Died (2)	Vomiting. Nausea. Headache. Dizziness. Lethargy. Confusion. Coma. Pulmonary edema. Diffuse brain stem edema. Death from disseminated sepsis and cardiac arrest. Autopsy showed diffuse cerebral and brain stem edema.	Drank 16 L fluid in 4 hr while on shooting range.	Gardner, 2002; Garigan and Ristedt, 1999; O'Brien, Montain, et al., 2001
1041-1072			1997 U.S. military	116-133			Survived	Treated in U.S. military hospitals.	TBW increased 3-5 L to achieve such low serum sodium.	Craig, 1999; Montain, Latzka, et al., 1999; O'Brien, Montain, et al., 2001
1073	49	F	1997 U.S. military	118	Fluid restriction	10 hr	Survived	Nausea. Lightheadedness. Confusion.	Drank large volume ice water.	Reynolds, Schumaker, et al., 1998
1074	23	M	1997 U.S. military	134	0.9	8 hr	Survived	Dizziness. Weakness.		Reynolds, Schumaker, et al., 1998
1075	36	F	1997 U.S. military	121	Fluid restriction	24 hr	Survived	Nausea. Vomiting. Altered LOC.		Reynolds, Schumaker, et al., 1998

(continued)

Number	Age	Sex	Event or service	Blood [Na$^+$] (mmol/L)	TREATMENT IV [Na$^+$] (%)	Diuretic	Recovery time	Outcome	Presentation	Documented weight gain (kg) or fluid retention (L)	Reference
1076	52	F	1997 U.S. military	121	0.9		12 hr	Survived	Nausea. Altered LOC. Delirium.	Drank >7.6 L water to avoid heat exhaustion.	Reynolds, Schumaker, et al., 1998
1077	22	F	1997 U.S. military	134	0.9		24 hr	Survived	Nausea. Weakness. Dizziness. Loose stools.	Overdrank to prevent dehydration.	Reynolds, Schumaker, et al., 1998
1078	25	M	1997 U.S. military	131	Fluid restriction		24 hr	Survived	Weak. Unable to stand.	Given much water.	Reynolds, Schumaker, et al., 1998
1079		M	1997 U.S. military	124			4 days	Survived	Nausea. Vomiting. Generalized seizures.	Drank 1.9 L per hr and then 1.7 L in a short time.	O'Brien, Montain, et al., 2001
1080		M	1997 U.S. military	127			Several days	Survived	Lightheadedness. Weakness. Generalized seizure.	Consumed much fluid to prevent heat symptoms.	O'Brien, Montain, et al., 2001
1081		F	1997 U.S. military	121			3 days	Survived	Headache. Nausea. Vomiting. Fatigue.	Drank 17-19 L water in 8 hr before hospitalization.	O'Brien, Montain, et al., 2001
1082		M	1997 U.S. military	123			Several days	Survived	Nausea. Fatigue. Disorientation. Generalized seizure.	Drank 9.5 L water in 4 hr period.	O'Brien, Montain, et al., 2001
1083		M	1997 U.S. military	128				Survived	Weakness. Blurred vision. Bloating	Drank 0.95 L water per hr, then 3.5 L in 30 min.	O'Brien, Montain, et al., 2001
1084-1108			1998 U.S. military	116-134				Survived	Treated in U.S. military hospitals.		Craig, 1999
1109-1147			1998 Ironman Hawaii Triathlon					Survived	Treated in medical facility at race finish.		Unpublished data
1148 RS		M	1998 Suzuki Rock 'n' Roll Marathon, San Diego	Hyponatremia diagnosed	Yes		5 days	Survived	Grand mal seizure. Pulmonary edema. Cerebral edema.	+7 L.	Public domain; *Richard Saffro vs Elite Racing, Inc.*

ID	Age	Sex	Event			Survived				Source
1149–1152				130–134				Treated in medical facility at race finish; 1 patient transferred to hospital.		Speedy, Rogers, et al., 2000b
1153 Kelley Barrett	43	F	1998 New Zealand Ironman Triathlon	121	Yes	**Died (3)**	Died after 3 days	Headache. Nausea. Vomiting. After running 38 km in 5 hr. Respiratory and cardiac arrest. Developed diabetes insipidus before death.	Passed an excess of 2.2 L during first 8 hr in hospital. For several weeks before race, was trying to drink enough to keep urine clear.	Public domain
1154	30	F	1998 Suzuki Rock 'n' Roll Marathon	119	0.9	Survived		Nausea. Confusion. Seizure.	Drank as much as possible.	Davis, Videen, et al., 2001
1155	31	F	1998 Suzuki Rock 'n' Roll Marathon	119	0.9	Survived		Vomiting. Weakness.	Drank as much as possible.	Davis, Videen, et al., 2001
1156	41	F	1998 Suzuki Rock 'n' Roll Marathon	120	0.9	Survived.		Vomiting. Confusion. Seizure.	Drank as much as possible.	Davis, Videen, et al., 2001
1157	45	F	1998 Suzuki Rock 'n' Roll Marathon	120	0.9	Survived		Vomiting. Seizure.	Drank as much as possible.	Davis, Videen, et al., 2001
1158	48	F	1998 Suzuki Rock 'n' Roll Marathon	121	0.9	Survived		Nausea. Weakness. Confusion.	Drank as much as possible.	Davis, Videen, et al., 2001
1159	39	F	1998 Suzuki Rock 'n' Roll Marathon	122	0.9	Survived		Weakness. Dizziness. Nausea.	Drank as much as possible.	Davis, Videen, et al., 2001
1160	39	F	1998 Suzuki Rock 'n' Roll Marathon	123	0.9	Survived		Weakness. Vomiting.	Drank as much as possible.	Davis, Videen, et al., 2001
1161	52	M	1998 Suzuki Rock 'n' Roll Marathon	124	0.9	Survived		Nausea. Weakness. Dizziness. Headache.	Drank as much as possible.	Davis, Videen, et al., 2001
1162	48	F	1998 Suzuki Rock 'n' Roll Marathon	124	0.9	Survived		Vomiting. Weakness.	Drank as much as possible.	Davis, Videen, et al., 2001
1163	47	F	1998 Suzuki Rock 'n' Roll Marathon	124	0.9	Survived		Nausea. Dizziness. Confusion.	Drank as much as possible.	Davis, Videen, et al., 2001
1164	56	F	1998 Suzuki Rock 'n' Roll Marathon	124	0.9	Survived		Nausea. Weakness.	Drank as much as possible.	Davis, Videen, et al., 2001

(continued)

Number	Age	Sex	Event or service	Blood [Na⁺] (mmol/L)	TREATMENT IV [Na⁺] (%)	TREATMENT Diuretic	TREATMENT Recovery time	Outcome	Presentation	Documented weight gain (kg) or fluid retention (L)	Reference
1165	35	M	1998 Suzuki Rock 'n' Roll Marathon	126	0.9			Survived	Nausea. Vomiting. Weakness.	Drank as much as possible.	Davis, Videen, et al., 2001
1166	24	F	1998 Suzuki Rock 'n' Roll Marathon	126	0.9			Survived	Nausea. Dizziness.	Drank as much as possible.	Davis, Videen, et al., 2001
1167	39	F	1998 Suzuki Rock 'n' Roll Marathon	126	0.9			Survived	Nausea. Vomiting.	Drank as much as possible.	Davis, Videen, et al., 2001
1168	31	F	1998 Suzuki Rock 'n' Roll Marathon	130	0.9			Survived	Weakness. Nausea.	Drank as much as possible.	Davis, Videen, et al., 2001
1169	37	F	1998 Suzuki Rock 'n' Roll Marathon	130	0.9			Survived	Vomiting. Weakness.	Drank as much as possible.	Davis, Videen, et al., 2001
1170	24	F	1998 Suzuki Rock 'n' Roll Marathon	131	0.9			Survived	Nausea. Vomiting.	Drank as much as possible.	Davis, Videen, et al., 2001
1171	39	F	1998 Suzuki Rock 'n' Roll Marathon	132	0.9			Survived	Headache. Dizziness. Headache.	Drank as much as possible.	Davis, Videen, et al., 2001
1172	37	M	1998 Suzuki Rock 'n' Roll Marathon	133	0.9			Survived	Vomiting.	Drank as much as possible.	Davis, Videen, et al., 2001
1173	50	F	1998 Suzuki Rock 'n' Roll Marathon	134	0.9			Survived	Nausea. Vomiting.	Drank as much as possible.	Davis, Videen, et al., 2001
1174	49	F	1998 Suzuki Rock 'n' Roll Marathon	134	0.9			Survived	Weakness.	Drank as much as possible.	Davis, Videen, et al., 2001
1175	29	F	1999 Suzuki Rock 'n' Roll Marathon	117	3.0			Survived	Nausea. Vomiting. Dizziness.	Similar drinking attitudes as patients from 1998 race.	Davis, Videen, et al., 2001
1176	51	F	1999 Suzuki Rock 'n' Roll Marathon	119	3.0			Survived	Weakness. Dizziness.	Similar drinking attitudes as patients from 1998 race.	Davis, Videen, et al., 2001
1177	55	F	1999 Suzuki Rock 'n' Roll Marathon	122	3.0			Survived	Vomiting. Weakness. Confusion.	Similar drinking attitudes as patients from 1998 race.	Davis, Videen, et al., 2001
1178	24	F	1999 Suzuki Rock 'n' Roll Marathon	123	3.0			Survived	Nausea. Vomiting.	Similar drinking attitudes as patients from 1998 race.	Davis, Videen, et al., 2001

1179	51	F	1999 Suzuki Rock 'n' Roll Marathon	131			Survived	Vomiting. Weakness.	Similar drinking attitudes as patients from 1998 race.	Davis, Videen, et al., 2001
1180	37	M	1995-1998 North American Marathon	119	5.0	12–24 hr	Survived	Nausea. Vomiting. Pulmonary edema. Cerebral edema.		Ayus, Varon, et al., 2000
1181	37	F	1995-1999 North American Marathon	120	5.0	12–24 hr	Survived	Nausea. Vomiting. Pulmonary edema. Cerebral edema.		Ayus, Varon, et al., 2000
1182	44	F	1995-1999 North American Marathon	121	5.0	12–24 hr	Survived	Nausea. Vomiting. Pulmonary edema. Cerebral edema.		Ayus, Varon, et al., 2000
1183	29	M	1995-1999 North American Marathon	127	5.0	12–24 hr	Survived	Nausea. Vomiting. Pulmonary edema. Cerebral edema.		Ayus, Varon, et al., 2000
1184	31	F	1995-1999 North American Marathon	125	5.0	12–24 hr	Survived	Nausea. Vomiting. Pulmonary edema. Cerebral edema.		Ayus, Varon, et al., 2000
1185	46	F	1995-1999 North American Marathon	120	5.0	12–24 hr	Survived	Nausea. Vomiting. Pulmonary edema. Cerebral edema.		Ayus, Varon, et al., 2000
1186	20	M	1999 U.S. Marine Corps	113		5 days	Survived	Cough. Generalized seizure.	Drank 6 canteens water in 2-3 hr. Passed 6.5 L urine in first 14 hr.	Gardner, 2002
1187	19	M	1999 U.S. Air Force	Hyponatremia diagnosed			**Died (4)**	Heatstroke. Vomiting. Cerebellar tonsillar herniation.	Recent excessive water intake.	Gardner, 2002
1188		M	After 2.5 hr laboratory cycling trial	128			Survived	Exhaustion. Incoordination.	Was drinking at a rate to prevent weight loss during exercise. Passed little urine during exercise.	Vrijens and Rehrer, 1999
1189 DM	49	M	1999 Boston Marathon	122	0.9	1 day	Survived	Ran 1 hr slower than usual time. Fatigued. Altered LOC.		Personal communication

(continued)

| Number | Age | Sex | Event or service | Blood [Na⁺] (mmol/L) | TREATMENT | | Recovery time | Outcome | Presentation | Documented weight gain (kg) or fluid retention (L) | Reference |
					IV [Na⁺] (%)	Diuretic					
1190-1213			2000 Houston Marathon	119-134	0.9			Survived	Nausea. Vomiting. Lightheadedness.		Hew, Chorley, et al., 2003
1214-1217	32-48	F	2000 Houston Marathon	114-128	5.0; 0.9			Survived	Nausea. Vomiting. Headache. Grand mal seizures.		Ayus, Varon, et al., 2000
1218	23	F	2000 Pittsburgh Marathon	122	0.9			Survived	Vomiting. Headache. Dizziness.		Hsieh, Roth, et al., 2002
1219	47	M	2000 Pittsburgh Marathon	126	0.9			Survived	Vomiting.		Hsieh, Roth, et al., 2002
1220	35	M	2000 Pittsburgh Marathon	129				Survived	Vomiting.		Hsieh, Roth, et al., 2002
1221-1232			2000 Pittsburgh Marathon	130-134				Survived	Asymptomatic. Part of surveillance study.		Hsieh, Roth, et al., 2002
1233	34	M	2000 South African Ironman Triathlon	129		Yes	24 hr	Survived	Altered LOC.	+4.5 L.	Noakes, Sharwood, et al., 2004
1234	28	F	2000 Hiking East Nepal	122	0.9 Ringer's lactate				Headache. Dizziness. Altered LOC.		Basnyat, Sleggs, et al., 2000
1235 JA		F	2000 Western States 100-mile (160 km) race						Weight gain of 5 kg by mile 80 of race. Seizure.	+5 kg.	Personal communication
1236 JD	48	M	2000 Walt Disney World Marathon, Orlando, Florida		Yes		6 days	Survived	Altered LOC. Coma. Generalized seizure. Cardiac arrest.	Drank ~700 ml fluid before race. Drank 9-10 L during race. Thought he was dehydrated.	Personal communication
1237 CJ	46	F	2000 42 km marathon		Yes		1 day	Survived	Muscle cramps. Altered LOC. Loss of coordination. Disorientation.	Drank 350 ml at start line and 200 ml at each of 13 aid stations during race. Drank another 350 ml water at finish.	Personal communication

Case	Age	Sex	Event	Serum Na			Duration	Outcome	Symptoms	Notes	Reference
1238–1244†	36 ± 10	M 5 F 2	2000 Iditasport 100-mile race	133 ± 2				Survived	Nausea. Vomiting. Malaise.	−0.8 ± 1.0 kg.	Stuempfle, Lehmann, et al., 2002
1245	20	M	2000 U.S. military 9 hr continuous exercise	113	3.0	Yes	5 days	Survived	Thirst. Generalized seizure lasting 2 min × 2.	Drank 5.8 L fluid in 2–3 hr before collapse but still felt thirsty during first 14 hr of treatment with 3% saline infusion. Total urine output exceeded intake by 6.55 L indicating profound overhydration.	Flinn and Sherer, 2000
1246–1254†			2001 246 km Spartathlon	<130				Survived	Asymptomatic. Part of surveillance study.	−0.6 ± 2.1 kg. Changes in BW negatively related to serum sodium.	Kavouras, Anastasiou, et al., 2003
1255–1261†			2001 48 hr adventure race	<135				Survived	Asymptomatic. Part of surveillance study.	Mean hourly fluid intake 310 ml. Consumption was less than recommended by ACSM.	Abbott and Nichols, 2003
1262	19	M	2001 U.S. military 42 km march	128			1 day	Died (5)	Vomiting. Excessive fatigue. Altered LOC. Coma. Brain death.	Reportedly drank 3.8 L fluid night before.	Gardner, 2002
1263 PB		M	2001 200-mile (320 km) bicycle race	114				Survived	Altered LOC. Coma. Generalized seizures.		Personal communication (K. Williamson)
1264	43	F	2001 Hotter 'n' Hell Hundred Cycling Race	130	0.9		2 hr	Survived	Nausea. Vomiting. Headache.		Personal communication (K. Williamson)
1265	36	F	2001 Hotter 'n' Hell Hundred Cycling Race	129	Fluid restriction		3 hr	Survived	Nausea. Vomiting.	Initially treated with 3 L IV fluids in the field. No improvement with treatment.	Personal communication (K. Williamson)

(continued)

Number	Age	Sex	Event or service	Blood [Na+] (mmol/L)	TREATMENT IV [Na+] (%)	TREATMENT Diuretic	Recovery time	Outcome	Presentation	Documented weight gain (kg) or fluid retention (L)	Reference
1266	29	F	2001 Hotter 'n' Hell Hundred Cycling Race	130	0.9		1 hr	Survived	Nausea. Vomiting. Muscle cramps.		Personal communication (K. Williamson)
1267	35	M	2001 Hotter 'n' Hell Hundred Cycling Race	126	0.9		3 hr	Survived			Personal communication (K. Williamson)
1268	29	M	2001 Hotter 'n' Hell Hundred Cycling Race	124	0.9		3 hr	Survived	Nausea. Vomiting. Muscle cramps.		Personal communication (K. Williamson)
1269	47	M	2001 Hotter 'n' Hell Hundred Cycling Race	127	0.9		2 hr	Survived	Nausea. Vomiting. Muscle cramps.		Personal communication (K. Williamson)
1270	61	F	2001 Hotter 'n' Hell Hundred Cycling Race	117			1 day	Survived	Fatigue.		Personal communication (K. Williamson)
1271	59	F	2001 Hotter 'n' Hell Hundred Cycling Race	134	0.9		1 hr	Survived	Shortness of breath.		Personal communication (K. Williamson)
1272	34	F	2001 Hotter 'n' Hell Hundred Cycling Race	124			3 hr	Survived	Weakness. Nausea. Vomiting. Disorientation.		Personal communication (K. Williamson)
1273	19	M	2001 Hotter 'n' Hell Hundred Cycling Race	134	0.9		2 hr	Survived	Headache. Dizziness. Muscle cramps.		Personal communication (K. Williamson)
1274	49	F	2001 Hotter 'n' Hell Hundred Cycling Race	125	0.9		24 hr	Survived	Nausea. Vomiting. Headache. Weakness.		Personal communication (K. Williamson)
1275	45	M	2001 Hotter 'n' Hell Hundred Cycling Race	122	0.9		2 hr	Survived			Personal communication (K. Williamson)
1276	46	F	2001 Hotter 'n' Hell Hundred Cycling Race	122			1 day	Survived			Personal communication (K. Williamson)

Case	Age	Sex	Event					Outcome	Description		Reference
1277		M	2001 Hotter 'n' Hell Hundred Cycling Race	123			2 days	Survived	Generalized seizure at race finish. Mild brain edema.		Personal communication (K. Williamson)
1278–1327			2001-2008 Boston Marathon	<135				Survived	Part of surveillance study. Excludes subjects also reported in cases 949 and 1040.		Siegel, d'Hemecourt, et al., 2009
1328	25	F	2002 London Marathon	122	0.9; 1.8		48 hr	Survived	Altered LOC. Collapse.		Goudie, Tunstall-Pedoe, et al., 2006
1329	27	F	2002 London Marathon	124	0.9		24 hr	Survived	Vomiting. Headache.		Goudie, Tunstall-Pedoe, et al., 2006
1330	31	F	2002 London Marathon	116	0.9; 1.8		24 hr	Survived	Grand mal seizures × 2.		Goudie, Tunstall-Pedoe, et al., 2006
1331	25	F	2002 London Marathon	124	0.9		24 hr	Survived	Altered LOC. Collapse.		Goudie, Tunstall-Pedoe, et al., 2006
1332	27	F	2002 London Marathon	122	0.9; 1.8		24 hr	Survived	Altered LOC. Collapse.		Goudie, Tunstall-Pedoe, et al., 2006
1333	32	F	2002 London Marathon	126	0.9		24 hr	Survived	Vomiting. Altered LOC.		Goudie, Tunstall-Pedoe, et al., 2006
1334	30	M	2002 London Marathon	129	0.9		24 hr	Survived	Altered LOC.		Goudie, Tunstall-Pedoe, et al., 2006
1335	25	F	2002 London Marathon	122	0.9; 1.8		24 hr	Survived	Vomiting. Altered LOC.		Goudie, Tunstall-Pedoe, et al., 2006
1336	56	M	2002 London Marathon	133	0.9		24 hr	Survived	Collapse.		Goudie, Tunstall-Pedoe, et al., 2006

(continued)

Number	Age	Sex	Event or service	Blood [Na+] (mmol/L)	TREATMENT IV [Na+] (%)	TREATMENT Diuretic	Recovery time	Outcome	Presentation	Documented weight gain (kg) or fluid retention (L)	Reference
1337	27	M	2002 London Marathon	127	0.9; 1.8		24 hr	Survived	Altered LOC.		Goudie, Tunstall-Pedoe, et al., 2006
1338	51	M	2002 London Marathon	127	0.9		24 hr	Survived	Vomiting.		Goudie, Tunstall-Pedoe, et al., 2006
1339	23	M	2002 London Marathon	122	0.9; 1.8		24 hr	Survived	Vomiting. Altered LOC.		Goudie, Tunstall-Pedoe, et al., 2006
1340	26	M	2002 London Marathon	128	0.9		24 hr	Survived	Vomiting. Altered LOC.		Goudie, Tunstall-Pedoe, et al., 2006
1341	27	M	2002 London Marathon	128	0.9		24 hr	Survived	Vomiting. Altered LOC. Headache.	Drank 13 L during race.	Goudie, Tunstall-Pedoe, et al., 2006
1342 Cynthia Lucero	28	F	2002 Boston Marathon	113	0.9		3 days	**Died (6)**	Altered LOC. Collapse. Diabetes insipidus.	Drank 1.2 L/hr for 5 hr during race. Evidence of SIADH.	Siegel, Verbalis, 2007
1343			2002 Boston Marathon	119				Survived	Part of surveillance study.		Almond, Shin, et al., 2005
1344			2002 Boston Marathon	118				Survived	Part of surveillance study.		Almond, Shin, et al., 2005
1345			2002 Boston Marathon	114				Survived	Part of surveillance study.		Almond, Shin, et al., 2005
1346-1415			2002 Boston Marathon	<135				Survived	Part of surveillance study.	EAH associated with substantial weight gain, consuming >3 L fluid during race, racing time of >4:00 hr, female sex, low BMI.	Almond, Shin, et al., 2005

1416 Hilary Bellamy	35	F	2002 Marine Corps Marathon	123	0.9; 3.0	24 hr	**Died (7)**	Altered LOC. Collapse. Brain stem herniation. Evidence of SIADH: serum AVP/ADH concentration at time of collapse was profoundly elevated (6.7 pm/ml).	Had been advised to drink as much as she could hold.	Thompson and Wolff, 2003; Siegel, Verbalis, et al., 2007
1417-1448			2000-2003 Houston Marathon	133 ± 2			Survived	Part of surveillance study.	–0.1 kg ± 3.2. Runners with EAH drank significantly more fluid and lost less weight during race than those who did not develop EAH.	Hew, 2005
1449 VC		F	2002 Cincinnati Flying Pig Marathon		0.9	3 hr	Survived	Postrace nausea. Vomiting. Shortness of breath.	Before, during, and after race drank 8.5 L including 5 L Gatorade. During race she drank 3.5 L Gatorade.	Personal communication
1450 Michelle Burr		F	2002 100-mile (160 km) Vermont Ultramarathon	113		3 days	Survived.	Vomiting. Slurred speech. Abnormal running gait. Generalized seizure. Coma.	+5 kg. Drank ~17 L during race (500 ml every 5 km).	Personal communication
1451		M	2002 Half-Standard (26 km) Triathlon, Arkansas	128	0.9; 1-2 L		**Died (8)**	Headache. Coma. Fixed, dilated pupils.		Personal communication
1452 KG		F	2003 Boston Marathon				Survived	Nausea. Vomiting. Confusion.	+1 kg. Drank 3 L before race and continuously during race.	Personal communication
1453-1461		M	2003 Boston Marathon	<135			Survived	Asymptomatic. Part of surveillance study.		Kratz, Siegel, et al., 2005

(continued)

Number	Age	Sex	Event or service	Blood [Na+] (mmol/L)	TREATMENT IV [Na+] (%)	Diuretic	Recovery time	Outcome	Presentation	Documented weight gain (kg) or fluid retention (L)	Reference
1462	34	M	2003 Kepler Challenge 60 km Mountain Run, New Zealand	130				Survived	Asymptomatic. Part of surveillance study.	+1.6 kg.	Page, Reid, et al., 2007
1463	33	F	2003 Kepler Challenge 60 km Mountain Run, New Zealand	133				Survived	Asymptomatic. Part of surveillance study.	+1.1 kg.	Page, Reid, et al., 2007
1464	34	M	2003 Kepler Challenge 60 km Mountain Run, New Zealand	134				Survived	Asymptomatic. Part of surveillance study.	−1.5 kg. Used NSAIDs.	Page, Reid, et al., 2007
1465	33	M	2003 Kepler Challenge 60 km Mountain Run, New Zealand	133				Survived	Asymptomatic. Part of surveillance study.	+1.5 kg. Used NSAIDs.	Page, Reid, et al., 2007
1466	47	F	2003 Kepler Challenge 60 km Mountain Run, New Zealand	131				Survived	Asymptomatic. Part of surveillance study.	+1.0 kg. Used NSAIDs.	Page, Reid, et al., 2007
1467		M	2003 Ironman CDA, Idaho,		8L of 0.9 for treatment of EAPH		1 day	Survived	Nausea. Dizziness. Loss of consciousness on standing.	+12 kg.	Personal communication
1468 DP	37	M	2003 Lake Placid Ironman Triathlon		4.5L of 0.9 3 hr post-race		6 hr	Survived	Headache. Puffiness of hands, arms, and legs.	+5 kg.	Personal communication
1469 AJ		M	2003 London Marathon		1.8		5 days	Survived	Muscle cramps. Felt unwell. Grand mal epileptic seizure. Semicoma. Vomiting. Muscle cell breakdown.		Public domain

ID	Age	Sex	Event	Na		Time	Outcome	Symptoms/Presentation	Notes	Reference
1470 Carol Krucoff	50	F	2003 Reggae Marathon Jamaica	118		6 days	Survived.	Altered LOC. Coma. Grand mal seizures × 3. Atrial fibrillation × 3.	Followed advice that it was impossible to drink too much.	Public domain
1471–1472			2003 4 hr running trial	<130			Survived	Part of experimental trial.	Drank to prevent weight loss during exercise. Subjects gained weight during exercise since they drank ~1 L/hr yet sweated at only ~500 ml/hr.	Twerenbold, Knechtle, et al., 2003
1473 MR	27	M	2004 Boston Marathon		0.9		Survived	Nausea. Muscle cramping. Vomiting. Diarrhea. Weakness. Altered LOC. Grand mal seizure. Respiratory arrest.	Drank >3.8 L before race. Stopped at every aid station to drink. Drank 1.9 L immediately at finish. While unconscious he received IV fluids because medics thought he was dehydrated.	Public domain
1474–1489			2004 Boston Marathon	125-134			Survived	Treated in medical facility at race finish.	Increased blood AVP/ADH concentrations in 7 of 16 athletes with EAH.	Siegel, Verbalis, et al., 2007
1490–1495			2004 New Zealand Ironman	>135			Survived	Asymptomatic. Part of surveillance study.	NSAID use associated with increased risk of developing EAH.	Wharam, Speedy, et al., 2006
1496–1500	37 ± 10	M 1 F 4	2004 Marine Corps Marathon	Hyponatremia diagnosed	IV given	91 min	Survived	Treated in medical facility at race finish.	Slow running times of 4:49 ± 49 min.	O'Connor, Bunt, et al., 2006
1501		F	2004 Marine Corps Marathon	123			Survived	Confusion. Moving arms and legs as if still running ("phantom running").	Consumed large amounts of fluid during race.	Bunt and O'Connor, 2004

(continued)

Number	Age	Sex	Event or service	Blood [Na+] (mmol/L)	TREATMENT IV [Na+] (%)	TREATMENT Diuretic	Recovery time	Outcome	Presentation	Documented weight gain (kg) or fluid retention (L)	Reference
1502 MW		F	2004 Yukon Trail	119	0.9; 2 L			Survived	Seizure.		Personal communication
1503		M	2004 Austrian Ironman Triathlon				3 days	Survived	Muscle cramping. Altered LOC. Seizure.	Increased fluid intake to treat cramps that developed during bike leg.	Personal communication
1504	57	F	2004 109 km Cape Town Argus Cycling Race	129	Fluid restriction		6 hr	Survived	Altered LOC. Headache.	+2.4 kg.	Dugas and Noakes, 2005
1505-1506			2005 Comrades Marathon	134	Fluid restriction			Survived	Nausea. Vomiting. Treated in medical facility at race finish.		Hew-Butler, Sharwood, et al., 2007
1507	41	M	2005 South African Ironman Triathlon	132	3.0		2 hr	Survived	Diarrhea. Altered LOC.	Drank to stay ahead of thirst during race.	Hew-Butler, Anley, et al., 2007
1508	32	M	2005 95-mile West Highlands Way Race	120	0.9		5 days	Survived	Fatigue. Confusion. Generalized seizure.		Cuthill, Ellis, et al., 2009; Ellis, Cuthill, et al., 2009
1509	47	F	2005 95-mile West Highlands Way Race	127	0.9; 3 L		3 days	Survived	Generalized seizure.		Cuthill, Ellis, et al., 2009; Ellis, Cuthill, et al., 2009
1510	35	M	2005 95-mile West Highlands Way Race	134	0.9; >11 L in 24 hr	Yes	5 days	Survived	Persistent vomiting postrace.		Cuthill, Ellis, et al., 2009; Ellis, Cuthill, et al., 2009
1511 VV	49	F	2005 Chicago Marathon	120			2 days	Survived	Weakness. Altered LOC. Nausea.	5 kg. Drank vigilantly before, during, after race, including 7 bottles fluid during first hr after race. Continued to drink voraciously at home. On hospital admission was treated as another dehydrated runner.	Personal communication

1512	F		2005 Ironman Canada	125	Survived	Muscle cramping. Confusion. Altered LOC.	Drank 16 L during race, including 9.5 L on bike leg.	Personal communication (D.A. Brooks)
1513-1526			2005 Ironman Canada	<126	Survived			Personal communication (D.A. Brooks)
1527-1546			2005 Ironman Canada	>126 but <135	Survived			Personal communication (D.A. Brooks)
1547 JM	M	25	2005 U.S. police		**Died (9)**	Dizziness. Nausea. Vomiting. Seizure.	Reportedly drank 11 L fluid before and during 20 km bike ride.	Public domain
1548-1551	3 M 1 F		2005 Argus Pick 'n' Pay 109 km Cycle Tour	<135	Survived	Asymptomatic. Part of surveillance study.	Two cyclists gained weight (0.2 and 0.8% BW) while 2 lost weight (−1 and −3%).	Hew-Butler, Noakes, et al., 2010
1552	F	65	2005 laboratory study	126; 131	Survived	Headache. Extreme tiredness.	Gained 2.4 kg while drinking 2.8 kg water during 60 min exercise (interspersed with 75 min rest) in a laboratory trial to determine whether a sports drink could prevent EAH. When she drank 2.7 L Gatorade her serum sodium fell to 131 mmol/L (vs 125 mmol/L when she drank water). Drinking Gatorade to excess did not prevent development of EAH.	Baker, Munce, et al., 2005

(continued)

Number	Age	Sex	Event or service	Blood [Na⁺] (mmol/L)	TREATMENT IV [Na⁺] (%)	TREATMENT Diuretic	Recovery time	Outcome	Presentation	Documented weight gain (kg) or fluid retention (L)	Reference
1553-1557		4 F 1 M	2006 Zurich Marathon	129-134				Survived	Asymptomatic. Part of surveillance study.	Weight gains of 0-2% BW.	Mettler, Rusch, et al., 2008
1558	45	F	2006 Frankfurt Ironman Triathlon	111	0.9; 2.5 L	Yes	7 days	Survived	Somnolence. Convulsions. Swollen face and ankles. Pulmonary edema. Respiratory failure requiring mechanical ventilation.	Evidence of SIADH. Subsequently finished another Ironman Triathlon with a normal blood sodium concentration when advised not to drink excessively.	Richter, Betz, et al., 2007
1559	33	F	2006 35 km cross country race	119	5.0		18 hr	Survived	Vomiting. Nausea. Pulmonary edema.		Kashyap, Anand, et al., 2006
1560	19	F	2006 23.4 km triathlon	127				Survived	Grand mal seizures.		Shapiro, Ejaz, et al., 2006
1561-1562		2 M	2006 Comrades Marathon	<135				Survived	Treated in medical facility at race finish.		Hew-Butler, Boulter, et al., 2008
1563	25	M	2006 Hotter 'n' Hell Hundred Cycling Race	129	3.0		2 hr	Survived	Exhaustion. Weakness. Nausea. Vomiting. Apathy. Bloating. Puffiness.	Drank 10 L during race.	Personal communication (K. Williamson)
1564	25	F	2006 Hotter 'n' Hell Hundred Cycling Race	134	3.0		6 hr	Survived	Headache. Nausea. Vomiting. Confusion. Withdrawn, lying in fetal position.		Personal communication (K. Williamson)
1565	63	F	2006 Hotter 'n' Hell Hundred Cycling Race	123	3.0		3 days	Survived	Headache. Nausea. Vomiting. Diarrhea. Confusion.	Drank >7.6 L during race. Passed 6.9 L fluid in first 48 hr after race.	Personal communication (K. Williamson)
1566	32	F	2006 Hotter 'n' Hell Hundred Cycling Race	123			3 hr	Survived	Syncopy. Headache. Nausea. Puffiness.		Personal communication (K. Williamson)

ID	Age	Sex	Event	Na	Vol	Duration	Outcome	Symptoms	Fluid intake	Reference
1567 TL	35	F	2006 Hotter 'n' Hell Hundred Cycling Race	118	3.0		Survived	Nausea. Bloating.	Drank 750 ml before race start, 9 L during race.	Personal communication (K. Williamson)
1568	35	M	2006 Hotter 'n' Hell Hundred Cycling Race	134	0.9; 1 L	2 hr	Survived	Agitation.		Personal communication (K. Williamson)
1569			2006 North Idaho Ironman Triathlon	120	3.0		Survived			Personal communication (R. Evans)
1570			2006 North Idaho Ironman Triathlon	131	3.0		Survived			Personal communication (R. Evans)
1571			2006 North Idaho Ironman Triathlon	130	3.0		Survived			Personal communication (R. Evans)
1572			2006 North Idaho Ironman Triathlon	126	3.0		Survived			Personal communication (R. Evans)
1573 DS	38	M	2006 Madison Ironman Triathlon			3 days	Survived	Fatigue. Weakness. Seizure.	Began hydrating 7 days before race	Personal communication
1574 Stacy Forster	33	F	2006 21 km Madison Half Marathon	117		3 days	Survived	Muscle cramping. Headache. Nausea. Vomiting. Repeated grand mal seizures.	Drank at most, if not all, refreshment stations during race. Self-treated postrace muscle cramps by continuing to drink despite development of progressive nausea, vomiting, headache culminating in grand mal epileptic seizure and coma.	Public domain; Hew-Butler, Noakes, et al., 2008
1575	43	M	2006 8-day Kokoda Trail, Papua, New Guinea	107	0.9	7 days	Survived	Weakness. Ataxia. Collapse. Generalized seizures.	Night before and day of collapse, fellow trekkers and guides encouraged him to drink excessively.	Rothwell and Rosengren, 2008

(continued)

Number	Age	Sex	Event or service	Blood [Na⁺] (mmol/L)	IV [Na⁺] (%)	Diuretic	Recovery time	Outcome	Presentation	Documented weight gain (kg) or fluid retention (L)	Reference
1576	27	M	2006 National Football League	116	0.9		2 days	Survived	Nausea. Fatigue. Headache. Vomiting. Disorientation. Grand mal seizure. Coma.	Drank up to 11.4 L per day based on advice during football career.	Public domain
1577–1587	37 (9)	4 M 7 F	2006 London Marathon	128-134				Survived	Asymptomatic. Part of surveillance study.	Those with EAH drank significantly more (3,683 vs 1,924 ml) during race and at a faster rate (843 ml/hr vs 451 ml/hr) than runners who did not develop EAH. Runners with EAH gained weight (1.65 kg) during race, whereas those who maintained normal blood sodium concentrations lost weight (1.46 kg).	Kipps, Sharma, et al., 2011
1588 TL	29	M	2007 Austrian Ironman Triathlon	115	0.9; Mannitol		Coma for 4 days; 10 days in hospital	Survived	Collapsed after 32 km of run section of triathlon. Altered LOC. Coma. Pulmonary edema.	Drank 8 L fluid (1.5 L/hr) during bike leg and 7.3 g sodium. Could not understand why sodium levels were so low with sodium supplements.	Personal communication; Hew-Butler, Noakes, et al., 2008

1589	37	F	2007 London Marathon	121	1.8		1 day		Diarrhea. Vomiting. Confusion. Altered LOC. Agitated. Legs moving continuously mimicking running motion. No recollection of race.	Consumed large volumes of fluid at each refreshment station because she thought it was necessary in high heat. Runners were advised to drink large volumes in the heat but were not warned of dangers of water intoxication.	Draper, Mori, et al., 2009; Hew-Butler, Noakes, et al., 2008
1590	"30's"	M	2007 London Marathon	133	0.9; 1 L; 5 dextrose; 1 L		12 hr	Died (10)	Faintness and dizziness. Headache. Coma. Respiratory arrest. Hydrocephalus. Midbrain herniation through foramen magnum.	Death due to inappropriate treatment of EAH in a person with a preexisting brain condition that reduced brain's ability to increase in volume in response to inappropriate IV fluids.	Petzold, Keir, et al., 2007
1591	22	M	2007 London Marathon	123	1.8; Mannitol	Yes	2 days	Died (11)	Collapse. Lethargy. Confusion. Coma. Respiratory arrest. Cardiac arrest.	Evidence of SIADH.	Doberenz, Nalla, et al., 2009
1592	28	M	2007 London Marathon	118	0.9 Hartmann's solution; 1 L; 1.8; 1.2 L		7 days	Survived	Nausea. Muscle twitching. Headache. Confusion. Slurred speech. Generalized seizure. Altered LOC. Repeated convulsions.	Drank much water and 1-1.5 L sports drink during race.	Doberenz, Nalla, et al., 2009
1593	28	F	2007 London Marathon	116	1.8		2 days	Survived	Collapsed after running 38.5 km. Confused. Altered LOC. Vomiting. Agitation.		Doberenz, Nalla, et al., 2009

(continued)

Number	Age	Sex	Event or service	Blood [Na⁻] (mmol/L)	IV [Na⁻] (%)	Diuretic	Recovery time	Outcome	Presentation	Documented weight gain (kg) or fluid retention (L)	Reference
					TREATMENT						
1594	29	F	2007 London Marathon	<122	1.8		3 days	Survived	Collapsed after finishing race. Generalized seizure. Respiratory failure.		Doberenz, Nalla, et al., 2009
1595	28	F	2007 London Marathon	116	3.0		3 days	Survived	Vomiting. Confusion. Altered LOC. Coma. Respiratory failure.		Doberenz, Nalla, et al., 2009
1596	31	F	2007 Chicago Marathon	125	3.0		2 days	Survived	Increasing abdominal pain. Nausea. Confusion. Lethargy beginning 48 hr after marathon.	Gained 0.8 kg during race despite suspension of race due to inadequate availability of fluid. Drank 8 L and 13 L on first 2 days after race on advice of race medical staff for treatment of postrace muscle soreness.	Rawlani and Noakes, 2008
1597	47	M	2007 Lake Placid Ironman Triathlon	112	3.0		48 hr	Survived	Altered LOC. Involuntary leg movements as if cycling. Grand mal seizure.	+1.5 kg.	Hew-Butler, Noakes, et al., 2008; personal communication
1598	34	F	2007 Half Marathon, New York	119	3.0; 0.9; 2.8 L		8 days	Survived	Nausea. Chest pain. Altered LOC. Grand mal seizure. Coma.	Drank much water before race and another ~4 L during race. Passed 5.4 L urine after receiving 2.8 L 0.9% saline for treatment of dehydration/hyponatremia.	Glace and Murphy, 2008

ID / Name	Age	Sex	Event	Na / Diagnosis	Fluid (L)		Duration	Outcome	Symptoms	Notes	Reference
1599	41	M	2007 95-mile West Highlands Way Race	128	0.9; 12 L	Yes	6 days	Survived	Vomiting. Unwell 24 hr postrace.		Cuthill, Ellis, et al., 2009; Ellis, Cuthill, et al., 2009
1600–1603			2007 Nijmegen Four-Day Marches					Survived	Asymptomatic. Part of surveillance study.	Average fluid intake 2.6–3.3 L. EAH predicted by fluid intake, change in BW, walking time.	Eijsvogels, Thijssen, et al., 2008
1604	36	M	2008 Australian Ironman Triathlon	120	0.9; 3		4 days	Survived	Alert. No change in LOC. Shortness of breath. Cough. Pulmonary edema. Generalized seizure 30 hr after hospital admission.	Evidence of SIADH.	Stefanko, Lancashire, et al., 2009
1605 Nate Bundy	22	M	2008 U.S. military	Diagnosed with water intoxication				Survived	Coma. Respiratory failure.		Public domain
1606–1609			2008 210 km Audax Challenge Cycle Race, Victoria, Australia	120–134				Survived			Personal communication (I. Rogers)
1610–1611	18 50		2008 marathon Spinning event	118–122	0.9		2 days	Survived	Nausea. Vomiting. Faintness. Confusion. Altered LOC.	One athlete drank 8 L during event.	Lorraine–Lichtenstein, Albert, et al., 2008
1612 Debra Paver	44	F	2008 8-day Kokoda Trail, Papua, New Guinea	Hyponatremia diagnosed				Survived	Altered LOC. Seizures. Coma. Respiratory failure.		Public domain
1613 Patrick Allen	17	M	2008 U.S. football	Hyponatremia diagnosed				**Died (12)**		Drank excessive fluid to avoid heat illness during football practice.	Public domain

(continued)

Number	Age	Sex	Event or service	Blood [Na+] (mmol/L)	TREATMENT IV [Na+] (%)	Diuretic	Recovery time	Outcome	Presentation	Documented weight gain (kg) or fluid retention (L)	Reference
1614–1634		M	2008 Rio del Lago 100-Mile (161 km) Endurance Run, Granite Bay, California	123–134				Survived	16 runners with asymptomatic EAH and 5 with clinical symptoms of EAHE.	Postrace blood sodium concentrations were not related to extent of BW loss during race. This study is unusual because all subjects with EAH lost weight during race. Explanation is currently unclear.	(3725) Personal communication (M. Van Loan)
1635–1637	M		2009 Singapore Night Marathon and 84 km Ultramarathon	117–134				Survived	Lethargy. Confusion.	Drank excessively.	Lee, 2011
1638	36	M	2009 Australian Ironman Triathlon	117	3; 200 ml followed by 0.9	Yes	5 days	Survived	Presented with acute pulmonary edema. Developed a seizure 30 hr after admission when serum sodium concentration was 124 mmol/L.		Stefanko, Lancashire, et al., 2009
1639–1643	39 (7)	M	2009 Western States 100-mile race	126–134				Survived		All athletes developed rhabdomyolysis and 3 acute renal failure.	Bruso, Hoffman, et al., 2010; personal communication T. Hew-Butler
1644–1657		10 M 4 F	2009 Western States 100-mile race	131–134				Survived	Asymptomatic. Participating in surveillance study.	−6% BW loss to 2% BW gain.	Hoffman, Stuempfle, et al., 2011
1658 Darren Baker	39	M	2009 222 km 5-day Amazon Jungle Marathon	Diagnosed with severe hyponatremia			2 days	Survived	Collapsed and lost consciousness 3 hr after the first day's stage, which he completed in 4 hr.		

				Survived	Asymptomatic. Participating in surveillance study.	Postrace blood sodium concentrations were linear function with negative slope of extent of BW change during race as is usually found.	Knechtle, Knechtle, et al., 2010
1659-1665	47.7	2007-2009 100 km Race Biel, Switzerland	133				
1666-1673		2010 Ironman Hawaii Triathlon	3 <130; 5 >131-134			Treated in medical facility at race finish.	Ironman Hawaii 2010 Medical Report

Key	
LOC	Loss of consciousness
[Na⁺]	Sodium concentration
SIADH	Syndrome of inappropriate secretion of antidiuretic hormone (SADH). Evidence includes elevated urine osmolality (>300 mOsm/kg) and presence of sodium in urine (>20 mmol/L) in the presence of hyponatremia.
†	Data are mean ± SD

APPENDIX C

Reported Cases of Heatstroke in Long-Distance Events

Cases of heatstroke reported in the scientific literature in marathon and ultra-marathon running and professional cycling.

APPENDIX C TABLE

Number	Date	Race	Time of day	Environmental conditions	Outcome	Comment	Reference
0	1908	London Olympic Games Marathon	5:23 p.m.	25.5 °C.	Survived	Dorando Pietri collapsed 5 times in the final 365 m of race. Removed from the track on a stretcher, he was revived quickly at a hospital. No medical records were released. Diagnosis uncertain.	Martin and Gynn, 2000
1	1912	Stockholm Olympic Games Marathon	3:45 p.m.	32 °C (shade temperature).	Died	Francisco Lazaro collapsed at 30 km and was taken to the hospital where he died the following day despite the doctors doing their best to treat him. Diagnosis uncertain.	Martin and Gynn, 2000
2	1954	Vancouver Commonwealth and Empire Games Marathon	2:25 p.m.	28 °C, windless, cloudless.	Survived	Jim Peters had rectal temperature of 39.0 °C 1 hr postrace. Recovered without active cooling. Diagnosis uncertain.	Noakes, Mekler, et al., 2008
3	1960	Rome Olympic Games 100 km cycling team time trial			Died	Knud Enemark was 8 km from finish when he complained of dizziness and fell behind his teammates; 5 km from finish he fell unconscious from his bicycle. Taken to the race finish where he was treated in a medical tent, the inside temperature of which was estimated at 50 °C. Died at 3:30 p.m.	Moller, 2005
4	1960	191 km French Amateur Cycling Championships	4:30 p.m.	25.9 °C, 56% RH, wind speed 5 km/hr.	Died	25-year-old cyclist fell unconscious from bicycle just before finish line. Rectal temperature was 43 °C. Admitted to hospital. Epileptic seizure. Cooled with ice. Died at 9:00 p.m. Had ingested 21 amphetamine tablets (Stenamine) before and during race. Diagnosis exercise-induced heatstroke associated with amphetamine ingestion.	Bernheim and Cox, 1960
5	1967	13th stage of Tour de France starting at Marseille and finishing on summit (1,829 m) of Mount Ventoux, 13 July.	4:00 p.m.	Reportedly 45 °C.	Died	Tommy Simpson fell from bicycle 1,600 m from summit of Mount Ventoux. Conscious at the time and asked to be helped back on his bicycle. Removed unconscious from bicycle 500 m from summit. Flown to hospital where he was pronounced dead at 5:40 p.m. Three tubes of amphetamines were found in the cycling jersey in which he died. A carton containing drugs (Stenamina and Tonedin) was found in his luggage. Presumptive diagnosis exercise-induced heatstroke associated with amphetamine ingestion. Other predisposing factors included illness (diarrhea) for some days and alcohol consumption at the start of the climb up Mount Ventoux.	Fotheringham, 2002
6	1979	42 km marathon		24 °C, 66% RH.	Survived	32-year-old male drank approximately 1.5 L during race. Rectal temperature 40.5 °C.	Hanson and Zimmerman, 1979a; Hanson and Zimmerman, 1979b

(continued)

APPENDIX C TABLE *(continued)*

Number	Date	Race	Time of day	Environmental conditions	Outcome	Comment	Reference
7	2006	Twin Cities Marathon, Minnesota	11:15 a.m.	6-9 °C, 62% RH, cloudless.	Survived	30-year-old collapsed 10 m short of finish line. Rectal temperature 40.7 °C reduced to <37.0 °C within 72 min. Muscle cell breakdown during recovery. Viral illness for 7 days before race. Drank appropriately during race. No evidence of dehydration. No cases of heatstroke reported in race from 1982 to 1994 involving 60,757 race finishers. Diagnosis exercise-induced heatstroke in an athlete running in cool conditions, likely due to excessive endogenous heat production as a result of recent viral infection.	Roberts, 2006
8	2008	Two Oceans 56 km Marathon	2:00 p.m.	7-24 °C, 93-36% RH. Wind speed 2.8-10.8 km/hr.	Survived	32-year-old male collapsed after running 55 km in 7 hr (8 km/hr) in cool conditions. Rectal temperature 41.8 °C. Patient required cooling for 10 hr before his temperature stabilized. Diagnosis exercise-induced heatstroke due to excessive endogenous heat production (likely due to an undiagnosed abnormality in skeletal muscle metabolism) in an athlete running slowly in cool conditions.	Rae, Knobel, et al., 2008

Introduction

Fixx JF. *The complete book of running.* 1977; pp. 1-314. New York: Random House.

Fotheringham W. *Put me back on my bike: In search of Tom Simpson.* 2002; pp. 1-242. London: Yellow Jersey Press.

Katz D. *Just do it: The Nike spirit in the corporate world.* 1994; pp. 1-336. Massachusetts: Adams Media.

Milvy P. *The marathon: Physiological, medical, epidemiological and psychological studies.* (edited by P. Milvy), 1977; pp. 1-1090. New York: New York Academy of Sciences.

Nevill AM, Whyte G. Are there limits to running world records? *Med. Sci. Sports Exerc.* 2005; 37, 1785-1788.

Noakes TD. *Lore of running.* 2003; pp. 1-930. Champaign, IL: Human Kinetics.

Pendergrast M. *For God, country and Coca-Cola.* 2000; pp. 1-621. New York: Basic Books.

Rushkoff D. *Coercion.* 2000; pp. 1-321. London: Little, Brown.

Introduction Notes

Noakes TD. *Lore of running.* 2003; pp. 1-930. Champaign, IL: Human Kinetics.

Chapter 1   Perspectives on Human Physiology and Hydration

ACSM. ACSM clarifies indicators for fluid replacement. www.acsm-msse.org; 12 February: 1-2. 2004.

Adams WC, Mack GW, Langhans GW, et al. Effects of varied air velocity on sweating and evaporative rates during exercise. *J. Appl. Physiol.* 1992; 73, 2668-2674.

Adolph EF, Dill DB. Observations on water metabolism in the desert. *Am. J. Physiol.* 1938; 123, 369-378.

Aiello LC, Wheeler P. The expensive-tissue hypothesis: The brain and the digestive system in human and primate evolution. *Curr. Anthropol.* 1995; 36, 199-221.

Armstrong LE, Curtis WC, Hubbard RW, et al. Symptomatic hyponatremia during prolonged exercise in heat. *Med. Sci. Sports Exerc.* 1993; 25, 543-549.

Armstrong LE, Epstein Y, Greenleaf JE, et al. American College of Sports Medicine position stand. Heat and cold illnesses during distance running. *Med. Sci. Sports Exerc.* 1996; 28, i-x.

Arnold D. "To the end, marathon was at center of student's life." *Boston Globe* April 18, 2002, p. A1.

Ayus JC, Varon J, Arieff AI. Hyponatremia, cerebral edema, and noncardiogenic pulmonary edema in marathon runners. *Ann Intern. Med.* 2000; 132, 711-714.

Brace CL, Montagu A. *Human evolution: An introduction to biological anthropology.* 1977; pp. 1-493. New York: Macmillan.

Brain CK. *The hunters or the hunted? An introduction to African cave taphonomy.* 1981; pp. 1-365. Chicago: University of Chicago Press.

Bramble DM, Lieberman DE. Endurance running and the evolution of Homo. *Nature* 2004; 432, 345-352.

Carrier DR. The energetic paradox of human running and hominid evolution. *Curr. Anthropol.* 1984; 25, 483-495.

Convertino VA, Armstrong LE, Coyle EF, et al. American College of Sports Medicine position stand. Exercise and fluid replacement. *Med. Sci. Sports Exerc.* 1996; 28, i-vii.

Dart R. The predatory transition from ape to man. *Int. Anthropol. Linguist. Rev.* 1953; 1, 201-219.

Dennis SC, Noakes TD. Advantages of a smaller bodymass in humans when distance-running in warm, humid conditions. *Eur. J. Appl. Physiol. Occup.Physiol.* 1999; 79, 280-284.

Diamond J. Evolutionary design of intestinal nutrient absorption enough but not too much. *News Physiol. Sci.* 1991; 6, 92-96.

Dill DB. *Life, heat and altitude.* 1938; pp. 1-211. Cambridge: Harvard University Press.

Duchman SM, Ryan AJ, Schedl HP, et al. Upper limit for intestinal absorption of a dilute glucose solution in men at rest. *Med. Sci. Sports Exerc.* 1997; 29, 482-488.

Finch VA. Thermoregulation and heat balance of the East African eland and hartebeest. *Am. J. Physiol.* 1972; 222, 1374-1379.

Folk GE. Responses to a hot environment. In *Introduction to Environmental Physiology* 1966; pp. 138-181. London: Kimpton.

Fowkes Godek S, Bartolozzi AR, Godek JJ. Sweat rate and fluid turnover in American football players compared with runners in a hot and humid environment. *Br. J. Sports Med.* 2005; 39, 205-211.

"Fred." Remembering Cynthia. N.d. www.remembercynthia.com/Carole.htm.

"From Rick Wasserboehr." Remembering Cynthia. N.d. www.remembercynthia.com/From_Rick_Wasserboehr.htm.

Grande F, Taylor HL, Anderson JT, et al. Water exchange in men on a restricted water intake and a low calorie carbohydrate diet accompanied by physical work. *J. Appl. Physiol.* 1958; 12, 202-210.

Greenleaf JE, Sargent F. Voluntary dehydration in man. *J. Appl. Physiol.* 1965; 20, 719-724.

GSSI. Drinking 101 (advertisement). *New York Runner.* 2002; 47, n.p.n.

Hanna JM, Brown DE. Human heat tolerance: An anthropological perspective. *Ann. Rev. Anthropol.* 1983; 12, 259-284.

Hart D, Sussman RW. *Man the hunted.* 2005; pp. 1-357. Boulder, CO: Westview Press.

Heinrich B. Endurance predator. In *The anthropology of sport and human movement.* R.R. Sands and L.R. Sands, eds. 2010; pp. 95-101. Lanham, MD: Lexington Books.

Heinrich B. *The hot-blooded insects*. 1993; pp. 1-601. Cambridge, MA: Harvard University Press.

Heinrich B. *Racing the antelope*. 2001; pp. 1-292. New York: Harper Collins.

Heinrich B. *The thermal warriors*. 1996; pp. 1-221. Cambridge: Harvard University Press.

Hew-Butler T, Noakes TD, Siegel AJ. Practical management of exercise-associated hyponatremic encephalopathy: The sodium paradox of non-osmotic vasopressin secretion. *Clin. J. Sport Med.* 2008; 18, 350-354.

Hohler B. A lesson in giving: After tragedy, Lucero's donation lets seven other women live. *Boston Globe.* 2005.

Hoyt DF, Taylor CR. Letter to editor: Gait and energetics of locomotion in horses. *Nature* 1981; 292, 239-240.

Johnson GS, Elizondo RS. Thermoregulation in Macaca mulatta: a thermal balance study. *J. Appl. Physiol.* 1979; 46, 268-277.

Jouffroy FK, Médina MF. A hallmark of humankind: The gluteus maximus muscle: Its form, action and function. In *Human origins and environmental backgrounds*. H. Ishida, ed. 2007; pp. 135-148. New York: Springer.

Kenney WL, DeGroot DW, Holowatz LA. Extremes of human heat tolerance: Life at the precipice of thermoregulatory failure. *J. Therm. Biol.* 2004; 29, 479-485.

Krantz GS. Brain size and hunting ability in earliest man. *Curr. Anthropol.* 1968; 9, 450-451.

Liebenberg L. Persistence hunting by modern hunter-gatherers. *Curr. Anthropol.* 2006; 47, 1017-1025.

Liebenberg L. *The art of tracking: The origin of science.* 1990; pp. 3-176. Claremont, South Africa: Philip.

Lieberman DE, Bramble DM. The evolution of marathon running capabilities in humans. *Sports Med.* 2007; 37, 288-290.

Lieberman DE, Raichlen DA, Pontzer H, et al. The human gluteus maximus and its role in running. *J. Exp. Biol.* 2006; 209, 2143-2155.

Marino FE, Mbambo Z, Kortekaas E, et al. Advantages of smaller body mass during distance running in warm, humid environments. *Pflugers Arch.* 2000; 441, 359-367.

Massachusetts School of Professional Psychology. Annual report. www.mspp.edu/files/mspp_2004_annual_report.pdf. 2004; p. 9.

McDougall C. *Born to run: A hidden tribe, superathletes, and the greatest race the world has never seen.* 2009; pp. 3-287. New York: Knopf.

McGee WJ. Desert thirst as disease. *J. Southwest* 1988; 30, 222-253.

Morris C. *Man and his ancestors.* 1900; pp. 1-238. New York: Macmillan.

Newman RW. Why man is such a sweaty and thirsty naked animal: A speculative review. *Hum. Biol.* 1970; 42, 12-27.

Nielsen B, Hales JR, Strange S, et al. Human circulatory and thermoregulatory adaptations with heat acclimation and exercise in a hot, dry environment. *J. Physiol.*1993; 460, 467-485.

Nolte HW, Noakes TD, Van Vuuren B. Trained humans can exercise safely in extreme dry heat when drinking water ad libitum. *J. Sports Sci.* 2011; 29: 1233-41.

Noakes TD, Adams BA, Myburgh KH, et al. The danger of an inadequate water intake during prolonged exercise: A novel concept re-visited. *Eur. J. Appl. Physiol. Occup. Physiol.* 1988; 57, 210-219.

Nummela AT, Heath KA, Paavolainen LM, et al. Fatigue during a 5-km running time trial. *Int. J. Sports Med.* 2008; 29, 738-745.

Nummela AT, Paavolainen LM, Sharwood KA, et al. Neuromuscular factors determining 5 km running performance and running economy in well-trained athletes. *Eur. J. Appl. Physiol.* 2006; 97, 1-8.

Palma R, Vidon N, Bernier JJ. Maximal capacity for fluid absorption in human bowel. *Dig. Dis. Sci.* 1981; 26, 929-934.

Read C. *The origin of man and of his superstitions.* 1925; pp. 1-98. Cambridge: University Press.

Richards SA. The biology and comparative physiology of thermal panting. *Biol. Rev. Camb.Philos.Soc* 1970; 45, 223-264.

Rolian C, Lieberman DE, Hamill J, et al. Walking, running and the evolution of short toes in humans. *J. Exp. Biol.* 2009; 212, 713-721.

Sands RR. Homo cursor: Running into the pleistocene. In *The anthropology of sport and human movement.* R.R. Sands and L.R. Sands, eds. 2010; pp. 143-181. Lanham, MD: Lexington Books.

Saunders AG, Dugas JP, Tucker R, et al. The effects of different air velocities on heat storage and body temperature in humans cycling in a hot, humid environment. *Acta Physiol. Scand.* 2005; 183, 241-255.

Schmidt-Nielsen K. *Desert animals.* 1964; pp. 1-270. London: Oxford University Press.

Schmidt-Nielsen K. The physiology of the camel. *Sci. Am.* 1959; 201, 140-151.

Shi X, Summers RW, Schedl HP, et al. Effects of solution osmolality on absorption of select fluid replacement solutions in human duodenojejunum. *J. Appl. Physiol.* 1994; 77, 1178-1184.

Smeaton Chase J. *California desert trails.* 2004; pp. 1-476. Long Riders' Guild Press.

Smith S. Marathon runner's death linked to excessive fluid intake. *Boston Globe.* 13 August. 2002; p. A1.

Stern JT, Jr. Anatomical and functional specializations of the human gluteus maximus. *Am. J. Phys. Anthropol.* 1972; 36, 315-339.

Stuempfle KJ, Lehmann DR, Case HS, et al. Change in serum sodium concentration during a cold weather ultradistance race. *Clin. J. Sport Med.* 2003; 13, 171-175.

Szlyk PC, Hubbard RW, Matthew WT, et al. Mechanisms of voluntary dehydration among troops in the field. *Mil. Med.* 1987; 152, 405-407.

Taylor CR. The eland and the oryx. *Sci. Am.* 1969; 220, 88-95.

Taylor CR. Exercise and environmental heat loads: Different mechanisms for solving different problems? *Int. Rev. Physiol.* 1977; 15, 119-146.

Taylor CR, Lyman CP. Heat storage in running antelopes: Independence of brain and body temperatures. *Am. J. Physiol.* 1972; 222, 114-117.

Taylor CR, Rowntree VJ. Temperature regulation and heat balance in running cheetahs: A strategy for sprinters? *Am. J. Physiol.* 1973; 224, 848-851.

Tucker R, Marle T, Lambert EV, et al. The rate of heat storage mediates an anticipatory reduction in exercise intensity during cycling at a fixed rating of perceived exertion. *J. Physiol.* 2006; 574, 905-915.

Tucker R, Rauch L, Harley YX, et al. Impaired exercise performance in the heat is associated with an anticipatory reduction in skeletal muscle recruitment. *Pflugers Arch.* 2004; 448, 422-430.

Twerenbold R, Knechtle B, Kakebeeke TH, et al. Effects of different sodium concentrations in replacement fluids during prolonged exercise in women. *Br. J. Sports Med.* 2003; 37, 300-303.

Watanabe H. Running, creeping and climbing: A new eco-logical and evolutionary perspective on human locomotion. *Mankind* 1971; 8, 1-13.

Watkins RG, Dennis S, Dillin WH, et al. Dynamic EMG analysis of torque transfer in professional baseball pitchers. *Spine* 1989; 14, 404-408.

Wheeler PE. The evolution of bipedality and loss of functional body hair in hominids. *J. Hum. Evol.* 1984; 13, 91-98.

Wheeler PE. The influence of bipedalism on the energy and water budgets of early hominids. *J. Hum. Evol.* 1991a; 21, 117-136.

Wheeler PE. The influence of the loss of functional body hair on the water budgets of early hominids. *J. Hum. Evol.* 1992; 23, 379-388.

Wheeler PE. The influence of stature and body form on hominid energy and water budgets; a comparison of Australopithe-cus and early Homo physiques. *J. Hum. Evol.* 1993; 24, 13-28.

Wheeler PE. The loss of functional body hair in man: The influ-ence of thermal environment, body form and bipedality. *J. Hum. Evol.* 1985; 14, 23-28.

Wheeler PE. Stand tall and stay cool. *New Scientist* 1988; May 12, 62-65.

Wheeler PE. The thermoregulatory advantages of hominid bipedalism in open equatorial environments: The contri-bution of increased convective heat loss and cutaneous evaporative cooling. *J. Hum. Evol.* 1991b; 21, 107-115.

Chapter 1   Notes

Below PR, Mora-Rodriguez R, Gonzalez-Alonso J, et al. Fluid and carbohydrate ingestion independently improve per-formance during 1 h of intense exercise. *Med. Sci. Sports Exerc.* 1995; 27, 200-210.

Costill DL, Kammer WF, Fisher A. Fluid ingestion during dis-tance running. *Arch. Environ. Health* 1970; 21, 520-525.

Dart R. The predatory transition from ape to man. *Int. Anthropol. Linguist. Rev.* 1953; 1, 201-219.

Darwin C. *The descent of man.* 1877; pp. 1-727. London: Folio Society.

Dennis SC, Noakes TD. Advantages of a smaller bodymass in humans when distance-running in warm, humid conditions. *Eur. J. Appl. Physiol. Occup. Physiol.* 1999; 79, 280-284.

Dill DB. *Life, heat and altitude.* 1938; pp. 1-211. Cambridge: Harvard University Press.

Heinrich B. *Racing the antelope.* 2001; pp. 1-292. New York: Harper Collins.

Montain SJ, Coyle EF. Influence of graded dehydration on hyperthermia and cardiovascular drift during exercise. *J. Appl. Physiol.* 1992; 73, 1340-1350.

Noakes TD, Wilson G, Gray DA, et al. Peak rates of diuresis in healthy humans during oral fluid overload. *S. Afr. Med. J.* 2001; 91, 852-857.

Robinson TA, Hawley JA, Palmer GS, et al. Water ingestion does not improve 1-h cycling performance in moderate ambient temperatures. *Eur. J. Appl. Physiol. Occup. Physiol.* 1995; 71, 153-160.

Sawka MN, Burke LM, Eichner ER, et al. American College of Sports Medicine position stand: Exercise and fluid replace-ment. *Med. Sci. Sports Exerc.* 2007; 39, 377-390.

Schmidt-Nielsen K. *Desert animals.* 1964; pp. 1-270. London: Oxford University Press.

Wheeler PE. The influence of stature and body form on hominid energy and water budgets: A comparison of

Australopithecus and early Homo physiques. *J. Hum. Evol.* 1993; 24, 13-28.

Chapter 2   Thirst as a Signal for Fluid Intake

Abrahams A. The nutrition of athletes. *Brit. J. Nutrit.* 1948; 2, 266-269.

Adolph, EF, and Dill, DB. Observations on water metabolism in the desert. *Am. J. Physiol.* 1938; 23, 369-378.

Armstrong LE, Maresh CM, Gabaree CV, et al. Thermal and circulatory responses during exercise: Effects of hypohydra-tion, dehydration, and water intake. *J. Appl. Physiol.* 1997; 82, 2028-2035.

Adolph EF. Signs and symptoms of desert dehydration. In *Physi-ology of man in the desert.* 1947b. New York: Interscience.

Bean WB, Eichna LW. Performance in relation to environmental temperature. *Fed. Proc.* 1943, 144-158.

Beis LY, Wright-Whyte M, Fudge B, Noakes T, Pitsiladis YP. Drinking behaviors of elite male runners during marathon competition. *Clin. J. Sport Med.* 2012 (in press).

Berry H. *From L.A. to New York, from New York to L.A.* 1990. Chorley: Author.

Bock AV, Dill DB. A resume of some physiological reactions to high external temperature. *N. Engl. J. Med.* 1933; 209, 442-444.

Brown AH. Water shortage in the desert. In *Physiology of man in the desert* 1947a. New York: Interscience.

Brown AH. Dehydration exhaustion. In *Physiology of man in the desert* 1947b. New York: Interscience.

Cheuvront SN, Ely BR, Kenefick RW, et al. Biological variation and diagnostic accuracy of dehydration assessment mark-ers. *Am. J. Clin. Nutr.* 2010; 92, 565-573.

Dill DB, Soholt LF, Oddershede IB. Physiological adjustments of young men to five-hour desert walks. *J. Appl. Physiol.* 1976; 40, 236-242.

Eichna LW, Bean WB, Ashe WF, et al. Performance in relation to environmental temperature. *Bull. Johns Hopkins Hospital* 1945; 76, 25-58.

Eichna LW, Horvath SM. Post-exertional orthostatic hypoten-sion. *Am. J. Med. Sci.* 1947; 213, 641-654.

Engell DB, Maller O, Sawka MN, et al. Thirst and fluid intake following graded hypohydration levels in humans. *Physiol. Behav.* 1987; 40, 229-236.

Gisolfi CV, Summers RW, Lambert GP, et al. Effect of beverage osmolality on intestinal fluid absorption during exercise. *J. Appl. Physiol.* 1998; 85, 1941-1948.

Gisolfi CV, Summers RD, Schedl HP, et al. Effect of sodium con-centration in a carbohydrate-electrolyte solution on intestinal absorption. *Med. Sci. Sports Exerc.* 1995; 27, 1414-1420.

Goulet ED. Effect of exercise-induced dehydration on time-trial exercise performance: A meta-analysis. *Br. J. Sports Med.* 2011; 45:1149-56.

Hanna JM, Brown DE. Human heat tolerance: An anthropologi-cal perspective. *Ann. Rev. Anthropol.* 1983; 12, 259-284.

Harrer H. *The white spider.* 1959; pp. 5-312. Norwich, England: Fletcher.

Hew-Butler T, Verbalis JG, Noakes TD. Updated fluid recom-mendation: position statement from the International Mara-thon Medical Directors Association (IMMDA). *Clin. J. Sport Med.* 2006; 16, 283-292.

Hew-Butler T, Collins M, Bosch A, et al. Maintenance of plasma volume and serum sodium concentration despite body weight loss in ironman triathletes. *Clin. J. Sport Med.* 2007; 17, 116-122.

Hughes T. *Tom Brown at Oxford*. EBook #26851. 1861/2008. www.manybooks.net/titles/hughesth2685126851.html.

King JHT. Brief account of the suffering of a detachment of United States Cavalry, from deprivation of water, during a period of eighty-six hours, while scouting on the "Llano Estacado" or "Staked Plains," *Am. J. Med. Sci.* 1878; 75, 404-408.

Leyton, RNA. Some practical aspects of the nutrition of athletes. *Br. J. Nutr.* 1948; 2, 269-273.

Maresh CM, Gabaree-Boulant CL, Armstrong LE, et al. Effect of hydration status on thirst, drinking, and related hormonal responses during low-intensity exercise in the heat. *J. Appl. Physiol.* 2004; 97, 39-44.

Martin DE, Gynn RWH. *The marathon footrace*. 1979. Springfield, IL: Thomas.

McGarvey J, Thompson J, Hanna C, et al. Sensitivity and specificity of clinical signs for assessment of dehydration in endurance athletes. *Br. J. Sports Med.* 2010; 44, 716-719.

Newton AFH. Drinks and the marathon. *Athl. Rev.* 1948, 14-16.

Newton AFH. Rations and athletes. *Athl. Rev.* 1947; Sept 1947, 2, 19.

Noakes T. *Lore of running*. 2003. Champaign, IL: Human Kinetics.

Nolte H, Noakes TD, Van Vuuren B. Ad libitum fluid replacement in military personnel during a 4 hour route march. *Med. Sci. Sports Exerc.* 2010; 42, 1675-1680.

Nolte H, Noakes TD, Van Vuuren B. Protection of total body water content and absence of hyperthermia despite 2% body mass loss ('voluntary dehydration') in soldiers drinking ad libitum during prolonged exercise in cool environmental conditions. *Br. J. Sports Med.* 2011a; 45, 1106-1112.

Nolte HW, Noakes TD, Van Vuuren B. Trained humans can exercise safely in extreme dry heat when drinking water ad libitum. *J. Sports Sci.* 2011b; 29, 1233-1241.

Peters, J.H., Johnston, J., Edmundson, J. *Modern middle and long distance running*. 1957. Kaye, London.

Pugh LG, Corbett JL, Johnson RH. Rectal temperatures, weight losses, and sweat rates in marathon running. *J. Appl. Physiol.* 1967; 23, 347-352.

Sawka MN, Noakes TD. Does dehydration impair exercise performance? *Med. Sci. Sports Exerc.* 2007; 39, 1209-1217.

Sharwood KA, Collins M, Goedecke JH, et al. Weight changes, medical complications, and performance during an Ironman triathlon. *Br. J. Sports Med.* 2004; 38, 718-724.

Sullivan JE. *Marathon Running*. 1909; pp. 3-110. New York: American Sports.

Szlyk PC, Sils IV, Francesconi RP, et al. Patterns of human drinking: Effects of exercise, water temperature, and food consumption. *Aviat. Space Environ.Med* 1990; 61, 43-48.

Wharam PC, Speedy DB, Noakes TD, et al. NSAID use increases the risk of developing hyponatremia during an Ironman triathlon. *Med. Sci. Sports Exerc.* 2006; 38, 618-622.

Wyndham CH, Strydom NB. The danger of an inadequate water intake during marathon running. *S. Afr. Med. J.* 1969; 43, 893-896.

Chapter 2 Notes

Adolph EF. *Physiology of man in the desert*. 1947a. New York: Interscience.

Brown AH. Dehydration exhaustion. In *Physiology of man in the desert* 1947a; pp. 208-225. New York: Interscience.

Irving RA, Noakes TD, Raine RI, et al. Transient oliguria with renal tubular dysfunction after a 90 km running race. *Med. Sci. Sports Exerc.* 1990; 22, 756-761.

Sallis R. Collapse in the endurance athlete. *GSSI Sports Sci. Exch.* 2004; 17, 1-6.

Chapter 3 Water's Role in Thermoregulation

Adams WC, Fox RH, Fry AJ, et al. Thermoregulation during marathon running in cool, moderate, and hot environments. *J. Appl. Physiol.* 1975; 38, 1030-1037.

American College of Sports Medicine. Position statement on the prevention of thermal injuries during distance running. *Med. Sci. Sports Exerc.* 1985; 17, ix-xiv.

American College of Sports Medicine. Position stand on the prevention of thermal injuries during distance running. *Med. Sci. Sports Exerc.* 1987; 19, 529-533.

Blake JB, Larrabee RC. Observations upon long-distance runners. *Boston Med. Surg. J.* 1903; 148, 195-206.

Buskirk ER, Beetham WPJ. Dehydration and body temperature as a result of marathon running. *Med. Sportiva* 1960; XIV, 493-506.

Byrne C. Response to study findings challenge core components of a current model of exercise thermoregulation. *Med. Sci. Sports Exer.* 2007; 39, 744.

Byrne C, Lee JK, Chew SA, et al. Continuous thermoregulatory responses to mass-participation distance running in heat. *Med. Sci. Sports Exer.* 2006; 38, 803-810.

Cheuvront SN, Carter RW, III, Sawka MN. Fluid balance and endurance exercise performance. *Curr. Sports Med. Rep.* 2003; 2, 202-208.

Christensen CL, Ruhling RO. Thermoregulatory responses during a marathon. A case study of a woman runner. *Br. J. Sports Med.* 1980; 14, 131-132.

Clark HR, Barker ME, Corfe BM. Nutritional strategies of mountain marathon competitors—an observational study. *Int. J. Sport Nutr. Exerc. Metab.* 2005; 15, 160-172.

Convertino VA, Armstrong LE, Coyle EF, et al. American College of Sports Medicine position stand. Exercise and fluid replacement. *Med. Sci. Sports Exer.* 1996; 28, i-vii.

Costill DL, Kammer WF, Fisher A. Fluid ingestion during distance running. *Arch. Environ. Health* 1970; 21, 520-525.

Costill DL. Physiology of marathon running. *JAMA* 1972; 221, 1024-1029.

Craig FN, Cummings EG. Dehydration and muscular work. *J. Appl. Physiol.* 1966; 21, 670-674.

Davies CT, Thompson MW. Physiological responses to prolonged exercise in ultramarathon athletes. *J. Appl. Physiol.* 1986; 61, 611-617.

Dugas JP, Oosthuizen U, Tucker R, Noakes TD. Rates of fluid ingestion alter pacing but not thermoregulatory responses during prolonged exercise in hot and humid conditions with appropriate convective cooling. *Eur. J. Appl. Physiol.* 2009;105:69-80.

Ebert TR, Martin DT, Stephens B, et al. Fluid and food intake during professional men's and women's road-cycling tours. *Int. J. Sports Physiol. Perform.* 2007; 2, 58-71.

Ely BR, Ely MR, Cheuvront SN, et al. Evidence against a 40 degrees C core temperature threshold for fatigue in humans. *J. Appl. Physiol.* 2009; 107, 1519-1525.

Fox RH. Heat stress and athletics. *Ergonomics* 1960; 3, 307-313.

Goulet ED. Effect of exercise-induced dehydration on time-trial exercise performance: A meta-analysis. *Br. J. Sports Med.* 2011; 45:1149-56.

Greenhaff PL, Clough PJ. Predictors of sweat loss in man during prolonged exercise. *Eur. J. Appl. Physiol. Occup. Physiol.* 1989; 58, 348-352.

Hiller WDB, O'Toole ML, Massimino F, et al. Plasma electrolyte and glucose changes during the Hawaiian Ironman Triathlon. *Med. Sci. Sports Exerc.* 1985; 17(suppl), 219.

Hoffer R. *Something in the Air.* 2009; pp. 1-258. New York: Free Press.

Hughson RL, Staudt LA, Mackie JM. Monitoring road racing in the heat. *Phys. Sportsmed.* 1983; 11, 94-105.

Irving RA, Noakes TD, Buck R, et al. Evaluation of renal function and fluid homeostasis during recovery from exercise-induced hyponatremia. *J. Appl. Physiol.* 1991; 70, 342-348.

Jardon OM. Physiologic stress, heat stroke, malignant hyperthermia—a perspective. *Mil.Med* 1982; 147, 8-14.

Judah T. *Bikila: Ethiopia's barefoot Olympian.* 2008; pp. 13-175. London: Reportage Press.

Kao WF, Shyu CL, Yang XW, et al. Athletic performance and serial weight changes during 12- and 24-hour ultra-marathons. *Clin. J. Sport Med.* 2008; 18, 155-158.

Kyle CR. Improving the racing bicycle. *Mech, Eng.* 1984; Sept: pp. 34-45.

Kyle CR. How wind affects cycling. *Bicycling.* 1988; May; pp. 194-204.

Ladell WS, Waterlow JC, Hudson MF. Desert climate: Physiological and clinical observations. *Lancet* 1944a; 2, 491-497.

Ladell WS, Waterlow JC, Hudson MF. Desert climate: Physiological and clinical observations: Heat exhaustion type II. *Lancet* 1944b; 2, 527-531.

Ladell WS. Disorders due to heat. *Trans. R. Soc. Trop. Med. Hyg.* 1957; 51, 189-207.

Ladell WS. Water and salt (sodium chloride) intakes. In *The physiology of human survival.* O.G. Edholm and A. Bacharach, eds. 1965; pp. 235-289. New York: Academic.

Laursen PB, Suriano R, Quod MJ, et al. Core temperature and hydration status during an Ironman triathlon. *Br. J. Sports Med.* 2006; 40, 320-325.

Leakey R, Lewin R. *Origins reconsidered: In search of what makes us human.* 1992; pp. 1-375. London: Abacus.

Lebus DK, Casazza GA, Hoffman MD, Van Loan MD. Can changes in body mass and total body water accurately predict hyponatremia? *Clin. J. Sport Med.* 2010: 20, 193-199.

Lee JK, Nio AQ, Lim CL, et al. Thermoregulation, pacing and fluid balance during mass participation distance running in a warm and humid environment. *Eur. J. Appl. Physiol.* 2010; 109, 887-898.

Lind AR. Physiological effects of continuous or intermittent work in the heat. *J.Appl.Physiol.* 1963; 18, 57-60.

Magazanik A, Shapiro Y, Meytes D, et al. Enzyme blood levels and water balance during a marathon race. *J.Appl.Physiol.* 1974; 36, 214-217.

Maron MB, Horvath SM, Wilkerson JE. Acute blood biochemical alterations in response to marathon running. *Eur.J.Appl. Physiol. Occup.Physiol* 1975; 34, 173-181.

Maron MB, Wagner JA, Horvath SM. Thermoregulatory responses during competitive marathon running. *J.Appl. Physiol.* 1977; 42, 909-914.

Maughan RJ. Thermoregulation in marathon competition at low ambient temperature. *Int.J Sports Med.* 1985; 6, 15-19.

Maughan RJ, Goodburn R, Griffin J, Irani M, Kiruran JP, Leiper JB, MacLaren DP, McLatchie G, Tsinkas K, Williams C. Fluid replacement in sport and exercise—a consensus statement. *Br. J. Sports Med.* 1993; 27, 34.

Maughan RJ, Leiper JB, Thompson J. Rectal temperature after marathon running. *Br. J. Sports Med.* 1985; 19, 192-195.

Morrow L. *Introduction:* 1968 a pictorial history. *Time* 1968. 1989; Spring: Special Collector's Edition. pp. 5-9.

Morrow L. United States: 1968. *Time.* 1988; 131:2. pp. 4-15.

Muir AL, Percy-Robb IW, Davidson IA, et al. Physiological aspects of the Edinburgh Commonwealth Games. *Lancet* 1970; 2, 1125-1128.

Myhre LG, Hartung GH, Tucker DM. Plasma volume and blood metabolites in middle-aged runners during a warm-weather marathon. *Eur. J. Appl. Physiol. Occup. Physiol.* 1982; 48, 227-240.

Myhre LG, Hartung GH, Nunneley SA, et al. Plasma volume changes in middle-aged male and female subjects during marathon running. *J.Appl.Physiol.* 1985; 59, 559-563.

Nielsen B. Die regulation der körpertemperatur bei muskelarbeit. *Skand. Archiv. für Physiol.* 1938; 79, 195-230.

Nielsen B, Nielsen M. Body temperature during work at different environmental temperatures. *Acta Physiol. Scand.* 1962; 56, 120-129.

Noakes TD. Letter: Heatstroke during the 1981 national cross-country running championships. *S. Afr. Med. J.* 1982; 61, 145.

Noakes TD. Fluid replacement during marathon running. *Clin. J. Sport Med.* 2003a; 13, 309-318.

Noakes TD. The dehydration myth and carbohydrate replacement during prolonged exercise. *Cycling Sci.* 1990; June, 23-29.

Noakes TD. Dehydration during exercise: what are the real dangers? *Clin. J. Sport Med.* 1995; 5, 123-128.

Noakes TD. Why marathon runners collapse. *S. Afr. Med. J.* 1988a; 73, 569-571.

Noakes TD. Fluid replacement during exercise. *Exerc. Sport Sci. Rev.* 1993; 21, 297-330.

Noakes TD, Adams BA, Myburgh KH, et al. The danger of an inadequate water intake during prolonged exercise. A novel concept re-visited. *Eur.J.Appl.Physiol.Occup.Physiol.* 1988; 57, 210-219.

Noakes TD, Goodwin N, Rayner BL, et al. Water intoxication: A possible complication during endurance exercise. *Med. Sci.Sports Exer.* 1985; 17, 370-375.

Noakes TD, Myburgh KH, du PJ, et al. Metabolic rate, not percent dehydration, predicts rectal temperature in marathon runners. *Med. Sci. Sports Exerc.* 1991; 23, 443-449.

Montain SJ, Coyle EF. Influence of graded dehydration on hyperthermia and cardiovascular drift during exercise. *J.Appl.Physiol.* 1992; 73, 1340-1350.

Owen MD, Kregel KC, Wall PT, et al. Effects of ingesting carbohydrate beverages during exercise in the heat. *Med. Sci. Sports Exerc.* 1986; 18, 568-575.

Pichan G, Gauttam RK, Tomar OS, et al. Effect of primary hypohydration on physical work capacity. *Int. J. Biometeorol.* 1988; 32, 176-180.

Popper K. *The logic of scientific discovery.* 1959; pp. 1-480. New York: Routledge.

Pugh LG, Corbett JL, Johnson RH. Rectal temperatures, weight losses and sweat rates in marathon running. *J.Appl.Physiol.* 1967; 23, 347-352.

Refsum HE, Tveit B, Meen HD, et al. Serum electrolyte, fluid and acid-base balance after prolonged heavy exercise at low environmental temperature. *Scand.J. Clin.Lab Invest.* 1973; 32, 117-122.

Robinson S. Temperature regulation in exercise. *Pediatrics* 1963; Suppl 32, 691-702.

Saltin B, Hermansen L. Esophageal, rectal, and muscle temperature during exercise. *J.Appl.Physiol.* 1966; 21, 1757-1762.

Saltin B. Aerobic work capacity and circulation at exercise in man. With special reference to the effect of prolonged exercise and/or heat exposure. *Acta Physiol. Scand. Suppl.* 1964; 230, 1-52.

Sawka MN, Burke LM, Eichner ER, et al. American College of Sports Medicine position stand. Exercise and fluid replacement. *Med. Sci. Sports Exerc.* 2007; 39, 377-390.

Sawka MN, Montain SJ, Latzka WA. Hydration effects on thermoregulation and performance in the heat. *Comp. Biochem. Physiol. A. Mol.Integr.Physiol.* 2001; 128, 679-690.

Sawka MN, Noakes TD. Does dehydration impair exercise performance? *Med. Sci. Sports Exerc.* 2007; 39, 1209-1217.

Sharwood K, Collins M, Goedecke J, et al. Weight changes, sodium levels, and performance in the South African Ironman Triathlon. *Clin. J. Sport Med.* 2002; 12, 391-399.

Sharwood KA, Collins M, Goedecke JH, et al. Weight changes, medical complications, and performance during an Ironman triathlon. *Br.J.Sports Med.* 2004; 38, 718-724.

Tucker R, Rauch L, Harley YX, et al. Impaired exercise performance in the heat is associated with an anticipatory reduction in skeletal muscle recruitment. *Pflugers Arch.* 2004; 448, 422-430.

Tucker R, Marle T, Lambert EV, et al. The rate of heat storage mediates an anticipatory reduction in exercise intensity during cycling at a fixed rating of perceived exertion. *J.Physiol.* 2006; 574, 905-915.

Wells CL, Schrader TA, Stern JR, et al. Physiological responses to a 20-mile run under three fluid replacement treatments. *Med. Sci. Sports Exerc.* 1985; 17, 364-369.

Wyndham CH, Strydom NB. The danger of an inadequate water intake during marathon running. *S. Afr. Med. J* 1969; 43, 893-896.

Wyndham CH, Strydom NB, Van Rensburg AJ, et al. Relation between VO_2max and body temperature in hot humid air conditions. *J.Appl.Physiol.* 1970; 29, 45-50.

Zouhal H, Groussard C, Vincent S, et al. Athletic performance and weight changes during the "Marathon of Sands" in athletes well-trained in endurance. *Int. J. Sports Med.* 2009; 30, 516-521.

Zouhal H, Groussard C, Minter G, et al. Inverse relationship between % weight change and finishing time in 643 42km marathon runners. *Br. J. Sports Med.* 2011; 45, 1101-1105.

Chapter 3   Notes

Benade AJ, Jansen CR, Rogers GG, et al. The significance of an increased RQ after sucrose ingestion during prolonged aerobic exercise. *Pflugers Arch.* 1973; 342, 199-206.

Burfoot A. Drink to your health. *Runner's World.* 2009; pp. 1-2.

Costill DL. Physiology of marathon running. *JAMA* 1972; 221, 1024-1029.

Marino FE. Anticipatory regulation and avoidance of catastrophe during exercise-induced hyperthermia. *Comp.Biochem. Physiol.B, Biochem.Mol.* 2004; 139, 561-569.

McGarvey J, Thompson J, Hanna C, et al. Sensitivity and specificity of clinical signs for assessment of dehydration in endurance athletes. *Br. J. Sports Med.* 2010; 44, 716-719.

Noakes TD. Study findings challenge core components of a current model of exercise thermoregulation. *Med. Sci. Sports Exerc.* 2007c; 39, 742-743.

Noakes TD, Mekler J, Pedoe DT. Jim Peters' collapse in the 1954 Vancouver Empire Games marathon. *S. Afr. Med. J.* 2008; 98, 596-600.

Noakes TD, St Clair Gibson A, Lambert EV. From catastrophe to complexity: A novel model of integrative central neural regulation of effort and fatigue during exercise in humans:

Summary and conclusions. *Br. J. Sports Med.* 2005; 39, 120-124.

Robinson S. Temperature regulation in exercise. *Pediatrics* 1963; Suppl 32, 691-702.

Strydom NB, Wyndham CH, Van Graan CH, et al. The influence of water restriction on the performance of men during a prolonged march. *S. Afr. Med. J.* 1966; 40, 539-544.

Tucker R, Rauch L, Harley YX, et al. Impaired exercise performance in the heat is associated with an anticipatory reduction in skeletal muscle recruitment. *Pflugers Arch.* 2004; 448, 422-430.

Wyndham CH. 1973 Yant Memorial Lecture: Research in the human sciences in the gold mining industry. *Am. Ind. Hyg. Assoc. J.* 1974; 35, 113-136.

Chapter 4   Salt Balance in the Body

Adolph EF. Urinary excretion of water and solutes. In *physiology of man in the desert* 1947; pp. 96-109. New York: Interscience.

Allsopp AJ, Sutherland R, Wood P, et al. The effect of sodium balance on sweat sodium secretion and plasma aldosterone concentration. *Eur. J. Appl. Physiol. Occup. Physiol.* 1998; 78, 516-521.

Armstrong LE, Casa DJ, Millard-Stafford M, et al. American College of Sports Medicine position stand: Exertional heat illness during training and competition. *Med. Sci. Sports Exerc.* 2007; 39, 556-572.

Armstrong LE. *Exertional heat illnesses* (edited by L.E. Armstrong), 2003; pp. 1-275. Champaign, IL: Human Kinetics.

Armstrong LE, Costill DL, Fink WJ. Changes in body water and electrolytes during heat acclimation: Effects of dietary sodium. *Aviat. Space Environ. Med* 1987; 58, 143-148.

Armstrong LE, Costill DL, Fink WJ, et al. Effects of dietary sodium on body and muscle potassium content during heat acclimation. *Eur. J. Appl. Physiol. Occup. Physiol.* 1985; 54, 391-397.

Armstrong LE, Hubbard RW, Askew EW, et al. Responses to moderate and low sodium diets during exercise-heat acclimation. *Int. J. Sport Nutr.* 1993; 3, 207-221.

Armstrong LE, Hubbard RW, Szlyk PC, et al.Voluntary dehydration and electrolyte losses during prolonged exercise in the heat. *Aviat. Space. Environ. Med.* 1985; 56, 765-770.

Asher R. Munchausen's syndrome. *Lancet* 1951; 1, 339-341.

Bergeron MF. Heat cramps during tennis: A case report. *Int. J. Sport Nutr.* 1996; 6, 62-68.

Bergeron MF. Heat cramps: Fluid and electrolyte challenges during tennis in the heat. *J. Sci. Med. Sport* 2003; 6, 19-27.

Bergeron MF. Muscle cramps during exercise: Is it fatigue or is it electrolyte deficit? *Current Sports Med. Reports* 2008; 7, S50-S55.

Bloch MR. The social influence of salt. *Sci. Amer.* 1963; 209, 89-99.

Brockbank EM. Miners' cramp. *Br. Med. J.* 1929; January 12, 65-66.

Bruso JR, Hoffman MD, Rogers IR, et al. Rhabdomyolosis and hyponatremia: A cluster of five cases at the 161-km 2009 Western States run endurance. *Wildern. Environ. Med.* 2010; 21, 301-308.

Conn JW, Johnston MW. The function of the sweat glands in the economy of NaCl under conditions of hard work in a tropical climate. *J. Clin. Invest.* 1944; 23, 933.

Conn JW. The mechanism of acclimatization to heat. *Adv. Intern. Med.* 1949a; 3, 373-393.

Conn JW. Electrolyte composition of sweat; clinical implications as an index of adrenal cortical function. *Arch. Intern. Med. (Chic.)* 1949b; 83, 416-428.

Conn JW. Primary aldosteronism. *J. Lab. Clin. Med.* 1955; 45, 661-664.

Conn JW. Some clinical and climatological aspects of aldosteronism in man. *Trans. Am. Clin. Climatol. Assoc.* 1962; 74, 61-91.

Convertino VA, Armstrong LE, Coyle EF, et al. American College of Sports Medicine position stand: Exercise and fluid replacement. *Med. Sci. Sports Exer.* 1996; 28, i-vii.

Costa F, Calloway DH, Margen S. Regional and total body sweat composition of men fed controlled diets. *Am. J. Clin. Nutr.* 1969; 22, 52-58.

Costill DL. Sweating: Its composition and effects on body fluids. In *The marathon: Physiological, medical, epidemiological and psychological studies* P. Milvy ed. 1977; pp. 160-174. New York: New York Academy of Sciences.

Costill DL, Coté R, Miller E, et al. Water and electrolyte replacement during repeated days of work in the heat. *Aviat. Space Environ. Med.* 1975; 46, 795-800.

Costill DL, Coté R, Fink W. Muscle water and electrolytes following varied levels of dehydration in man. *J. Appl. Physiol.* 1976; 40, 6-11.

Costill DL, Coté R, Fink WJ, et al. Muscle water and electrolyte distribution during prolonged exercise. *Int. J. Sports Med.* 1981; 2, 130-134.

Costill DL, Coté R, Fink WJ. Dietary potassium and heavy exercise: Effects on muscle water and electrolytes. *Am. J. Clin. Nutr.* 1982; 36, 266-275.

Daly C, Dill DB. Salt economy in humid heat. *Am. J. Physiol.* 1937; 118, 285-289.

Daniell HW. Simple cure for nocturnal leg cramps. *N. Eng. J. Med.* 1979; 310, 216.

Derrick EH. Heat cramps and uraemic cramps with special reference to their treatment with sodium chloride. *Med. J. Aust.* 1934; November 10, 612-616.

Dill DB, Bock AV, Edwards HT, et al. Industrial fatigue. *J. Ind. Hyg. Toxicol.* 1936; 18, 417-431.

Dill DB, Jones BF, Edwards HT, et al. Salt economy in extreme dry heat. *J. Biol. Chem.* 1933; 100, 755-767.

Drew N. Exercise associated muscle cramping (EAMC) in Ironman triathletes. A dissertation prepared by Nichola Drew in partial fulfillment of the requirements for the Master of Philosophy degree in Sports Medicine (MPhil Sports Medicine). 2006. South Africa: University of Cape Town.

Edelman IS, Leibman J, O'Meara MP, et al. Interrelations between serum sodium concentration, serum osmolarity and total exchangeable sodium, total exchangeable potassium and total body water. *J. Clin. Invest.* 1958; 37, 1236-1256.

Ellis C, Cuthill J, Hew-Butler T, et al. Case report: Exercise-associated hyponatremia with rhabdomyolysis during endurance exercise. *Phys. Sportsmed.* 2009; 37, 126-132.

Epstein Y, Sohar E. Fluid balance in hot climates: Sweating, water intake, and prevention of dehydration. *Pub. Health Rev.* 1985; 13, 115-137.

Fudge BW, Easton C, Kingsmore D, et al. Elite Kenyan endurance runners are hydrated day-to-day with ad libitum fluid intake. *Med. Sci. Sports Exerc.* 2008; 40, 1171-1179.

Fudge BW, Pitsiladis Y, Kingsmore D, et al. Outstanding performance despite low fluid intake: The Kenyan running experience. In *East African running: Towards a cross-disciplinary perspective* Y. Pitsiladis, J. Bale, C. Sharp and T.D. Noakes, eds. 2007; pp. 63-84. London: Routledge.

Glover DM. Heat cramps in industry: Their treatment and prevention by means of sodium chloride. *J. Ind. Hyg.* 1931; 13, 347-360.

Haldane JS. Heat cramp. *Br. Med. J.* 1928; April 7, 609-610.

Hancock W, Whitehouse AGR, Haldane JS. The loss of water and salts through the skin, and the corresponding physiological adjustments. *Proc. Roy. Soc. London.Series B, Biol.* 1929a; 105, 43-59.

Hew-Butler T, Verbalis JG, Noakes TD. Updated fluid recommendation: position statement from the International Marathon Medical Directors Association (IMMDA). *Clin. J. Sport Med.* 2006; 16, 283-292.

Horswill, CA, Stofan JR, Lacambra M, et al. Sodium balance during U.S. football training in the heat: cramp-prone vs. reference players. *Int. J. Sports Med.* 2009; 30, 789-794.

Hsu YD, Lee WH, Chang MK, et al. Blood lactate threshold and type II fibre predominance in patients with exertional heatstroke. *J. Neurol. Neurosurg. Psych.* 1997; 62, 182-187.

Hutton RS, Nelson DL. Stretch sensitivity of Golgi tendon organs in fatigued gastrocnemius muscle. *Med. Sci. Sports Exerc.* 1986; 18, 69-74.

Institute of Medicine of the National Academies. *Dietary reference intakes for water, potassium, sodium, chloride, and sulfate.* 2005; pp. 1-617. Washington, DC: National Academies Press.

Johnson RE, Pitts GC, Consolazio FC. Factors influencing chloride concentration in human sweat. *Am. J. Physiol.* 1944; 141, 575-589.

Jung AP, Bishop PA, Al-Nawwas A, et al. Influence of hydration and electrolyte supplementation on incidence and time to onset of exercise-associated muscle cramps. *J. Athl. Train.* 2005; 40, 71-75.

Kamoi K, Ebe T, Kobayashi O, et al. Atrial natriuretic peptide in patients with the syndrome of inappropriate antidiuretic hormone secretion and with diabetes insipidus. *J. Clin. Endocrinol. Metab.* 1990; 70, 1385-1390.

Kawai N, Baba A, Suzuki T, et al. Roles of arginine vasopressin and atrial natriuretic peptide in polydipsia-hyponatremia of schizophrenic patients. *Psych. Res.* 2001; 101, 39-45.

Khan SI, Burne JA. Reflex inhibition of normal cramp following electrical stimulation of the muscle tendon. *J. Neurophysiol.* 2007; 98, 1102-1107.

Knochel JP. Environmental heat illness: An eclectic review. *Arch. Intern. Med.* 1974; 133, 841-864.

Konikoff F, Shoenfeld Y, Magazanik A, et al. Effects of salt loading during exercise in a hot dry climate. *Biomed. Pharmacother.* 1986; 40, 296-300.

Ladell WS. Heat cramps. *Lancet* 1949; 2, 836-839.

Ladell WS. Disorders due to heat. *Trans. R. Soc. Trop. Med. Hyg.* 1957; 51, 189-207.

Ladell WS. Water and salt (sodium chloride) intakes. In *The physiology of human survival* O.G. Edholm and A. Bacharach, eds. 1965; pp. 235-289. New York: Academic.

Ladell WS, Shephard RJ. Aldosterone inhibition and acclimatization to heat. *J. Physiol.* 1962; 160, 19-20.

Ladell WS, Waterlow JC, Hudson MF. Desert climate: Physiological and clinical observations: Heat exhaustion type II. *Lancet* 1944a; 2, 527-531.

Ladell WS, Waterlow JC, Hudson MF. Desert climate: Physiological and clinical observations. *Lancet* 1944b; 2; 491-497.

Liebenberg L. *The art of tracking: The origin of science.* 1990; pp. 3-176. Claremont, South Africa: Philip.

Lonn E. *Salt as a factor in the confederacy.* 1965; pp. 1-324. Tuscaloosa: University of Alabama Press.

Malhotra MS. Salt and water requirement of acclimatized people working outdoors in severe heat. *Ind. J. Med. Res.* 1960; 48, 212-217.

Mange K, Matsuura D, Cizman B, et al. Language guiding therapy: the case of dehydration versus volume depletion. *Ann. Intern. Med.* 1997; 127, 848-853.

Marriott HL. Water and salt depletion: Part II. *Br. Med. J.* 1947; 1, 285-290.

Maughan RJ. Exercise-induced muscle cramp: A prospective biochemical study in marathon runners. *J. Sports Sci.* 1986; 4, 31-34.

McCance RA. Medical problems in mineral metabolism. *Lancet* 1936a; 1, 823-830.

McCance RA. Experimental sodium chloride deficiency in man. *Proc. Roy. Soc. B* 1936b; 119, 245-268.

McCance RA. The changes in the plasma and cells during experimental human salt deficiency. *Biochem.* 1937; 31, 1278-1284.

McCord CP. Fatigue in soldiers due to chlorine losses. *Mil. Surg.* 1931; 69, 608-614.

Meneely GR, Tucker RG, Darby WJ, et al. Chronic sodium chloride toxicity: Hypertension, renal and vascular lesions. *Ann. Intern. Med.* 1953; 39, 991-998.

Miller KC, Mack GW, Knight KL, et al. Three percent hypohydration does not affect threshold frequency of electrically induced cramps. *Med. Sci. Sports Exerc.* 2010a; 42, 2056-2063.

Miller KC, Mack GW, Knight KL, et al. Reflex inhibition of electrically induced muscle cramps in hypohydrated humans. *Med. Sci. Sports Exerc.* 2010b; 42, 953-961.

Miller KC, Mack G, Knight KL. Electrolyte and plasma changes after ingestion of pickle juice, water, and a common carbohydrate-electrolyte solution. *J. Athl. Train.* 2009; 44, 454-461.

Minetto MA, Botter A, Ravenni R, et al. Reliability of a novel neurostimulation method to study involuntary muscle phenomena. *Muscle Nerve* 2008; 37, 90-100.

Morse WR, McGill MD. Blood pressure amongst aboriginal ethnic groups of Szechwan Province, West China. *Lancet* 1937; 1, 966-967.

Moss KN. Some effects of high air temperatures and muscular exertion upon Colliers. *Proc. Roy. Soc. B* 1923; 95, 181-200.

Moss M. The hard sell on salt. *New York Times.* 29 May 2010.

Nelson DL, Hutton RS. Dynamic and static stretch responses in muscle spindle receptors in fatigued muscle. *Med. Sci. Sports Exerc.* 1985; 17, 445-450.

Noakes TD. The hyponatremia of exercise. *Int. J. Sport Nutr.* 1992; 2, 205-228.

Norris FH, Jr., Gasteiger EL, Chatfield PO. An electromyographic study of induced and spontaneous muscle cramps. *Electroenceph. Clin. Neurophysiol.* 1957; 9, 139-147.

Oswald RJW. Saline drink in industrial fatigue. *Lancet* 1925; 1, 1369-1370.

Pandolf KB, Burr RE. *Medical aspects of harsh environments.* (D.E. Lounsbury, R.F. Bellamy, R. Zajtchuk, eds.), 2010; pp. 1-609. Washington, DC: TMM.

Reinhardt HW, Seeliger E. Toward an integrative concept of control of total body sodium. *News Physiol. Sci.* 2000; 15, 319-325.

Robinson S, Nicholas JR, Smith JH, et al. Time relation of renal and sweat gland adjustments to salt deficiency in men. *J. Appl. Physiol.* 1955; 8, 159-165.

Rovner DR, Streeten DH, Louis LH, et al. Content and uptake of sodium and potassium in bone. Influence of adrenalectomy, aldosterone, desoxycorticosterone and sprionolactone. *J. Clin. Endocrinol. Metab.* 1963; 23, 938-944.

Rowntree LG. Water intoxication. *Arch. Int. Med.* 1923; 32, 157-174.

Sanders B, Noakes TD, Dennis SC. Water and electrolyte shifts with partial fluid replacement during exercise. *Eur. J. Appl. Physiol. Occup. Physiol.* 1999; 80, 318-323.

Sanders B, Noakes TD, Dennis SC. Sodium replacement and fluid shifts during prolonged exercise in humans. *Eur. J. Appl. Physiol.* 2001; 84, 419-425.

Schwellnus MP. Cause of exercise associated muscle cramps (EAMC)—altered neuromuscular control, dehydration or electrolyte depletion? *Br. J. Sports Med.* 2009; 43, 401-408.

Schwellnus MP. Muscle cramping in the marathon: Aetiology and risk factors. *Sports Med.* 2007; 37, 364-367.

Schwellnus MP, Derman EW, Noakes TD. Aetiology of skeletal muscle "'cramps'" during exercise: a novel hypothesis. *J. Sports Sci.* 1997; 15, 277-285.

Schwellnus MP, Drew N, Collins M. Increased running speed and previous cramps rather than dehydration or serum sodium changes predicts exercise associated muscle cramping (EAMC): A prospective cohort sutdy in 210 ironman triathletes. *Br. J. Sports Med.* 2011; 45: 650-656.

Schwellnus MP, Drew N, Collins M. Muscle cramping in athletes—risk factors, clinical assessment, and management. *Clin. Sports Med.* 2008; 27, 183-194.

Schwellnus MP, Nicol J, Laubscher R, et al. Serum electrolyte concentrations and hydration status are not associated with exercise associated muscle cramping (EAMC) in distance runners. *Br. J. Sports Med.* 2004; 38, 488-492.

Shem S. *The house of God.* 2003; pp. 1-397. New York: Bantam Dell.

Spital A. Dehydration versus volume depletion--and the importance of getting it right. *Am. J. Kidney Dis.* 2007; 49, 721-722.

Stofan JR, Zachwieja JJ, Horswill CA, et al. Sweat and sodium losses in NCAA football players: a precursor to heat cramps? *Int. J. Sport Nutr. Exerc. Metab.* 2005; 15, 641-652.

Stone MB, Edwards JE, Babington JP, et al. Reliability of an electrical method to induce muscle cramp. *Muscle Nerve* 2003; 27, 122-123.

Streeten DHP, Conn JW, Louis LH, et al. Secondary aldosteronism: Metabolic and adrenocortical responses of normal men to high environmental temperatures. *Metabolism* 1960; 9, 1071-1092.

Streeten DH, Rapoport A, Conn JW. Existence of a slowly exchangeable pool of body sodium in normal subjects and its diminution in patients with primary aldosteronism. *J. Clin. Endocrinol. Metab.* 1963; 23, 928-937.

Sulzer NU, Schwellnus MP, Noakes TD. Serum electrolytes in Ironman triathletes with exercise-associated muscle cramping. *Med. Sci. Sports Exerc.* 2005; 37, 1081-1085.

Talbott JH. Heat cramps. *Medicine* 1935; 14, 323-376.

Talbott JH, Michelsen J. Heat cramps: A clinical and chemical study. *J. Clin. Invest.* 1933; 12, 533-549.

Taylor HL, Henschel A, Mickelsen O, et al. The effect of the sodium chloride intake on the work performance of man during exposure to dry heat and experimental heat exhaustion. *Am. J. Physiol.* 1943; 140, 439-451.

Weiner JS, Van Heyningen RE. Salt losses of men working in hot environments. *Br. J. Ind. Med.* 1952; 9, 56-64.

Wyndham CH, Strydom NB, Benade AJ, et al. The effect on acclimatization of various water and salt replacement regimens. *S. Afr. Med. J.* 1973; 47, 1773-1779.

Chapter 4 Notes

Brockbank EM. Miners' cramp. *Br. Med. J.* 1929; January 12, 65-66.

Conn JW. Some clinical and climatological aspects of aldosteronism in man. *Trans. Am. Clin. Climatol. Assoc.* 1962; 74, 61-91.

Dancaster CP, Whereat SJ. Fluid and electrolyte balance during the Comrades Marathon. *S. Afr. Med. J.* 1971; 45, 147-150.

Noakes TD. Fluid replacement during marathon running. *Clin. J. Sport Med.* 2003c; 13, 309-318.

Simpson SA, Tait JF, Bush IE. Secretion of a salt-retaining hormone by the mammalian adrenal cortex. *Lancet* 1952; 2, 226-228.

Williams JS, Williams GH. 50th anniversary of aldosterone. *J. Clin. Endocrinol. Metab.* 2003; 88, 2364-2372.

Chapter 5 Emergence of the Sports Drink Industry

Aarseth HP, Eide I, Skeie B, et al. Heat stroke in endurance exercise. *Acta Med. Scand.* 1986; 220, 279-283.

Al-Harthi SS, Sharaf El-Deane MS, Akhtar J, et al. Hemodynamic changes and intravascular hydration state in heat stroke. *Annals Saudi Med.* 1989; 9, 378-383.

"James Robert Cade: September 26, 1927-November 27, 2007." American Physiological Society; 2007. www.the-aps.org/membership/obituaries/robert_cade.htm.

"When wife gave him lemons, doctor made Gatorade." University of Texas Southwestern; 1-2. 2004b.

"Gatorade celebrates 35 years of quenching thirst." Alligatoronline; 2002. www.alligator.org/edit/news/issues/02-spring/020321/b02gatorade21.html

"Gatorade returns to "'origins'" as legend continues." *Gatorade News*; 1-2. 2003.

"Dr Robert Cade: Preaching." Jan/Feb: 58-59. 1990. www.e-steeple.com/browse-by-topic/I/Income.html.

Armstrong LE, Casa DJ, Millard-Stafford M, et al. American College of Sports Medicine position stand: Exertional heat illness during training and competition. *Med. Sci. Sports Exerc.* 2007; 39, 556-572.

Austin MG, Berry JW. Observations on one hundred cases of heatstroke. *J. Am. Med. Assoc.* 1956; 161, 1525-1529.

Barr SI, Costill DL, Fink WJ. Fluid replacement during prolonged exercise: Effects of water, saline, or no fluid. *Med. Sci. Sports Exerc.* 1991; 23, 811-817.

Bartley JD. Heat stroke: is total prevention possible? *Mil. Med.* 1977; 142, 528, 533-528, 535.

Baxter CR, Teschan PE. Atypical heat stroke, with hypernatremia, acute renal failure, and fulminating potassium intoxication. *Arch. Intern. Med.* 1958; 101, 1040-1050.

Beller GA, Boyd AE, III. Heat stroke: A report of 13 consecutive cases without mortality despite severe hyperpyrexia and neurologic dysfunction. *Mil. Med.* 1975; 140, 464-467.

Bergeron MF, McKeag DB, Casa DJ, et al. Youth football: Heat stress and injury risk. *Med. Sci. Sports Exerc.* 2005; 37, 1421-1430.

Brodeur VB, Dennett SR, Griffin LS. Exertional hyperthermia, ice baths, and emergency care at the Falmouth Road Race. *J. Emerg. Nurs.* 1989; 15, 304-312.

Brown AH. Fluid intakes in the desert. In *Physiology of man in the desert* 1947a; pp. 110-114. New York: Interscience.

Brown AH. Water requirements of man in the desert. In *Physiology of man in the desert* 1947b; pp. 115-135. New York: Interscience.

Burgess ML, Robertson RJ, Davis JM, et al. RPE, blood glucose, and carbohydrate oxidation during exercise: Effects of glucose feedings. *Med. Sci. Sports Exerc.* 1991; 23, 353-359.

Cade JR, Free HJ, De Quesada AM, Shires DL, Roby L. Changes in body fluid composition and volume during vigorous exercise by athletes. *J. Sports Med. Phys. Fitness* 1971; 11, 172-178.

Cade R, Packer D, Zauner C, et al. Marathon running: Physiological and chemical changes accompanying late-race functional deterioration. *Eur. J. Appl. Physiol. Occup. Physiol.* 1992; 65, 485-491.

Cade R, Spooner G, Schlein E, Pickering M, Dean R. Department of Medicine, University of Florida Medical School. *J. Sports Med. Phys. Fit.* 12, 150-156, 1972.

Carter R, III, Cheuvront SN, Sawka MN. A case report of idiosyncratic hyperthermia and review of U.S. Army heat stroke hospitalizations. *J. Sport Rehabil.* 2007; 16, 238-243.

Carter R, III, Cheuvront SN, Williams JO, et al. Epidemiology of hospitalizations and deaths from heat illness in soldiers. *Med. Sci. Sports Exerc.* 2005; 37, 1338-1344.

Epstein Y, Moran DS, Shapiro Y, et al. Exertional heat stroke: A case series. *Med. Sci. Sports Exerc.* 1999; 31, 224-228.

Ferris EB, Blankenhorn MA, Robinson HW, et al. Heat stroke: Clinical and chemical observations on 44 cases. *J. Clin. Invest.* 1938; 17, 249-262.

Fowkes Godek S, Bartolozzi AR, Burkholder R, et al. Sweat rates and fluid turnover in professional football players: A comparison of national football league linemen and backs. *J. Athl. Train.* 2008; 43, 184-189.

Fowkes Godek S, Bartolozzi AR, Godek JJ. Sweat rate and fluid turnover in American football players compared with runners in a hot and humid environment. *Br. J. Sports Med.* 2005; 39, 205-211.

Fowkes GS, Godek JJ, Bartolozzi AR. Thermal responses in football and cross-country athletes during their respective practices in a hot environment. *J. Athl. Train.* 2004; 39, 235-240.

Gant N, Stinear CM, Byblow WD. Carbohydrate in the mouth immediately facilitates motor output. *Brain Res.* 2010; 1350, 151-158.

Gavva NR. Body-temperature maintenance as the predominant function of the vanilloid receptor TRPV1. *Trends Pharmacol. Sci.* 2008; 29, 550-557.

Gilat T, Shibolet S, Sohar E. The mechanism of heatstroke. *J. Trop. Med. Hyg.* 1963; 66, 204-212.

Gisolfi CV. Fluid balance for optimal performance. *Nutr. Rev.* 1996; 54, S159-S168.

Godek SF, Bartolozzi AR, Burkholder R, et al. Core temperature and percentage of dehydration in professional football linemen and backs during preseason practices. *J. Athl. Train.* 2006; 41, 8-14.

Hein K. Gatorade sues Powerade over ad claims. *Brandweek*; 13 April: 2009. www.brandweek.com/bw/content_display/news-and-features/packaged-goods/e3i98782c058bdfe7fd9b-d08a52ff906b70.

Henderson A, Simon JW, Melia WM, et al. Heat illness: A report of 45 cases from Hong Kong. *J. R. Army Med. Corps* 1986; 132, 76-84.

Hopkins PM, Wappler F. Is there a link between malignant hyperthermia and exertional heat illness? *Br. J. Sports Med.* 2007; 41, 283-284.

Johnson RJ, Perez-Pozo SE, Sautin YY, et al. Hypothesis: Could excessive fructose intake and uric acid cause type 2 diabetes? *Endocr. Rev.* 2009; 30, 96-116.

Kark JA, Burr PQ, Wenger CB, et al. Exertional heat illness in Marine Corps recruit training. *Aviat. Space Environ. Med.* 1996; 67, 354-360.

Kays J, Phillips-Han A. The idea that launched an industry. *Explore* 2003; 8: 1-4.

Kretsch A, Grogan R, Duras P, et al. 1980 Melbourne marathon study. *Med. J. Aust.* 1984; 141, 809-814.

Kochs E, Hoffman WE, Roewer N, et al. Alterations in brain electrical activity may indicate the onset of malignant hyperthermia in swine. *Anesthesiol.* 1990; 73, 1236-1242.

Malamud N, Haymaker W, Custer RP. Heat stroke: A clinicopathologic study of 125 fatal cases. *Mil. Surg.* 1946; 99, 397-449.

Malawer SJ, Ewton M, Fordtran JS, et al. Interrelation between Jejunal absorption of sodium glucose, and water in man. *J. Clin. Invest.* 1965; 44, pp. 1072-1073.

Molnar GW. Man in the tropics compared with man in the desert. In *Physiology of man in the desert* 1947; pp. 315-325. New York: Interscience.

Mudambo KS, Leese GP, Rennie MJ. Dehydration in soldiers during walking/running exercise in the heat and the effects of fluid ingestion during and after exercise. *Eur. J. Appl. Physiol. Occup. Physiol.* 1997; 76, 517-524.

Noakes TD, Mekler J, Pedoe DT. Jim Peters' collapse in the 1954 Vancouver Empire Games marathon. *S. Afr. Med. J.* 2008; 98, 596-600.

Nordlie T. UF honors Gatorade inventor Cade with evening of memories. 2004; 1-3. University of Florida.

O'Donnell TF, Jr. Acute heat stroke: Epidemiologic, biochemical, renal, and coagulation studies. *JAMA* 1975; 234, 824-828.

O'Donnell TF, Jr., Clowes GH, Jr. The circulatory abnormalities of heat stroke. *N. Engl. J. Med.* 1972; 287, 734-737.

Pettigrew RT, Galt JM, Ludgate CM, et al. Circulatory and biochemical effects of whole body hyperthermia. *Br. J. Surg.* 1974; 61, 727-730.

Porter AM. The death of a British officer-cadet from heat illness. *Lancet* 2000; 355, 569-571.

Rae DE, Knobel GJ, Mann T, et al. Heatstroke during endurance exercise: Is there evidence for excessive endothermy? *Med. Sci. Sports Exerc.* 2008; 40, 1193-1204.

Roberts WO. Exertional heat stroke during a cool weather marathon: A case study. *Med. Sci. Sports Exerc.* 2006; 38, 1197-1203.

Roberts WO. A 12-yr profile of medical injury and illness for the Twin Cities Marathon. *Med. Sci. Sports Exerc.* 2000; 32, 1549-1555.

Rovell D. *First in thirst: How Gatorade turned the science of sweat into a cultural phenomenon.* 2005; New York: Amacom.

Sargent F. Depression of sweating in man: So called "sweat gland fatigue." In *Advances in biology of skin* W. Montagna, R.A. Ellis and A.F. Silver, eds. 1962; p. 127. New York: Pergamon Press.

Sawka MN, Burke LM, Eichner ER, et al. American College of Sports Medicine position stand: Exercise and fluid replacement. *Med. Sci. Sports Exerc.* 2007; 39, 377-390.

Sawka MN, Montain SJ. Fluid and electrolyte supplementation for exercise heat stress. *Am. J. Clin. Nutr.* 2000; 72, 564S-572S.

Sawka MN, Young AJ, Latzka WA, et al. Human tolerance to heat strain during exercise: Influence of hydration. *J. Appl. Physiol.* 1992; 73, 368-375.

Schickele E. Environment and fatal heat stroke: An analysis of 157 cases occurring in the army in the US during World War II. *Milit. Surg.* 1947, 235-256.

Schrier RW, Henderson HS, Tisher CC, et al. Nephropathy associated with heat stress and exercise. *Ann. Intern. Med.* 1967; 67, 356-376.

Schwartz IL, Itoh S. Proceedings of the forty-eighth annual meeting of the American Society for Clinical Investigation held in Atlantic City, NJ, April 30, 1956. 1956; pp. 733-734.

Seraj MA, Channa AB, al Harthi SS, et al. Are heat stroke patients fluid depleted? Importance of monitoring central venous pressure as a simple guideline for fluid therapy. *Resuscitation* 1991; 21, 33-39.

Shibolet S, Coll R, Gilat T, et al. Heatstroke: its clinical picture and mechanism in 36 cases. *Q. J. Med.* 1967; 36, 525-548.

Strydom NB. The state of hydration and the physiological responses of men during work in heat. *Aust. J. Sports Med.* 1975; 7, 28-33.

Vassallo SU, Delaney KA. Pharmacologic effects on thermoregulation: mechanisms of drug-related heatstroke. *J. Toxicol. Clin. Toxicol.* 1989; 27, 199-224.

Wyndham CH. A survey of the causal factors in heat stroke and of their prevention in the gold mining industry. *J. S. A. Inst. Mining Metall.* 1965, 125-155.

Yu FC, Lu KC, Lin SH, et al. Energy metabolism in exertional heat stroke with acute renal failure. *Nephrol. Dial. Transplant* 1997; 12, 2087-2092.

Chapter 5   Notes

Bernard C. *An introduction to the study of experimental medicine.* 1957; pp. 1-226. New York: Dover.

Clark VR, Hopkins WG, Hawley JA, et al. Placebo effect of carbohydrate feedings during a 40-km cycling time trial. *Med. Sci. Sports Exerc.* 2000; 32, 1642-1647.

Fowkes GS, Godek JJ, Bartolozzi AR. Thermal responses in football and cross-country athletes during their respective practices in a hot environment. *J. Athl. Train.* 2004; 39, 235-240.

Irving RA, Noakes TD, Buck R, et al. Evaluation of renal function and fluid homeostasis during recovery from exercise-induced hyponatremia. *J. Appl. Physiol.* 1991; 70, 342-348.

Marino FE. Anticipatory regulation and avoidance of catastrophe during exercise-induced hyperthermia. *Comp. Biochem. Physiol. B. Biochem. Mol.* 2004; 139, 561-569.

Marino FE, Lambert MI, Noakes TD. Superior performance of African runners in warm humid but not in cool environmental conditions. *J. Appl. Physiol.* 2004; 96, 124-130.

Nassif C, Ferreira AP, Gomes AR, et al. Double blind carbohydrate ingestion does not improve exercise duration in warm humid conditions. *J. Sci. Med. Sport* 2008; 11, 72-79.

Rovell D. *First in thirst: How Gatorade turned the science of sweat into a cultural phenomenon.* 2005; pp. 1-243. New York: Amacom.

Tucker R, Marle T, Lambert EV, et al. The rate of heat storage mediates an anticipatory reduction in exercise intensity during cycling at a fixed rating of perceived exertion. *J. Physiol.* 2006; 574, 905-915.

Tucker R, Rauch L, Harley YX, et al. Impaired exercise performance in the heat is associated with an anticipatory reduction in skeletal muscle recruitment. *Pflugers Arch.* 2004; 448, 422-430.

Chapter 6 The Shaky Science of Hydration

Adams WC, Mack GW, Langhans GW, et al. Effects of varied air velocity on sweating and evaporative rates during exercise. *J. Appl. Physiol.* 1992; 73, 2668-2674.

Below PR, Mora-Rodriguez R, Gonzalez-Alonso J, et al. Fluid and carbohydrate ingestion independently improve performance during 1 h of intense exercise. *Med. Sci. Sports Exerc.* 1995; 27, 200-210.

Brotherhood JR. Heat stress and strain in exercise and sport. *J. Sci. Med. Sport* 2008; 11, 6-19.

Buskirk ER, Beetham WPJ. Dehydration and body temperature as a result of marathon running. *Med. Sportiva* 1960; XIV, 493-506.

Cade R, Packer D, Zauner C, et al. Marathon running: Physiological and chemical changes accompanying late-race functional deterioration. *Eur. J. Appl. Physiol. Occup. Physiol.* 1992; 65, 485-491.

Christensen EH, Hansen O. Hypoglykamie, arbeitsfahigkeit and Ernahrung. *Skand. Arch. Physiol.* 1939; 81, 172-179.

Coggan AR, Coyle EF. Reversal of fatigue during prolonged exercise by carbohydrate infusion or ingestion. *J. Appl. Physiol.* 1987; 63, 2388-2395.

Convertino VA, Armstrong LE, Coyle EF, et al. American College of Sports Medicine position stand: Exercise and fluid replacement. *Med. Sci. Sports Exerc.* 1996; 28, i-vii.

Costill DL. Physiology of marathon running. *JAMA* 1972; 221, 1024-1029.

Costill DL. *Inside running: Basics of sports physiology.* 1986; pp. 1-189. Indianapolis: Benchmark.

Costill DL, Kammer WF, Fisher A. Fluid ingestion during distance running. *Arch. Environ. Health* 1970a; 21, 520-525.

Coyle EF. Fluid and carbohydrate replacement during exercise: How much and why? *Sports Sci. Exch.* 1994; 7, 1-8. www.myclients.ca/customers/gprc/a_fluid_and_carbohydrate_replacement.pdf.

Coyle EF, Coggan AR, Hemmert MK, et al. Muscle glycogen utilization during prolonged strenuous exercise when fed carbohydrate. *J. Appl. Physiol.* 1986; 61, 165-172.

Crewe H, Tucker R, Noakes TD. The rate of increase in rating of perceived exertion predicts the duration of exercise to fatigue at a fixed power output in different environmental conditions. *Eur. J. Appl. Physiol.* 2008; 103, 569-577.

Ely BR, Ely MR, Cheuvront SN, et al. Evidence against a 40 degrees C core temperature threshold for fatigue in humans. *J. Appl. Physiol.* 2009; 107, 1519-1525.

Eston R, Faulkner J, St Clair Gibson A, et al. The effect of antecedent fatiguing activity on the relationship between perceived exertion and physiological activity during a constant load exercise task. *Psychophysiol.* 2007; 44, 779-786.

Eston R, Lambrick D, Sheppard K, et al. Prediction of maximal oxygen uptake in sedentary males from a perceptually regulated, sub-maximal graded exercise test. *J. Sports Sci.* 2008; 26, 131-139.

Fritzsche RG, Switzer TW, Hodgkinson BJ, et al. Water and carbohydrate ingestion during prolonged exercise increase maximal neuromuscular power. *J. Appl. Physiol.* 2000; 88, 730-737.

Gisolfi CV. Exercise, heat, and dehydration don't mix. *Rx Sports and Travel*; May-June: 23-25. 1975.

Gisolfi CV, Copping JR. Thermal effects of prolonged treadmill exercise in the heat. *Med. Sci. Sports* 1974; 6, 108-113.

González-Alonso J, Calbet JA. Reductions in systemic and skeletal muscle blood flow and oxygen delivery limit maximal aerobic capacity in humans. *Circulation* 2003; 107, 824-830.

González-Alonso J, Calbet JA, Nielsen B. Metabolic and thermodynamic responses to dehydration-induced reductions in muscle blood flow in exercising humans. *J. Physiol.* 1999; 520, 577-589.

González-Alonso J, Calbet JA, Nielsen B. Muscle blood flow is reduced with dehydration during prolonged exercise in humans. *J. Physiol.* 1998; 513, 895-905.

González-Alonso J, Crandall CG, Johnson JM. The cardiovascular challenge of exercising in the heat. *J. Physiol.* 2008; 586, 45-53.

González-Alonso J, Dalsgaard MK, Osada T, et al. Brain and central haemodynamics and oxygenation during maximal exercise in humans. *J. Physiol.* 2004; 557, 331-342.

González-Alonso J, Mora-Rodriguez R, Coyle EF. Stroke volume during exercise: interaction of environment and hydration. *Am. J. Physiol. Heart Circ. Physiol.* 2000; 278, H321-H330.

González-Alonso J, Mora-Rodriguez R, Coyle EF. Supine exercise restores arterial blood pressure and skin blood flow despite dehydration and hyperthermia. *Am. J. Physiol.* 1999; 277, H576-H583.

González-Alonso J, Mora-Rodriguez R, Below PR, et al. Dehydration markedly impairs cardiovascular function in hyperthermic endurance athletes during exercise. *J. Appl. Physiol.* 1997; 82, 1229-1236.

González-Alonso J, Mora-Rodriguez R, Below PR, et al. Dehydration reduces cardiac output and increases systemic and cutaneous vascular resistance during exercise. *J. Appl. Physiol.* 1995; 79, 1487-1496.

Johnson JM, Rowell LB. Forearm skin and muscle vascular responses to prolonged leg exercise in man. *J. Appl. Physiol.* 1975; 39, 920-924.

Kenefick RW, Sawka MN. Heat exhaustion and dehydration as causes of marathon collapse. *Sports Med.* 2007; 37, 378-381.

Kolata G. A career spent in study of training and exercise. *New York Times*; October 30, 2001: 1-3. 2001. www.alexandria-masters.com/articles/study.htm.

Montain SJ, Coyle EF. Influence of graded dehydration on hyperthermia and cardiovascular drift during exercise. *J. Appl. Physiol.* 1992; 73, 1340-1350.

Montain SJ, Coyle EF. Fluid ingestion during exercise increases skin blood flow independent of increases in blood volume. *J. Appl. Physiol.* 1997; 73: 903-910.

Morante SM, Brotherhood JR. Thermoregulatory responses during competitive singles tennis. *Br. J. Sports Med.* 2008; 42, 736-741.

Mora-Rodriguez R, Del Coso J, Aguado-Jimenez R, et al. Separate and combined effects of airflow and rehydration during exercise in the heat. *Med. Sci. Sports Exerc.* 2007; 39, 1720-1726.

Morrison P. Air-Cooled. *Sci. Am.* 1997; October 1997, 149-150.

Noakes TD. Testing for maximum oxygen consumption has produced a brainless model of human exercise performance. *Br. J. Sports Med.* 2008; 42, 551-555.

Noakes TD, Marino FE. Arterial oxygenation, central motor output and exercise performance in humans. *J. Physiol.* 2007; 585, 919-921.

Noakes TD, St. Clair Gibson A. Logical limitations to the "catastrophe" models of fatigue during exercise in humans. *Br. J. Sports Med.* 2004; 38, 648-649.

Rowell LB. Cardiovascular aspects of human thermoregulation. *Circ. Res.* 1983; 52, 367-379.

Rowell LB, Marx HJ, Conn RD, et al. Reduction in central blood volume and stroke volume with exercise and heat stress in normal man. *Clin. Res.* 1964; 14, 163-173.

Saunders AG, Dugas JP, Tucker R, et al. The effects of different air velocities on heat storage and body temperature in humans cycling in a hot, humid environment. *Acta Physiol. Scand.* 2005; 183, 241-255.

Speedy DB, Noakes TD, Boswell T, et al. Response to a fluid load in athletes with a history of exercise induced hyponatremia. *Med. Sci. Sports Exerc.* 2001; 33, 1434-1442.

Stachenfeld NS, Taylor HS. Sex hormone effects on body fluid and sodium regulation in women with and without exercise-associated hyponatremia. *J. Appl. Physiol.* 2009; 107, 864-872.

Wyndham CH. 1973 Yant Memorial Lecture: Research in the human sciences in the gold mining industry. *Am. Ind. Hyg. Assoc. J.* 1974; 35, 113-136.

Wyndham CH, Strydom NB. The danger of an inadequate water intake during marathon running. *S. Afr. Med. J.* 1969; 43, 893-896.

Chapter 6 Notes

Carter JM, Jeukendrup AE, Jones DA. The effect of carbohydrate mouth rinse on 1-h cycle time trial performance. *Med. Sci. Sports Exerc.* 2004; 36, 2107-2111.Carter JM, Jeukendrup AE, Mann CH, et al. The effect of glucose infusion on glucose kinetics during a 1-h time trial. *Med. Sci. Sports Exerc.* 2004; 36, 1543-1550.

Chambers ES, Bridge MW, Jones DA. Carbohydrate sensing in the human mouth: Effects on exercise performance and brain activity. *J. Physiol.* 2009; 587, 1779-1794.

Cordain L, Friel J. *The paleo diet for athletes.* 2005. Emmaus, PA: Rodale.

Johnson RJ, Perez-Pozo SE, Sautin YY, et al. Hypothesis: Could excessive fructose intake and uric acid cause type 2 diabetes? *Endocrine Rev.* 2009; 30, 96–116.

Kolata G. *Ultimate fitness: The quest for truth about exercise and health.* 2003; pp. 3-292. New York: Farrar.

Noakes TD, Adams BA, Myburgh KH, et al. The danger of an inadequate water intake during prolonged exercise: A novel concept re-visited. *Eur. J. Appl. Physiol. Occup. Physiol.* 1988a; 57, 210-219.

Taubes G. *Why we get fat and what to do about it.* 2011. New York: Alfred A. Knopf.

Taubes G. *Good calories, bad calories.* 2007. New York: Anchor Books.

Chapter 7 Early Drinking Guidelines

American College of Sports Medicine. The American College of Sports Medicine position statement on prevention of heat injuries during distance running. *Med. Sci. Sports* 1975; 7, VII-IX.

American College of Sports Medicine. Position stand on the prevention of thermal injuries during distance running. *Med. Sci. Sports Exerc.* 1987; 19, 529-533.

Armstrong LE, Crago AE, Adams R, et al. Whole-body cooling of hyperthermic runners: Comparison of two field therapies. *Am. J. Emerg.Med.* 1996; 14, 355-358.

Armstrong LE, Epstein Y, Greenleaf JE, et al. American College of Sports Medicine position stand: Heat and cold illnesses during distance running. *Med. Sci. Sports Exerc.* 1996; 28, i-x.

Armstrong LE, Maresh CM. Effects of training, environment, and host factors on the sweating response to exercise. *Int. J. Sports Med.* 1998; 19 Suppl 2, S103-S105.

Below PR, Mora-Rodriguez R, Gonzalez-Alonso J, et al. Fluid and carbohydrate ingestion independently improve performance during 1 h of intense exercise. *Med. Sci. Sports Exerc.* 1995; 27, 200-210.

Cade R, Spooner G, Schlein E, et al. Effect of fluid, electrolyte, and glucose replacement during exercise on performance, body temperature, rate of sweat loss, and compositional changes of extracellular fluid. *J. Sports Med. Phys. Fitness* 1972; 12, 150-156.

Cheuvront SN, Haymes EM. Thermoregulation and marathon running: Biological and environmental influences. *Sports Med.* 2001; 31, 743-762.

Convertino VA, Armstrong LE, Coyle EF, et al. American College of Sports Medicine position stand: Exercise and fluid replacement. *Med. Sci. Sports Exerc.* 1996; 28, i-vii.

Costill DL, Cote R, Miller E, et al. Water and electrolyte replacement during repeated days of work in the heat. *Aviat. Space Environ. Med.* 1975; 46, 795-800.

Costill DL, Kammer WF, Fisher A. Fluid ingestion during distance running. *Arch. Environ. Health* 1970; 21, 520-525.

Department of the Army. FM 21-10 Field hygiene and sanitation. 1988. Fort Sam Houston, TX: US Army Medical Center and School.

Gisolfi CV, Copping JR. Thermal effects of prolonged treadmill exercise in the heat. *Med. Sci. Sports* 1974; 6, 108-113.

Hubbard RW, Armstrong LE. Hyperthermia: New thoughts on an old problem. *Phys. Sportsmed.* 1989; 17, 97-113.

Hubbard RW, Mager M, Kerstein M. Water as a tactical weapon: A doctrine for preventing heat casualties. Defense Technical Information Center OAI-PMH Repository 1982, 1-19.

Hultman E. Studies on muscle metabolism of glycogen and active phosphate in man with special reference to exercise and diet. *Scand. J. Clin. Lab. Invest. Suppl.* 1967; 94, 1-63.

Jokl E, Melzer L. Acute fatal non-traumatic collapse during work and sport. *S. Afr. J. Med. Sci.* 1940; 5, 4-14.

Kerstein M, Mager M, Hubbard R, et al. Heat-related problems in the desert: The environment can be an enemy. *Mil. Med.* 1984; 149, 650-656.

Martin DE, Gynn RWH. *The Olympic Marathon.* 2000; pp. 1-511. Champaign, IL: Human Kinetics.

Montain SJ, Coyle EF. Influence of graded dehydration on hyperthermia and cardiovascular drift during exercise. *J. Appl. Physiol.* 1992; 73, 1340-1350.

Muir AL, Percy-Robb IW, Davidson IA, et al. Physiological aspects of the Edinburgh Commonwealth Games. *Lancet* 1970; 2, 1125-1128.

Murray B. Cooled & fueled: Helping your active kids stay in the play. Gatorade. 1999.

Murray B. Fluid replacement: The American College of Sports Medicine position stand. *Sports Sci. Exch.* 1996; 9, 1-5.

Nadel ER, Wenger CB, Roberts MF, et al. Physiological defenses against hyperthermia of exercise. *Ann. N.Y. Acad. Sci.* 1977; 301, 98-109.

Nash HL. Treating thermal injury: Disagreement heats up. *Phys. Sportsmed.* 1985; 13, 134-144.

Noakes, T.D. Changes in body mass alone explain almost all of the variance in the serum sodium concentrations during prolonged exercises: Has commercial influence impeded scientific endeavour? *Br. J. Sports Med.* 2011; 45: 475-477.

Noakes TD. Letter: Heatstroke during the 1981 National Cross-Country Running Championships. *S. Afr. Med. J.* 1982; 61, 145.

Noakes TD, Goodwin N, Rayner BL, et al. Water intoxication: a possible complication during endurance exercise. *Med. Sci. Sports Exerc.* 1985; 17, 370-375.

Pearlmutter EM. The Pittsburgh marathon: playing weather roulette. *Phys. Sportsmed.* 1986; 14, 132-138.

Robinson TA, Hawley JA, Palmer GS, et al. Water ingestion does not improve 1-h cycling performance in moderate ambient temperatures. *Eur. J. Appl. Physiol. Occup. Physiol.* 1995; 71, 153-160.

Saunders AG, Dugas JP, Tucker R, et al. The effects of different air velocities on heat storage and body temperature in humans cycling in a hot, humid environment. *Acta Physiol. Scand.* 2005; 183, 241-255.

Sullivan JE. *Marathon running.* 1909; pp. 3-110. New York: American Sports.

Sutton JR. Clinical implications of fluid imbalance. In *Perspectives in exercise science and sports medicine.* C.V. Gisolfi and D.R. Lamb, eds. 1990; pp. 425-455. Carmel, IN: Benchmark.

Twerenbold R, Knechtle B, Kakebeeke TH, et al. Effects of different sodium concentrations in replacement fluids during prolonged exercise in women. *Br. J. Sports Med.* 2003; 37, 300-303.

Wyndham CH. Heat stroke and hyperthermia in marathon runners. *Ann. N.Y. Acad. Sci.* 1977; 301, 128-138.

Wyndham CH, Strydom NB. The danger of an inadequate water intake during marathon running. *S. Afr. Med. J.* 1969; 43, 893-896.

Chapter 7 Notes

Below PR, Mora-Rodriguez R, Gonzalez-Alonso J, et al. Fluid and carbohydrate ingestion independently improve performance during 1 h of intense exercise. *Med. Sci. Sports Exerc.* 1995; 27, 200-210.

Convertino VA, Armstrong LE, Coyle EF, et al. American College of Sports Medicine position stand: Exercise and fluid replacement. *Med. Sci. Sports Exerc.* 1996; 28, i-vii.

Costill DL, Cote R, Miller E, et al. Water and electrolyte replacement during repeated days of work in the heat. *Aviat. Space Environ. Med.* 1975; 46, 795-800.

Costill DL, Kammer WF, Fisher A. Fluid ingestion during distance running. *Arch. Environ. Health* 1970; 21, 520-525.

Fowkes GS, Godek JJ, Bartolozzi AR. Thermal responses in football and cross-country athletes during their respective practices in a hot environment. *J. Athl. Train.* 2004; 39, 235-240.

Montain SJ, Coyle EF. Influence of graded dehydration on hyperthermia and cardiovascular drift during exercise. *J. Appl. Physiol.* 1992; 73, 1340-1350.

Noakes TD. Sodium ingestion and the prevention of hyponatraemia during exercise. *Br. J. Sports Med.* 2004; 38, 790-792.

Noakes TD. Sports drinks: Prevention of "voluntary dehydration" and development of exercise-associated hyponatremia. *Med. Sci. Sports Exerc.* 2006; 38, 193.

Chapter 8 Discovery of Exercise-Associated Hyponatremia (EAH)

Costill DL. Sweating: Its composition and effects on body fluids. *Ann. N.Y. Acad. Sci.* 1977; 301, 160-174.

Dancaster CP, Duckworth WC, Roper CJ. Nephropathy in marathon runners. *S. Afr. Med. J.* 1969; 43, 758-760.

Dancaster CP, Whereat SJ. Fluid and electrolyte balance during the Comrades Marathon. *S. Afr. Med. J.* 1971; 45, 147-150.

Dickson DN, Wilkinson RL, Noakes TD. Effects of ultra-marathon training and racing on hematologic parameters and serum ferritin levels in well-trained athletes. *Int. J. Sports Med.* 1982; 3, 111-117.

Gambaccini P. Unforgettable. The 40 most influential people and moments of the past four decades. *Runner's World*; Nov. 2006. www.runnersworld.com/article/1,712 4,s6-243-297--10545-0,00.html.

Goldberg M. Hyponatremia. *Med. Clin. North Am.* 1981; 65, 251-269.

Hiller WD. Dehydration and hyponatremia during triathlons. *Med. Sci. Sports Exerc.* 1989; 21, S219-S221.

Irving RA, Noakes TD, Irving GA, et al. The immediate and delayed effects of marathon running on renal function. *J. Urol.* 1986; 136, 1176-1180.

Kelly JC, Godlonton JD. The 1980 Comrades Marathon. *S. Afr. Med. J.* 1980; 58, 509-510.

Ladell WS. Water and salt (sodium chloride) intakes. In *The physiology of human survival* O.G. Edholm and A. Bacharach eds. 1965; pp. 235-289. New York: Academic.

Mink BD, Schwartz A. Immediate and delayed metabolic and cardiovascular effects of 1 100-mile trail run. *Houst. Med.* 1990; 6, 18-23.

Myhre LG, Hartung GH, Tucker DM. Plasma volume and blood metabolites in middle-aged runners during a warm-weather marathon. *Eur. J. Appl. Physiol. Occup. Physiol.* 1982; 48, 227-240.

Noakes TD. Comrades makes medical history—again. *S.A. Runner.* 1981b; 4: September. pp. 8-10.

Noakes TD. Dealing with the heat. In *The complete marathoner.* Joe Henderson, ed. 1978; pp. 247-256. Mountain ViewCA: World.

Noakes TD. Exercise-induced heat injury in South Africa. *S. Afr. Med. J.* 1973; 47, 1968-1972.

Noakes TD. Five ways to improve the 'imperfect' peak. *S.A. Sports Med.* 1981a; May, 10-12.

Noakes TD. Hot-weather marathons. In The complete runner. *Runner's World*, ed. 1974; pp. 185-189. Mountain View, CA: World.

Noakes TD. *Lore of running.* 2003a; pp. 1-930. Champaign, IL: Human Kinetics. Noakes TD. Fluid replacement during marathon running. *Clin. J. Sport Med.* 2003b; 13, 309-318.

Noakes TD, Goodwin N, Rayner BL, et al. Water intoxication: A possible complication during endurance exercise. *Med. Sci. Sports Exerc.* 1985; 17, 370-375.

Noakes TD, Sharwood K, Speedy D, et al. Three independent biological mechanisms cause exercise-associated hyponatremia: Evidence from 2,135 weighed competitive athletic performances. *PNAS* 2005; 102, 18550-18555.

Shem S. *The house of God.* 2003; pp. 1-397. New York: Bantam.

Shibolet S, Coll R, Gilat T, et al. Heatstroke: Its clinical picture and mechanism in 36 cases. *Q. J. Med.* 1967; 36, 525-548.

Wyndham CH, Strydom NB. The danger of an inadequate water intake during marathon running. *S. Afr. Med. J.* 1969; 43, 893-896.

Chapter 8 Notes

Taleb NN. *The black swan: The impact of the highly improbable.* 2007; pp. 1-366. London: Penguin Books.

Verbalis JG. Disorders of body water homeostasis. *Best Pract. Res. Clin. Endocrinol. Metab.* 2003; 17, 471-503.

Chapter 9 The Biology of EAH

Almond CS, Shin AY, Fortescue EB, et al. Hyponatremia among runners in the Boston Marathon. *N. Engl. J. Med.* 2005; 352, 1550-1556.

American College of Sports Medicine, American Dietetic Association, Dietitians of Canada. Joint position statement: Nutrition and athletic performance. *Med. Sci. Sports Exerc.* 2009; 32, 2130-2145.

American Football Monthly Research Staff. Maximizing player performance. *American Football Monthly.* August 2004, 1-7. www.americanfootballmonthly.com/Subaccess/printer_friendly.php?article_id=4228.

Armstrong LE. *Exertional heat illnesses.* L.E. Armstrong, ed., 2003; pp. 1-275. Champaign, IL: Human Kinetics.

Armstrong LE. Exertional hyponatremia. In *Performing in extreme environments.* L.E. Armstrong, ed. 2000b; pp. 103-135. Champaign, IL: Human Kinetics.

Armstrong LE, Casa DJ, Millard-Stafford M, et al. American College of Sports Medicine position stand: Exertional heat illness during training and competition. *Med. Sci. Sports Exerc.* 2007; 39, 556-572.

Armstrong LE, Casa DJ, Watson G. Exertional hyponatremia. *Curr. Sports Med. Rep.* 2006; 5, 221-222.

Armstrong LE, Curtis WC, Hubbard RW, et al. Symptomatic hyponatremia during prolonged exercise in heat. *Med. Sci. Sports Exerc.* 1993; 25, 543-549.

Armstrong LE, Epstein Y, Greenleaf JE, et al. American College of Sports Medicine position stand: Heat and cold illnesses during distance running. *Med. Sci. Sports Exerc.* 1996; 28, i-x.

Ayus JC, Varon J, Arieff AI. Hyponatremia, cerebral edema, and noncardiogenic pulmonary edema in marathon runners. *Ann. Intern. Med.* 2000; 132, 711-714.

Barr SI, Costill DL, Fink WJ. Fluid replacement during prolonged exercise: effects of water, saline, or no fluid. *Med. Sci. Sports Exerc.* 1991; 23, 811-817.

Baylis PH. The syndrome of inappropriate antidiuretic hormone secretion. *Int. J. Biochem. Cell. Biol.* 2003; 35, 1495-1499.

Bergstrom WH, Wallace WM. Bone as a sodium and potassium reservoir. *J. Clin. Invest.* 1954; 33, 867-873.

Convertino VA, Armstrong LE, Coyle EF, et al. American College of Sports Medicine position stand: Exercise and fluid replacement. *Med. Sci. Sports Exerc.* 1996; 28, i-vii.

Davis DP, Videen JS, Marino A, et al. Exercise-associated hyponatremia in marathon runners: A two-year experience. *J. Emerg. Med.* 2001; 21, 47-57.

Dugas JP, Noakes TD. Hyponatraemic encephalopathy despite a modest rate of fluid intake during a 109 km cycle race. *Br. J. Sports Med.* 2005; 39, e38.

Eichner ER. Pearls and Pitfalls: Six paths to hyponatremia. *Curr. Sports Med. Rep.* 2009; 8, 280-281.

Eichner ER, Laird R, Hiller D, et al. Hyponatremia in sport: Symptoms and prevention. *Sports Sci. Exch.;* 4: 1-4. 1993a. www.gssiweb.com.

Forbes GB, Lewis AM. Total sodium, potassium and chloride in adult man. *J. Clin. Invest.* 1956; 35, 596-600.

Garnett ES, Ford J, Golding PL, et al. The mobilizaton of osmotically inactive sodium during total starvation in man. *Clin. Sci.* 1968; 35, 93-103.

GSSI. Sodium: The forgotten nutrient: SSE#78. *Sports Sci. Exch.* 2000; 13:3. pp. 1-4.

Hew-Butler T. Arginine vasopressin, fluid balance and exercise: is exercise-associated hyponatraemia a disorder of arginine vasopressin secretion? *Sports Med.* 2010; 40, 459-479.

Hew-Butler TD, Almond CS, Ayus JC, et al. Consensus document of the 1st International Exercise-Associated Hyponatremia (EAH) Consensus Symposium, Cape Town, South Africa 2005. *Clin. J. Sport Med.* 2005; 15, 207-213.

Hew-Butler T, Ayus JC, Kipps C, et al. Statement of the Second International Exercise-Associated Hyponatremia Consensus Development Conference, New Zealand, 2007. *Clin. J. Sport Med.* 2008; 18, 111-121.

Hiller WD. Dehydration and hyponatremia during triathlons. *Med. Sci. Sports Exerc.* 1989; 21, S219-S221.

Hiller WDB. Hyponatremia and ultramarathons. *JAMA* 1986; 256, 213-214.

Hiller WDB. The United States Triathlon Series: Medical considerations. In *Ross Symposium on Medical Coverage of Endurance Athletic Events.* R.H. Laird, ed. 1988a; pp. 80-82. Columbus, OH: Ross Laboratories.

Hiller WD, O'Toole ML, Fortess EE, et al. Medical and physiological considerations in triathlons. *Am. J. Sports Med.* 1987; 15, 164-167.

Irving RA, Noakes TD, Buck R, et al. Evaluation of renal function and fluid homeostasis during recovery from exercise-induced hyponatremia. *J. Appl. Physiol.* 1991; 70, 342-348.

Irving RA, Noakes TD, Burger SC, et al. Plasma volume and renal function during and after ultramarathon running. *Med. Sci. Sports Exerc.* 1990a; 22, 581-587.

Irving RA, Noakes TD, Irving GA, et al. The immediate and delayed effects of marathon running on renal function. *J. Urol.* 1986; 136, 1176-1180.

Ladell WS. Effects of drinking small quantities of sea-water. *Lancet* 1943; 2, 441-444.

Ladell WS. Effects on man of restricted water supply. *Br. Med. Bull.* 1947; 5, 9-13.

Laird RH. Medical complications during the Ironman Triathlon World Championship, 1981-1986. In *Ross Symposium on Medical Coverage of Endurance Athletic Events* R.H. Laird, ed. 1988; pp. 83-88. Columbus, OH: Ross Laboratories.

Laird RH. Medical complications during the Ironman Triathlon World Championship 1981-1984. *Annal. Sports Med.* 1987; 3, 113-116.

Leaf A. The clinical and physiologic significance of the serum sodium concentration. *N. Engl. J. Med.* 1962a; 267, 24-30.

Leaf A. The clinical and physiologic significance of the serum sodium concentration (concluded). *N. Engl. J. Med.* 1962b; 267, 77-83.

Lind RH. The Western States 100 mile run. In *Ross Symposium on Medical Coverage of Endurance Athletic Events* 1988, pp. 26-35. Columbus, OH: Ross Laboratories.

McGarvey J, Thompson J, Hanna C, et al. Sensitivity and specificity of clinical signs for assessment of dehydration in endurance athletes. *Br. J. Sports Med.* 2010; 44, 716-719.

McRae D. *Every second counts: The race to transplant the first human heart.* 2006; pp. 1-356. London: Simon & Schuster.

Montain SJ. Strategies to prevent hyponatremia during prolonged exercise. *Curr. Sports Med. Rep.* 2008; 7, S28-S35.

Montain SJ, Cheuvront SN, Sawka MN. Exercise associated hyponatraemia: Quantitative analysis to understand the aetiology. *Br. J. Sports Med.* 2006; 40, 98-105.

Montain SJ, Coyle EF. Influence of graded dehydration on hyperthermia and cardiovascular drift during exercise. *J. Appl. Physiol.* 1992; 73, 1340-1350.

Montain SJ, Latzka WA, Sawka MN. Fluid replacement recommendations for training in hot weather. *Mil. Med.* 1999; 164, 502-508.

Montain SJ, Sawka MN, Wenger CB. Hyponatremia associated with exercise: Risk factors and pathogenesis. *Exerc. Sport Sci. Rev.* 2001; 29, 113-117.

Murray R. Exercise associated hyponatraemia: quantitative analysis to understand the aetiology: Commentary 3. *Br. J. Sports Med.* 2006; 40, 106.

Murray B. Manufactured arguments: Turning consensus into controversy does not advance science. *Br. J. Sports Med.* 2007; 41, 106-107.

Murray B, Eichner ER. Hyponatremia of exercise. *Curr. Sports Med. Rep.* 2004; 3, 117-118.

Murray B, Stofan J, Eichner ER. "Water intoxication" and subsequent death has become a "hot" topic. How dangerous is it? *Marathon & Beyond* Jan/Feb 2004; 77-92.

Nguyen MK, Kurtz I. New insights into the pathophysiology of the dysnatremias: A quantitative analysis. *Am. J. Physiol. Renal Physiol.* 2004; 287, F172-F180.

Noakes TD. Dealing with the heat. In *The complete marathoner,* Joe Henderson, ed. 1978; pp. 247-256. Mountain View, CA: World.

Noakes TD. Hot-weather marathons. In *The complete runner by Runner's World* ed. 1974; pp. 185-189. Mountain View, CA: World.

Noakes TD. Hyponatremia during endurance running: A physiological and clinical interpretation. *Med. Sci. Sports Exerc.* 1992b; 24, 403-405.

Noakes TD. Hyponatremia in distance runners: Fluid and sodium balance during exercise. *Curr. Sports Med. Rep.* 2002; 1, 197-207.

Noakes TD. Letter: Heatstroke during the 1981 National Cross-Country Running Championships. *S. Afr. Med. J.* 1982; 61, 145.

Noakes TD. *Lore of running.* 2003a; pp. 1-930. Champaign, IL: Human Kinetics.

Noakes TD. Overconsumption of fluids by athletes. *Br.Med.J.* 2003b; 327, 113-114.

Noakes TD. Running, the kidneys and drinking too much— the hyponatraemia of exercise. *S. Afr. Med. J.* 2001b; 91, 843-844.

Noakes TD. The hyponatremia of exercise. *Int. J. Sport Nutr.* 1992a; 2, 205-228.

Noakes TD, Carter JW. Biochemical parameters in athletes before and after having run 160 kilometres. *S. Afr. Med. J.* 1976; 50, 1562-1566.

Noakes TD, Goodwin N, Rayner BL, et al. Water intoxication: A possible complication during endurance exercise. *Med. Sci. Sports Exerc.* 1985; 17, 370-375.

Noakes TD, Nathan M, Irving RA, et al. Physiological and biochemical measurements during a 4-day surf-ski marathon. *S. Afr. Med. J.* 1985; 67, 212-216.

Noakes TD, Sharwood K, Collins M, et al. The dipsomania of great distance: Water intoxication in an Ironman triathlete. *Br. J. Sports Med.* 2004; 38, E16.

Noakes TD, Sharwood K, Speedy D, et al. Three independent biological mechanisms cause exercise-associated hyponatremia: Evidence from 2,135 weighed competitive athletic performances. *PNAS* 2005; 102, 18550-18555.

Noakes TD, Wilson G, Gray DA, et al. Peak rates of diuresis in healthy humans during oral fluid overload. *S. Afr. Med. J.* 2001; 91, 852-857.

O'Toole, ML. Prevention and treatment of electrolyte abnormalities. In *Ross Symposium on Medical Coverage of Endurance Athletic Events* 1988, pp. 93-96. Columbus, OH: Ross Laboratories.

O'Toole ML, Douglas PS, Laird RH, et al. Fluid and electrolyte status in athletes receiving medical care at an ultradistance triathlon. *Clin. J. Sport Med.* 1995; 5, 116-122.

Pahnke MD. Sodium and fluid balance in ultra-endurance triathletes. MSc thesis, University of Texas at Austin 2004; 1-122.

Pahnke MD, Trinity JD, Zachwieja JJ, et al. Serum sodium concentration changes are related to fluid balance and sweat sodium loss. *Med. Sci. Sports Exerc.* 2010; 42, 1669-1674.

Pahnke MD, Trinity JD, Zachwieja JJ, et al. Sodium balance and sweat loss during the Hawaii Ironman Triathlon. *Med. Sci. Sports Exerc.* 2005; 37, S347-S348.

Pasantes-Morales H, Franco R, Ordaz B, et al. Mechanisms counteracting swelling in brain cells during hyponatremia. *Arch. Med. Res.* 2002; 33, 237-244.

Pasteur L, Lister J. *Germ theory and its applications to medicine and on the antiseptic principle of the practice of surgery.* 1996; pp. 15-144. New York: Prometheus Books.

Richter S, Betz C, Geiger H. Severe hyponatremia with pulmonary and cerebral edema in an Ironman triathlete (article in German). *Dtsch. Med. Wochenschr.* 2007; 132: 1829 -1832.

Sallis R. Collapse in the endurance athlete. *GSSI Sports Sci. Exch.* 2004; 17, 1-6.

Sallis RE. Fluid balance and dysnatremias in athletes. *Curr. Sports Med. Rep.* 2008; 7, S14-S19.

Sawka MN, Burke LM, Eichner ER, et al. American College of Sports Medicine position stand: Exercise and fluid replacement. *Med. Sci. Sports Exerc.* 2007; 39, 377-390.

Speedy DB, Faris JG, Hamlin M, et al. Hyponatremia and weight changes in an ultradistance triathlon. *Clin. J. Sport Med.* 1997; 7, 180-184.

Speedy DB, Noakes TD, Boswell T, et al. Response to a fluid load in athletes with a history of exercise induced hyponatremia. *Med. Sci. Sports Exerc.* 2001a; 33, 1434-1442.

Speedy DB, Noakes TD, Kimber NE, et al. Fluid balance during and after an ironman triathlon. *Clin. J. Sport Med.* 2001b; 11, 44-50.

Speedy DB, Noakes TD, Rogers IR, et al. A prospective study of exercise-associated hyponatremia in two ultradistance triathletes. *Clin. J. Sport Med.* 2000; 10, 136-141.

Speedy DB, Noakes TD, Rogers IR, et al. Hyponatremia in ultradistance triathletes. *Med. Sci. Sports Exerc.* 1999; 31, 809-815.

Speedy DB, Noakes TD, Schneider C. Exercise-associated hyponatremia: A review. *Emerg. Med. (Fremantle)* 2001c; 13, 17-27.

Speedy DB, Rogers IR, Noakes TD, et al. Exercise-induced hyponatremia in ultradistance triathletes is caused by inappropriate fluid retention. *Clin. J. Sport Med.* 2000a; 10, 272-278.

Speedy DB, Rogers IR, Noakes TD, et al. Diagnosis and prevention of hyponatremia at an ultradistance triathlon. *Clin. J. Sport Med.* 2000b; 10, 52-58.

Strydom NB, Kielblock AJ, Schutte PC. Heatstroke: Its definition, diagnosis and treatment. *S. Afr. Med. J.* 1982; 61, 537.

Titze J, Lang R, Ilies C, et al. Osmotically inactive skin Na+ storage in rats. *Am.J. Physiol. Renal Physiol.* 2003; 285, F1108-F1117.

Verbalis JG. Vasopressin V2 receptor antagonists. *J. Molecular Endocrin.* 2002; 29: 1–9.

Weschler LB. Exercise-associated hyponatraemia: A mathematical review. *Sports Med.* 2005; 35, 899-922.

Weschler LB. Under what conditions is ingested sodium rendered osmotically inactive? *Am. J. Physiol. Regul. Integr. Comp. Physiol.* 2006; 291, R856-R857.

Chapter 9   Notes

Ladell WS. Effects of drinking small quantities of sea-water. *Lancet* 1943; 2, 441-444.

Ladell WS. Effects on man of restricted water supply. *Br. Med. Bull.* 1947; 5, 9-13.

Ladell WS. The effects of water and salt intake upon the performance of men working in hot and humid environments. *J. Physiol.* 1955; 127, 11-46.

Levine BD, Thompson PD. Marathon maladies. *N. Engl. J. Med.* 2005; 352, 1516-1518.

Macfarlane WV, Morris RJH, Howard B. Turn-over and distribution of water in desert camels, sheep, cattle and kangaroos. *Nature* 1963; 197, 270-271.

Olsson KE, Saltin B. Variation in total body water with muscle glycogen changes in man. *Acta Physiol. Scand.* 1970; 80, 11-18.

Chapter 10   EAH and EAHE on a Global Scale

Adner MM. The Boston Marathon. In *Ross Symposium on Medical Coverage of Endurance Athletic Events* R.H. Laird ed. 1988; pp.2-8. Columbus, OH: Ross Laboratories.

Adner MM, Gembarowicz R, Casey J, et al. Point-of-care biochemical monitoring of Boston Marathon runners. *Point of Care* 2002; 1, 237-240.

Adner MM, Scarlett JJ, Casey J, et al. The Boston Marathon medical care team: Ten years of experience. *Phys. Sportsmed.* 1988; 16, 99-106.

Almond CS, Shin AY, Fortescue EB, et al. Hyponatremia among runners in the Boston Marathon. *N. Engl. J. Med.* 2005; 352, 1550-1556.

Anastasiou CA, Kavouras SA, Arnaoutis G, et al. Sodium replacement and plasma sodium drop during exercise in the heat when fluid intake matches fluid loss. *J. Athl. Train.* 2009; 44, 117-123.

Armstrong LE, Curtis WC, Hubbard RW, et al. Symptomatic hyponatremia during prolonged exercise in heat. *Med. Sci. Sports Exerc.* 1993; 25, 543-549.

Armstrong LE, Casa DJ, Millard-Stafford M, et al. Exertional heat illness during training and competition. *Med. Sci. Sports Exerc.* 2007; 39, 556-572.

Au-Yeung KL, Wu WC, Yau WH, et al. A study of serum sodium level among Hong Kong runners. *Clin. J. Sport Med.* 2010; 20, 482-487.

Ayus JC, Varon J, Arieff AI. Hyponatremia, cerebral edema, and noncardiogenic pulmonary edema in marathon runners. *Ann. Intern. Med.* 2000; 132, 711-714.

Backer HD, Shopes E, Collins SL, et al. Exertional heat illness and hyponatremia in hikers. *Am. J. Emerg. Med.* 1999; 17, 532-539.

Backer H, Shopes E, Collins SL. Hyponatremia in recreational hikers in Grand Canyon National Park. *Wilderness Med.* 1993; 4, 391-406.

Baker J, Cotter JD, Gerrard DF, et al. Effects of indomethacin and celecoxib on renal function in athletes. *Med. Sci. Sports Exerc.* 2005; 37, 712-717.

Berning JR. Football coaches' guide to heat illness and hydration. The Clipboard, GSSI; 2008. www.gssiweb.com/Article_Detail.aspx?articleid=216.

Burr RE. *Heat illness: A handbook for medical officers.* 1991; Natick, MA: US Army Research Institute of Environmental Medicine.

Chorley J, Cianca J, Divine J. Risk factors for exercise-associated hyponatremia in non-elite marathon runners. *Clin. J. Sport Med.* 2007; 17, 471-477.

Convertino VA, Armstrong LE, Coyle EF, et al. American College of Sports Medicine position stand: Exercise and fluid replacement. *Med. Sci. Sports Exer.* 1996; 28, i-vii.

"Coroner: BCHS student died from chemical imbalance." www.bakersfieldnow.com/news/27633459.html. August 28, 2008.

Craig SC. Hyponatremia associated with heat stress and excessive water consumption: The impact of education and a new army fluid replacement policy. *MSMR* 1999; 5, 1-9.

Creamer M, Hagedorn E. Family in disbelief that drinking too much water killed football player. 2009. www.bakersfield.com/news/local/x1489917533/Family-in-disbelief-that-drinking-too-much-water-killed-football-player.

Davis C. High school football player dies from too much water. News Channel 7, South Carolina, 2008. www.wspa.com/spa/lifestyles/health_med_fit/medical/article/high_school_football_player_dies_from_too_much_water/7837.

Davis D, Marino A, Vilke G, et al. Hyponatremia in marathon runners: Experience with the inaugural Rock'n Roll Marathon. *Ann. Emerg. Med.* 1999; 34, S40.

Davis DP, Videen JS, Marino A, et al. Exercise-associated hyponatremia in marathon runners: a two-year experience. *J. Emerg. Med.* 2001; 21, 47-57.

Dimeff RJ. Seizure disorder in a professional American football player. *Curr. Sports Med. Rep.* 2006; 5, 173-176.

Doberenz DT, Nalla BP, Gillies M, et al. Exercise-associated hyponatraemia and encephalopathy following the 2007 London Marathon. Unpublished manuscript.

"Dr. Sean Rothwell." *60 Minutes*; 1-3. 2010. http://sixtyminutes.ninemsn.com.au/article.aspx?id=1066946.

Dugas JP, Noakes TD. Hyponatraemic encephalopathy despite a modest rate of fluid intake during a 109 km cycle race. *Br. J. Sports Med.* 2005; 39, e38.

Eichner ER, Laird R, Hiller D, et al. Hyponatremia in sport: symptoms and prevention. *Sports Sci. Exch.* 1993; 4: 1-4. www.gssiweb.com.

Eijsvogels TM, Thijssen DH, Poelkens F, et al. Physical risks whilst walking the Nijmegen Four Days Marches in 2007: Electrolyte imbalance in 1 in 5 walkers. *Ned. Tijdschr. Geneeskd.* 2008; 152, 1571-1578.

"Electrolyte imbalance blamed in death of football player: Coroner's office says athlete failed to replenish lost sodium." *Bakersfield News*; 29 August: 2008. www.turnto23.com/news/17338293/detail.html.

Frizzell RT, Lang GH, Lowance DC, et al. Hyponatremia and ultramarathon running. *JAMA* 1986; 255, 772-774.

Galun E, Tur-Kaspa I, Assia E, et al. Hyponatremia induced by exercise: A 24-hour endurance march study. *Miner. Electrolyte Metab.* 1991; 17, 315-320.

Gardner JW. Death by water intoxication. *Mil. Med.* 2002; 167, 432-434.

Gatorade. Gatorade and NFL launch annual beat the heat campaign to educate youth football players and coaches about heat-related illnesses. The Free Library; 2007. www.thefreelibrary.com/gatorade and NFL launch annual beat the heat campaign to educate...-a0166975945.

Glace B, Murphy C. Severe hyponatremia develops in a runner following a half-marathon. *JAAPA.* 2008; 21, 27-29.

Godlonton JD. The Comrades Marathon—setting the record straight. *S. Afr. Med. J.* 1985; 68, 291.

GSSI. Gatorade Sports Science Institute issues hydration recommendations for Boston Marathon runners. *PR Newswire* 2006; 11 April, 1-2.

GSSI. Gatorade Sports Science Institute refutes hydration guidelines in *British Journal of Medicine* [sic] report. Gatorade Sports Science Institute, 2003. http://www.pepsico.com/news/gatorade/2003/20030718g.shtml.

GSSI. Drinking 101 (advertisement). *New York Runner.* 2002; 47, n.p.n.

GSSI. GSSI guidelines on heat safety in football: Attacking heat-related death and illness in football players. *Sports Science Library;* 2002. www.gssiweb.com/Article_Detail.aspx?articleid=566.

Herfel R, Stone CK, Koury SI, et al. Iatrogenic acute hyponatraemia in a college athlete. *Br. J. Sports Med.* 1998; 32, 257-258.

Hew-Butler T, Anley C, Schwartz P, et al. The treatment of symptomatic hyponatremia with hypertonic saline in an Ironman triathlete. *Clin. J. Sport Med.* 2007; 17, 68-69.

Hew-Butler T, Noakes TD, Siegel AJ. Practical management of exercise-associated hyponatremic encephalopathy: the sodium paradox of non-osmotic vasopressin secretion. *Clin. J. Sport Med.* 2008; 18, 350-354.

Hew TD. Women hydrate more than men during a marathon race: Hyponatremia in the Houston Marathon: A report on 60 cases. *Clin. J. Sport Med.* 2005; 15, 148-153.

Hew TD, Chorley JN, Cianca JC, et al. The incidence, risk factors, and clinical manifestations of hyponatremia in marathon runners. *Clin. J. Sport Med.* 2003; 13, 41-47.

Hiller WDB, O'Toole ML, Massimino F, et al. Plasma electrolyte and glucose changes during the Hawaiian Ironman Triathlon. *Med. Sci. Sports Exerc.* 1985; 17(suppl), 219.

Honig C. Eating on the run: Proper nutrition for marathon running. *Inside Texas Running.* Endurance Sports Media Group. Texas. 2003; pp. 8-9.

Hsieh M, Roth R, Davis DL, et al. Hyponatremia in runners requiring on-site medical treatment at a single marathon. *Med. Sci. Sports Exerc.* 2002; 34, 185-189.

Irving RA, Noakes TD, Buck R, et al. Evaluation of renal function and fluid homeostasis during recovery from exercise-induced hyponatremia. *J. Appl. Physiol.* 1991; 70, 342-348.

Kashyap AS, Anand KP, Kashyap S. Sudden collapse of a young female cross country runner. *Br. J. Sports Med.* 2006; 40, e11.

Kavouras SA, Anastasiou C, Yiannakouris N, et al. Incidence of hyponatremia after a 246 km continuous foot race. *Med. Sci. Sports Exerc.* 2003; 35, S246.

Kipps C, Sharma S, Tunstall PD. The incidence of exercise-associated hyponatraemia in the London Marathon. *Br. J. Sports Med.* 2011; 45, 14-19.

Knechtle B, Knechtle P, Rosemann T. No exercise-associated hyponatremia found in an observational field study of male ultra-marathoners paticipating in a 24-hour ultra-run. *Phys. Sportsmed.* 2010; 38, 94-100.

Knechtle B, Senn O, Imoberdorf R, et al. Maintained total body water content and serum sodium concentrations despite body mass loss in female ultra-runners drinking ad libitum during a 100 km race. *Asia Pac. J. Clin. Nutr.* 2010; 19, 83-90.

Kolata G. Study cautions runners to limit their water intake. *New York Times* April 14, 2005: 1-3. 2005. www.nytimes.com/2005/04/14/health...partner=MYWAY&pagewanted=print&position. Last accessed: 2005.

Kratz A, Lewandrowski KB, Siegel AJ, et al. Effect of marathon running on hematologic and biochemical laboratory parameters, including cardiac markers. *Am. J. Clin. Pathol.* 2002; 118, 856-863.

Kratz A, Siegel AJ, Verbalis JG, et al. Sodium status of collapsed marathon runners. *Arch. Pathol. Lab. Med.* 2005; 129, 227-230.

Laird R. Ironman Kona 2010: Medical treatment guidelines. Kona, HI: 2010.

Lebus DK, Casazza GA, Hoffman MD, et al. Can changes in body mass and total body water accurately predict hyponatremia after a 161-km running race? *Clin. J. Sport Med.* 2010; 20, 193-199.

Lorraine-Lichtenstein E, Albert J, Hjelmqvist H. Vattenar ett farligt gift ... Tva fall av hyponatremi i samband med maratonsport och stort vatskeintag. *Lakartidningen* 2008; 105, 1650-1652.

Marino FE, King M. Limitations of hydration in offsetting the decline in exercise performance in experimental settings: Fact or fancy? In M.R. Bishop (2010) *Chocolate, fast foods and sweeteners: Consumption and health.* (pp. 63-83). Hauppauge, NY: Nova.

Montain SJ, Latzka WA, Sawka MN. Fluid replacement recommendations for training in hot weather. *Mil. Med.* 1999; 164, 502-508.

Murray B. Fluid replacement: The American College of Sports Medicine position stand. *Sports Sci. Exch.* 1996; 9, 1-5.

Murray B. Fluid replacement: The American College of Sports Medicine position stand. GSSI; 1-11. 1999. www.gssiweb.com/references/s0000000200000128/s000.../d00000002000002c2.htm.

Nash HL. Exploring the medical aspects of sport: One man's goal. *Physcn. Sportsmed.* 1986; 14, 205-219.

Nearman S. Drinking too much water can kill you: Death of a marathon runner. *Metro Competitor.* 2003; 24 October.

Nelson PB, Ellis D, Fu F, et al. Fluid and electrolyte balance during a cool weather marathon. *Am. J. Sports Med.* 1989; 17, 770-772.

Nelson PB, Robinson AG, Kapoor W, et al. Hyponatremia in a marathoner. *Phys. Sportsmed.* 1987; 16, 78-87.

Noakes TD. Fluid replacement during marathon running. *Clin. J. Sport Med.* 2003; 13, 309-318.

Noakes TD, Goodwin N, Rayner BL, et al. Water intoxication: A possible complication during endurance exercise. *Med. Sci. Sports Exer.* 1985; 17, 370-375.

Noakes TD, Martin DE. IMMDA-Aims advisory statement on guidelines for fluid replacement during marathon running. *New. Stud. Athlet.* 2002; 17, 15-24.

Noakes TD, Norman RJ, Buck RH, et al. The incidence of hyponatremia during prolonged ultraendurance exercise. *Med. Sci. Sports Exerc.* 1990; 22, 165-170.

Noakes TD, Sharwood K, Collins M, et al. The dipsomania of great distance: water intoxication in an Ironman triathlete. *Br. J. Sports Med.* 2004; 38, E16.

O'Brien KK, Montain SJ, Corr WP, et al. Hyponatremia associated with overhydration in U.S. Army trainees. *Mil. Med.* 2001; 166, 405-410.

Pacelli LD. Overhydration: Is it possible? *Phys. Sportsmed.* 1990; 18, 29-30.

Pahnke MD. Sodium and fluid balance in ultra-endurance triathletes. MSc thesis, University of Texas at Austin 2004; 1-122.

Pahnke MD, Trinity JD, Zachwieja JJ, et al. Serum sodium concentration changes are related to fluid balance and sweat sodium loss. *Med. Sci. Sports Exerc.* 2010; 42, 1669-1674.

Petzold A, Keir G, Appleby I. Marathon related death due to brainstem herniation in rehydration-related hyponatraemia: A case report. *J. Med. Case Reports* 2007; 1, 186.

Ratliff D, Youngblood D. Coroner: Water overdose killed H.S. football player. 17KGet.com; 2008. www.kget.com/

mostpopular/story/Coroner-Water-Overdose-Killed-H-S-Football-Player/zLCscuDxQk-jc88oEDyZ4g.cspx.

Rawlani V, Noakes TD. Hyponatremic encephalopathy 72 hours after a marathon footrace. Unpublished manuscript. 2008.

Richter S, Betz C, Geiger H. Severe hyponatremia with pulmonary and cerebral edema in an Ironman triathlete (article in German). *Dtsch. Med. Wochenschr.* 2007; 132, 1829-1832.

Rothwell SP, Rosengren DJ. Severe exercise-associated hyponatremia on the Kokoda Trail, Papua New Guinea. *Wilderness Environ. Med.* 2008; 19, 42-44.

Rovell D. *First in thirst: How Gatorade turned the science of sweat into a cultural phenomenon.* 2005; New York: Amacom.

Sharwood KA, Collins M, Goedecke JH, et al. Weight changes, medical complications, and performance during an Ironman triathlon. *Br. J. Sports Med.* 2004; 38, 718-724.

Sharwood K, Collins M, Goedecke J, et al. Weight changes, sodium levels, and performance in the South African Ironman Triathlon. *Clin. J. Sport Med.* 2002; 12, 391-399.

Shem S. *The house of God.* 2003; pp. 1-397. New York: Bantam Dell.

Stuempfle KJ, Lehmann DR, Case HS, et al. Change in serum sodium concentration during a cold weather ultradistance race. *Clin. J. Sport Med.* 2003; 13, 171-175.

Stuempfle KJ, Lehmann DR, Case HS, et al. Hyponatremia in a cold weather ultraendurance race. *Alaska Med.* 2002; 44, 51-55.

Surgenor S, Uphold RE. Acute hyponatremia in ultra-endurance athletes. *Am. J. Emerg. Med.* 1994; 12, 441-444.

Thompson J-A, Wolff AJ. Hyponatremic encephalopathy in a marathon runner. *Chest* (Supplement) 2003; 124, 313S.

Verbalis JG. Renal function and vasopressin during marathon running. *Sports Med.* 2007; 37, 455-458.

Weiler-Ravell D, Shupak A, Goldenberg I, et al. Pulmonary oedema and haemoptysis induced by strenuous swimming. *Br. Med. J.* 1995; 311, 361-362.

Wharam PC, Speedy DB, Noakes TD, et al. NSAID use increases the risk of developing hyponatremia during an Ironman triathlon. *Med. Sci. Sports Exerc.* 2006; 38, 618-622.

Young M, Sciurba F, Rinaldo J. Delirium and pulmonary edema after completing a marathon. *Am. Rev. Respir. Dis.* 1987; 136, 737-739.

Zelingher J, Putterman C, Ilan Y, et al. Case series: Hyponatremia associated with moderate exercise. *Am. J. Med. Sci.* 1996; 311, 86-91.

Zorn E. Runner's demise sheds light on deadly myth. *Chicago Tribune.* MetroChicago. 11 October, 1999a; p. 1.

Zorn E. Water intoxication rare, but runners should pay heed. *Chicago Tribune.* 12 October, 1999b; p. 1.

Chapter 10   Notes

Beltrami F, Hew-Butler T, Noakes T. Drinking policies and exercise-associated hyponatraemia: Is anyone still promoting overdrinking? *Br. J. Sports Med.* 2008; 42, 496-501.

Noakes TD, Goodwin N, Rayner BL, et al. Water intoxication: A possible complication during endurance exercise, 1985. *Wilderness Environ. Med.* 2005; 16, 221-227. (Rogers I.R., 2005).

Thompson J-A, Wolff AJ. Hyponatremic encephalopathy in a marathon runner. *Chest (Supplement)* 2003; 124, 313S.

Zorn E. Water intoxication rare, but runners should pay heed. *Chicago Tribune.* MetroChicago. 12 October. Chicago. 1999b; p.1.

Chapter 11   Guidelines for Fluid Intake and Diagnosis of EAH

Adolph EF. *Physiology of man in the desert.* 1947; pp. 1-357. New York: Interscience.

Armstrong LE, Casa DJ, Millard-Stafford M, et al. American College of Sports Medicine position stand: Exertional heat illness during training and competition. *Med. Sci. Sports Exerc.* 2007; 39, 556-572.

Beis LY, Wright-Whyte M, Fudge B, Noakes T, Pitsiladis YP. Drinking behaviours of elite male runners during marathon competition. *Clin. J. Sport Med.* 2012 (in press).

Bethell H, Jewell D, Burke P. Medical hazards of a four-km fun run. *Br. J. Sports Med.* 1991; 25, 181-182.

Brown AH. Water shortage in the desert. In *Physiology of man in the desert* 1947; pp. 136-159. New York: Interscience.

Bruso JR, Hoffman MD, Rogers IR, et al. Rhabdomyolosis and hyponatremia: A cluster of five cases at the 161-km 2009 Western States run endurance. *Wilderness Environ. Med.* 2010; 21, 303-308.

Cannon WB. *The wisdom of the body.* 1939; pp. 19-333. New York: Norton.

Carter R, III, Cheuvront SN, Williams JO, et al. Epidemiology of hospitalizations and deaths from heat illness in soldiers. *Med. Sci. Sports Exerc.* 2005; 37, 1338-1344.

Claassen A, Lambert EV, Bosch AN, et al. Variability in exercise capacity and metabolic response during endurance exercise after a low carbohydrate diet. *Int. J. Sport Nutr. Exerc. Metab.* 2005; 15, 97-116.

Cheuvront SN, Ely BR, Kenefick RW, et al. Biological variation and diagnostic accuracy of dehydration assessment markers. *Am. J. Clin. Nutr.* 2010; 92, 565-573.

Convertino VA, Armstrong LE, Coyle EF, et al. American College of Sports Medicine position stand: Exercise and fluid replacement. *Med. Sci. Sports Exer.* 1996; 28, i-vii.

Currell K, Jeukendrup AE. Superior endurance performance with ingestion of multiple transportable carbohydrates. *Med. Sci. Sports Exerc.* 2008; 40, 275-281.

Epstein Y, Moran DS, Shapiro Y, et al. Exertional heat stroke: A case series. *Med. Sci. Sports Exerc.* 1999; 31, 224-228.

Fowkes GS, Godek JJ, Bartolozzi AR. Thermal responses in football and cross-country athletes during their respective practices in a hot environment. *J. Athl. Train.* 2004; 39, 235-240.

GSSI. Gatorade Sports Science Institute issues hydration recommendations for Boston Marathon runners. *PR Newswire* 2006; 11 April, 1-2.

Gisolfi CV, Summers RW, Lambert GP, et al. Effect of beverage osmolality on intestinal fluid absorption during exercise. *J. Appl. Physiol.* 1998; 85, 1941-1948.

Hawking S. *Black holes and baby universes and other essays.* 1993; pp. 1-173. London: Bantam Press.

Heinrich B. *The hot-blooded insects.* 1993; pp. 1-601. Cambridge, MA: Harvard University Press.

Hew-Butler TD, Almond CS, Ayus JC, et al. Consensus Document of the 1st International Exercise-Associated Hyponatremia (EAH) Consensus Symposium, Cape Town, South Africa, 2005. *Clin. J. Sport Med.* 2005; 15, 207-213.

Hew-Butler T, Anley C, Schwartz P, et al. The treatment of symptomatic hyponatremia with hypertonic saline in an Ironman triathlete. *Clin. J. Sport Med.* 2007; 17, 68-69.

Hew-Butler T, Ayus JC, Kipps C, et al. Statement of the Second International Exercise-Associated Hyponatremia Consensus Development Conference, New Zealand, 2007. *Clin. J. Sport Med.* 2008; 18, 111-121.

Hew-Butler T, Noakes TD, Siegel AJ. Practical management of exercise-associated hyponatremic encephalopathy: The sodium paradox of non-osmotic vasopressin secretion. *Clin. J. Sport Med.* 2008; 18, 350-354.

Hew-Butler TD, Sharwood KA, Collins M, et al. Sodium supplementation is not required to maintain serum sodium concentrations during an Ironman triathlon. *Br. J. Sports Med.* 2006; 40, 255-259.

Holtzhausen LM, Noakes TD. Collapsed ultraendurance athlete: Proposed mechanisms and an approach to management. *Clin. J. Sport Med.* 1997; 7, 292-301.

Holtzhausen LM, Noakes TD, Kroning B, et al. Clinical and biochemical characteristics of collapsed ultra-marathon runners. *Med. Sci. Sports Exer.* 1994; 26, 1095-1101.

Irving RA, Noakes TD, Buck R, et al. Evaluation of renal function and fluid homeostasis during recovery from exercise-induced hyponatremia. *J. Appl. Physiol.* 1991; 70, 342-348.

Jentjens RL, Jeukendrup AE. High rates of exogenous carbohydrate oxidation from a mixture of glucose and fructose ingested during prolonged cycling exercise. *Br. J. Nutr.* 2005; 93, 485-492.

Jentjens RL, Shaw C, Birtles T, et al. Oxidation of combined ingestion of glucose and sucrose during exercise. *Metabolism* 2005; 54, 610-618.

Jentjens RL, Underwood K, Achten J, et al. Exogenous carbohydrate oxidation rates are elevated after combined ingestion of glucose and fructose during exercise in the heat. *J. Appl. Physiol.* 2006; 100, 807-816.

Jeukendrup AE, Currell K, Clarke J, et al. Effect of beverage glucose and sodium content on fluid delivery. *Nutr. Metab. (Lond)* 2009; 6, 9.

Lamb DR, Williams MH. Perspectives in exercise science and sports medicine: Ergogenics: Enhancement of performance in exercise and sport. 1991; pp. 1-422. Traverse City: MI: Cooper.

Malawer SJ, Ewton M, Fordtran JS, et al. Interrelation between jejunal absorption of sodium glucose, and water in man. *J. Clin. Invest.* 1965:44, pp. 1072-1073.

Mayers LB, Noakes TD. A guide to treating Ironman triathletes at the finish line. *Phys. Sportsmed.* 2000; 28, 35-50.

McGarvey J, Thompson J, Hanna C, et al. Sensitivity and specificity of clinical signs for assessment of dehydration in endurance athletes. *Br. J. Sports Med.* 2010; 44, 716-719.

Montain SJ, Cheuvront SN, Sawka MN. Exercise associated hyponatraemia: Quantitative analysis to understand the aetiology. *Br. J. Sports Med.* 2006; 40, 98-105.

Noakes TD. A contemporary understanding of the exercise-related heat illnesses. In *Exercise physiology: From a cellular to an integrative approach.* P. Connes, O. Hue and S. Perrey, eds. 2010; pp. 456-467. Amsterdam: IOS Press.

Noakes TD. Drinking guidelines for exercise: What evidence is there that athletes should drink "as much as tolerable," "to replace the weight lost during exercise" or "ad libitum"? *J. Sports Sci.* 2007b; 25, 781-796.

Noakes TD. Fluid replacement during marathon running. *Clin. J. Sport Med.* 2003a; 13, 309-318.

Noakes TD. *Lore of Running.* 2003b; pp. 1-930. Champaign, IL: Human Kinetics.

Noakes TD. Medical coverage of endurance events. In *Clinical sports medicine.* P. Brukner, ed. 2000; pp. 865-871. Australia: McGraw-Hill.

Noakes TD. Reduced peripheral resistance and other factors in marathon collapse. *Sports Med.* 2007a; 37, 382-385.

Noakes TD. Why endurance athletes collapse. *Phys. Sportsmed.* 1988b; 16, 23-26.

Noakes TD. Why marathon runners collapse. *S. Afr. Med. J.* 1988a; 73, 569-571.

Noakes TD, Adams BA, Myburgh KH, et al. The danger of an inadequate water intake during prolonged exercise. A novel concept re-visited. *Eur. J. Appl. Physiol. Occup. Physiol.* 1988; 57, 210-219.

Noakes TD, Martin DE. IMMDA-Aims Advisory statement on guidelines for fluid replacement during marathon running. *New Stud. Athlet.* 2002; 17, 15-24.

Noakes TD, Myburgh KH, du PJ, et al. Metabolic rate, not percent dehydration, predicts rectal temperature in marathon runners. *Med. Sci. Sports Exerc.* 1991; 23, 443-449.

Noakes TD, Rehrer NJ, Maughan RJ. The importance of volume in regulating gastric emptying. *Med. Sci. Sports Exerc.* 1991; 23, 307-313.

Sawka MN, Burke LM, Eichner ER, et al. American College of Sports Medicine position stand: Exercise and fluid replacement. *Med. Sci. Sports Exerc.* 2007; 39, 377-390.

Sawka MN, Noakes TD. Does dehydration impair exercise performance? *Med. Sci. Sports Exerc.* 2007; 39, 1209-1217.

Sharwood KA, Collins M, Goedecke J, et al. Weight changes, sodium levels, and performance in the South African Ironman Triathlon. *Clin. J. Sport Med.* 2002; 12, 391-399.

Sharwood KA, Collins M, Goedecke JH, et al. Weight changes, medical complications, and performance during an Ironman triathlon. *Br. J. Sports Med.* 2004; 38, 718-724.

Shi X, Summers RW, Schedl HP, et al. Effects of carbohydrate type and concentration and solution osmolality on water absorption. *Med. Sci. Sports Exerc.* 1995; 27, 1607-1615.

Sheehan GA. *Dr. Sheehan on running.* 1975; pp. 1-204. Mountain View, CA: World.

Siegel AJ, Verbalis JG, Clement S, et al. Hyponatremia in marathon runners due to inappropriate arginine vasopressin secretion. *Am. J. Med.* 2007; 120, 461-467.

Sole CC, Noakes TD. Faster gastric emptying for glucose-polymer and fructose solutions than for glucose in humans. *Eur. J. Appl. Physiol. Occup. Physiol.* 1989; 58, 605-612.

Speedy DB, Noakes TD, Holtzhausen LM. Exercise-associated collapse. *Phys. Sportsmed.* 2003; 31, 23-29.

Speedy DB, Rogers IR, Noakes TD, et al. Exercise-induced hyponatremia in ultradistance triathletes is caused by inappropriate fluid retention. *Clin. J. Sport Med.* 2000; 10, 272-278.

Speedy DB, Thompson JM, Rodgers I, et al. Oral salt supplementation during ultradistance exercise. *Clin. J. Sport Med.* 2002; 12, 279-284.

Stuempfle KJ, Lehmann DR, Case HS, et al. Change in serum sodium concentration during a cold weather ultradistance race. *Clin. J. Sport Med.* 2003; 13, 171-175.

Tatterson AJ, Hahn AG, Martin DT, et al. Effects of heat stress on physiological responses and exercise performance in elite cyclists. *J. Sci. Med. Sport* 2000; 3, 186-193.

Tucker R, Marle T, Lambert EV, et al. The rate of heat storage mediates an anticipatory reduction in exercise intensity during cycling at a fixed rating of perceived exertion. *J. Physiol.* 2006; 574, 905-915.

Tucker R, Rauch L, Harley YX, et al. Impaired exercise performance in the heat is associated with an anticipatory reduction in skeletal muscle recruitment. *Pflugers Arch.* 2004; 448, 422-430.

USATF. USATF announces major change in hydration guidelines. USA Track & Field; 1-3. 2003. www.usatf.org/news/showRelease.asp?article=/news/releases/2003-04-19-2.xml.

Chapter 11 Notes

Ayus JC, Arieff A, Moritz ML. Hyponatremia in marathon runners. *N. Engl. J. Med.* 2005; 353, 427-428.

Ayus JC, Arieff AI. Chronic hyponatremic encephalopathy in postmenopausal women: association of therapies with morbidity and mortality. *JAMA* 1999; 281, 2299-2304.

Ayus JC, Arieff AI. Hyponatremia and myelinolysis. *Ann. Intern. Med.* 1997; 127, 163.

Bryant J. *The London Marathon: The history of the greatest race on earth.* 2005; pp. 1-280. London: Hutchinson.

Cluitmans FH, Meinders AE. Management of severe hyponatremia: Rapid or slow correction? *Am.J. Med.* 1990; 88, 161-166.

Cordain, L. *The paleo diet.* John Wiley and Sons. Hoboken, NJ, 2011.

Cordain L, Brand Miller J, Eaton SB, Mann N, Holt SHA, Speth JD. Plant-animal subsistence ratios and macronutrient energy estimations in worldwide hunter-gatherer diets. *Am. J. Clin. Nutr.* 2000; 71: 682-692.

Cordain L and Friel J. *The paleo diet for athletes.* Emmaus, PA: Rodale Press, 2005.

Dugas JP, Noakes TD. Hyponatraemic encephalopathy despite a modest rate of fluid intake during a 109 km cycle race. *Br. J. Sports Med.* 2005; 39, e38.

Montain SJ, Cheuvront SN, Sawka MN. Exercise associated hyponatraemia: Quantitative analysis to understand the aetiology. *Br. J. Sports Med.* 2006; 40, 98-105.

Rae DE, Knobel GJ, Mann T, et al. Heatstroke during endurance exercise: Is there evidence for excessive endothermy? *Med. Sci. Sports Exerc.* 2008; 40, 1193-1204.

Speedy DB, Noakes TD, Kimber NE, et al. Fluid balance during and after an ironman triathlon. *Clin. J. Sport Med.* 2001; 11, 44-50.

Strydom NB, Wyndham CH, Cooke HM, et al. Effect of heat on work performance in the gold mines of South Africa. *Fed. Proc.* 1963; 22, 893-896.

Volek JS, Phinney SD. *The art and science of low carbohydrate living.* Beyond Obesity, LLC. 2011.

Wyndham CH. 1973 Yant Memorial Lecture: Research in the human sciences in the gold mining industry. *Am. Ind. Hyg. Assoc. J.* 1974; 35, 113-136.

Appendixes

Abbott KD, Nichols JF. Hyponatremia and adventure racing. *Med. Sci. Sports Exerc.* 2003; 35, S246.

Almond CS, Shin AY, Fortescue EB, et al. Hyponatremia among runners in the Boston Marathon. *N. Engl. J. Med.* 2005; 352, 1550-1556.

Armstrong LE, Curtis WC, Hubbard RW, et al. Symptomatic hyponatremia during prolonged exercise in heat. *Med. Sci. Sports Exerc.* 1993; 25, 543-549.

Ayus JC, Varon J, Arieff AI. Hyponatremia, cerebral edema, and noncardiogenic pulmonary edema in marathon runners. *Ann. Intern. Med.* 2000; 132, 711-714.

Backer HD, Shopes E, Collins SL. Hyponatremia in recreational hikers in Grand Canyon National Park. *Wilderness Med.* 1993; 4, 391-406.

Backer HD, Shopes E, Collins SL, et al. Exertional heat illness and hyponatremia in hikers. *Am. J. Emerg. Med.* 1999; 17, 532-539.

Baker LB, Munce TA, Kenney WL. Sex differences in voluntary fluid intake by older adults during exercise. *Med. Sci. Sports Exerc.* 2005; 37, 789-796.

Basnyat B, Sleggs J, Spinger M. Seizures and delirium in a trekker: the consequences of excessive water drinking? *Wilderness Environ. Med.* 2000; 11, 69-70.

Bernheim J, Cox JN. [Heat stroke and amphetamine intoxication in a sportsman.] *Schweiz. Med. Wochenschr.* 1960; 90, 322-331.

Bruso JR, Hoffman MD, Rogers IR, et al. Rhabdomyolosis and hyponatremia: A cluster of five cases at the 161-km 2009 Western States run endurance. *Wildern. Environ. Med.* 2010; 21, 301-308.

Bunt C, O'Connor H. The "Phantom Runner." *Phys. Sportsmed.* 2004; 32, 32.

Craig SC. Hyponatremia associated with heat stress and excessive water consumption: The impact of education and a new army fluid replacement policy. *MSMR* 1999; 5, 1-9.

Cuthill JA, Ellis C, Inglis A. Hazards of ultra-marathon running in the Scottish Highlands: Exercise-associated hyponatraemia. *Emerg. Med. J.* 2009; 26, 906-907.

Davis DP, Videen JS, Marino A, et al. Exercise-associated hyponatremia in marathon runners: A two-year experience. *J. Emerg. Med.* 2001; 21, 47-57.

Doberenz DT, Nalla BP, Gillies M, et al. Exercise-associated hyponatraemia and encephalopathy following the 2007 London Marathon. Unpublished manuscript.

Draper SB, Mori KJ, Lloyd-Owen S, et al. Overdrinking-induced hyponatraemia in the 2007 London Marathon. *Br. Med. J. Case Reports* 2009, 1-5.

Dugas JP, Noakes TD. Hyponatraemic encephalopathy despite a modest rate of fluid intake during a 109 km cycle race. *Br. J. Sports Med.* 2005; 39, e38.

Eijsvogels TM, Thijssen DH, Poelkens F, et al. Physical risks whilst walking the Nijmegen Four Days Marches in 2007: Electrolyte imbalance in 1 in 5 walkers. *Ned. Tijdschr. Geneeskd.* 2008; 152, 1571-1578.

Ellis C, Cuthill J, Hew-Butler T, et al. Case report: Exercise-associated hyponatremia with rhabdomyolysis during endurance exercise. *Phys. Sportsmed.* 2009; 37, 126-132.

Flinn SD, Sherer RJ. Seizure after exercise in the heat: Recognizing life-threatening hyponatremia. *Phys. Sportsmed.* 2000; 28, 61-67.

Fotheringham W. *Put me back on my bike: In search of Tom Simpson.* 2002; pp. 1-242. London, UK: Yellow Jersey Press.

Frizzell RT, Lang GH, Lowance DC, et al. Hyponatremia and ultramarathon running. *JAMA* 1986; 255, 772-774.

Gardner JW. Death by water intoxication. *Mil. Med.* 2002; 167, 432-434.

Garigan TP, Ristedt DE. Death from hyponatremia as a result of acute water intoxication in an Army basic trainee. *Mil. Med.* 1999; 164, 234-238.

Glace B, Murphy C. Severe hyponatremia develops in a runner following a half-marathon. *JAAPA.* 2008; 21, 27-29.

Godlonton JD. The Comrades Marathon: Setting the record straight. *S. Afr. Med. J.* 1985; 68, 291.

Goudie AM, Tunstall-Pedoe DS, Kerins M, et al. Exercise-associated hyponatraemia after a marathon: Case series. *J. R. Soc. Med.* 2006; 99, 363-367.

Hanson PG, Zimmerman SW. Exertional heatstroke in novice runners. *JAMA* 1979a; 242, 154-157.

Hanson PG, Zimmerman SW. Heatstroke in road races. *N. Engl. J. Med.* 1979b; 300, 96-97.

"Hawaiian Ironman 2010 medical report." Paper presented at the 2010 Hawaiian Ironman Medical Conference. Kona, Hawaii. October 2010.

Hew TD. Women hydrate more than men during a marathon race: Hyponatremia in the Houston Marathon: A Report on 60 Cases. *Clin. J. Sport Med.* 2005; 15, 148-153.

Hew TD, Chorley JN, Cianca JC, et al. The incidence, risk factors, and clinical manifestations of hyponatremia in marathon runners. *Clin. J. Sport Med.* 2003; 13, 41-47.

Hew-Butler T, Anley C, Schwartz P, et al. The treatment of symptomatic hyponatremia with hypertonic saline in an Ironman triathlete. *Clin. J. Sport Med.* 2007; 17, 68-69.

Hew-Butler T, Boulter J, Mbchb JG, Phd RT, Mbchb TN. Hypernatremia and intravenous fluid resuscitation in collapsed ultramarathon runners. *Clin. J. Sport Med.* 2008; 18, 273-278.

Hew-Butler T, Noakes TD, Siegel AJ. Practical management of exercise-associated hyponatremic encephalopathy: The sodium paradox of non-osmotic vasopressin secretion. *Clin. J. Sport Med.* 2008; 18, 350-354.

Hew-Butler T, Noakes TD, Soldin SJ, Verbalis JG. Acute changes in arginine vasopressin, sweat, urine and serum sodium concentrations in exercising humans: Does a coordinated homeostatic relationship exist? *Br. J. Sports Med.* 2010; 44, 710-715.

Hew-Butler T, Sharwood K, Boulter J, Collins M, Tucker R, Dugas J, Shave R, George K, Cable T, Verbalis JG, Noakes T. Dysnatremia predicts a delayed recovery in collapsed ultramarathon runners. *Clin. J. Sport Med.* 2007; 17, 289-296.

Hoffman MD, Stuempfle KJ, Rogers IR, Weschler LB, Hew-Butler T. Hyponatremiain the 2009 161-km Western States Endurance Run. *Int. J. Sports Physiol. Perform.* 2011; Aug 30 [Epub ahead of print].

Hsieh M, Roth R, Davis DL, et al. Hyponatremia in runners requiring on-site medical treatment at a single marathon. *Med. Sci. Sports Exerc.* 2002; 34, 185-189.

Irving RA, Noakes TD, Buck R, et al. Evaluation of renal function and fluid homeostasis during recovery from exercise-induced hyponatremia. *J. Appl. Physiol.* 1991; 70, 342-348.

Kashyap AS, Anand KP, Kashyap S. Sudden collapse of a young female cross country runner. *Br. J. Sports Med.* 2006; 40, e11.

Kavouras SA, Anastasiou C, Yiannakouris N, et al. Incidence of hyponatremia after a 246km continuous foot race. *Med. Sci. Sports Exerc.* 2003; 35, S246.

Kipps C, Sharma S, Tunstall PD. The incidence of exercise-associated hyponatraemia in the London Marathon. *Br. J. Sports Med.* 2011; 45, 14-19.

Knechtle B, Knechtle P Rosemann T. No exercise-associated hyponatremia found in an observational field study of male ultra-marathoners participating in a 24-hour ultra-run. *Phys. Sportsmed.* 2010; 38, 94-100.

Kratz A, Siegel AJ, Verbalis JG, et al. Sodium status of collapsed marathon runners. *Arch. Pathol. Lab. Med.* 2005; 129, 227-230.

Laird RH. Medical complications during the Ironman Triathlon World Championship 1981-1984. *Annal. Sports Med.* 1987; 3, 113-116.

Laird RH. Medical complications during the Ironman Triathlon World Championship, 1981-1986. In *Ross Symposium on Medical Coverage of Endurance Athletic Events.* R.H. Laird ed. 1988; pp. 83-88. Columbus, OH: Ross Laboratories.

Lee JK, Nio AQ, Ang WH, Johnson C, Aziz AR, Lim CL, Hew-Butler T. First cases of exercise-associated hyponatremia in Asia. *Int. J. Sports Med.* 2011; 32, 297-302.

Lorraine-Lichtenstein E, Albert J, Hjelmqvist H. Vattenar ett farligt gift . . . Tva fall av hyponatremi i samband med maratonsport och stort vatskeintag. *Lakartidningen* 2008; 105, 1650-1652.

Martin DE, Gynn RWH. *The Olympic Marathon.* 2000; pp. 1-511. Champaign, IL: Human Kinetics.

Mettler S, Rusch C, Frey WO, et al. Hyponatremia among runners in the Zurich Marathon. *Clin. J. Sport Med.* 2008; 18, 344-349.

Moller V. Knud Enemark Jensen's death during the 1960 Rome Olympics: A search for truth? *Sport Hist.* 2005; 25, 452-471.

Montain SJ, Latzka WA, Sawka MN. Fluid replacement recommendations for training in hot weather. *Mil. Med.* 1999; 164, 502-508.

Noakes TD, Goodwin N, Rayner BL, et al. Water intoxication: A possible complication during endurance exercise. *Med. Sci. Sports Exerc.* 1985; 17, 370-375.

Noakes TD, Norman RJ, Buck RH, et al. The incidence of hyponatremia during prolonged ultraendurance exercise. *Med. Sci. Sports Exerc.* 1990; 22, 165-170.

Noakes TD, Mekler J, Pedoe DT. Jim Peters' collapse in the 1954 Vancouver Empire Games marathon. *S. Afr. Med. J.* 2008; 98, 596-600.

Noakes TD, Sharwood K, Collins M, et al. The dipsomania of great distance: Water intoxication in an Ironman triathlete. *Br. J.Sports Med.* 2004; 38, E16.

Novak D. Ironman Canada Triathlon Championship: Medical coverage of an ultradistance event. In *Ross Symposium on Medical Coverage of Endurance Athletic Events.* R.H. Laird ed. 1988; pp. 69-73. Columbus, OH: Ross Laboratories.

O'Brien KK, Montain SJ, Corr WP, et al. Hyponatremia associated with overhydration in U.S. Army trainees. *Mil. Med.* 2001; 166, 405-410.

O'Toole, ML. Prevention and treatment of electrolyte abnormalities. In *Ross Symposium on Medical Coverage of Endurance Athletic Events* 1988, pp. 93-96. Columbus, OH: Ross Laboratories.

O'Toole ML, Douglas PS, Laird RH, et al. Fluid and electrolyte status in athletes receiving medical care at an ultradistance triathlon. *Clin. J. Sport Med.* 1995; 5, 116-122.

Page AJ, Reid SA, Speedy DB, Mulligan GP, Thompson J. Exercise-associated hyponatremia, renal function, and nonsteroidal antiinflammatory drug use in an ultraendurance mountain run. *Clin. J. Sport Med.* 2007; 17, 43-48.

Petzold A, Keir G, Appleby I. Marathon related death due to brainstem herniation in rehydration-related hyponatraemia: A case report. *J. Med. Case Reports* 2007; 1, 186.

Putterman C, Levy L, Rubinger D. Transient exercise-induced water intoxication and rhabdomyolysis. *Am. J. Kidney Dis.* 1993; 21, 206-209.

Rae DE, Knobel GJ, Mann T, et al. Heatstroke during endurance exercise: Is there evidence for excessive endothermy? *Med. Sci. Sports Exerc.* 2008; 40, 1193-1204.

Rawlani, V, Noakes, TD. Hyponatremic encephalopathy 72 hours after a marathon footrace, Unpublished manuscript. 2008.

Reynolds NC, Jr., Schumaker HD, Feighery S. Complications of fluid overload in heat casualty prevention during field training. *Mil. Med.* 1998; 163, 789-791.

Richter S, Betz C, Geiger H. Severe hyponatremia with pulmonary and cerebral edema in an Ironman triathlete (article in German). *Dtsch. Med. Wochenschr.* 2007; 132, 1829-1832.

Roberts WO. A 12-yr profile of medical injury and illness for the Twin Cities Marathon. *Med. Sci. Sports Exerc.* 2000; 32, 1549-1555.

Rothwell SP, Rosengren DJ. Severe exercise-associated hyponatremia on the Kokoda Trail, Papua New Guinea. *Wilderness Environ. Med.* 2008; 19, 42-44.

Shapiro SA, Ejaz AA, Osborne MD, et al. Moderate exercise-induced hyponatremia. *Clin. J. Sport Med.* 2006; 16, 72-73.

Siegel AJ, d'Hemecourt P, Adner MM, Shirey T, Brown JL, Lewandrowski KB. Exertional dysnatremia in collapsed marathon runners: a critical role for point-of-care testing to guide appropriate therapy. *Am. J. Clin. Pathol.* 2009; 132, 336-340.

Siegel AJ, Verbalis JG, Clement S, et al. Hyponatremia in marathon runners due to inappropriate arginine vasopressin secretion. *Am. J. Med.* 2007; 120, 461-467.

Stefanko G, Lancashire B, Coombes J, et al. Pulmonary oedema and hyponatremia after an ironman triathlon. *BMJ Case Reports* 2009, 1-11.

Speedy DB, Faris JG, Hamlin M, et al. Hyponatremia and weight changes in an ultradistance triathlon. *Clin. J. Sport Med.* 1997; 7, 180-184.

Speedy DB, Noakes TD, Rogers IR, et al. Hyponatremia in ultradistance triathletes. *Med. Sci. Sports Exerc.* 1999; 31, 809-815.

Speedy DB, Noakes TD, Rogers IR, et al. A prospective study of exercise-associated hyponatremia in two ultradistance triathletes. *Clin. J. Sport Med.* 2000; 10, 136-141.

Speedy DB, Rogers IR, Noakes TD, et al. Exercise-induced hyponatremia in ultradistance triathletes is caused by inappropriate fluid retention. *Clin. J. Sport Med.* 2000a; 10, 272-278.

Speedy DB, Rogers IR, Noakes TD, et al. Diagnosis and prevention of hyponatremia at an ultradistance triathlon. *Clin. J. Sport Med.* 2000b; 10, 52-58.

Speedy DB, Rogers IR, Safih S, et al. Hyponatremia and seizures in an ultradistance triathlete. *J. Emerg. Med.* 2000; 18, 41-44.

Stuempfle KJ, Lehmann DR, Case HS, et al. Hyponatremia in a cold weather ultraendurance race. *Alaska Med.* 2002; 44, 51-55.

Surgenor S, Uphold RE. Acute hyponatremia in ultra-endurance athletes. *Am. J. Emerg. Med.* 1994; 12, 441-444.

Thompson J-A, Wolff AJ. Hyponatremic Encephalopathy in a Marathon Runner. *Chest (Supplement)* 2003; 124, 313S.

Twerenbold R, Knechtle B, Kakebeeke TH, et al. Effects of different sodium concentrations in replacement fluids during prolonged exercise in women. *Br. J. Sports Med.* 2003; 37, 300-303.

Vrijens DM, Rehrer NJ. Sodium-free fluid ingestion decreases plasma sodium during exercise in the heat. *J. Appl. Physiol.* 1999; 86, 1847-1851.

Wharam PC, Speedy DB, Noakes TD, et al. NSAID use increases the risk of developing hyponatremia during an Ironman triathlon. *Med. Sci. Sports Exerc.* 2006; 38, 618-622.

Young M, Sciurba F, Rinaldo J. Delirium and pulmonary edema after completing a marathon. *Am. Rev. Respir. Dis.* 1987; 136, 737-739.

Zelingher J, Putterman C, Ilan Y, et al. Case series: Hyponatremia associated with moderate exercise. *Am. J. Med. Sci.* 1996; 311, 86-91.

INDEX

Note: The italicized *f* and *t* following page numbers refer to figures and tables, respectively.

ABOUT THE AUTHOR

Known throughout the academic community for the high-caliber nature of his scientific insights and work, **Dr. Timothy Noakes** is the Discovery Health professor of exercise and sport science at the University of Cape Town in South Africa. He is also director of the Medical Research Council/University of Cape Town Research Unit for Exercise Science and Sports Medicine at the Sports Science Institute of South Africa in Newlands. Noakes was awarded a doctorate in science (DSc) in 2002, the highest degree awarded by the University of Cape Town. Publishing the first scientific article on exercise-associated hyponatremia (EAH) is considered among his greatest achievements.

Noakes is a veteran of more than 70 marathons and ultramarathons, and his book *Lore of Running* (Human Kinetics, 2003) is considered a classic by serious distance runners. In addition, Noakes is an editorial board member for many international sport science journals and a former president of the South African Sports Medicine Association. In 1996, he presented the prestigious J.B. Wolffe Memorial Lecture at the American College of Sports Medicine's annual meeting. In 1999 he was elected as one of 22 founding members of the International Olympic Committee's Olympic Science Academy. The National Research Foundation of South Africa considers Noakes an A1-rated scientist, and in 2008 he received the Order of Mapungubwe (Silver) from the president of South Africa for "excellent contribution in the field of sport and the science of physical exercise."

Noakes and his wife, Marilyn Anne, reside in Cape Town.

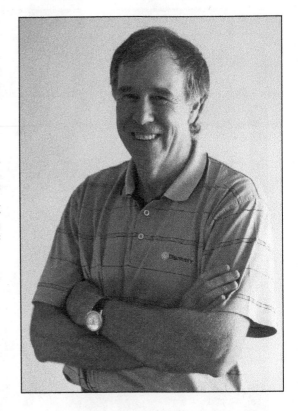

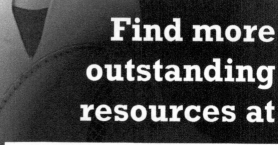